ONCOLOGY
NURSING
SECRETS

ONCOLOGY NURSING SECRETS

ROSE A. GATES, RN, MSN, CNS
Oncology Clinical Nurse Specialist
Department of Pediatrics
Tripler Army Medical Center
Honolulu, Hawaii

REGINA M. FINK, RN, PhD(c), AOCN
Acute Pain Clinical Nurse Specialist
Department of Anesthesiology
University Hospital
Denver, Colorado

HANLEY & BELFUS, INC./Philadelphia

Publisher: HANLEY & BELFUS, INC.
Medical Publishers
210 South 13th Street
Philadelphia, PA 19107
(215) 546-7293; 800-962-1892
FAX (215) 790-9330

United States sales and distribution:

Mosby
11830 Westline Industrial Drive
St. Louis, MO 63146

Note to the reader: Although the information in this book has been carefully reviewed for correctness of dosage and indications, neither the authors nor the editors nor the publisher can accept any legal responsibility for any errors or omissions that may be made. Neither the publisher nor the editors make any warranty, expressed or implied, with respect to the material contained herein. Experimental compounds and off-label uses of approved products are discussed. Before prescribing any drug, the reader must review the manufacturer's current product information (package inserts) for accepted indications, absolute dosage recommendations, and other information pertinent to the safe and effective use of the product described. This is especially important when drugs are given in combination or as an adjunct to other forms of therapy.

Library of Congress Cataloging-in-Publication Data

Oncology Nursing Secrets / |edited by| Rose A. Gates, Regina M. Fink.
    p.   cm. — (The Secrets Series®)
    Includes bibliographical references and index.
    ISBN 1-56053-210-6 (alk. paper)
    1. Cancer—Nursing—Miscellanea. I. Gates, Rose A., 1952–
II. Fink, Regina M., 1955–   . III. Series.
    |DNLM: 1. Neoplasms—nursing—examination questions. 2. Oncologic
Nursing—methods—examination questions. WY 18.2 058 1997|
RC266.057 1997
610.73'698—dc21
DNLM/DLC
for Library of Congress   97-3107
                                           CIP

ONCOLOGY NURSING SECRETS   ISBN 1-56053-210-6

Last digit is the print number: 9 8 7 6 5 4 3 2 1

CONTENTS

IV. SOLID TUMORS

V. SYMPTOM MANAGEMENT

VI. ONCOLOGIC EMERGENCIES AND COMPLICATIONS

VII. CARING FOR THE PERSON WITH CANCER

CONTRIBUTORS

Lowell A. Anderson-Reitz, RN, MS, ANP, OCN
Nurse Practitioner, Bone Marrow Transplant Program, University of Colorado Health Sciences Center and University Hospital, Denver, Colorado

Maude Becker, RN, OCN
Oncology Nurse Clinician, University of Colorado Cancer Center, Denver, Colorado

Mona Bernaiche Bedell, RN, BSN, MSPH, OCN
Epidemiology Nurse, Denver Public Health Department, Denver, Colorado

Anne Elizabeth Belcher, PhD, RN, FAAN
Chairperson, Department of Acute and Long-term Care, School of Nursing, University of Maryland at Baltimore, Baltimore; Associate Professor, Program in Oncology, Greenebaum Cancer Center, University of Maryland Medical Center, Baltimore, Maryland

Jeffrey L. Berenberg, MD, COL, MC
Clinical Associate Professor, and Chief, Division of Medical Oncology, John A. Burns School of Medicine, University of Hawaii; Associate Researcher, Cancer Research Center of Hawaii; Chief, Hematology-Oncology Service, Tripler Army Medical Center, Honolulu, Hawaii

Charlene Berlam, RN, MS, ANP, OCN
Oncology Case Manager, Professional Resources, University Hospital, Denver, Colorado

Janelle McCallum Betley, RN, BSN, MSM
Process Leader for Quality Facilitation, Hospice of MetroDenver, Denver, Colorado

Rocky L. Billups, RN
Bone Marrow Transplant Program, University of Colorado Health Sciences Center and University Hospital, Denver, Colorado

Deborah McCaffrey Boyle, RN, MSN, OCN
Oncology Clinical Nurse Specialist, The Cancer Center at Fairfax Hospital, Falls Church, Virginia

Jane Saucedo Braaten, RN, MS, CCRN
Clinical Nurse Specialist, St. Anthony's Hospital North, Westminster, Colorado

Harri Brackett, RN, BSN, OCN
Oncology Nurse Clinician, University Hospital, Denver, Colorado

Mary Alice Browning, RN, MSN, OCN
Breast Cancer Nurse Coordinator, Penrose Cancer Center, Colorado Springs, Colorado

Carol M. Brueggen, MS, RN, OCN
Surgical Clinical Nurse Specialist, St. Marys Hospital, Mayo Medical Center, Rochester, Minnesota

Richard D. Callahan, MD
Consulting Physician, Medical Oncology, Haywood Regional Medical Center, Clyde, North Carolina

Dawn Camp-Sorrell, RN, MSN, FNP, AOCN
Oncology Nurse Practitioner, University of Alabama at Birmingham, Birmingham, Alabama

Mary Jo Cleaveland, RN, MS, CNS
Director of Complementary Healing, Children's Hospital, Denver, Colorado

Susanne K. Cook, RN, BSN, OCN
Oncology Nurse Clinician, University of Colorado Health Sciences Center, Denver, Colorado

Susan A. Davidson, MD
Assistant Professor and Director of Gynecologic Oncology, Department of Obstetrics and Gynecology, University of Colorado Health Sciences Center, Denver, Colorado

Ann Marie Dose, MS, RN, OCN
Surgical Clinical Nurse Specialist, Rochester Methodist Hospital and Mayo Medical Center, Rochester, Minnesota

Constance Engelking, RN, MS, OCN
Executive Director, Zalmen A. Arlin Cancer Institute, Westchester County Medical Center, Valhalla, New York

Lynn Kendrick Erdman, RN, MN, OCN
Director, Presbyterian Cancer Center, Charlotte, North Carolina

David C. Faragher, MD
Rocky Mountain Cancer Centers, Columbia Aurora Medical Center, Aurora, Colorado

Kyle M. Fink, MD
Rocky Mountain Cancer Centers, Columbia Presbyterian–St. Lukes Hospital, Denver, Colorado

Regina M. Fink, RN, PhD(c), AOCN
Acute Pain Clinical Nurse Specialist, Department of Anesthesiology, University Hospital, Denver, Colorado

Joan E. Foley, RN, BSN
Head Nurse, Radiation Oncology Clinic, Tripler Army Medical Center, Honolulu, Hawaii

Mary T. Garcia, RN, BSN, MPH, CCRA
Research Nurse, Clinical Investigations Core, University of Colorado Cancer Center, Denver, Colorado

Robert H. Gates, MD, FACP
Associate Clinical Professor of Medicine, University of Hawaii; Chief, Department of Medicine, Tripler Army Medical Center, Honolulu, Hawaii

Rose A. Gates, RN, MSN, CNS
Oncology Clinical Nurse Specialist, Department of Pediatrics, Tripler Army Medical Center, Honolulu, Hawaii

Colleen Gill, MS, RD
Clinical Dietitian, Nutrition Services, University of Colorado Health Sciences Center and University Hospital, Denver, Colorado

Michelle Goodman, RN, MS
Oncology Clinical Nurse Specialist, Rush Cancer Institute, Rush Presbyterian–St. Luke's Medical Center; Assistant Professor of Nursing, Rush University, Chicago, Illinois

Elder Granger, MD, FACP
Staff Hematologist/Oncologist, Dunham Army Health Clinic, Carlisle Barracks, Pennsylvania

Rebecca Hawkins, RN, MSN, ANP, AOCN
Oncology Nurse Practitioner, St. Mary Regional Cancer Center, Walla Walla, Washington

Ioana M. Hinshaw, MD
Rocky Mountain Cancer Centers, Columbia Presbyterian–St. Luke's Medical Center, Denver, Colorado

Brenda M. Hiromoto, RN, MS, CETN, OCN
Oncology/Hospice Coordinator, Kaiser Foundation Medical Center, Honolulu, Hawaii

Priscilla A. Ingebrigtsen, MSW
Licensed Clinical Social Worker, University Hospital, Denver, Colorado

R. Lee Jennings, MD
Surgical Oncologist, Colorado Surgical Oncology Associates, Denver, Colorado

Gari Jensen, RN, BSN, OCN
Staff Oncology Nurse, University Hospital, Denver, Colorado

Patrick H. Judson, MD
Great Plains Regional Medical Center, North Platte, Nebraska

Judy J. Kadlec-Fuller, RN, MSN, AOCN
Oncology Clinical Nurse Specialist, Lutheran Medical Center, Wheat Ridge, Colorado

Leigh K. Kaszyk, RN, MS, OCN
Staff Oncology Nurse, University Hospital, Denver, Colorado

Janet E. Kemp, RN, MSN
Lecturer, School of Nursing, University of Colorado Health Sciences Center, Denver; Associate Chief, Nursing Service/Education, Denver Veterans Affairs Medical Center, Denver, Colorado

Linda U. Krebs, RN, PhD, AOCN
Senior Instructor, University of Colorado School of Nursing; Nursing Oncology Focus Group Leader, University of Colorado Cancer Center, University of Colorado Health Sciences Center, Denver, Colorado

Scott Kruger, MD
Virginia Oncology Associates, Newport News, Virginia

Susan A. Leigh, RN, BSN
Cancer Survivorship Consultant, Tucson, Arizona

Kevin Owen Lillehei, MD
Associate Professor Neurosurgery, University of Colorado Health Sciences Center, Denver, Colorado

Kelly C. Mack, RN, MSN, OCN
Clinical Nurse Specialist, Rocky Mountain Cancer Centers, Denver, Colorado

Heidi A. Mahay, PharmD
Assistant Professor, School of Pharmacy, and Clinical Pharmacist, University of Colorado Health Sciences Center, Denver, Colorado

Michael T. McDermott, MD
Professor of Medicine, University of Colorado Health Sciences Center, Denver, Colorado

Beth E. Mechling, RN, MS, OCN
Clinical Nurse Specialist, Bone Marrow Transplant Program, University of Colorado Health Sciences Center and University Hospital, Denver, Colorado

Susan K. Morgan, MD
Department of Hematology/Oncology, Tripler Army Medical Center, Honolulu, Hawaii

Lillian M. Nail, PhD, RN, FAAN
Associate Professor, Associate Dean for Research, University of Utah School of Nursing, Salt Lake City, Utah

Diane K. Nakagaki, RN, BSN, ET
Hematology/Oncology Outpatient Clinic, Level III RN, Kaiser Foundation Medical Center, Honolulu, Hawaii

Patrice Y. Neese, MSN, RN, CS, ANP
Nurse Practitioner, Breast and Melanoma Teams, University of Virginia Cancer Center, Charlottesville, Virginia

Paula Nelson-Marten, RN, PhD, AOCN
Assistant Professor, Oncology Nursing, School of Nursing, University of Colorado Health Sciences Center, Denver, Colorado

Patricia W. Nishimoto, BSN, MPH, DNS
Adult Oncology Clinical Nurse Specialist, Department of Hematology/Oncology, Tripler Army Medical Center; Associate Professor, School of Nursing, Graduate Division, University of Hawaii, Honolulu, Hawaii

Mark Nishiya, MD
Urology Fellow, University of Colorado Health Sciences Center, Denver, Colorado

Patricia Novak-Smith, RN, MS, OCN
Gynecologic Oncology Case Manager, Oncology Administration, University Hospital, Denver, Colorado

Betty M. Owens, RN, MS
Formerly, Neuro-oncology Nurse Specialist, Division of Neurosurgery, University of Colorado Health Sciences, Denver, Colorado; Currently, Clinical Research Associate, Clinimetrics Research Associates, Inc., San Jose, California

Jennifer Petersen, RN, MS
Oncology Clinical Nurse Specialist, Rush Cancer Institute, Rush Presbyterian–St. Luke's Medical Center, Chicago, Illinois

Linda Marie Petersen-Rivera, RN, MSN, OCN
Clinical Nurse Specialist, Tripler Army Medical Center, Honolulu, Hawaii

Cathy E. Pickett, RN, BSN
Oncology Nurse Clinician, University of Colorado Health Sciences Center and University Hospital, Denver, Colorado

Karyn P. Prochoda, RN, MD
Assistant Clinical Professor of Medicine, Department of Internal Medicine, University of Colorado Health Sciences Center, Denver, Colorado

Mary Roach, MS, RN, OCN
Clinical Nurse Specialist, Hematology-Oncology Clinic, Lahey-Hitchcock Clinic, Windsor, Vermont

Brenda Ronk, RN, MS, OCN
Oncology Clinical Nurse Specialist, Salisbury, Maryland

Pamela A. Rosse, RN, MS, CCRA
Outreach Coordinator, Clinical Investigations Core, University of Colorado Cancer Center, Denver, Colorado

Kimberly A. Rumsey, RN, MSN, OCN
Clinical Nurse Specialist, Tomball, Texas

Deborah M. Rust, MSN, CRNP, OCN
Instructor, Oncology Nurse Practitioner Program, University of Pittsburgh; Nurse Practitioner, Adult Bone Marrow Transplant Program, University of Pittsburgh Cancer Institute, Pittsburgh, Pennsylvania

Diana L. Ruzicka, RN, MSN, MAJ, AN
Clinical Coordinator, Pain Management Service, Tripler Army Medical Center, Honolulu, Hawaii

Ida A. Sansoucy, RN, BSN, MS, MEd, OCN
Field Nurse, Columbia Homecare, Denver, Colorado

Paul A. Seligman, MD
Professor of Medicine, University of Colorado Health Sciences Center, Denver, Colorado

Jean K. Smith, RN, MS, OCN
Breast Cancer Nurse Coordinator and Lymphedema Case Manager, Penrose Cancer Center of Centura Health, Colorado Springs, Colorado

Meribeth Wallio Smith, MSW
Adjunct Faculty, Graduate School of Social Work, University of Denver, Denver, Colorado

Merle S. Sprague, MD
Chief of Radiation Oncology, Tripler Army Medical Center, Honolulu, Hawaii

Julie R. Swaney, MDiv
Chaplain, Associate Department of Pastoral Care; Associate Faculty, Program in Healthcare Ethics, Humanities and the Law; Clinical Faculty, Department of Medicine; Clinical Faculty, Department of Psychiatry; University of Colorado Health Sciences Center, Denver, Colorado

Daniel I. Tell, DO, FACP
Clinical Assistant Professor of Medicine, University of Colorado School of Medicine, Denver; Oncology Clinic P.C., Colorado Springs, Colorado

Debra K. Thaler-DeMers, BSN, RN, OCN, PHN
Staff Oncology Nurse, Columbia Good Samaritan Hospital; IV Infusion Nurse Specialist, Advanced Infusion Systems, San Jose, California

Marion Tolch, RN, BSN, CETN
Ostomy and Wound Specialist/Case Manager, Department of Educational Resources, University Hospital, Denver, Colorado

Elizabeth Folk Tracey, RN, PhDc, OCN
Clinical Nurse Specialist, Rocky Mountain Cancer Centers, Denver, Colorado

Leslie Tuchmann, RN, MSN
Oncology Clinical Nurse Specialist, and Head Nurse, Specialized Nursing Care Center, Tripler Army Medical Center, Honolulu, Hawaii

Carol S. Viele, RN, MS
Clinical Nurse Specialist, University of California at San Francisco, San Francisco, California

Michael R. Watters, MD, FAAN
Associate Professor of Medicine, Division of Neurology, University of Hawaii School of Medicine; Chief, Neurology Service, Tripler Army Medical Center, Honolulu, Hawaii

Marie B. Whedon, MS, RN, AOCN, FAAN
Instructor, Dartmouth Medical School; Hematology/Oncology Clinical Nurse Specialist, Dartmouth-Hitchcock Medical Center, Lebanon, New Hampshire

Rita S. Wickham, RN, PhD(c), AOCN
Assistant Professor and Teacher-Practitioner, Medical-Surgical Nursing, Rush University College of Nursing, Rush Presbyterian–St. Luke's Medical Center, Chicago, Illinois

Pamela Williams, RN, BSN, OCN
Oncology Nurse Clinician, University of Colorado Cancer Center, University Hospital, Denver, Colorado

Anne Marie Zobec, MS, RN, CS, ANP, AOCN
Oncology/Pain Clinical Nurse Specialist, Penrose-St. Francis Health Care System, Colorado Springs, Colorado

DEDICATION

To our husbands, Rob and Kyle, who participate in the ultimate collaboration by staying married to us, and to our children, Brandon, Melissa, and Brian, for their gifts of love and understanding.

PREFACE

With over 40 years of combined oncology nursing experience, we were motivated to create this book in order to share knowledge that we wished had been at our fingertips when we began our careers. We have often heard new oncology staff nurses say: "I don't know enough to even ask a question"; "I don't know where to begin looking for the answers", "I don't have time to look up something in a book that weighs 50 pounds"; or "I'm embarassed to ask a question." The Secrets Series® is an ideal format for presenting questions and answers in a convenient, readable, and concise manner. *Oncology Nursing Secrets* includes questions and answers appropriate for novices as well as advanced practitioners. As Socrates exemplified, the best way to teach is to ask questions.

Since oncology nursing derives "secrets" from many areas of medicine, we made full use of our collaborative ties with physicians and other disciplines. The authors range from staff nurses to oncologists to nurse academicians, all of whom are actively contributing to the care of oncology patients. This book is not meant to be a complete reference or comprehensive textbook. Rather it is intended to focus on commonly asked questions and to stimulate further discussion and research. The reader is encouraged to make full use of the excellent oncology textbooks and references cited throughout the book. With so many facts to present, it is impossible to express the complex human dimensions and love that permeate every aspect of oncology nursing care. We hope that you will discover those secrets for yourself. We invite you to share your secrets and to always ask questions. May you find wisdom and compassion in the answers.

We are grateful to all our patients and their families, who have been our best teachers. They have taught us to make the most of each day and to live even as we are dying. A special thanks to our husbands, who not only gave us their loving support, but also contributed their medical expertise in answering our questions and reviewing many chapters. We would like to express our appreciation to all the contributors for their time and work. We also acknowledge the oncologists, nurses, pharmacists, and other health care providers who have been our partners, as well as our teachers. Special recognition is extended to Becky Gossert for her phenomenal secretarial skills, diligence, and caring in the preparation of many of the manuscripts. Finally, we would like to thank Linda Belfus and her staff for their editorial assistance, support, and willingness to believe in *Oncology Nursing Secrets*.

We hope that this book will provide information and secrets to enhance nursing care and symptom management for patients with cancer.

Rose A. Gates, RN, MSN, CNS
Regina M. Fink, RN, PhD(c), AOCN

I. General Overview of Cancer

1. BIOLOGY OF CANCER

Richard D. Callahan, MD, and David C. Faragher, MD

While there are several chronic diseases more destructive to life than cancer, none is more feared.

Charles H. Mayo (1865–1939)
Annals of Surgery 83:357, 1926

1. What are the chances of getting cancer?

Approximately one of three Americans will develop a malignancy at some time in their lives, and one of five will die of cancer. Cancer is second to heart disease as the most common cause of death in the U.S. For 1997, there will be an estimated 1,382,400 new cases of invasive cancer in the U.S. and 560,000 deaths from cancer (1500 people/day). The good news is that relative survival rates for almost every major site, except non-Hodgkin's lymphoma, are showing improvement, and data from 1995 suggest that overall mortality from cancer is declining.

2. How are cancer cells different from normal cells?

The first rule for cancers is that they follow no rules. Cancer cells exhibit dysplasia (disorganized growth), hyperplasia (increased cellularity), metaplasia (abnormal appearing cells that are not yet identified as malignant), and pleomorphism (variations in size and shape not seen in normal cell lines). The basic features of cancer cells are summarized below:

- **Unregulated cell growth.** Cancer cells continue to divide and proliferate as long as space and nutrients allow.
- **Poor cellular differentiation.** Although cancer cells are derived from normal tissues, they do not reach full differentiation. Differentiation refers to the maturation of a cell and its ability to perform functions based on the tissue of origin. As cells become more differentiated, their potential is restricted and they lose their replicating ability, eventually dying (e.g. neurons, muscle cells). Well-differentiated cancer cells are more like the original tissue's normal cells. In contrast, undifferentiated cells are not totally committed cells (e.g. precursor or stem cells). Many cancer cells resemble undifferentiated cells, retaining the ability to divide. Undifferentiated or anaplastic cancer cells are disorganized, exhibit few features of the normal tissue, and may express antigens (e.g., alpha-fetoprotein) not normally possessed by the adult cell.
- **Ability to invade other tissues.** Cancer cells lack contact inhibition, meaning they are not inhibited in either growth or movement by contact with other cells. Many metastatic cancer cells have altered surface enzymes and can secrete enzymes (e.g., hyaluronidase) that dissolve their way through other cells. Cancer cells observed in vitro (grown in culture) are not attached as firmly to neighboring cells and lack the adhesiveness of normal cells.
- **Ability to initiate new growth at distant sites.** The lack of contact inhibition and lack of adhesiveness allow cancer cells to grow and spread without the restraint exhibited by normal cells.
- **Ability to escape detection and destruction by the immune system.** Carcinogenesis and the metastatic potential of tumor cells may be a balance between effective immunosurveillance and evasion by tumor cells from cell-mediated destruction.

1

3. Explain carcinogenesis. In other words, how do cancers get started?

Many environmental, chemical, and viral factors can cause cancer or contribute to the transformation of a cell from normal to malignant. This transformation involves a complex series of essential steps. The first step, called **initiation**, begins with production of altered DNA in the cell, which leads to mutation of certain genes, protooncogenes, and tumor suppressor genes. This mutation may result in preneoplastic cells, which are converted to neoplastic cells in a process called **promotion**. Promoters facilitate clonal expansion and subsequent cancerous neoplasms. **Protooncogenes** are normal genes that control cellular division and proliferation. Alterations or mutations of protooncogenes result in activated oncogenes (genes that can transform normal cells into malignant cells) and subsequently carcinogenesis. Approximately 60 protooncogenes have been identified. One of the best-described classes of protooncogenes that is significant in the progression of human cancers is *ras*. Cancer growth is stimulated by oncogenes because they encode growth factors or other proteins that result in excessive cellular proliferation.

Tumor suppressor genes arrest cell proliferation and allow cells with DNA damage (result of initiation) to undergo self-repair. One of the best-described tumor suppressor genes is called P53. When P53 is inactivated by gene deletion or mutation, the restraint on proliferation is lost, and malignancy is likely to result.

4. How do cancers grow? Why is it so difficult to detect a cancer?

Cancers begin when a single cell mutates and loses the capacity for regulated growth. Cancers grow by reproducing cells. The malignant cell may be a breast cell, lung cell, or white blood cell that can grow to become a life-threatening disease. The initial cancer cell must duplicate its DNA, which is the blueprint for all of the biochemical processes necessary to sustain the cell. Once the DNA is duplicated, the cell is able to divide into two daughter cells. The two daughter cells divide to become four cells. These four cells divide to become eight cells, and so on.

Tumor doubling times (time it takes for tumor to double in size) vary from hours to months according to the type of cancer (primary and metastatic). It may take years for a tumor to double 20 times. Once the cancer goes through about 30 doublings, it has reached roughly the size of a marble, about 1 cm in diameter. A tumor of this size contains approximately 1 billion cancer cells. This is about the earliest stage at which we can detect developing cancers with screening x-ray studies. At this stage the cancer needs to go through only about 10 more doublings to reach 1 trillion cells, which is usually the amount of cancer that leads to death. Thus, much of the life span of the cancer is "silent" and takes place before the cancer is large enough to be detected, as depicted in the diagram (top of next page).

5. What is the influence of immunosurveillance on cancer development?

The greatest risk for developing cancer is older age because the aging process may diminish the vigor of the immune response. It is believed that we all have single cell mutations that could develop into cancers if the immune system did not attack the tumor cells. The carcinogens in cigarette smoke, chemical agents, or viruses may transform cells to malignant potential, but the immune system effectively nips it in the bud before the cancer can grow large enough to fend off the body's immune system. The immune system works best against a very small number of cells. As people get older, the immune system is probably assaulted by malignant changes with greater frequency, and the immune system itself may temporarily drop its guard when people are under great emotional stress or receive inadequate nutrition.

6. What is tumor heterogeneity?

Tumor heterogeneity refers to the subpopulations of biologically diverse cancer cells present in tumors. A key point is that not all of the cells which make up a malignant tumor are the same. A tumor mass may contain multiple clones with different chromosomal numbers and different characteristics. Some cells within a malignant tumor may be sensitive to one chemotherapy drug,

Growth Curve for Cancers (either Primary or Metastatic Tumor Masses)
and the Effect of Surgery, Radiation, or Chemotherapy

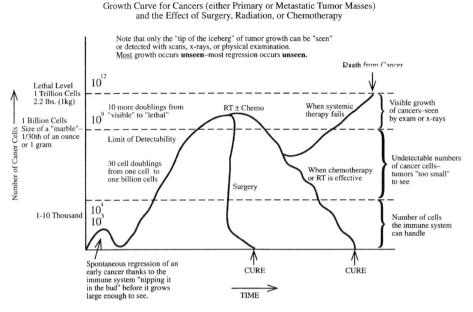

Growth curve for cancers. (Adapted from DeVita VT, et al: Principles of chemotherapy. In DeVita VT, et al: (eds): Cancer: Principles and Practice of Oncology, 1982, p 149.)

whereas other cells are resistant (hence the rationale for combination chemotherapy). Some cells are growing and others are dormant, only to emerge years later. This lack of uniformity makes it difficult to eradicate every last cell in treating cancers.

7. How do cancer cells invade tissues and metastasize to distant sites?

The most unique characteristic of malignant cells that results in the morbidity and mortality of cancer is their capability to invade tissues and to metastasize to other sites. A cancer cell's ability to metastasize requires multiple steps: (1) invasion of adjacent tissues through basement membranes, (2) entrance into nearby vessels (lymph or blood), (3) evasion of the immune system, (4) reentrance into distant tissues, and (5) implantation of malignant cell in new tissue.

Invasive tumor cells secrete enzymes that degrade basement membranes, which normally bar access to adjacent tissues. After access to adjacent tissue, malignant cells erode through vessel walls and circulate as individual cells or small aggregate of tumor cells (tumor embolus). These tumor cells may be coated by fibrin or circulate in aggregates of platelets, thereby escaping the immune cells in the blood. This process is relatively inefficient, because only about 0.1% of tumor cells that reach the circulation survive more than 24 hours. It is not known for certain why tumor cells of different malignancies prefer to metastasize to specific organs—in a process called **homing.** In some cases, this process is simply a result of anatomic blood circulation—as in the spread of colon cancer to the liver via the portal venous circulation. In other cases, tumor cells home to specific target organs as a result of specific chemotactic signals released by certain cells. Specific receptors have been identified on the surface of certain circulating tumor cells that recognize sites on endothelial cells of specific organs.

For tumor cells ultimately to develop into organ metastasis, they must develop their own vascular supply—in a process called **neovascularization** or **angiogenesis.** The tumor cells and neighboring normal cells synthesize and secrete angiogenic molecules that produce capillary networks for tumors at least 1–2 mm in size.

8. How do you explain to a patient that cancer has spread to another site?

Patients and families frequently misunderstand the concept of cancer spreading to another site. For example, if breast cancer spreads to the bone, the patient may believe that she has a new bone cancer. It is important to point out to the patient that the bone metastasis is still breast cancer, not bone cancer. Bone metastases from breast cancer are breast cancer cells that have spread through the blood stream to another site. This can happen long before the original tumor mass in the breast is large enough to be felt on physical examination or picked up on screening mammograms. A metastatic lesion may start as one cell or a small number of cells that have migrated through the blood stream to a distant organ or site. When the surgeon does a lumpectomy or mastectomy for breast cancer and tells the patient he "got it all," he means that he removed all of the cancer that could be seen. Currently there are no good tests to pick up micrometastases, which are small colonies of cancer growing away from the primary site.

9. Can the metastatic process be halted or prevented?

Experimental treatments to block various aspects of the metastatic process are under investigation, but as of 1997, no proven therapies of this nature are available for common clinical use. Perhaps the closest treatment is the use of agents that inhibit angiogenesis, the growth of blood vessels within a tumor mass to supply its nutrient needs.

10. Can cancer cells be induced to differentiate into more mature or less malignant cells?

Yes. Residual tumors that survive chemotherapy contain differentiated cells. Because growth of malignant tumors results from uncontrolled expansion of immature cells, attempts have been made to stimulate the cells to grow up or mature. In the laboratory, cultures of acute leukemia cells (HL-60 cells) have responded to differentiating agents, thereby becoming mature or differentiated. When malignant cells transform to differentiated cells, it is theorized that they lose their cancerous characteristics and thus become incapable of invasion or metastatic spread. Another benefit to differentiation of malignant cells is induction of programmed cell death; in other words, the cancer cells are no longer immortal. Many clinical studies have focused on the use of differentiating agents in various cancers. Fortunately, there have been some remarkable strides in areas such as leukemia, head and neck cancers, and lung cancers.

Retinoids, which are vitamin A analogs, have been studied most intensively. The most significant clinical breakthrough is in the treatment of acute promyelocytic leukemia (APL). All-transretinoic acid (ATRA) can induce complete remission in APL. The remission is a result of induced differentiation of leukemic cells. The resulting cells in the peripheral blood and bone marrow are intermediate in maturation between promyelocytes and normal mature white blood cells. Other retinoids, such as 13-cis-retinoic acid, have been studied extensively for primary prevention (prevention of the initial cancer) in high-risk patients as well as secondary prevention (prevention of recurrence). Numerous clinical studies are in progress.

11. How do you answer patients who ask, "How much time do I have?"

We are frequently asked to predict outcomes and often respond by quoting statistics. Patients and their families hear the statistics and commonly interpret them as a prediction of outcome for themselves or their loved ones. An explanation that the average survival for advanced, non-small cell lung cancer is 6 months should not be interpreted by the patient that he or she will live exactly 6 months. If it is carefully explained that statistical figures are averages and that no one can predict the outcome for a specific individual, it is reasonable to give patients or family members an idea of usual outcome. It is appropriate to try to leave a little room for hope. There is nothing wrong with saying, "I don't know," when patients ask, "Exactly how long does Dad have?" There is a tendency among healthcare workers, especially those just out of training, to feel that they should have all of the answers. We do not. We have far more questions than answers. One of the most difficult concepts to get across to patients is that we do not have all the answers. The hope of curing cancer lies in our ability to understand its biology more accurately and precisely.

BIBLIOGRAPHY

1. Appelbaum JW: The role of the immune system in the pathogenesis of cancer. Semin Oncol Nurs 8:51–62, 1992.
2. DeVita VT, et al: Principles of chemotherapy. In DeVita VT, et al: (eds): Cancer: Principles and Practice of Oncology, 1987.
3. Hwu P: The gene therapy of cancer. Prin Pract Oncol 9:1–10, 1995.
4. Lind J: Tumor cell growth and cell kinetics. Semin Oncol Nurs 8:3–9, 1992.
5. Lydon J: Metastasis. Part I: Biology and prevention. In Hubbard SM, Goodman M, Knobf MT (eds): Oncology Nursing. Philadelphia, Lippincott-Raven Publishers, 1995, pp 1–13.
6. Olopade O: Genetic counseling for cancer. Prin Pract Oncol 10:1–11, 1996.
7. Parker SL, Tong T, Bolden S, Wingo PA: Cancer Statistics 1997. CA Cancer J Clin 47:5–27, 1997.
8. Reilly JA: The biology of metastasis: Basic science of oncology. Contemp Oncol 11:32–46, 1993.

2. CANCER PREVENTION AND DETECTION

Mona Bernaiche Bedell, RN, BSN, MSPH, OCN

1. Which risk factors for cancer can be modified?

Over 70% of all cancers are associated with lifestyle choices. Adopting a healthy lifestyle and changing risky personal habits and behaviors can reduce the risk for cancer. Examples include elimination of both smoking and chewing tobacco, modification of alcohol intake, limiting exposure to ultraviolet light, adoption of sexual practices that limit exposure to sexually transmitted viruses (such as abstinence, limited number of sexual partners, use of condoms), stress reduction, eating foods high in fiber and low in fat, and regular exercise.

2. Which single lifestyle factor, if eliminated, would have the greatest impact on reducing the incidence of cancer?

Cigarette smoking is the most preventable cause of cancer-related death in the United States. Smoking is not only responsible for more than 85% of lung cancer cases, but is also the leading cause of head and neck cancers and is associated with cancers of the stomach, bladder, kidney, pancreas, liver, and cervix. Smoking also contributes to deaths from cardiovascular disease, pneumonia, stroke, emphysema, and bronchitis.

3. Are vaccines available to prevent cancer?

Vaccines are not yet available to prevent cancer directly. A highly effective vaccine is currently available to prevent hepatitis B virus (HBV) infection. Approximately 10% of patients infected with HBV become chronic carriers, which is a significant risk factor for the development of hepatocellular carcinoma. At present there are over one million chronic carriers of HBV in the U.S., or about 1 in every 250 Americans.

4. How useful is the Papanicolaou (Pap) test?

The Pap test is highly effective in detecting precancerous cells of the cervix. This simple, painless, and inexpensive test has reduced deaths from cervical cancer by 70% in the past 40 years. Screening efforts must be made to reach high-risk women in lower socioeconomic groups and elderly women. In both groups the incidence of advanced disease at diagnosis remains high. Over one-half of all American women with newly diagnosed cervical cancer have never had a Pap test.

5. Describe primary and secondary levels of cancer prevention.

Primary prevention refers to simple measures taken early to avoid the development of cancer. Primary cancer prevention can be achieved by making changes in lifestyles that eliminate risky behavior before cancers occur. Examples of primary prevention activities include smoking cessation, dietary changes to reduce fat and increase fiber, and limiting exposure to ultraviolet light and sexually transmitted viruses. Secondary prevention targets specific populations and refers to activities such as testing or screening to identify high-risk groups with cancer or precursors to cancer. Mammography, Papanicolaou testing, sigmoidoscopy, and prostate-specific antigen (PSA) testing are examples of secondary prevention activities.

6. How successful is screening for lung cancer in high-risk populations?

Extensive studies have failed to show a decrease in mortality even when patients at high risk for lung cancer were screened with chest radiography and sputum cytology. Currently, primary prevention offers the only hope for reducing the incidence of lung cancer. Routine screening is not recommended.

7. When is cancer screening most beneficial?

The greatest benefit from screening occurs when a certain cancer is highly prevalent in the population and early diagnosis and treatment result in a reduced mortality. Screening tests must be simple, inexpensive, and safe as well as clinically acceptable to the patient. Tests must be sensitive (able to identify cancer when it is present) and specific (able to determine when cancer is not present).

8. Does exposure to environmental tobacco smoke increase a nonsmoker's risk for lung cancer?

Passive cigarette smoke, involuntary smoke, and sidestream smoke refer to environmental exposure to tobacco smoke, which is responsible for about 30% of lung cancers. Risk of lung cancer is higher for nonsmokers who have lived or worked for years among heavy smokers. Second-hand smoke has significantly higher concentrations of carcinogenic compounds than mainstream smoke. A burning cigarette gives off at least 43 known carcinogens.

9. What is the most common cancer?

Skin cancer is the most common cancer; basal cell and squamous cell carcinomas account for more than 800,000 cases annually. Melanoma accounts for just over 38,000 cases annually, but the incidence of this deadly cancer is rising more rapidly than the incidence of any other cancer in the United States. Skin cancers are highly curable when diagnosed early and surgically excised.

10. Are tanning booths a safer way to obtain a tan?

Avoid tanning booths or salons! There is no such thing as a safe tan. Damage from sunlight or artificial sources of sunlight is cumulative over a lifetime and increases risk for the development of skin cancer. Tanning is the skin's response to injury. Excessive exposure also contributes to skin changes that cause wrinkles, premature aging, and rough, leathery skin.

11. Are sunscreens effective in protecting against skin cancer?

The lifetime incidence of skin cancer can be reduced by as much as 78% with regular use of sunscreen with sun protection factor (SPF) of at least 15 during the first 18 years of life. It is never too late to start using sunscreen.

12. How can the rising incidence of prostate cancer be explained?

The number of men diagnosed with prostate cancer has doubled in the past 10 years. This increase is most likely the result of mass screening programs, improved detection techniques, and increased public awareness.

13. Why is the widespread use of PSA screening for early detection of prostate cancer so controversial?

There is little consensus about screening guidelines for prostate cancer, and debate continues over routine widespread use of PSA alone. Because PSA is not specific for cancer of the prostate, its use in screening is limited. Elevated levels are found with prostate cancer as well as benign hypertrophy, prostatitis, and prostatic trauma. PSA may identify prostate cancers early, when they are small and localized. Unfortunately PSA cannot distinguish latent from aggressive prostate cancers that require treatment. Mass screening of asymptomatic men may identify too many low-grade tumors that may never become clinically significant or require treatment. Scientific evidence is insufficient to establish that PSA, alone or in combination with digital rectal examination or transrectal ultrasonography, has had any impact on reducing the mortality rates of prostate cancer.

14. Which tests are required for complete screening for colorectal cancer in asymptomatic individuals?

Digital rectal examination (DRE), fecal occult blood testing (FOBT), and flexible sigmoidoscopy are the primary screening tools. The American Cancer Society recommends an annual

DRE beginning at age 40, annual FOBT beginning at age 50, and flexible sigmoidoscopy every 3–5 years after age 50. Studies show that early stage colorectal cancer can be detected by these tests; however, randomized control trials have yet to show a decrease in mortality.

15. What are serum tumor markers?

Tumor markers are biochemical indicators of neoplastic activity found in the blood; they are produced by a tumor or by other cells in response to a tumor. Tumor markers are not sufficiently sensitive or specific to be used as screening tools in the general population, but they are helpful in monitoring response to therapy. Some of the commonly used serum tumor markers are listed below.

Tumor Marker	Malignancies Associated with Elevation
Alpha-fetoprotein (AFP)	Hepatocellular carcinoma
	Choriocarcinoma, teratoma
	Embryonal cell tumors of ovary or testis
Carcinoembryonic antigen (CEA)	Colon, rectum, pancreas, stomach, lung, breast, ovary
CA-125	Epithelial ovarian neoplasms, breast, colorectal
CA 19-9	Colorectal, pancreas, stomach, liver
Human chorionic gonadotropin (HCG)	Choriocarcinoma, germ cell, testicular teratoma, hydatidiform mole
Prostate-specific antigen (PSA)	Adenocarcinoma of prostate

16. What is carcinoembryonic antigen (CEA)? How is it used?

CEA is a protein normally found in small quantities in the blood of healthy people. It is elevated in over one-half of patients who have cancer of the colon, pancreas, stomach, lung, or breast. Elevations also have been associated with noncancerous conditions such as ulcerative colitis, liver disease, lung infections, and smoking (20% of smokers); therefore, elevated CEA is not specific enough to be used for screening or diagnosis. CEA testing is most useful for monitoring response to therapy and detecting disease recurrence.

17. List foods and drugs that may give false-positive reactions to guaiac-based tests for fecal occult blood.

Rare red meat, broccoli, turnips, cauliflower, parsnips, cabbage, horseradish, potatoes, and melons should be avoided for 3 days before and during testing. Aspirin, vitamin C, iron tablets, nonsteroidal antiinflammatory drugs, and cimetidine also should be avoided.

18. What factors help to identify families at increased risk for hereditary forms of cancer?

Hereditary cancer accounts for 5–10% of all cancers diagnosed. Families at high risk have some of the following features in their history and should be referred for genetic or cancer-risk counseling:
1. Two or more generations diagnosed with the same or related forms of cancer
2. Early age of onset
3. Occurrence of rare tumors
4. Bilateral, multifocal, or multiple primary tumors in one or more family members.

19. At what age should screening for breast cancer be started?

Clearly, women aged 50 years and over derive the greatest benefit from screening. The American Cancer Society recommends monthly breast self-examinations and yearly clinical breast examinations and mammography for women older than 50 years. Many randomized, controlled trials have evaluated the effectiveness of mammography and clinical breast examination; they found a reduction in mortality among women in this age group. Evidence of benefit for women aged 40–49 years is less clear, and recommendations from scientific organizations are varied. Potential risks and benefits should be discussed with women under age 50 when screening is considered.

20. List the general dietary recommendations of the American Cancer Society to reduce cancer risk.

1. Avoid overeating and maintain an ideal body weight.

2. Reduce total fat intake to less than 30% of caloric intake. Excessive fat intake and obesity increase the risk of developing cancers of the breast, colon, and prostate.

3. Include a variety of fruits and vegetables that provide fiber, vitamins, minerals, and other chemicals known to have a protective effect. Lower cancer rates have been associated with higher intake of fruits and vegetables.

4. Increase fiber intake by eating whole grain cereals, legumes, fresh fruits, and vegetables. Fiber decreases transit time of fecal material through the bowel and reduces contact between carcinogens and intestinal mucosa.

5. Minimize the intake of foods that are salt-cured, smoked, and nitrite-cured, such as luncheon meats, bacon, and hot dogs. Stomach and esophageal cancers are associated with consumption of smoked and pickled foods. Nitrates and nitrites, used as food preservatives, are believed to enhance carcinogenic nitrosamine formation.

6. Limit consumption of alcoholic beverages. Heavy drinkers are at increased risk for cancers of the oral cavity, larynx, esophagus, breast, and liver.

BIBLIOGRAPHY

1. Doherty K, Breslin S: Prostate cancer: An update on screening and management. Oncol Nurs Updates 3:1–13, 1996.
2. Groenwald SL, Frogge MH, Goodman M, Yarbro CH (eds): Cancer Nursing: Principles and Practice, 3rd ed. Boston, Jones & Bartlett, 1995.
3. Kibarian MA, Hruza GJ: Nonmelanoma skin cancer: Risks, treatment options, and tips on prevention. Postgrad Med 98: 39–58, 1995.
4. McPhee SJ: Screening for cancer: Useful despite its limitations. West J Med 163:169–172, 1995.
5. Murphy GP, Lawrence W, Lenhard R: American Cancer Society Textbook of Clinical Oncology, 2nd ed. Atlanta, American Cancer Society, 1995.
6. Parker SL, Tong T, Bolden S, Wingo PA: Cancer statistics, 1996. CA Cancer J Clin 65:5–27, 1996.
7. Potanovich LM: Lung cancer: Prevention and detection update. Semin Oncol Nurs 9:174–179, 1993.
8. Waldman AR, Osborne DM: Screening for prostate cancer. Oncol Nurs Forum 21:1512–1516, 1994.

3. DIAGNOSIS AND STAGING

Daniel T. Tell, DO, FACP

1. How is cancer diagnosed?

Cancer may be diagnosed clinically or by looking at a sample of tissue suspected of being cancerous under a microscope. A clinical diagnosis is the physician's best educated guess at the most likely diagnosis. A patient may be asymptomatic or present with a group of signs and symptoms that suggest a diagnosis of cancer. Most signs and symptoms, however, are nonspecific and can be seen in a wide variety of illnesses. A diagnosis of cancer requires a diagnostic test—and that test is the biopsy.

2. What is a biopsy?

A biopsy is a surgical procedure that involves removing all or part of the tissue suspected of being cancerous. There are several different types of biopsy: needle, incisional, and excisional. A needle biopsy involves inserting a needle into a suspicious lesion and removing individual cells (aspiration biopsy) or a core of tissue (core biopsy). If a lesion is large or accessible only by endoscopy, a surgeon may remove only a small portion of the lesion with a scalpel or forceps (incisional biopsy). Lastly, the surgeon may remove the entire lesion (excisional biopsy).

Another sampling method is to obtain cytology specimens. Malignant cells can be found in body fluids (e.g., ascites, spinal fluid, pleural effusions) or exfoliated from organs (e.g., cervical Papanicolaou smears, sputum).

3. Why is it important to establish a tissue (pathologic) diagnosis?

Cytology or biopsy specimens establish with certainty a diagnosis of cancer. A tissue diagnosis (tissue procurement and identification) eliminates all of the other diseases in the differential diagnoses originally considered by the clinician when the patients' signs and symptoms were first evaluated. With a firm diagnosis, accurate and specific treatment can be administered, and the patient can be given a prognosis.

4. What does the pathologist do with the biopsy?

Specimens are sent to the laboratory to identify the histopathology (tumor type, classification, and grade) of the malignancy. Examples of tumor types are carcinoma, sarcoma, germ cell tumor, lymphoma, and glioma. Classification is the subtype of the malignancy, such as a squamous or adenocarcinoma. Grade refers to the degree to which a malignant tumor is similar to normal tissue. For example, poorly differentiated or high-grade tumors contain few features of normal tissue.

Biopsied tissue may be processed in many different ways, depending on the suspected diagnosis. Initially, all tissue is fixed in a preservative solution and embedded in wax (tissue block). This method of processing the tissue allows thin slices to be cut from the block for staining and subsequent viewing under a microscope. Standard stains allow the pathologist to identify features specific to the biopsied organ as well as individual cells, nuclei, and nucleoli. Results from a biopsy should be available in 24 hours.

5. What if standard stains do not help?

If the pathologist cannot make a diagnosis with standard tissue stains, a wide variety of stains and techniques is available to define the cancer further. In general, a pathologist is able to diagnose cancer from the standard fixation and tissue stains. It is not unusual for the pathologist to have some difficulty in giving a final diagnosis without further testing. Additional testing often includes special stains as well as specialized studies (e.g., flow cytometry, monoclonal antibody testing, cytogenetics, and electronmicroscopy).

6. What are special stains?

Like the clinician, the pathologist generates a differential diagnosis when looking at the biopsy. The pathologist may not be sure of what he or she is looking at but usually has a good idea. Probabilities are ranked, and various tests are ordered to rule in (or out) the most likely diagnosis. The tests that the pathologist orders in this situation are collectively known as "special stains." The test may be as simple as a stain for mucin to differentiate a squamous carcinoma from an adenocarcinoma. Alternatively, immunoperoxidase techniques may be used to identify prostate-specific antigen in an otherwise nonspecific adenocarcinoma. Special stains generally take another 24–48 hours to complete. Considering the differential diagnosis obtained by looking at the biopsy, a pathologist generally orders several special stains at once.

7. What is flow cytometry?

Flow cytometry is a technique that allows analysis of individual cells based on specific characteristics or characteristics identified by specific stains. The cells are placed in suspension and are analyzed as they flow through a port or laser source that separates the cells on the basis of the selected characteristic. As a diagnostic technique, it is generally used to characterize the various types of lymphoma and leukemia. Cells can be labeled with antibodies directed at various antigens specific for certain types of lymphoma. The cells are then sorted by this characteristic. An example is the selection and sorting of the CD5 antigen, which is present in most cases of chronic lymphatic leukemia. A suspension of lymphoma cells is exposed to an antibody directed at the CD5 antigen. The antibody is labeled to allow detection as the cells pass through the port. The CD5 cells are detected and counted separately, as is the total number of cells. The results are generally reported as a percentage of the number of CD5 cells relative to the total number of cells counted. It is, therefore, most useful in refining rather than establishing a diagnosis. Occasionally, an otherwise undiagnosible lymphoma may exhibit a characteristic flow cytometric pattern, thereby yielding a specific diagnosis.

Flow cytometry is used to determine the chromosomal content and growth fraction of various tumors, most commonly breast cancer. Although neither a diagnostic nor a staging procedure, this ancillary test is often used to assess prognosis and guide treatment. Flow cytometry provides the clinician with the percentage of tumor cells in "S" phase (dividing cells) and an indicator for the presence of tumor cells with abnormal DNA content. High percentages of cells in S phase and with abnormal DNA content are generally believed to confer a worse prognosis in breast cancer, and often more aggressive treatment is prescribed.

8. What are monoclonal antibodies?

All cells possess surface antigens that may be detected by antibodies directed against them. The antibodies are labeled to facilitate detection. The label may be radioactive or designed to fluoresce or change color so that it can be seen. Cancer cells often possess antigens unique to that particular type of cancer.

The pathologist may request a wide variety of monoclonal antibody tests to evaluate a biopsy, depending on the suspected diagnosis. Some examples of commonly used monoclonal antibodies are anti-LCA (leukocyte common antigen) and anti-cytokeratin. Both tests are often used in the evaluation of a poorly differentiated malignancy.

During routine staining, a pathologist may be able to say that a tissue specimen is malignant but unable to determine whether the cancer is a lymphoma or a carcinoma. This distinction is important with respect to both treatment and prognosis. Such a biopsy probably would be tested for both LCA and cytokeratin. An LCA-positive biopsy is consistent with lymphoma, whereas a cytokeratin-positive biopsy is consistent with carcinoma.

9. What are cytogenetic studies?

Some tumors are associated with specific genetic abnormalities, which often can be detected by cytogenetic studies. The chromosomes from individual cells are cultured and isolated during cell division. They are fixed, stained, and magnified so that rearrangements (translocations) and deletions can be seen. Probably the best known translocation is the Philadelphia chromosome, which is associated with and is usually diagnostic of chronic myelogenous leukemia. Further refinements of cytogenetic techniques have allowed the identification of individual mutations.

10. What is electronmicroscopy?

Just as light is used to view microscopic structures, electrons can be used to visualize the extremely small cell components. Because the wavelength of electrons is much shorter than visible light, resolution and magnification are much greater. Electronmicroscopy (EM) can be used to visualize cellular organelles, cellular inclusions, and intercellular bridges, which are often characteristic of various malignancies. The limit of magnification with light microscopy is about 1000×. EM can enlarge into the tens of thousands and even higher with specialized techniques.

11. What happens after the pathologist decides that the diagnosis is cancer?

Usually, the pathologist calls the patient's physician, who has to tell the patient. In most cases, the patient has been advised that a malignant diagnosis is likely and is mentally prepared to deal with the news. Preparing a patient to receive the news and actually delivering the news are an art that requires compassion, awareness of the patient's personality, and, to a certain extent, experience. The physician most qualified to inform the patient is the primary care physician; it is most important that he or she be involved. However, many physicians are uncomfortable in this role—which is why God made oncologists. Effective collaboration and communication between physicians and nurses are essential in assisting the patient through this initial crisis.

The nurse's role in this setting is critical; it is not only supportive but also informative. The nurse should be able to address issues that invariably arise after the patient has been told the diagnosis. Because most patients are anxious, they hear little of the physician's discussion after they hear the diagnosis or are confused about what they did hear. Patients may not be comfortable with questioning the physician or may be afraid that they are taking up too much of the physician's time. The nurse should be prepared to address the patient's questions and have general information about the disease process, prognosis, further testing, potential complications, and available treatments. If a specific question cannot be answered, the nurse should say so and obtain the answer or refer the patient to an oncology clinical nurse specialist or other appropriate health care provider. It is always better to admit that the answer is not known than to provide incorrect information. The patient may not necessarily be interested in specific answers at this point. Listening, support, guidance, and reassurance may be more important at this stage than statistics and technical information.

12. After the patient has been told, what's next?

Once a patient has been given the diagnosis of cancer, a series of tests is performed to determine the extent of the disease. This process is known as staging. Patients need to be informed about why the tests are done and instructed about preparation procedures and possible complications. Other instructions include description of physical sensations or discomfort that may be anticipated, when results are available, and identification of who will report the results. Patients should be assessed for contraindications or hypersensitivities to iodine or other radioactive agents.

13. What is staging?

Staging is used to determine the extent of disease in an individual patient. The TNM system of the American Joint Committee on Cancer (AJCC) is preferred for the solid tumors (e.g., breast, lung, colon):

T = characteristics of a given tumor (size, depth of invasion, involvement of surrounding structures)

N = presence or absence of involved nodes and size or number of involved nodes

M = presence or absence of metastases.

A typical TNM classification for a 3-cm breast cancer with one involved lymph node and bone metastases would be as follows: T2N1M1 (bone).

TNM results can be incorporated into larger groupings, called stages, in which various Ts, Ns, and Ms with similar prognoses are collected. Most tumors proceed from stage I through stage IV. Prognosis worsens with stage progression for any given disease. Stage IV disease is generally metastatic, whereas stage I disease is generally confined to the organ of origin. A T2N1M1 breast cancer is stage IV, whereas a T2N1M0 breast cancer is stage II. Such a system allows the clinician to assign a prognosis for a given clinical situation and usually guides treatment. It also allows health professionals to discuss individual clinical situations and to exchange information about prognosis and management. The detail provided by such a system allows retrospective (or prospective) investigations, which may reveal differences in prognosis for certain situations. These differences may justify moving a particular TNM combination to a different stage or provide new information about its management.

The system is specific for all of the different anatomic sites with respect to T and many Ns; as a result, it is complicated. Fortunately, *The Manual for Staging of Cancer*, published by the AJCC, lists all of the anatomic sites and the accepted staging schema for each. If a staging manual is not available, most oncology texts will explain TNM staging in the chapter for each tumor.

14. Why is staging important?

There are three main reasons to stage a patient:
1. The extent to which a disease has spread is prognostic.
2. Extent of disease often dictates treatment.
3. Accurate staging allows collection of data that eventually provide information about treatment outcomes for each type of cancer and each stage of disease. Staging information is collected by a tumor registry.

15. What is a tumor registry?

Most hospitals have a tumor registry. Hospitals with an accredited cancer program are required by the American College of Surgeons to have a registry that collects data about all malignant diagnoses made at the institution. When a patient is entered into the registry, the cancer diagnosis, stage, and treatment are recorded. The registry follows the patient for life. Follow-up information is collected from the patient, the patient's medical records, and the treating physician. If the patient is no longer under treatment or has not seen the physician in the preceding year, a letter is sent to the patient requesting information about the status of the disease.

The American College of Surgeons periodically collects data about an individual disease from all of the tumor registries in the country. This information is then analyzed and published. These data allow a hospital to determine whether treatment provided for its patients is comparable to other hospitals around the country.

16. Is there a different staging system for the lymphomas?

Yes. Sometimes the term *liquid tumor* is used to distinguish the lymphomas and leukemias from the solid tumors. For most lymphomas, the Ann Arbor classification is used. It has a number of advantages over the TNM system: (1) clinicians are comfortable with it; (2) it is easy to remember; and (3) it provides generally accurate information for prognosis and treatment.

In the Ann Arbor system, stage I disease is confined to one nodal group. Stage II disease involves more than one nodal group on the same side of the diaphragm. Stage III disease is present on both sides of the diaphragm, and stage IV disease is disseminated (i.e., present in nonlymphoid organs). This system also includes modifiers to denote the presence or absence of constitutional or "B" symptoms (e.g., fevers, sweats, weight loss). The system is further modified to denote whether the disease involves a nonlymphoid organ by contiguity. Such involvement is referred to as "E" disease (extralymphatic) and is distinguished from disseminated disease. A patient with a non-Hodgkin's lymphoma involving the liver is classified as stage IV. A patient with mediastinal adenopathy and direct extension to the surrounding lung is classified as stage I_E (lung). If the same patient also had a greater than 10% loss in body weight or unexplained fever or sweats, the patient would be classified as stage IB$_E$ (lung). This system is in common usage among oncology health professionals and is worth knowing.

17. Is there a separate staging system for the leukemias?

Chronic lymphatic leukemia (CLL) is the only leukemia to which a staging system is applied on a regular basis. The rationale is simple in that staging of CLL has prognostic implications. CLL is a chronic disease that lends itself well to a staging system. A patient with only an absolute lymphocytosis may live 7–10 years or more, whereas a patient with thrombocytopenia may live only 2 years. The most commonly used classification is the Rai system:

Stage 0   > 10,000 lymphocytes
Stage I   Enlarged lymph nodes
Stage II   Enlarged liver and/or spleen
Stage III   Anemia
Stage IV   Thrombocytopenia

Lack of staging systems for other leukemias does not mean that prognostic indicators do not exist or that extent of disease (tumor burden) is not important. Other leukemias are disseminated at diagnosis and have a short clinical course if not treated promptly and effectively. This fact somewhat lessens the value of a staging system. Staging systems with widespread acceptance may eventually be formulated for the acute leukemias as more information becomes available. The presence or absence of certain genes or immunophenotypes, certain ages, and certain locations are of known prognostic importance for various forms of leukemia. This information is often used to formulate a treatment plan. Eventually, these variables may be organized into a clinically useful staging system.

18. How are cancers staged?

All staging begins with a history and physical examination. Usually both have been done by the time a patient is diagnosed with cancer. More specific questions and more thorough physical testing may be performed after diagnosis to assess the presence of signs or symptoms peculiar to the diagnosed cancer. This information may make a physician suspect the presence of disease at another site, and other tests may be ordered to confirm such suspicions.

The physician generally orders a complete blood count, chemistry tests of liver and kidney function, and urinalysis when a patient is first suspected of having cancer. These tests help to detect the presence of metastatic disease and to assess organ function in preparation for treatment. Tumor markers may be ordered to serve as a point of reference for subsequent treatment. In some diseases, elevated tumor markers may suggest the extent of disease and tumor burden as well as have prognostic implications.

Besides the history, physical examination, and screening laboratory studies, a wide variety of tests is available to evaluate the extent of a particular disease. The most commonly used tests are radiographs (plain film, CAT scans, MRI, and nuclear medicine scans). Biopsies are sometimes used to confirm a suspicious radiograph or scan abnormalities and to evaluate tissue that cannot be evaluated in any other way (e.g., bone marrow).

19. What are tumor markers?

Tumor markers are substances secreted by tumors that can be found in the blood. In general, they are used to evaluate response to therapy and to monitor for recurrence. These tests are somewhat organ-specific, although overlap with other diseases is common. Many tumor markers can also be elevated in benign conditions.

Carcinoembryonic antigen (CEA) was the first tumor marker to be described and remains a useful test. CEA is elevated in many tumors of epithelial origin but is most commonly used to evaluate colon malignancies. It is often elevated in breast and lung cancer but may be abnormal in benign conditions such as bronchitis, hepatitis, and ulcerative colitis. It is mildly elevated in patients who smoke cigarettes. CEA is ordered preoperatively in patients with colon cancer. In this setting, an elevated CEA implies a worse prognosis. The test is repeated postoperatively, and levels should return to normal if all disease is resected. The test is repeated at periodic intervals to detect recurrence.

Many tumor markers are available to monitor various tumors. The most commonly used markers include CEA (colon), PSA (prostate cancer), CA-125 (ovarian cancer), CA-15-3 and CA-27-29 (breast cancer), and CA-19-9 (pancreatic cancer). All of these tests may be abnormal in benign conditions and may be useful to monitor other malignancies. CA-19-9 may be used to follow gastric or biliary tract cancers; CEA may be abnormal in breast and lung cancer.

Tumor markers are more likely to be elevated in patients with metastatic disease and tend to rise progressively with worsening disease. No test is perfect, however, and some patients with metastatic disease may have normal tumor markers.

20. Are tumor markers useful for cancer screening?

This is as much an economic as a scientific question. Screening asymptomatic patients for various cancers with tests that lack sensitivity and, of greater importance, specificity may be a waste of valuable health care dollars. Screening for prostate cancer with an annual PSA test is considered useful, although PSA is elevated in patients with benign prostatic hypertrophy. How much is society willing to spend for PSA tests that yield normal results and for evaluations in patients with abnormal results to detect cancer? Put another way, how much does it cost to diagnose one cancer in a population of asymptomatic adult men? As a corollary, what is the benefit to the patient diagnosed with cancer? Is the patient curable, or does a patient diagnosed in this manner require treatment at all? Should the test be restricted to a high-risk population or a certain age range? Such questions apply to all available tumor markers; they will assume increasing importance as economic pressures on medicine become more intense.

Currently, a screening PSA test is performed annually for all men over the age of 50. Screening CA-125 for ovarian cancer is used on a more selective basis for women at higher than average risk for disease.

21. What are CAT scans?

Computerized axial tomography (CAT) is a radiographic procedure in which a patient is exposed to x-rays and an image is generated based on the differential absorption of x-rays by different tissues in the body. In this respect the technique is similar to plain radiographs. In CAT scanning, the images are manipulated by a computer to provide cross-sectional images (or images in any plane, for that matter). The result is multiple cross-sectional images, usually several centimeters apart, depicted from head to toe. CAT is usually ordered for a general anatomic area such as head, chest, abdomen, or pelvis. It allows visualization of most internal organs in great detail and may spare the patient a surgical procedure. It is useful in the staging of a wide variety of cancers. In lung cancer, CAT visualizes the mediastinum, which may show enlarged lymph nodes not apparent on plain chest radiograph. Such a patient would not undergo surgical treatment; instead, the patient would be treated with radiation and chemotherapy. In pancreatic cancer, a CAT scan of the abdomen may show liver metastases. Again, surgery would not be an option; the patient would receive chemotherapy. In either of these cases, a biopsy probably would be performed to confirm the presence of disease in the lymph nodes or liver; the presence of disease in either location would radically affect treatment and prognosis.

22. What is an MRI scan?

In magnetic resonance imaging (MRI), the area of the patient to be visualized is exposed to a strong magnetic field, which aligns all of the atoms of the organ in question in one direction. When the magnet is deactivated, the atoms return to their normal alignment and in so doing release energy. Different tissues with varying water content release energy at different times. This energy is monitored and can be imaged. The result is a scan that at first glance appears similar to a CAT scan but provides different information. MRI may be used to image a suspicious area on a CAT scan, such as an area of fibrosis or an enlarged lymph node. Tumor within a scar or enlarged lymph node emits a different signal, allowing the radiologist to detect its presence.

MRI also may be used to detect lesions that are isodense. Such lesions have the same density as the tissue in which they grow and may not be seen on CAT scanning. Brain and liver metastases are occasionally isodense; when an MRI scan is performed, the lesions become obvious as bright white masses. Because isodense lesions are relatively uncommon, MRI scanning is not a routine part of staging. Generally a negative CAT scan is accepted as normal unless the patient displays symptoms suggesting the presence of disease. In this situation an MRI may be ordered to exclude isodense metastases.

MRI also has proved useful in the diagnosis of carcinomatous meningitis. Before the availability of MRI, patients often required myelography, which is invasive, uncomfortable, and potentially dangerous.

23. What are nuclear medicine scans?

Nuclear medicine scans are radiographic studies in which a radioactive label is administered to the patient intravenously. The radioactive isotope concentrates within the target organ, where it is temporarily trapped. The label emits radiation that can be imaged. Before the advent of CAT scanning, brain and liver scans were commonly used for staging. However, CAT scans have far better resolution than nuclear medicine scans and have largely replaced nuclear medicine scanning of the brain and liver.

A bone scan is often used to stage patients with lymphoma and various solid tumors such as lung and breast cancer. Gallium scans are often used to assess the extent of lymphoma, because gallium is often taken up by lymphomatous tissue. Gallium scans are considered part of the staging evaluation of Hodgkin's disease, and some authors find them useful in the evaluation of lymphoma. Like all staging studies, these studies are often repeated after treatment to assess response.

A multiple-gated acquisition (MUGA) or heart scan is often ordered during staging to assess cardiac function in patients who may need potentially cardiotoxic chemotherapy. This scan provides information about cardiac wall motion, contractility, and ejection fraction; it is used to determine whether the patient's heart is functioning well enough to tolerate specific drugs (e.g., Adriamycin). It is not part of staging per se.

24. What is a bone marrow biopsy?

Bone marrow biopsy is a commonly used minor surgical procedure that determines the presence or absence of marrow involvement by tumor. The posterior iliac crest is the site most commonly chosen. It may be seen in most patients when viewed from the back as the two dimples on either side of the lower lumbar spine at the belt line. In most patients, the iliac bone is close to the surface at this point and separated from the surface of the skin only by fat. The patient may be sedated for the procedure. After local anesthetic infiltration, a small stab incision is made. A needle is then inserted through the bone cortex into the marrow cavity and a small amount of liquid marrow is aspirated into a syringe. A biopsy needle is then inserted into the bone to remove a core or cylinder of bone marrow, usually about 2 cm long and a few millimeters wide. In patients in whom sedation is not possible, the procedure is moderately uncomfortable. The dominant sensation is an intense pressure punctuated by brief periods of toothache-like pain. The only major complication of a correctly performed bone marrow biopsy is the remote possibility of infection in the bone. Postprocedural pain is generally mild and resolves within a few days. An occasional patient develops a subperiostial hematoma, which may cause point tenderness for several weeks. In the bone marrow involved by tumor, collections of tumor cells may be seen in scattered areas throughout the marrow cavity, or tumor may completely fill the space.

25. How is bone marrow biopsy used in staging?

A bone marrow biopsy is a diagnostic procedure for leukemia, whereas it is generally a part of the staging evaluation of lymphomas. It is also used in small cell lung cancer when the likelihood of marrow involvement is substantial and when marrow involvement changes treatment. In most other diseases, marrow biopsy is used selectively. In solid tumors and lymphomas, marrow involvement often changes treatment and always changes prognosis. As a result, bone marrow biopsy may be used to stage a patient in whom bone marrow involvement is suspected. For example, the complete blood count (CBC) of a patient with breast cancer may show mild anemia and thrombocytopenia. The differential may show a small number of immature white cells and an occasional nucleated red blood cell. This constellation of CBC findings is highly suspicious for marrow involvement by tumor. In the absence of another good explanation, bone marrow biopsy would be recommended. Treatment will be affected dramatically if the bone marrow is involved. Local measures such as mastectomy become secondary to systemic treatment, and bone marrow transplantation may even be considered. Prognosis, of course, is also changed.

26. When does it all end?

Staging is complete when the doctor and patient know the diagnosis, prognosis, and correct treatment. Every attempt is made to make the process safe, comfortable, informative, efficient, and cost-effective.

27. Are there any cancers that cannot be diagnosed? What are cancers of unknown primaries?

In occasional patients who present with metastatic cancer, a careful search reveals no obvious primary tumor. This situation, which is known as adenocarcinoma–unknown primary (AUCP) or simply unknown primary, accounts for about 5–10% of all patients with cancer. Most commonly such tumors are poorly differentiated carcinomas or adenocarcinomas. AUCP is approached carefully by the oncologist, because the "carcinoma" in fact may be a lymphoma or germ cell tumor, both of which are highly responsive to treatment and even curable in many cases. The oncologist generally collaborates closely with the pathologist to make sure that both lymphoma and germ cell tumor are considered and looked for with special stains.

Once the pathologist and oncologist are sure that both have been excluded and that the patient has a carcinoma, other considerations come into play. One approach is to look for treatable tumors, or cancers that have high response rates to treatment with tolerable toxicity and reasonable duration of remission. In men, prostate cancer would be considered, and a tissue stain for PSA would be ordered. Prostate cancer can be treated with orchiectomy or chemical castration with minimal toxicity and response rates in the range of 70%. In women, one would attempt to diagnose breast cancer. No tissue stain is specific for breast cancer, but the finding of estrogen and progesterone receptors in the biopsy may suggest the diagnosis. A mammogram certainly would be ordered as well. Breast cancer is also responsive to hormonal therapy, and chemotherapy induces remission in about 50% of patients.

If germ cell tumors, lymphoma, and breast and prostate cancer are excluded, the prognosis is dismal. The average survival in such patients is about 4 months, and few treatments are successful or well tolerated. Tumors are often approached as lung cancers, if the dominant disease is above the diaphragm, or pancreatic tumors, if below the diaphragm. They are often treated empirically on this basis in patients desirous or capable of treatment.

28. What is scintigraphy?

In scintigraphy, a radioactive isotope is injected around a primary tumor and the isotope is then imaged after it has traveled to the lymph node group that serves as primary drainage for the tumor site. This technique is useful in evaluating tumors with ambiguous lymph node drainage, such as melanomas on the trunk. A melanoma on the back, for instance, may drain to either axilla or groin or even the cervical region. Demonstrating lymph node involvement in melanoma has become highly important, because effective adjuvant treatment has been discovered for patients with metastatic lymph nodes.

Scintigraphy is also gaining popularity in the evaluation of breast cancer. The first lymph node draining the breast cancer, known as the sentinel node, is biopsied rather than performing an axillary node dissection. The assumption is that a negative sentinel lymph node is predictive of a negative axillary lymphadenectomy. At present, this approach remains experimental, but if preliminary studies are confirmed, it may become standard care for patients with breast cancer. This procedure is often referred to as sentinel lymph node mapping.

29. Are there any controversies in the diagnosis of cancer?

No. A tissue diagnosis must always be made. Physicians may argue about the best way to obtain a diagnosis, but none would argue against making the diagnosis. The implications of a diagnosis of cancer and the potential for harm during the treatment of cancer are too great to assume the diagnosis. A clinical diagnosis, if incorrect, exposes the patient to great emotional, physical, and financial stress. The cardinal rule of oncology is simple: no D_x (diagnosis)—no R_x (treatment).

30. Are there any controversies in the staging of cancer?

Yes. For most diseases, staging procedures and tests are standard. Controversy arises when technologic advances and new or ancillary tests become available. Patient risk, inconvenience, and cost enter the equation, and there is a period of uncertainty until the new technology is perceived or proved to be indispensable or ancillary. In the future, advancing technology will clash with increasing cost consciousness, and the manner in which cancer is diagnosed and staged will change—hopefully for the better.

BIBLIOGRAPHY

1. Beahrs OH, Henson DE, Hutter RVP, Kennedy BJ (eds): Manual for Staging of Cancer, 4th ed. Philadelphia, J.B. Lippincott, 1992.
2. Madeya ML, Pfab-Tokarsky JM: Flow cytometry: An overview. Oncol Nurs Forum 19:459–463, 1992.

II. Treatment of Cancer

4. PRINCIPLES OF THERAPY

Kyle M. Fink, MD, and Ioana Hinshaw, MD

1. How is cancer treated? What therapies are currently being studied?

The major treatment modalities for cancer are surgery, radiation therapy, chemotherapy, and hormonal therapy; each may be used alone or in combination with other modalities. Studies are ongoing to evaluate the effectiveness of other modalities, such as gene therapy, novel drugs, cryotherapy, immunotherapy, hyperthermia, photodynamic therapy, bone marrow and stem cell transplantations, and differentiation therapy as well as to improve strategies and reduce toxicities of standard therapies.

2. What are some strategies to establish rapport and trust when interacting with a patient presenting with a new diagnosis of cancer or for follow-up care?

First you must listen to patients and maintain open communication to understand their concerns about cancer and treatments and their fears about the future. Two of the most worrisome problems for patients are fear of the unknown and probable survival time. You need to understand their perspective and their level of knowledge, making sure that you talk **with** them, not at them. In a busy setting, it is important for the health care provider to be centered and focused on the patient. Try to ensure that outside interruptions, such as phone calls and paging, are kept to a minimum.

Always try to connect with your patients, even in the smallest manner. Find out something personal about them—what kind of work they do, their support system, their interests, their children. Try to find something in common in a nonmedical area. For instance, you may be from the same town or state or have gone to the same school; both of you may play tennis, have an interest in movies or books, or like cats.

"Compassionate" disclosure of information requires that you communicate a new diagnosis of cancer or bad test results as directly and as soon as possible. Do not "beat around the bush" for the first half of the visit. Patients are unable to focus on your discussion until they know specifically with what they are dealing and until anxiety and fear of the unknown have been relieved.

Honesty about the diagnosis or test results increases the patient's level of trust. Whenever possible, the physician should enlist the collaborative assistance of a nurse or oncology clinical nurse specialist. By being present in the room, the nurse will know what has been said and will be able to offer support, compassion, and follow-up information to clarify what the physician has said.

Make sure that the patient initially understands the treatment objective, whether it is curative, adjuvant, or palliative. Some patients, especially if they are to receive palliative care, may not wish to acknowledge the fact after the initial discussion. Sometimes they cope better by using denial—and this strategy is all right. However, the oncologist, nurse, patient, and family can be reassured that the subject has been broached openly and honestly.

Incorporate patients into the treatment plan by giving them options from which to choose. By being able to help determine their treatment program, patients are better able to accept and comply with therapy. Nurses can offer options such as timing of chemotherapy and choice of antiemetic.

Try to leave the room with a positive note, no matter how dismal the information. The only positive element may be reassuring a terminal patient that great medications are available to control pain or that the health care team will do everything possible to help quality of life.

3. What are the most important steps before initiating therapy for cancer?

All decisions in oncology are based on understanding the natural history of the disease, treated or untreated. Before initiating any therapy, important points need to be considered:

1. The diagnosis needs to be confirmed, almost always by tissue biopsy. Do not diagnose unconfirmed cancer.

2. The disease needs to be staged by appropriate diagnostic means (e.g., physical examination, computed tomography [CT] scans, bone scan). Extent or stage of disease critically determines prognosis and treatment.

3. The goal of therapy needs to be defined: curative, adjuvant, or palliative.

4. A treatment plan must be chosen from many therapeutic options, depending on the stage of the disease and patient characteristics such as age, performance status, and comorbid disease as well as the patient's wishes.

4. What is the difference between curative and palliative treatment?

Curative treatment is given with the intent of eradicating measurable, discernible malignant disease. Some cancers, such as lymphomas and testicular cancers, can be cured despite extensive disease at diagnosis. In this curative setting, therapy should be aggressive, and some treatment-related morbidity and even risk of death may be justified. To increase the chance for cure, the dose intensity of any chemotherapy regimen should be maintained and dose reductions avoided. **Palliative treatment** is given when the disease is not curable and survival time is limited. The goals of palliative treatment are to alleviate symptoms and to improve quality of life while also extending survival. In this setting, care must be taken to keep toxicity at a minimum, and drug dose reductions are often necessary.

5. What is adjuvant therapy? When is it given?

Adjuvant therapy refers to the use of therapy, usually chemotherapy, along with another treatment modality. Adjuvant therapy is given with curative intent. The primary treatment (surgery) may have already cured the patient; the adjuvant therapy is added to increase the cure rate. Adjuvant treatments are given to patients who may or may not have cancer. It can cure only a microscopic tumor load. If the tumor becomes discernible or macroscopic, the treatment strategy must be adjusted, because adjuvant therapy is not strong enough to cure a larger tumor burden.

The best example is adjuvant chemotherapy for breast cancer given after mastectomy to a patient with positive nodes. The patient with breast cancer may be "cured" by the mastectomy, but the positive lymph nodes are an indication of possible microscopic disease somewhere in the body that may later develop into recurrent cancer; thus, adjuvant therapy is indicated. In contrast, adjuvant chemotherapy is not used in non-small cell lung cancer because, even if microscopic disease is present after surgical removal, chemotherapy is not effective in killing these microscopic tumor cells.

6. What cancers are responsive to chemotherapy?

Responsiveness of Various Cancer Types to Chemotherapy

Cancers with macroscopic disease that can be cured with chemotherapy	
Testicular cancer	Acute leukemias
Hodgkin's disease	Small cell lung cancer (nonmetastatic)
High-grade non-Hodgkin's lymphoma	Ovarian cancer

Cancers with microscopic disease that can be cured with adjuvant chemotherapy	
Breast cancer	Osteosarcoma
Colorectal cancer	Bladder cancer

Table continued on following page.

Responsiveness of Various Cancer Types to Chemotherapy (Continued)

Cancers with metastatic disease that can be controlled but not cured with chemotherapy

Breast cancer	Endometrial cancer
Colorectal cancer	Cervical cancer
Prostate cancer	Head and neck cancer
Lung cancer (non-small cell and small cell)	Bladder cancer
Low-grade non-Hodgkin's lymphoma	Stomach cancer
Multiple myeloma	Esophageal cancer
Chronic leukemias	Soft tissue sarcoma
Ovarian cancer	Osteosarcoma

Cancers that have low response rates or are unresponsive to chemotherapy

Brain tumors	Thyroid cancer
Renal cell cancer	Cholangiocarcinoma
Malignant melanoma	Mesothelioma
Hepatoma	Carcinoid tumors
Pancreatic cancer	

7. How can the concept of adjuvant therapy be explained to patients?

Explain to patients that the detectable limit of cancer with currently available tests is 1 cubic centimeter of tumor, which equals one billion cancer cells (10^9). Patients may be told that if they have cancer, they have anywhere from 1 to 1 billion cancer cells; it is the objective of adjuvant chemotherapy to destroy the microscopic cancer cells. Always emphasize the positive: the patient may have zero cancer cells and already be cured.

8. What is the difference between adjuvant therapy and neoadjuvant therapy?

Neoadjuvant chemotherapy is adjuvant therapy given before primary treatment (surgery or radiation) in patients with localized tumor. Neoadjuvant therapy reduces the extensiveness of surgery. For example, patients with breast cancer who initially are not surgical candidates because of tumor size may be able to undergo surgery after tumor size is reduced by adjuvant chemotherapy. Response to neoadjuvant therapy is also useful in establishing tumor chemosensitivity and prognosis. After removal of the residual tumor, the viability of the remaining tumor cells is examined to classify patients into complete responders, partial responders, or nonresponders; all have different prognoses.

9. In addition to the oral and parenteral routes, how else can chemotherapy be given?

- Instillation into the cerebrospinal fluid (CSF) for control of meningeal carcinomatosis
- Intrapleural or intrapericardial administration for control of malignant effusions
- Intraperitoneal administration as postsurgical therapy for ovarian carcinoma
- Intraarterial administration for isolated liver metastases due to colon carcinoma; also selected arterial infusion for sarcomas of the extremities

10. Why is performance status important in making treatment decisions?

In general, performance status predicts how the patient will tolerate therapy. Patients with poor performance status have an increased risk of chemotherapy-related toxicity.

Karnofsky and American Joint Committee on Cancer (AJCC) Performance Status Scales

DESCRIPTION	KARNOFSKY SCALE (%)	AJCC SCALE	DESCRIPTION
Normal; no complaints; no evidence of disease	100	H0	Normal activity
Able to carry on normal activity; minor signs or symptoms of disease	90		

Table continued on following page.

Karnofsky and American Joint Committee on Cancer (AJCC) Performance Status Scales (Continued)

DESCRIPTION	KARNOFSKY SCALE	AJCC SCALE	DESCRIPTION
Normal activity with effort; some signs or symptoms of disease	80	H1	Symptomatic and ambulatory; cares for self
Cares for self; unable to carry on normal activity or do active work	70		
Requires occasional assistance but is able to care for most of own needs	60	H2	Ambulatory > 50% of time; occasionally needs assistance
Requires considerable assistance and frequent medical care	50		
Disabled; requires special care and assistance	40	H3	Ambulatory ≤ 50% of time; nursing care needed
Severely disabled; hospitalization indicated, although death not imminent	30		
Very sick; hospitalization with active supportive treatment necessary	20	H4	Bedridden; may need hospitalization
Moribund, fatal processes progressing rapidly	10		
Dead	0		

Adapted from Beahrs OH (ed): American Joint Committee on Cancer: Manual for Staging of Cancer, 4th ed. Philadelphia, J.B. Lippincott, 1992.

11. What are some of the most useful prognostic factors in cancer?

Prognostic factors are both tumor-related and patient-related. Important tumor-related prognostic factors are histologic type, grade, and stage of disease. Other factors include expression of hormone receptors, cytogenetic abnormalities, and tumor-associated markers. Important patient-related prognostic factors are performance status, age, and associated systemic symptoms (weight loss, fevers, night sweats). Certain cancers have defined prognostic groups associated with specific survival rates.

12. How is response to therapy defined?

The response is usually quantified into complete response, partial response, stable disease, and progressive disease. **Complete response** means the disappearance of all measurable disease for at least 1 month. This response is clinically the most important indicator of effectiveness of chemotherapy and is the prerequisite for cure. **Partial response** is defined as at least 50% reduction in measurable tumor mass without appearance of new lesions for at least 2 months. **Stable disease** is characterized as either a decrease or increase of tumor by less than 25%. **Progressive disease** means an increase of tumor mass by more than 25% or appearance of new tumor lesions.

13. What are mixed responses to therapy?

If chemotherapy is effective in shrinking disease at one site, it usually has the same affect on all disease-involved sites; thus, the response is uniform. In rare cases, however, there may be tumor shrinkage at one site with tumor growth at another site. This is called a mixed response.

14. Why are multiple cycles of chemotherapy necessary?

Based on observations in experimental systems of animal tumors, it is believed that tumor cell killing is fractional in humans. According to the log cell kill hypothesis, at any given exposure chemotherapy drugs kill only a fraction of the cells. Because visible tumors are usually larger than 10^9 cells and one chemotherapy cycle is of the order of 2–5 log cell kill, it is apparent that treatment must be repeated many times to achieve control.

15. What are the major advantages of combination chemotherapy?

Most successful chemotherapy programs involve the use of multiple drugs, sometimes following complex schedules of administration. This approach is commonly referred to as combination chemotherapy. By using combinations of drugs, one can get maximal cell kill for each drug within a tolerated range of toxicity, broader range of activity against different subgroups or a heterogeneous tumor population, and prevent or retard the development of new resistant cell lines.

16. What principles govern the use of combination chemotherapy?

1. Only drugs that are active against the tumor to be treated are included in the combination.
2. The drugs should have a different mechanism of action to minimize the possibility of drug resistance.
3. The drugs should have different toxic side effects, thus allowing administration of full or nearly full doses of each active agent.
4. Each drug should be given at an optimal dose and schedule and at consistent intervals.

17. How is a patient's progress with chemotherapy assessed?

Because chemotherapy agents are potentially toxic, one should strive to follow objective markers of response in patients with metastatic disease. Objective markers may include decrease in size of a tumor, disappearance of hypercalcemia or other paraneoplastic syndrome, or decrease or disappearance of a tumor marker such as prostate-specific antigen (PSA) or carcinoembryonic antigen (CEA). Subjective responses such as tumor-related pain or weight gain are less reliable indicators of drug action. An objective determination of performance status gives an accurate estimation of the patient's overall condition and quality of life.

18. What does 5-year survival mean? When is a cancer considered cured?

National statistics about cancer are based on 5-year survival rates. For the most part, patients who are still alive 5 years after initial diagnosis are considered cured. With common tumors such as breast, lung, and colon cancer, recurrences usually follow a bell-curve; the incidence of recurrence peaks at 18–24 months after diagnosis, with few recurrences after 5 years.

19. What is chemoprevention?

Chemoprevention refers to the use of specific chemical agents to prevent the development of a premalignant or malignant lesion or to cause regression of a premalignant lesion. Many large chemoprevention trials are in progress. Examples include prevention of breast cancer with tamoxifen, prevention of lung cancer with the retinoid Accutane, and prevention of prostate cancer with the testosterone inhibitor finasteride (Proscar).

20. What is biochemical modulation?

The activity of some drugs may be increased or decreased by the presence of other drugs or normal metabolites. This process is called biochemical modulation and is best illustrated by studies of 5-fluorouracil (5-FU). Several chemicals potentiate the activity of 5FU, including methotrexate, thymidine, PALA, allopurinol, uridine, and leucovorin. Leucovorin best modulates 5-FU with beneficial effect for the patient. This combination is commonly used in the adjuvant or palliative treatment of colon cancer. 5-FU works by binding to the enzyme thymidilate synthetase, which leads to depletion of thymidine, a necessary ingredient for DNA synthesis. Reduced folate is a cofactor for 5-FU binding to the enzyme; leucovorin enhances this binding, thus potentiating 5-FU activity. The combination of the two drugs is more potent but also more toxic with increased incidence of mucositis and diarrhea.

21. How is chemotherapy dosed?

Information about dosage is derived from prior empirical dose-escalating trials in patients. Drug dosage is determined as a function of body surface area (BSA) rather than body weight. This convention was adopted because of research relating the maximal tolerated dose of chemotherapy in multiple species to body weight and BSA; it became apparent that interspecies comparison of dose were far more accurate using BSA than weight. Patients who are grossly obese require higher doses of chemotherapy, and their dosing is not calculated on ideal body weight. The chemotherapy dose must be adjusted according to renal, liver, cardiac, and pulmonary function.

22. Does BSA need to be recalculated with weight changes?
Because chemotherapy dosing is based on body surface area, recent weight loss or gain (> 10 pounds) requires recalculation of doses.

23. What is the concept of dose intensity?
The concept of dose intensity is significant because a major factor limiting the ability to cure cancer is adequate dosing. Dose intensity is defined as the amount of drug given per unit of time ($mg/m^2/week$), regardless of the schedule used. Generally, to cure cancer, it is best to give chemotherapy drugs at the highest dose at the shortest intervals; however, this is often difficult because of the low therapeutic index (toxicity to normal tissues) of many chemotherapy agents. There has been increasing concern that cancer patients may be receiving inadequate doses of chemotherapy because of inappropriate dose reductions by physicians concerned about drug toxicity. A positive relation between dose intensity and response rate has been observed in advanced ovarian, breast, and colon cancers and in lymphomas.

BIBLIOGRAPHY

1. Beahrs OH (ed): American Joint Committee on Cancer: Manual for Staging of Cancer, 4th ed. Philadelphia, J.B. Lippincott, 1992.
2. DeVita VT Jr: Principles of cancer management: Chemotherapy. In DeVita VT, Hellman S, Rosenberg SA (eds): Cancer: Principles and Practice of Oncology, 5th ed. Philadelphia, Lippincott-Raven, 1997, p 333.
4. Lenhard RE, Lawrence W, McKenna RJ: General approach to patients. In Murphy GP, Lawrence W Jr, Lenhard RE Jr (eds): American Cancer Society Textbook of Clinical Oncology, 2nd ed. Atlanta, American Cancer Society, 1995, pp 64–74.

5. SURGICAL ONCOLOGY

Ann Marie Dose, MS, RN, OCN, and Carol Brueggen, MS, RN, OCN

1. What is the role of surgery in the prevention of cancer?

Certain people may be at higher risk for development of cancer because of underlying health conditions or congenital or genetic traits. If an organ with potential for development of cancer is not crucial for ongoing survival, surgery may be necessary or desirable to prevent malignancy. Surgery may be performed to prevent colon cancer (in cases of familial polyposis), breast cancer, or testicular cancer.

Other cancers, such as cervical cancer, develop from a premalignant phase and, even in early stages of malignancy, remain locally confined. Limited surgical excision, laser or cryotherapy techniques may effectively obliterate or reduce spread of disease.

2. What are the goals of surgery in the treatment of cancer?

1. **Prophylactic** (see question 1).

2. **Diagnostic.** Tissue biopsy is necessary to validate the diagnosis and to identify the histology or specific type of cancer (see questions 4 and 5).

3. **Staging.** The extent of disease can be determined by surgical staging, which identifies tumor type, extent of growth, size, nodal involvement, and regional and distant spread. Exploratory surgery is sometimes required to stage Hodgkin's disease or ovarian cancer. Sentinel node biopsy can be done for breast cancer or malignant melanoma.

4. **Definitive or curative.** The primary goal of cancer surgery is cure. Definitive or curative surgery involves removing the entire tumor, associated lymph nodes, and a 2–5 cm margin of surrounding tissue. The amount of surrounding tissue removed is determined by the type of cancer. Early diagnosis is essential when the goal is cure. Surgery for early-stage cervical, breast, skin, renal cell, prostate, and colon cancer may be curative. Surgical placement of brachytherapy for cervical and prostate cancers is for curative intent.

5. **Palliative.** Surgical intervention for palliation is most commonly done to minimize symptoms of advanced disease and relieve distress. For example, palliative surgeries include cytoreductive surgery; ablative procedures; surgery to relieve gastrointestinal, respiratory, and urinary obstructions or fistulas; and neurosurgical procedures for pain control. Decompressive laminectomy may be done to relieve spinal cord compression secondary to malignancy.

6. **Adjuvant or supportive.** Surgical procedures that are performed in addition to other treatment modalities are called adjuvant or supportive. Adjuvant surgery is a secondary therapy. Examples include surgery to implant a vascular access device, feeding tube, or tracheostomy.

7. **Reconstructive or rehabilitative.** Advances in plastic and reconstructive surgery have made it possible to repair anatomic defects and to improve function and cosmetic appearance after radical surgery. The goal is to minimize deformity and improve the quality of life. Breast and head and neck reconstruction are examples.

3. What patient and cancer/tumor factors need to be assessed before undertaking surgery?

Tumor factors to consider include growth rate, invasiveness, metastatic potential, and location. In general, tumors that are slow-growing and have cells with prolonged cell cycles lend themselves best to local control by surgery. Surgeons need to know the pattern of local invasion for a specific tumor to be able to remove it as an entire mass with adequate normal surrounding tissue to minimize seeding or local recurrence. Some tumor invasions may necessitate more radical surgery; other tumors may not need total resection if additional chemotherapy and radiation therapy have been demonstrated to improve survival. Metastatic potential of a tumor determines the amount and appropriate combination of multimodal therapies. Location of the tumor and spread into adjacent tissue and vital organs or structures also need to be considered in weighing the risks and benefits of surgical intervention and effect on functional status and overall quality of life.

Patient factors include overall health status and comorbidities such as diabetes and cardiac, pulmonary, or kidney disease. General health habits, nutritional status, rehabilitation potential, and use of prior oncologic treatment modalities are other issues to explore. Age may be a factor, but it is relevant only in the face of overall general health status and quality of life.

4. Why are biopsies important in cancer care?
A biopsy is performed to confirm or diagnose cancer correctly. A biopsy consists of removing a tissue sample from an organ or other part of the body for histologic examination by a pathologist. A positive biopsy indicates the presence of cancer, whereas a negative biopsy may indicate that no cancer is present or that the biopsy specimen was not adequate. When a biopsy is negative but cancer is still suspected, further investigation is required.

5. What different types of biopsies can be performed?
The ideal biopsy method should be relatively inexpensive and noninvasive, convenient for patients, and easy to perform while providing enough information to deliver a preliminary cancer diagnosis. Numerous types of biopsies are available, each with different uses and advantages and disadvantages, as outlined in the table below.

Surgical Biopsy Techniques

TECHNIQUE	USES	ADVANTAGES	DISADVANTAGES
Fine-needle aspiration (20–22 gauge)	Retrieves cells vs. tissue For solid, palpable lesions Examples: breast, thyroid, cervical adenopathy	Quick Avoids surgical scar Local anesthesia Outpatient	Needs trained cytologist False-negative results Cannot be used to diagnose lymphoma or sarcoma
Percutaneous needle aspiration (20–23 gauge)	Retrieves cells vs. tissue For solid, nonpalpable lesions Radiologic localization (MRI, US, mammogram) Examples: lung, breast	May avoid need and cost of surgery Local anesthesia Outpatient	False-negative results Cannot be used to diagnose lymphoma or sarcoma Special stain procedures cannot be done
Core needle biopsy (14–20 gauge Trucut automated biopsy gun)	Retrieves tissue For both palpable and nonpalpable lesions through radiographic approach Examples: pancreas, liver, stereotactic breast biopsy, retroperitoneum	Avoids surgical scar Local anesthesia Outpatient	Needs technically trained and skilled personnel Risk of injury to adjacent structures Minimal risk of tumor cell seeding along biopsy tract
Incisional biopsy	Obtains wedge of tissue for solid, large mass Example: head and neck tumors, liver	For tissue diagnosis of mass too large for easy surgical removal Local and/or IV sedation	Necessitates scar Requires OR time Bleeding at site Risk of infection
Excisional biopsy	Solid, palpable mass Removal of complete lump with little or no planned margin	Day surgery Removes all gross disease	Risk of infection Requires scar

Continued on following page.

Surgical Biopsy Techniques (Continued)

TECHNIQUE	USES	ADVANTAGES	DISADVANTAGES
Endoscopic biopsy	For solid mass in lumen Obtains cytologic brushings and/or tissue	Avoids surgical procedure May place scar cosmetically Day surgery	Pain and trauma associated with scope
Laparoscopic biopsy	To sample tissue—abdomen, pelvis, lymphadenopathy, pancreas, liver	May avoid need for more major surgery Decreased length of stay	Decreased ability to assess complete abdomen

From McCorkle R, Grant M, Frank-Stromberg M, Baird SB: Cancer Nursing: A Comprehensive Textbook, 2nd ed. Philadelphia, W.B. Saunders, 1996, p. 320, with permission.

6. What is fine-needle aspiration?

Fine-needle aspiration (FNA) is a noninvasive approach for the diagnosis and evaluation of potential tumors of the breast, thyroid, salivary glands, and lymph nodes. CT imaging extends the range of FNA by making it feasible to biopsy lung, liver, pancreas, kidney, and adrenal glands. Pathologists are able to examine the sample cells to determine the level of discohesion (tendency of cells to separate from each other), nuclear atypia, and extracellular components (which may assist in identifying the tissue of origin).

7. Why is surgery sometimes done when metastasis is present?

In certain situations, when the primary tumor has been resected or is in remission, resecting solitary metastatic tumors may be appropriate. In patients with evidence of multiple metastatic lesions or aggressive tumors, resection is not indicated. The following factors must be considered before surgical intervention is attempted: (1) histology of the tumor, (2) disease-free interval, (3) tumor doubling time, (4) tumor size and location, (5) rate of metastasis, and (6) patient's performance status. Studies have reported successful resection of solitary metastatic tumors of the lung, liver, brain, and bone.

8. How does surgical staging differ from clinical staging?

Clinical staging includes findings acquired before definitive treatment: physical examinations, imaging, endoscopy, biopsy, and some surgical exploration. Surgical evaluative and pathologic staging is done after surgery, including lymph node studies.

Staging of Cancer

TYPE	METHOD	DATABASE	COMMENT
Clinical diagnosis	Physical exam X-rays and scans Biopsy	All information available before definitive treatment	Almost all cancers are clinically staged Accuracy limited
Surgical evaluation	Biopsy Exploratory surgery with intraoperative palpation ± biopsies Sentinel node biopsy	All clinical information Histology from biopsies	More information needed for definitive treatment decision (e.g., laparotomy for Hodgkin's disease, mediastinoscopy for lung primary)
Postsurgical pathology	Resection of tumor, often including nodes	Histologic information on all resected tissues	Comprehensive histologic information of tumor ± regional nodes or organs

Adapted from Knobf MKT: Surgery. In Gross J, Johnson BL: Handbook of Oncology Nursing, 2nd ed. Boston, Jones & Bartlett, 1994.

9. What nursing issues should be considered preoperatively?

Preoperatively the nurse provides education and psychosocial support to the patient and family. Preoperative teaching should include a discussion of the extent of the planned surgery and of any expected functional limitations. Issues of concern should be clarified, and sources of support should be identified and discussed. Instructions about the use of any equipment, pulmonary exercises, coughing techniques, and pain management options should be provided. Because of shortened postoperative hospital stays, it is also beneficial to do an initial discharge assessment preoperatively. Factors that may influence discharge planning include the home environment, financial status, self-care abilities, anticipated postoperative self-care abilities, available family and agency support, and employment status and type of work.

It is common for patients and families to experience anxiety. As the nurse interacts with patients and families preoperatively, their concerns related to the uncertainty of long-term survival and the possible need for further treatment should be assessed and addressed. Because anxiety reduces a patient's ability to understand and retain information, teaching should be reinforced as appropriate.

10. What nursing issues should be considered postoperatively?

Because of decreased hospital stays and the potential for fragmentation of care as patients are seen by the primary care provider, surgeon, and other specialists, it is even more imperative for nurses to communicate and collaborate with one another. Generic components of postoperative nursing care include assessment, patient education, emotional support, physical care, and rehabilitation.

11. What topics should be included in postoperative patient education?

The challenges of teaching patients and family members what they need to know to provide care after hospital discharge are increased by shortened hospital stays and increased complexities of surgical interventions. Patients and families need to know about any prescribed medications, ongoing wound care, signs and symptoms of infection, appropriate nutrition, proper balance of rest and exercise, care of catheters or ostomies (if present), and where and when to return for postoperative examinations. Communication with agencies providing care after hospitalization, such as home care agencies or nursing homes, is key to providing continuity in provision of care. If there is to be additional chemotherapy or radiation therapy, basic baseline teaching can be done if the patient/family are ready and receptive. Use of anatomical models to enhance patient learning are particularly helpful for patients receiving surgery.

12. Discuss the important aspects of physical care in the postoperative period.

Physical care centers on general surgical nursing principles, with specific focus on pain management, wound care, nutrition, and hemostasis. Good pain control can improve patient satisfaction, promote healing, reduce recovery time, and decrease postoperative complications. Postoperative pain can be managed in many ways, including administration of opioids by patient-controlled analgesia (PCA) and continuous epidural analgesia; addition of injectable nonsteroidal anti-inflammatory drugs (NSAIDs), such as ketorolac (Toradol), to traditional intravenous opioids; and various nondrug methods to decrease anxiety and pain (see chapter on Pain.)

13. Does Toradol increase the risk of bleeding?

Ketorolac tromethamine (Toradol) is a parenteral NSAID that is useful for acute postoperative pain. It is also especially helpful for bone pain, chest tube pain, or inflammation. Although surgeons vary in their acceptance of ketorolac because of concern with bleeding, it has been shown that ketorolac is associated with a small increased risk for overall operative-site bleeding only in elderly patients or with higher doses. Ketorolac has also not been associated with an increased risk for gastrointestinal bleeding when its use has been restricted to patients less than age 65 at an average dose of 105 mg/day or lower for 5 or less days of therapy. The adult dose usually given is 30 mg intravenously or intramuscularly every 6 hours as needed. Patients who are older than 65 years, frail, or renally impaired may not be candidates for ketorolac or should receive a smaller dose (15 mg IV or IM). The contraindications for its use are an active GI ulcer, bleeding, renal impairment, volume depletion, aspirin or NSAID allergy, coagulopathy, pregnancy, or lactation.

14. What factors should be considered in the assessment and care of surgical wounds?

Wound assessment should include such factors as length, width, depth, location, and direction of the wound as well as descriptions of the base, edges, and any exudate. Factors that can delay wound healing include age, obesity, prior chemotherapy or radiation therapy, malnutrition, and diabetes. If the surrounding tissue is compromised or a deep pocket of infection exists, wounds may be left to heal on their own (from the inside out). Dressings may be used to protect the wound, to promote comfort, to immobilize wound edges, and to maintain a moist environment.

15. Does nutritional status affect surgical outcome?

Nutritional status before surgery can significantly affect outcome. Protein/calorie malnutrition, a problem seen in cancer patients with prior treatment and compromised immune status, may lead to wound dehiscence, ileus, sepsis, and increased hospital length of stay. Perioperative and postoperative support in the form of high protein/calorie oral diets, enteral tube feedings, and total parenteral nutrition (TPN) can significantly decrease morbidity and mortality.

16. Are patients with cancer at increased risk for hemostatic or bleeding problems?

Altered hemostasis in the form of hypercoagulability and thrombosis can put the patient with cancer at higher risk for postoperative complications. Some patients have been reported to have elevated clotting factors and shortened partial thromboplastin time or hemorrhage. Common cancer types include adenocarcinoma of the lung, pancreas, and colon. Early postoperative ambulation is imperative to prevent thrombophlebitis.

17. What factors should be considered in postoperative rehabilitation?

Rehabilitation centers on meeting the following needs: physical, psychosocial, sexual, spiritual, educational, vocational, and financial. It begins preoperatively, and the plan of care continues postoperatively. Nursing interventions should be individualized according to patients' needs and priorities. Common nursing diagnoses include body image disturbance related to disfigurement, impaired tissue integrity, and self-esteem disturbance. For example, some patients may have no desire to address workplace issues and concerns in the first few days after surgery; others may have increased pain and/or lack of sleep related to anxieties and worries about how they will continue to provide for their families. Thorough and ongoing assessment is imperative to discover the "real" issues or questions.

18. How soon after surgery can adjuvant chemotherapy and radiation therapy begin?

Certain antineoplastic agents and radiation doses interfere with wound healing; thus, special consideration must be given to the timing sequence of adjuvant therapy. Adjuvant therapy can be started as early as a few days after surgery, but in many instances a 3–6 week postoperative recovery time is standard. Some patients with cancer are at greater risk for postoperative complications such as bleeding and infection.

19. What has changed in cancer surgery over the past 25–30 years?

Surgeries that originated as radical procedures to remove tumors with adequate tissue margins have become more conservative, enhancing overall quality of life and promoting rehabilitation. In addition, as more is understood about how cancers originate and metastasize, the proper combination of surgery, chemotherapy, and radiation therapy has emerged. Multimodal therapy has improved cure and control rates for many cancers.

Surgery has played a major role in the cure of breast, colorectal, and thyroid cancers and melanoma. Technologic advances in surgery, such as the use of lasers, stapling devices, and microsurgery, have further contributed to the array of surgical options.

20. If a tumor is exposed to air during surgery, will the cancer spread?

A common unproven myth is that surgery may cause cancer to spread by exposing the cancerous cells to air. This is not true. Cancer does not spread because it has been exposed to the air. It is true that patients sometimes feel worse after surgery than before surgery because of incisional discomfort and organ manipulation. This feeling is normal. Surgery also can lower the patient's immune response, and if the cancer is found to be more advanced at the time of surgery than originally thought, the patient may be more susceptible to postoperative complications. Because early removal of all cancer cells provides the best chance of cure, it is important that people do not allow this myth to prevent them from seeking surgery.

21. What is "seeding"?

Seeding means that the cancer has spread, with the occurrence of small nodules in the peritoneum or wound. Seeding may occur in an area where surgery has been performed previously.

22. What types of surgeries are indicated for rehabilitation?

Often, after radical surgery, wounds may not close adequately, or enough skin, muscle, or subcutaneous tissue may not be available for satisfactory results. Reconstructive surgery may also be indicated to promote self-esteem and body image, to enhance quality of life, and to improve certain physical functions. Examples include breast reconstruction, facial reconstruction for head and neck cancers, and skin grafting after removal of melanomas.

23. Should a surgeon say, "I got it all"?

In general, when a surgeon says, "I got it all," it means that the tumor was removed in its entirety, the margins were clean or free of cancer cells, and there was no evidence of lymph node or metastatic spread. Because approximately 70% of patients have evidence of micrometastases at the time of diagnosis, this statement should be made with caution.

It may be less misleading to the patient if the surgeon says, "Apparently there is no evidence of cancer left behind. In one to two days, we'll have a pathology report that will give us more information. If the pathology is clear at the margins, there is a good chance that it's all been removed. There is a chance, however, that microscopic disease has already spread. That is why it is important to see a medical oncologist to talk about chemotherapy."

Surgery alone can be curative in patients with localized disease, but often it is necessary to combine surgery with other treatment modalities to achieve higher response rates.

24. What is a second-look procedure?

Second-look surgery is an exploratory laparotomy performed to stage cancer more accurately after completion of initial treatment, to determine treatment response, and to plan for possible further therapy. Its use may be less common with advances in diagnostic imaging. It may be used in ovarian cancer and other solid tumors in the face of rising tumor markers and negative clinical work-ups for metastasis.

25. What does it mean when a surgeon says, "We got adequate margins"?

The surgeon needs to remove not only the tumor but also enough surrounding tissue to prevent local spread of disease. The amount of surrounding tissue that needs to be removed varies with the type of cancer and site of involvement. Margins range from 2–5 cm of "normal" tissue in solid tumors to wide excision for primary melanomas in the skin. How to define "adequate margins" is an area still under question.

ACKNOWLEDGMENT

The authors thank William R. Nelson, MD, Clinical Professor, Department of Surgery, University of Colorado Health Sciences Center, for his critical review of this chapter.

BIBLIOGRAPHY

1. Alavassevich M, McKibbon A, Thomas S: Information and needs of patients who undergo surgery for head and neck cancer. Can Oncol Nurs 5:9–11, 1995.
2. American Joint Commission on Cancer, TNM Committee of the International Union Against Cancer: Handbook for Staging of Cancer. Philadelphia, J.B. Lippincott, 1993.

3. DeVita VT, Hellman S, Rosenberg SA: Cancer: Principles and Practice of Oncology, 4th ed. Philadelphia, J.B. Lippincott, 1993.

4. Groenwald SL, Frogge M, Goodman M, Yarbro C: Cancer Nursing: Principles & Practice, 2nd ed. Boston, Jones & Bartlett, 1992.

5. Knobf MKT: In Gross J, Johnson BL: Handbook of Oncology Nursing, 2nd ed. Boston, Jones & Bartlett, 1994.

6. McCaffrey M: Nursing Practice Theories Related to Cognition, Bodily Pain, and Man-Environment Interactions. Los Angeles, University of California at Los Angeles, 1968.

7. McCorkle R, Grant M, Frank-Stromberg M, Baird SB: Cancer Nursing: A Comprehensive Textbook, 2nd ed. Philadelphia, W.B. Saunders, 1996.

8. Srom BL, Berlin JA, Kinman JA, et al: Parenteral ketorolac and risk of gastrointestinal and operative-site bleeding: A postmarketing surveillance study. JAMA 275:376–382, 1996.

9. U.S. Dept. of Health and Human Services, Agency for Health Care Policy and Research: Clinical Practice Guideline for Acute Pain Management: Operative or Medical Procedures and Trauma. AHCPR Pub. No. 92-0032. Rockville, MD, Agency for Health Care Policy and Research, Public Health Service, U.S. Dept. of Health and Human Services, 1992.

6. RADIATION THERAPY

Joan Foley, RN, BSN, and Merle Sprague, MD

1. How does radiation therapy work?

Radiation therapy, if given in a high enough dose, can kill any cell or tissue. In patients with cancer, the goal of radiation therapy is to destroy tumor cells while sparing normal cells. Over 60% of patients with various types of cancers receive radiation therapy alone or in combination with another modality for cure, control, or palliation of disease. Radiation is delivered from a distance by a machine (teletherapy) or close to the patient via an implanted or injected radioactive source (brachytherapy).

Radiation therapy uses x-rays just like the x-rays used for chest films or CT scans. The difference is that low-energy radiation is used to visualize anatomy, whereas a high-energy x-ray beam from a linear accelerator is used to destroy malignant tissues. The high-energy beam causes breaks in the chromosomes of the cells transgressed by the beam and alters the cells' ability to divide. DNA cross-linkages result from free radical interactions, and unless the cellular damage is repaired, the cells lose protein synthesis functions and die. Cells affected by the radiation ultimately are injured, destroyed, or repaired. Basically, tumor cells cannot repair radiation damage as efficiently as healthy cells.

2. What is involved in planning radiation treatments?

The radiation oncologist works with a professional team, usually consisting of radiation technologists, dosimetrists, radiation physicists, computer scientists, radiobiologists, and nurses, to create an optimal and individualized treatment strategy. Factors taken into consideration include the histology and characteristics of the tumor (stage, size, location, routes of spread) and the patient's general condition and prognosis. The multidisciplinary planning process includes the following aspects:

- **Delineation of tumor volume and evaluation of field arrangements.** Physical examination and diagnostic imaging outline the tumor volume to be targeted. The treatment volume is usually slightly larger than the tumor target volume to take into account any local microscopic extension of the tumor or microscopic drainage into regional lymph nodes. Patient movement, such as respiratory variation, is also taken into account.
- **Simulation.** An x-ray machine resembling the treatment machine is used to simulate and make necessary measurements or modifications for aiming the beam and to immobilize the patient. This step is necessary to plan the most precise way to deliver each treatment. The goal is to maximize tumor coverage with the best combination of beams while minimizing exposure to normal structures. Marks are made on the patient's skin to delineate the targeted field or "radiation port." There is often no more than 2 mm difference between daily treatments. It is important to explain the significance of the marks to the patient during education about skin care.
- **Construction of patient immobilization or positioning devices.** To ensure consistency in treatment areas, patients may need to use devices, such as casts, arm boards, or plastic masks, to immobilize body parts.
- **Organ shielding and beam modification.** The beam is emitted from the linear accelerator in a square or rectangle. Individualized blocks made of lead alloy are created to conform the beam to each patient's anatomy and tumor. The blocks slide into a tray on the treatment machine between the beam exit port and the patient. The blocks absorb the radiation and cast a shadow that protects as much normal tissue as possible.

Treatments are started after simulation is completed (one to several days). Time is required for the dosimetrist and physicist to input information into a computer and to make plans to optimize beam combinations consistent with the radiation oncologist's treatment strategy. Time is also needed to construct individualized shielding or blocking devices.

3. What are portal films?

A portal or beam film is an x-ray film of the treatment target site, usually obtained weekly on the treatment machine, to verify accuracy of the daily treatment field size and location as well as positioning.

4. How are doses expressed? What is fractionation?

Before 1985, radiation doses were expressed in units called rads (radiation absorbed doses). Currently, doses are expressed in grays (Gy) or centigrays (cGy). One gray equals 100 rads or one joule per kilogram; one rad equals one cGy.

Radiation oncologists divide the total radiation dose into daily "fractions" to preserve normal cellular growth and function. Different doses are used for different tumor volumes. For squamous cell and adenocarcinomas, total doses may range from 4500–5000 cGy for subclinical disease to 6000–8000 cGy for clinically palpable tumors. Minimal and maximal tolerated doses for various organs have been determined. For example, the maximal tolerated dose to the spinal cord is 4500 cGy. Patients usually get one treatment per day, Monday through Friday, over a period ranging from 2–8 weeks, depending on tumor type and location.

5. What are the four Rs of radiobiology?

Fractionation of radiation therapy attempts to exploit differences between tumor cell and normal cell responses and thus to maximize tumor cell kill as reflected in the four R's:

Repair is the ability of cells to recover from radiation injury between treatments. Normal cells are able to repair better than tumor cells.

Repopulation refers to the mitosis and proliferation of cells after repair of damage. Tumor cells are less successful in undergoing mitosis because of inadequate repair.

Redistribution refers to how the cycle delay of radiation therapy will catch more tumor cells in the mitotic stage, which is more sensitive to radiation. Normal cells are less likely to be delayed or redistributed.

Reoxygenation occurs between fractionated doses in previously radioresistant hypoxic tumor cells. As a radiosensitizer, oxygen enhances tumor cell kill.

6. Which tissues are most sensitive to radiation therapy?

The cells most sensitive to radiation therapy are bone marrow stem cells, germ cells, and intestinal epithelial cells. The least sensitive cells are found in the bone, muscle, cartilage, and central nervous system.

7. Can radiation therapy alone cure anything?

Radiation therapy alone is curative for many types of cancers, such as Hodgkin's disease and tumors of the cervix or upper airway. It is often the only adjuvant treatment necessary for many other types of cancers, particularly tumors of the head and neck or male and female genital systems. Radiation therapy and chemotherapy are often used together, as in early-stage breast cancer, to provide the best chances for cancer cure and control.

8. How do people who work around radiation protect themselves from exposure?

Regulatory agencies have established the maximum permissible dose (MPD) for radiation workers. Each institution has a radiation safety officer whose purpose is to ensure that the regulations and restrictions related to radiation use are maintained according to state and federal law. Radiation safety principles are based on the **ALARA** concept: exposure should be **A**s **L**ow **A**s **R**easonably **A**chievable. Radiation workers wear film badges that record exposure. The badges are checked monthly to maintain the worker within safe parameters. Key components of radiation safety include attention to the following:

- Time: minimize time of exposure
- Distance: maximize distance from exposure
- Shielding: use protection between radiation source and exposed person

9. What is brachytherapy?

Brachytherapy is the placement of sealed radioactive sources close to the tumor to provide a high dose of radiation directly to the tumor while creating a rapid drop-off gradient in surrounding normal tissues. It is used alone or in combination with external beam therapy or other treatment modalities. The radioactive source may be placed into a hollow body organ (endo- or intracavitary) with tandem or ovoids, cylinders, or catheters; it may be threaded with needles, wires, seeds, or catheters into tissue (interstitial) or placed on external body surfaces, as for superficial eye tumors. Brachytherapy can be "low-dose rate," staying in place for several days, or "high-dose rate," when extremely active sources stay in place for only several minutes. The advantage of brachytherapy is that high doses are delivered to tumors without causing irreparable damage to radiosensitive normal tissues, such as the small bowel, bladder, or rectum. Brachytherapy is currently used for cancers of the cervix, prostate, lung, breast, and brain and melanomas of the eye. Patients need instructions and precautions about the procedure to allay fears about isolation and radioactivity. Adequate anesthesia and analgesia are also necessary, particularly for tandem and ovoid placement for gynecologic cancers.

10. How do you answer family members or health care providers who ask, "Is the patient radioactive or dangerous to be around?"

Patients receiving external beam radiation therapy are not radioactive, and radiation precautions for others are not necessary. However, patients receiving brachytherapy are sources of radiation, and precautions are warranted. Removal of the internal radiation source removes the radioactivity. Precautions with brachytherapy include universal precautions, private room with radiation precaution sign, radiation film badges for personnel, and shields in the patient's room, if indicated. Visitors are allowed for limited periods (30 minutes/day), according to institutional policies, and should stay at least 6 feet from the radioactive source. Children younger than 18 years and pregnant visitors are not allowed.

11. Discuss the acute side effects of radiation therapy.

Side effects from radiation therapy vary according to the dose and are site-specific, occurring only in tissues included in the treatment field or "port." For example, a patient whose pelvis is radiated may develop diarrhea or bladder irritation but not hair loss. Generalized side effects include fatigue, anorexia, skin reactions, and bone marrow depression.

Acute side effects occur during treatment and can be predicted from the volume of normal tissue exposed to the beam, the total dose delivered, and the sensitivity of the normal tissue to radiation. Age, nutritional status, and chemotherapy also contribute to predicting severity of acute side effects. The larger the treated volume of normal tissue, the more likely the patient is to develop the respective side effect. Most acute side effects are transient and are managed symptomatically with appropriate medications. Acute side effects usually abate rapidly after completion of therapy. If side effects, such as nausea or diarrhea, persist after 1 or 2 weeks, other causes should be sought. Examples of site-specific acute side effects include alopecia, xerostomia, mucositis, taste alterations, pharyngitis, esophagitis, gastritis, nausea and vomiting, cystitis, diarrhea, sexual dysfunction (vaginal dryness, erectile dysfunction), edema, lymphedema, and cerebral edema.

12. Discuss the chronic side effects of radiation therapy.

Chronic or late side effects are local, usually permanent reactions that may develop several months to years after the radiation is completed. The daily fraction dose tends to predict the severity of chronic side effects. As the daily dose increases, the normal tissue loses its ability to maintain adequate repair and long-term damage tends to be worse. Late-reacting tissues include skin, spinal cord, bone, and organs such as lung, liver, and gonads. Examples of site-specific late effects include eye cataracts, xerostomia, dental caries, taste changes, head and neck flap necrosis, esophageal stricture or fistula, hypothyroidism, pneumonitis or pulmonary fibrosis, pericarditis, gastric atrophy or ulcers, cirrhosis, bowel adhesions, proctitis or enteritis, cystitis, vaginal fibrosis, infertility, osteoradionecrosis, myelopathies, permanent epilation, skin pigmentation changes, and secondary malignancies.

13. How do you encourage patients to comply with treatments and the interventions for acute side effects?

It is important to acknowledge each patient's feelings of being "out of control." Patients should not be forced or made to do anything. People diagnosed with cancer often feel like all control of their life has been ripped away. Patients can be empowered to make good decisions about their care and treatments by:

- Educating them about the disease and treatment, including honest expectations of outcome
- Acknowledging their feelings
- Including them as primary members or planners in their health care
- Providing nonjudgmental support, even when they test what they have been told

14. How often does radiation therapy cause a second cancer?

The incidence of second tumor induction in radiated normal tissue is usually estimated as < 5 per 1000 patients. To be declared a radiation-induced second cancer, the tumor must be different from the primary, must arise within the previously irradiated tissue, and must occur 10–15 years after the original tumor. Examples of radiation-induced second malignancies are high-grade sarcomas, meningiomas, and thyroid tumors. Genetic considerations, immune status and other treatment modalities also must be weighed in predicting an individual patient's risk of a second malignancy. Secondary malignancies have been reported in people who were treated with radiation therapy for nonmalignant processes such as ankylosing spondylitis, tuberculosis, or tinea capitis. Statistics about children and young adults who received radiation therapy show a higher rate of second malignancies in comparison with similarly aged people without radiation therapy, although it is not clear whether radiation therapy is the only inciting cause.

15. Why not radiate every bone in the body to prevent bone metastases?

This question is frequently asked once bone metastasis is discovered; however, side effects must always be anticipated and weighed carefully so that the risk is not higher than the expected benefit. Unfortunately, radiation of too much bone marrow leads to serious immunosuppression because the blood-forming elements of the bone marrow are among the most radiosensitive cells. The central skeleton, such as the pelvis, spine, sternum, and proximal long bones, have the highest marrow activity in adults; the amount of marrow depression can be roughly predicted by the amount of active bone marrow that is radiated. Bone marrow depression may last up to 1 year when a bone is given 2000 cGy; the usual treatment dose for bone metastasis is 3000 cGy. Hemi-body radiation can be done for multiple metastases if confined to the upper or lower body. Currently, there is great interest to see whether radioactive strontium will be as effective and less toxic than hemi-body radiation for multiple bone metastases, as in prostate cancer.

16. Can a previously irradiated site be retreated for recurrent cancer?

If the cancer recurs in another part of the body, radiation therapy can be used; however, previously radiated sites usually cannot be retreated. Retreatment is usually too risky because it may cause irreparable damage to the surrounding normal tissues, which have already received close to or the maximal tolerated dose. In certain instances, it is possible to approach a recurrent tumor from a different angle, exposing a different area of normal tissue.

17. Why are people who cannot be cured and may even be close to death treated with radiation?

Palliative radiation is given with the goal of providing comfort or increasing quality of life even when a cure cannot be achieved. The relief that the treatment offers must be weighed against side effects and the time that the treatment requires. In palliative radiation therapy, daily doses are larger, but fewer treatments are given and total doses are lower. Although the toxicity

risks of a larger daily fraction are higher for late or chronic side effects, the risk is balanced by
the patient's terminal prognosis. Indications for palliative radiation therapy include:
- To reduce tumor volume and provide pain control
- To open an airway or esophagus
- Radiation to the brain to provide relief from incapacitating headaches, seizures, or loss of
  motor control
- Radiation to a vertebral metastasis to relieve pain and prevent paralysis for the last few
  days or weeks of life
- To relieve bleeding or obstruction from advanced bowel, bladder, prostate, or cervical cancers

18. What is the role of radiation in pain control?

Tumor pain is caused by pressure of the tumor on an adjacent structure, invasion of an
organ, tumor growth within an enclosed area, tissue necrosis that exposes nerves, or muscle
spasms in adjacent areas. Radiation is particularly effective in controlling pain from bone or
lymph node metastases. Radiation therapy can give long-term relief or partial relief, thereby improving quality of life or making death more comfortable. Patients who subsequently need
smaller doses of opioids may have a greater sense of well-being and control. Adequate, aggressive medical interventions are necessary for pain control until the radiation takes effect, which
may be as long as 2 weeks.

19. Do certain drugs interfere with radiation? What are radiosensitizers?

Most drugs that patients take for other problems do not interfere with radiation therapy.
Radiosensitizers are various classes of drugs that make radiation cell-killing more efficient.
Certain chemotherapy agents, such as 5-fluorouracil, cisplatin, or mitomycin C, are specifically
used before, during, or after the radiation sequence to improve the efficacy of tumor cell kill.
These agents may cause worse side effects than radiation alone.

20. What is the best skin care regimen during and after treatment?

Skin in the treatment field can be expected to show some response to most courses of radiation. An unexpected site of skin reaction is the exit site, which should receive the same monitoring and care as the treatment field. Before initiation of treatment, the skin in the area should be
inspected to note areas of irritation or thinning.

Inform the patient not to remove lines or ink marks until instructed. During radiation, a thin,
soothing moisturizing cream should be consistently applied twice a day and washed off before
each day's treatment. Many commercial agents are available for skin care, and it is wise to check
the patient's or family's choice of product. Advise patients and their families to avoid creams
with alcohol or anything that may be irritating. Caution the patient about the use of abrasive or
strong soaps and suggest that they avoid extremes in temperature (cold and sun). Patients should
also avoid clothing that is constrictive or causes friction. Men should shave with an electric razor.

After about 2–4 weeks, erythema may be seen in the treatment ports, and dry desquamation
may develop. The skin becomes dry and rough, sometimes unpleasantly so. If the patient
scratches the area, the danger of secondary infection is increased. If the changes progress to wet
desquamation, we usually use a mild drying agent such as Domeboro's solution, which is usually
effective and cheap. When the course of radiation is finished, skin reactions usually clear in 2
weeks. At this time, if the skin is intact, an aloe-based moisturizing cream may be used.

21. Discuss the management of acute oral side effects.

On initiating treatment, a basic mouth care regimen of saline and baking soda mouth rinses
every 2 hours are encouraged. As side effects increase, Benmylid (benadryl, Mylanta, and lidocaine) and a liquid nonsteroidal antiinflammatory drug (NSAID) can be added for swelling and
pain. Patients should evaluate oral intake for three points of possible irritation: physical, chemical, and temperature. Some patients appreciate the opportunity to help control the severity of
side effects and have been highly creative in developing recipes that they offer to share.

22. Are dietary supplements helpful?

Patients undergoing radiation therapy are particularly affected by nutritional issues. They must be able to take in adequate calories and protein to maintain weight and promote healing. It is estimated that two extra calories per pound are needed each day during radiation therapy. Assessment of the patient's intake history and present diet is essential. Dietary supplements that offer high calories and high protein may help the patient to achieve a sense of well-being by maintaining weight, immune status, and positive nitrogen balance. Some supplements are difficult for patients to tolerate because of smell, taste, or consistency. Patients can prepare their own supplements with a blender or food processor. The clinical dietitian can offer invaluable help.

23. What is the role of radiation therapy in childhood cancers?

The role of radiation therapy in children is limited as much as possible because growing tissues and organs are more severely affected by doses that would be easily tolerated in adults. In general, the younger the child, the greater the toxicity. Radiation can retard bone growth, contribute to neuropsychiatric dysfunction, impair normal organ growth and development, cause endocrine dysfunction, permanently impair muscles and nerves, and increase the risk of second cancers. Careful baseline testing of organ functions in the proposed field should be done before radiation therapy and as part of routine follow-up care. Parents must be counseled about the functional losses or effects that may continue to occur even if the child's cancer is cured.

Children under age 3 years usually require sedation or anesthesia to hold still long enough to cooperate with treatment. If the parents understand the goals of therapy and the likely side effects, they are more likely to feel like full partners in the treatment regimen and to share a calmer, more positive attitude with the child. Educating children requires a good understanding of age-appropriate interventions. Role playing with stuffed animals, coloring books, and modeling work well to prepare most children from 3–5 years old for the radiation experience and to explore their fears.

24. What is hyperthermia?

Hyperthermia is the use of devices for selective heating of tumors to destroy cancer cells or to enhance the cytotoxicity of chemotherapy or radiation. Current technology makes heat delivery difficult to control precisely. More research is necessary to improve technology and efficacy.

25. When is total body irradiation used?

Total body irradiation (TBI) is used to eradicate cancer cells throughout the body and to enhance engraftment of stem cells by suppressing the body's immune response. TBI is usually used as part of the conditioning regimens to prepare patients with certain leukemias for bone marrow transplantation.

26. What new techniques of radiation therapy are under investigation?

Proton or heavy-particle beams are being used at a few research institutions in an attempt to exploit the different physical properties of different beams for better tumor control with fewer or more acceptable effects on normal tissue. The machines used to generate these beams are currently too expensive to find a place in mainstream treatment centers.

Radioimmunotherapy is being explored at several research institutions. Tumor-specific antigens are isolated, and various techniques are used to develop radiolabeled antibodies to the particular antigen. Antibody tagged with isotope can then be injected back into the patient with the hope of selective tumor cell targeting and killing.

Photodynamic therapy exploits laser technology delivered to body surfaces after the patient is injected with light-sensitizing compounds that are selectively retained by tumor cells. This strategy may be helpful for tumors that cause seeding throughout body cavities, such as gastrointestinal or ovarian cancers that stud peritoneal surfaces.

The views contained in this manuscript are solely those of the author and do not reflect the views or policies of Tripler Army Medical Command, the Department of Defense, or the U.S. Government.

BIBLIOGRAPHY

1. Baird SB, McCorkle R, Grant M: Cancer Nursing: A Comprehensive Textbook. Philadelphia, W.B. Saunders , 1991.
2. Bruner DW, Iwamoto R, Keane K, Strohl R (eds): Manual for Radiation Oncology Nursing: Practice and Education. Pittsburgh, PA, Oncology Nursing Society, 1992.
3. Coia LR, Moylan DJ: Introduction to Clinical Radiation Oncology. Madison, WI, Medical Physics Publishing, 1991.
4. Dose AM: The symptom experience of mucositis, stomatitis, and xerostomia. Semin Oncol Nurs 11:248–255, 1995.
5. Dow KH, Hilderly LJ (eds): Nursing Care in Radiation Oncology. Philadelphia, W.B. Saunders, 1992.
6. Fleming ID, Brady LW, Mieszkalski GB, et al: Basis for current therapies for cancer. In Murphy GP, Lawrence W, Lenhard RE (eds): American Cancer Society Textbook of Clinical Oncology, 2nd ed. Atlanta, American Cancer Society, 1995, pp 102–110.
7. Gallagher J: Management of cutaneous symptoms. Semin Oncol Nurs 11:239–247, 1995.
8. Groenwald SL, Frogge MH, Goodman M, Yarbro CH: Cancer Nursing: Principles and Practice. Boston, Jones & Bartlett, 1992.

7. PRINCIPLES OF CHEMOTHERAPY

Jennifer Petersen, RN, MS, and Michelle Goodman, RN, MS

1. How successful is chemotherapy in treating cancers?

Chemotherapy, the use of drugs to kill cells, has its origins in antibacterial research. The theoretical approach to management of patients with systemic infection and patients with cancer is strikingly similar. Combination drug therapy, importance of scheduling, timing of therapy, monitoring of toxicity, and the overwhelming problem of drug-resistant tumor cells or microorganisms are excellent examples of the challenges involved in treating cancers and infections alike.

Chemotherapy was not successful in treating cancer until nitrogen mustard was used in the treatment of lymphomas in the 1940s. The use of nitrogen mustard as chemotherapy was discovered accidentally when seamen developed marrow and lymphoid hypoplasia after exposure to mustard gas made for chemical warfare in World War II. Currently, chemotherapy is responsible for increasing the survival time of many patients with cancer (see chapter 4).

2. How does chemotherapy work?

Chemotherapy drugs interfere with steps of the cell cycle specifically involved in synthesis of DNA and replication of tumor cells. The cell cycle, the process whereby both normal and cancerous cells replicate, involves five basic phases:

G0 Resting stage in which cells are out of cycle temporarily
G1 RNA and protein synthesis; the gap between resting and DNA synthesis
S   DNA synthesis
G2 Second gap, during which the cell constructs the mitotic apparatus
M   Mitosis

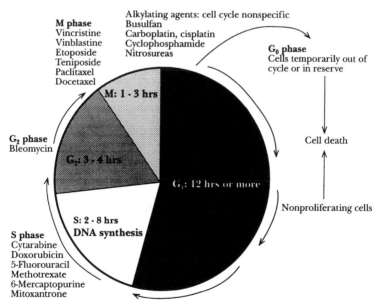

Cell cycle and cytotoxic targets of common antineoplastic agents. (Adapted from Tannock IF: Biological properties of anticancer drugs. In Tannock IF, Hill RP (eds): The Basic Science of Oncology, 2nd ed. New York, McGraw-Hill, 1992, pp. 302–316.)

3. How are chemotherapeutic agents classified?

Most antineoplastic agents in current use may be categorized into three groups based on their biochemical activity or origins:

1. The **alkylating agents** exert their lethal activity by interacting with bases in DNA. They are predominantly cycle nonspecific but are also effective against resting cells. Examples include nitrogen mustard, cyclophosphamide, ifosfamide, melphalan, the nitrosoureas, and busulfan.

2. The **antimetabolites** resemble normal metabolites and compete as substrates for enzyme activity, thereby inhibiting critical biochemical pathways and preventing DNA or RNA synthesis. The antimetabolites are phase-specific; that is, they act during a specific phase of the cell cycle and are therefore most effective against cancers that are highly proliferative. Examples include methotrexate, 5-fluorouracil (5-FU), cytarabine, and 6-thioguanine.

3. **Drugs derived from natural products** include antitumor antibiotics, the taxanes, and synthesized chemicals. The antitumor antibiotics (doxorubicin, daunorubicin) appear to act during the S phase of the cell cycle, binding to DNA and causing the DNA helix partially to unwind. The vinca alkaloids (vincristine, vinblastine) are specific for the M phase of the cell cycle and act by binding to protein tubulin, disrupting the formation of the mitotic spindle so that the cell dies as it attempts division. The taxanes (paclitaxel and docetaxel) are M phase-specific and promote microtubule formation, resulting in a stable but nonfunctional microtubule. Synthesized chemicals such as cisplatin and carboplatin are similar in that they bind to DNA, causing intrastrand cross-linking and interstrand adducts. In this way they act similarly to the alkylating agents.

The topoisomerase 1 inhibitors (topotecan, irinotecan) are the newest drugs in the plant alkaloid category. Topoisomerase is an enzyme that relaxes coiled DNA during replication and transcription and repairs broken DNA strands. If topoisomerase 1 is inhibited, the coiled DNA is unable to relax during synthesis. The DNA strands break and are unable to repair themselves.

4. What is the effect of tumor growth on responsiveness to chemotherapy?

Tumor growth rate is one of the major factors affecting response to chemotherapy. A tumor grows exponentially, with growth rates varying among tumor types; for example, colon cancer takes about 90 days to double its volume, whereas breast cancer takes about 60 days and testicular cancer about 30 days. The higher the proliferative rate of a tumor, the more effective the chemotherapy. Tumors are most likely to be responsive to chemotherapy early, when the tumor is small and vascular rather than later when cell proliferation slows. Exposure to chemotherapy is limited when the rate of cancer cell proliferation is decreased by limited diffusion of nutrients, accumulation of toxic metabolites, and poor vascularization of tumors.

5. How does flow cytometry help to predict response to chemotherapy?

By providing information about the percentage of dividing cells and ratio of DNA content, flow cytometry is useful in identifying patients who may benefit from more aggressive treatment or adjuvant chemotherapy. Flow cytometry is used to estimate the growth fraction, cell cycle phase distribution, and kinetic properties of cell populations. Tumors that contain a higher percentage of proliferating cells (cells in S phase) are more sensitive to cycle-dependent chemotherapy and have a better prognosis than tumors with a low S phase fraction. Ploidy refers to the ratio of DNA content of tumor cells in G1 phase. Patients with diploid tumors (DNA index < 1 or normal DNA content) tend to have a better prognosis than those with aneuploid tumors (DNA index > 1 or abnormal DNA content). In patients with an aneuploid tumor with a high S phase fraction, the likelihood of subclinical dissemination and tumor recurrence is greater.

6. Why are certain cancers resistant to chemotherapy?

Drug resistance is one of the major barriers to cure. Drug resistance may be intrinsic or acquired over time, because each cancer cell has the ability to mutate spontaneously. Many cancers (e.g., melanoma, renal cell, pancreatic cancer) are intrinsically resistant to most if not all chemotherapeutic agents. Cancers that are intrinsically resistant to chemotherapy contain the multidrug resistant gene, known as the MDR pump, which contains P-glycoprotein. The MDR pump resides within the cellular membrane and actively pumps out certain drugs as they are given, thus preventing accumulation of the drug within the cell. In the presence of overexpression of P-glycoprotein, drugs such as doxorubicin, mitoxantrone, daunorubicin, vincristine, vinblastine, paclitaxel, etoposide, and dactinomycin are readily extruded from the cell.

Cancer cells may be resistant to drugs by other mechanisms, such as decreased drug uptake, reduced drug activation, impaired drug transport into cells, increased catabolism of the drug, alterations in target enzymes to reduce drug binding, and increased DNA repair, all of which reduce therapeutic efficacy.

In the past decade, resistance to programmed cell death (apoptosis) and presence of telomerase have been described as significant properties that permit cancer cells not to die or age despite appropriate signals. Apoptosis refers to the cell death that normally follows cellular damage. When cancer cells lack apoptosis, they survive despite damage from chemotherapy drugs or other mechanisms that initiate programmed cell death, thus contributing to malignant transformation and chemotherapy resistance. Normally, cell senescence (process of aging) results when telomeres shorten with each division and chromosomes are not able to replicate their DNA. Unlike normal somatic cells, most cancer cells possess telomerase, an enzyme that lengthens telomeres to sustain DNA replication. Telomerase permits cells to ignore the biologic clock, thereby promoting tumor cell growth and possible chemotherapy resistance.

7. How can drug resistance be overcome?

Research suggests that tamoxifen, cyclosporine, verapamil, and quinidine may be effective in reversing the MDR pump mechanism. Other important strategies in overcoming resistance are combination chemotherapy and dose-intensive chemotherapy, which kill the cells before they have the chance to become resistant. Further chemotherapy may be developed to target cancer cell resistance to apoptosis and the presence of telomerase.

8. What factors affect response to chemotherapy?

- Tumor burden (the larger the primary tumor, the greater the risk for metastatic disease)
- Tumor cell heterogeneity
- Drug resistance
- Dose reductions
- Duration of exposure to chemotherapy
- Treatment delays due to toxicity and patient compliance
- Depressed immune system

9. Does circadian rhythm affect the patient's response to chemotherapy?

Certain variations in drug metabolism and tissue sensitivity correlate with circadian rhythm. The goals of chronotherapy, the administration of chemotherapy in accordance with the patient's circadian rhythm, are to reduce drug toxicity and to permit increased dose intensity, which results in higher cancer cell kill. Circadian chemotherapy is directed toward the administration of intensive doses of chemotherapy during specific times of the day when normal organ and cellular function are least affected. For example, the cells of the gut and bone marrow divide most actively during the first half of the working day. Chemotherapy such as 5-FU, which targets the gut and bone marrow, therefore may be best tolerated if given in the evening. This schedule may reduce the incidence and severity of specific toxicities, such as stomatitis, diarrhea and myelosuppression, while allowing maximal dose and therapeutic benefit.

Chronobiology has been widely studied in use with administration of floxuridine (FUDR), 5-FU, cytarabine, doxorubicin, cisplatin, carboplatin, interferon, and methotrexate. As chronobiology becomes more commonly used, nurses may find that chemotherapy will be administered according to a predetermined schedule based on the patient's circadian rhythm. This goal can be achieved by the use of portable programmable infusion pumps (e.g., Disetronic, CADD micropump, Medtronic) designed to deliver a chemotherapy bolus or infusion at varying times.

10. What is the advantage of combination chemotherapy?

Cell kill is maximized by combining drugs that are synergistic and act at different phases of the cell cycle. Combination drug therapy further minimizes the proliferation of resistant tumor stem cells. Because the drugs act differently, their toxicities are not additive and maximal doses of each can be given.

11. Does the sequence of administering certain drugs affect the patient's response?

The sequence in which drugs are given may enhance efficacy and/or minimize toxicity. When paclitaxel is given in combination with carboplatin or cisplatin, it is always given first. Giving paclitaxel after carboplatin or cisplatin not only decreases efficacy but possibly enhances myelosuppression of paclitaxel. When paclitaxel is combined with doxorubicin, paclitaxel is given after the doxorubicin. If paclitaxel is given before doxorubicin, the clearance of doxorubicin is significantly reduced, resulting in dose-limiting (grade 3) mucositis without increased efficacy. For combination methotrexate and 5-FU in patients with breast cancer, the methotrexate is given intravenously 1 hour before 5-FU. The dose of methotrexate is escalated to promote synergism between the two drugs. The methotrexate sensitizes the cell membrane to enhance the transport of 5-FU into the cell, thereby promoting intracellular concentration and presumably cell kill.

12. What agents can be given to minimize the toxicity of chemotherapy?

The following protective agents have the potential to minimize toxicity and maximize treatment options.

- High-dose methotrexate may be given only with leucovorin rescue, which blocks the action of the methotrexate and thus rescues normal cells from toxicity. Leucovorin is started 24 hours after the methotrexate and continued according to blood levels of methotrexate.
- Doxorubicin is known to damage the myocytes of the heart, causing it to function less efficiently as a pump once the maximal dose is reached. Administering the doxorubicin along with a cardioprotective agent such as Zinecard may permit longer courses of treatment with doxorubicin beyond the traditional recommendation of 550 mg/m². Zinecard is dosed at a 10:1 ratio (i.e., 1,000 mg of Zinecard and 100 mg of doxorubicin) and given by intravenous push (IVP) or intravenous piggy-back (IVPB) within 30 minutes before doxorubicin. Zinecard is an important option for many patients who continue to respond to doxorubicin and have few other effective options for treatment but risk the long-term effects of congestive heart failure as a consequence of continued therapy.
- Ethyol (Amifostine) has been well studied and commercially released to prevent the nephrotoxicity associated with cisplatin therapy. Other platinum side effects such as neurotoxicity, ototoxicity, and myelosuppression also have been minimized by this drug. Amifostine has a special affinity for normal body cells, to which it binds and detoxifies the chemotherapy. It also acts as a scavenger of oxygen free radicals caused by chemotherapy and radiation. The potential protective role of Amifostine with paclitaxel, carboplatin, doxorubicin, and radiation therapy is under investigation. The standard dose of Amifostine is 910 mg/m² by IVPB over 15 minutes immediately before administration of chemotherapy. Patients need to be monitored for side effects of nausea and hypotension.
- Mesna is given along with ifosfamide. After administration, ifosfamide is broken down into the toxic metabolite acrolein, which binds to and damages urinary tract epithelium. Mesna lacks any antitumor activity but binds directly to acrolein and blocks its ability to damage the cells of the bladder.

13. How and when is mesna administered with ifosfamide?

Because mesna has a shorter plasma half-life than ifosfamide, the two drugs are usually given concomitantly. Mesna is continued for 12–24 hours after the ifosfamide is administered. Typically mesna is given at 0 (before), 4, and 8 hours after ifosfamide has been given.

Route	Dose	Administration
Oral	40% of ifosfamide dose	Give at 0, 4, and 8 hours
IVP	20% of ifosfamide dose	Give at 0, 4, and 8 hours
Continuous IV infusion	Dose = ifosfamide dose	Give continuously

Oral mesna tastes and smells of sulfur and may not be well tolerated by patients prone to nausea and vomiting. Administration in 7-Up or Coca-Cola helps to mask the taste. Patients should be advised to push fluids, empty the bladder frequently, and report symptoms of irritation or pain during voiding.

14. What are the most common side effects of chemotherapy?

In general, adverse effects from chemotherapy result from damage to the rapidly dividing stem cells or drug toxicity to cells or tissues of specific organs unrelated to cell growth rate. The degree or severity of effects varies according to chemotherapy dosage, timing or duration, route of administration, prior chemotherapy or radiation therapy, co-administration of other agents, condition of patient, and individual sensitivities. Acute, late, and chronic effects ranging from mild to dose-limiting or fatal toxicities can occur that may or may not be predictable. See table for common side effects and toxicities; refer to chapter 40 for specific organ toxicities and late effects.

Quick Facts: Cancer Chemotherapy Side Effects

CHEMOTHERAPEUTIC AGENT (TRADE NAME)	NAUSEA/ VOMIT- ING	MUCO- SITIS	DIAR- RHEA/ CONSTI- PATION	ALO- PECIA	BONE MARROW SUPPRES- SION	HSR	VESI- CANT/ IRRI- TANT	ORGAN AND OTHER TOXICITIES
L-Asparaginase (Elspar)	±	0	0	0	0	++	0	Hepatic, neuro, hyperglycemia, pancreatitis
Bleomycin (Blenoxane)	±	+	0	±	0	+	I	Derm, fever, pulm, Raynaud's phenomenon
Busulfan (Myleran)	±	0	D±	±	++	0	0	Derm, gonadal, hepatic, ocular, pulm
Carboplatin (Paraplatin)	±	0	0	0	+	+	I	Hepatic, neuro, hypomag- nesemia
Carmustine, BCNU (BiCNU)	+	+	D±	0	++	0	I	Gonadal, hepatic, neuro*, pulm*, renal
Chlorambucil (Leukeran)	±	0	0	0	±	0	0	Gonadal, pulm*
Cisplatin, CDDP (Platinol)	++	0	D±	0	±	+	I	Gonadal, neuro, ototoxic, renal, hypomagnesemia
Cladribine, 2-CdA (Leustatin)	±	0	0	0	+	0	0	Derm, neuro, renal*
Cyclophosphamide, Cytoxan (Neosar)	+	0	0	++	++	0	0	Cardiac*, gonadal, SIADH*, hemorrhagic cystitis
Cytarabine, Ara-C (Cytosar-U)	+	++	D+	±	++	0	0	Derm*, flu-like syndrome, neuro*, ocular*, pulm
Dacarbazine (DTIC)	++	0	0	±	+	0	I	Derm, hepatic, flu-like illness
Dactinomycin, actino- mycin D (Cosmegen)	+	++	D±	+	++	0	V	Derm, fever, hepatic
Daunorubicin, dauno- mycin (Cerubidine)	+	+	0	++	++	+	V	Cardiac, red urine, derm
Docetaxel (Taxotere)	±	+	D±	+	++	++	I	Derm, neuro, fluid retention syndrome, fatigue
Doxorubicin, ADR (Adriamycin, Rubex)	+	+	0	++	++	+	V	Cardiac, derm, red urine
Epirubicin (Epidoxorubicin)	+	+	D±	+	++	+	V	Cardiac, red-orange urine
Estramustine (Emcyt)	+	0	D±	±	±	0	0	Cardiac, gynecomastia
Etoposide, VP-16-213 (VePesid)	±	0	C±	+	+	+	I	Hypotension (rapid infusion), neuro
Floxuridine (FUDR)	±	+	D+	±	±	0	0	Derm, hepatic
Fludarabine (Fludara)	±	0	D±	±	+	0	0	Neuro*, decreased T-cells
5-Fluorouracil, 5-FU (Adrucil)	±	++	D++	±	+	0	I	Cardiac, derm, neuro, ocular
Gemcitabine (Gemzar)	±	0	0	±	+	0	0	Derm, fever, flu-like syndrome
Hydroxyurea (Hydrea)	±	±	D±/C±	±	+	0	0	Derm, megaloblastosis
Idarubicin HCl (Idamycin)	+	+	D±	+	++	0	V	Cardiac, derm
Ifosfamide (Ifex)	+	±	D/C±	+	++	0	I	Neuro*, hemorrhagic cystitis, renal*

Table continued on following page.

Quick Facts: Cancer Chemotherapy Side Effects (Continued)

CHEMOTHERAPEUTIC AGENT (TRADE NAME)	NAUSEA/ VOMIT- ING	MUCO- SITIS	DIAR- RHEA/ CONSTI- PATION	ALO- PECIA	BONE MARROW SUPPRES- SION	HSR	VESI- CANT/ IRRI- TANT	ORGAN AND OTHER TOXICITIES
Irinotecan HCl (Camptosar)	++	±	D+	+	+	0	I	Pulmonary
Lomustine, CCNU (CeeNu)	+	±	D±	±	++	0	0	Gonadal, hepatic, pulm, renal
Mechlorethamine, nitrogen mustard, HN2 (Mustargen)	++	0	0	+	++	0	V	Derm, fever, gonadal
Melphalan, L-PAM (Alkeran)	±	0	0	±	+	+ (IV)	0	Derm, hepatic*, gonadal
Mercaptopurine, 6MP (Purinethol)	±	+	D±	0	+	0	0	Hepatic, derm
Methotrexate, MTX (Folex, Rheumatrex)	±	++	D±	±	+	0	0	Derm, hepatic*, neuro*, ocular, pulm*, renal*
Mitomycin C (Mutamycin)	+	+	0	+	++	0	V	Derm, hemolytic uremic syndrome, hepatic*, pulm
Mitoxantrone HCl (Novantrone)	±	+	D±	+	++	0	I	Cardiac, blue-green discoloration (nails, sclera, urine)
Paclitaxel (Taxol)	±	±	D±	+	+	++	I	Bradycardia, derm, neuro
Procarbazine (Matulane)	+	±	D±	±	+	+	0	Gonadal*, neuro, MAO inhibitory effect
Thiotepa (Thioplex)	±	±	0	0	+	0	0	Derm*, gonadal, neuro*
Topotecan (Hycamtin)	+	+	D±	+	+	0	0	Derm, fever, flu-like illness, neuro
Vinblastine, VLB (Velban)	±	+	C+	±	+	0	V	Neuro, jaw pain
Vincristine, VCR (Oncovin)	±	±	C+	±	±	0	V	Neuro, SIADH
Vinorelbine tartrate (Navelbine)	±	±	C+	±	+	0	V	Neuro

Disclaimer: This table illustrates principal or unique toxicities, but is not all-inclusive. It may not list rare, occasional, or late effects. Side effect profiles change with dosage, timing, route and duration of administration, prior chemotherapy or radiation therapy, co-administration of other therapies, as well as the patient's condition and sensitivities.

* = high dose, C = constipation, D = diarrhea, derm = dermatologic, HSR = hypersensitivity reaction, neuro = neurologic, pulm = pulmonary, SIADH = syndrome of inappropriate antidiuretic hormone, I = irritant, V = vesicant; 0 = none or rare; ± = mild, + = moderate to moderately high, ++ = severe.

Developed by Fink R, Gates R, Goodman M, Petersen J, 1997.

BIBLIOGRAPHY

1. Berg DT: New chemotherapy treatment options and implications for nursing care. Oncol Nurs Forum 24(Suppl):5–12, 1997.
2. Donehower RC, Abeloff MD, Perry MC: Chemotherapy. In Abeloff MD, Armitage JO, Lichter AS, Niederhuber JE (eds): Clinical Oncology, New York, Churchill Livingstone, 1995, pp 201–218.
3. Dorr RT, Von Hoff DD: Cancer Chemotherapy Handbook. Norwalk, CT, Appleton & Lange, 1994.
4. Erlichman C: Pharmacology of anticancer drugs. In Tannock IF, Hill RP (eds): The Basic Science of Oncology, 2nd ed. New York, McGraw-Hill, 1992, pp 317–337.
5. Fischer DS, Knobf MT, Durivage HJ: The Cancer Chemotherapy Handbook. St. Louis, Mosby, 1993.
6. Goodman M, Riley MB: Principles of chemotherapy administration. In Groenwald S, Frogge M, Goodman M, Yarbro C (eds): Cancer Nursing Principles and Practice, 4th ed. Boston, Jones & Bartlett, 1997.
7. Hrushesky W, Bjanason G: Circadian cancer therapy. J Clin Oncol 11:1403–1417, 1993.
8. Kemp G, Rose P, Turain J, et al: Amifostine pretreatment for protection against cyclophosphamide-induced and cisplatin-induced toxicities: Results of a randomized control trial in patients with advanced ovarian cancer. J Clin Oncol 14: 2101–2112. 1996.
9. Miaskowski C: Oncology Nursing: An Essential Guide for Patient Care. Philadelphia, W.B. Saunders, 1997.
10. Perry MC (ed): The Chemotherapy Source Book. Baltimore, Williams & Wilkins, 1996.
11. Powel LL, Fishman M, Mrozek-Orlowski M (eds): Cancer Chemotherapy Guidelines and Recommendations for Practice. Pittsburgh, Oncology Nursing Society, 1996.
12. Tannock IF: Biological properties of anticancer drugs. In Tannock IF, Hill RP (eds): The Basic Science of Oncology, 2nd ed. New York, McGraw-Hill, 1992, pp 302–316.

8. TIPS FOR ADMINISTERING CHEMOTHERAPY

Michelle Goodman, RN, MS, and Jennifer Petersen, RN, MS

1. What qualifications are needed to administer chemotherapy?

Patients with cancer receive complicated drug regimens and schedules with the potential for severe side effects and reactions. Chemotherapy should be administered only by nurses and physicians with advanced educational preparation. Such preparation includes certification in chemotherapy administration, which consists not only of didactic instruction but also of clinical application and skill supervision. The practitioner also should be knowledgeable about the proper procedures for drug preparation, handling and alternate methods of drug delivery, including various vascular access devices and ambulatory infusion pumps and their associated complications.

Currently no official credentialing programs are endorsed by professional nursing organizations; however, guidelines are available from the Oncology Nursing Society (ONS). The ONS guidelines cover course content for chemotherapy classes as well as administration and handling of chemotherapeutic drugs.

2. What are the most important precautions for preventing errors in chemotherapy administration?

Serious errors in chemotherapy administration are relatively rare considering the number of patients treated. Although mistakes can be made by even the most knowledgeable practitioner, they are most likely when untrained personnel are asked to perform tasks beyond their expertise or when an order is written in an unclear way that allows misinterpretation. Important precautions include the following:

- The administration of chemotherapy should be delayed until a properly trained practitioner is available. With rare exceptions (e.g., high-grade lymphoma), the administration of chemotherapy is not an emergency procedure.
- Only qualified personnel should write orders or administer chemotherapy.
- All orders should be double checked by personnel preparing and administering the drugs.
- The patient should be cared for by only one or two nurses who communicate and work together to chart which drugs have been given and repeatedly check that they have *the right dose of the right drug for the right patient via the right route according to the right schedule.*
- Nurses need to question any aspect of the order that is contrary to customary practice or to what has been done for the patient in the past, especially when unusually high doses or unusual schedules are involved.
- Nurses should be careful not to permit distractions while checking an order or administering treatment. Too often the nurse is treating 4 or 5 patients at one time and forgets to check an order or to identify a patient properly. Distractions such as telephones, beepers, and physicians' requests for assistance should be kept to a minimum in the treatment area.

3. Who should write chemotherapy orders? How should they be written?

Only the attending physician or oncology fellow (**not the resident or intern**) responsible for the patient's care and most familiar with the drug regimen and dosing schedule should write the order for chemotherapy. Orders should be written according to the following guidelines:

- The order should be written clearly and without abbreviations.
- The dose should be written first as it is to be calculated (mg/m^2 or mg/kg), and the total dose should be indicated along with route and length of time of the injection or infusion. When carboplatin is dosed based upon area under the curve (AUC), it will be expressed as total milligrams, not milligrams per square meter (mg/m^2), and will be correlated to a desired AUC level. (AUC dosing for carboplatin correlates better with toxicity than BSA

dosing and is calculated with the Calvert formula: total dose = target AUC x [glomerular filtration rate + 25].)

- If one drug in a combination is to be given for 1 day only and the other(s) for more than 1 day, this distinction should be clearly indicated.

Example: Patient is 72 cm tall and weighs 150 lbs; m^2 = 2.

Order: Cisplatin 75 mg/m^2 = 150 mg in 250 cc normal saline IV over 1 hour (day 1 only)
Etoposide 75 mg/m^2 = 150 mg in 250 cc normal saline IV over 1 hour on days 1, 2, 3. Etoposide total dose = 450 mg over 3 days.

4. Should a nurse take a verbal order for chemotherapy?

No. *Verbal orders for chemotherapy should not be given or taken.* The risk of confusion about drug names and dosages is too great. People unfamiliar with chemotherapy may mistake carboplatin for cisplatin, vincristine for vinblastine, or Taxol for Taxotere. Mitoxantrone may be easily mistaken for mitomycin because both have a similar dosage range, both are used for breast cancer, both have an unusual color (mitomycin is light purple, mitoxantrone is dark blue), and both can be given by intravenous push. However, mitoxantrone is given more commonly as an infusion over 15 minutes; it is potentially dangerous to give mitomycin as an infusion because it is a vesicant. An error such as giving the wrong drug or wrong dose can be fatal.

5. I work alone in an oncology office, where I mix and administer my own chemotherapy. Is this arrangement safe?

Nurses commonly work in solo practice, preparing as well as administering chemotherapy. Although the nurse may be skilled in both tasks, it is not optimal for anyone to mix and administer the drug without having someone else doublecheck the order. In a solo practice, the physician should be asked to doublecheck the drug.

6. In a busy practice, is it okay to prepare drugs before the patient arrives for treatment?

It is not uncommon for drugs to be prepared in advance and placed on trays until the patient arrives for treatment. Often the treatment involves 3 or 4 drugs plus hydration and antiemetics. Trays should be large enough to contain the patient's medicines, or all medicines should be placed in a large plastic Ziploc bag to prevent confusing one patient's drugs with another's.

7. Can small frail veins that may have been adequate for methotrexate and 5-fluorouracil be used for doxorubicin, a known vesicant?

Small veins do not necessitate use of a vascular access device (VAD) to administer a vesicant. However, the vein must be properly selected and prepared before venipuncture is attempted. The nurse should take time, avoid distraction, and be focused on the patient.

Selection of arm veins
- Begin exam at dorsum of hand and move up.
- Avoid the antecubital fossa for vesicant administration.
- Distal forearm is best site to avoid nerve and tendon damage.
- Avoid veins that have been used in past 24 hours.
- Avoid veins with compromised circulation.
- Evaluate the patient for need of a VAD if multiple cycles of chemotherapy are planned.

Before attempting venipuncture
- Apply warm compresses.
- Use gravity.
- Have the patient squeeze a handball.
- Offer a hot drink.

8. How can I distinguish among extravasation, irritation, and flare reaction?

Extravasation, although rare, is probably one of the most worrisome findings a nurse may encounter. It is characterized by swelling, erythema, pain at the IV site, and inability to obtain blood return (usually). **Vein irritation** manifests as complaints of achiness and tightness along the vein accompanied by redness and darkness. Blood return usually is present. **Flare reaction**

almost always has blood return and is not characterized by pain; it is associated with immediate blotches around the needle site and streaking or itching along the vein.

9. As long as I have blood return, I do not need to worry about extravasation. True or false?

False. Extravasations of vesicant agents may occur in the presence of perfect blood return. Evidence of good blood return is not the only measure of safe and trouble-free injection of a vesicant. If pain, swelling, or tension is evident in the surrounding tissue, the drug probably has infiltrated despite adequate blood return. Do not ignore the patient's complaint of pain—it may be the first sign of extravasation.

10. What can I do if I am giving a vesicant and lose blood return?

The main problem with small veins is that blood return may be intermittent during drug injection. The saying, "if in doubt, pull it out," is appropriate but sometimes not practical. Because presumably the best vein has already been chosen, removal of the needle without cause is not only unnecessary but also may diminish the chance of safe delivery of the drug. If any of the cardinal symptoms of extravasation (pain or swelling at the site) is present, the nurse should stop injecting the drug and attempt to aspirate. If it is not possible to aspirate blood or drug, the needle is removed and the site is treated as an extravasation (see form below).

Documentation Record for Suspected or Actual Chemotherapy Drug Extravasation

Patient: _____ **Date** infiltration occurred: _____

Drug: _____ Dilution mg/ml _____ Vesicant _____ Irritant _____

Amount of drug infiltrated: < 1 ml _____ 1–3 ml _____ 3–5 ml _____ 5–10 ml _____ > 10 ml _____

Method of drug administration:
_____ Two-syringe technique IV push
_____ Side-arm with IV freely running
_____ Continous infusion: Rate ___ cc/hour Peristaltic pump: ____ Yes ____ No
_____ VAD: ____ Port ____ Tunneled catheter Type of needle _____
_____ Other: _____

Description of site:
Size _____ Color _____ Texture _____
(Indicate site on diagram)

Process documentation: Describe the events   Right arm   Left arm
that occurred during the drug administration   (Attach photograph)
S (patient's symptoms): _____
_____
_____

O (clinical symptoms): _____
_____
_____

A (assessment): _____ Suspected extravasation _____ Definite extravasation _____

P (plan of care): Initial actions: _____
_____

Physician notified _____ Instruction _____
_____

Follow-up instructions: _____
_____

Additional comments: _____
Consultations: _____ Plastic surgery _____ Physical therapy _____ Other _____
Date of referral: _____ Follow-up _____
Return appointment: _____ Written instructions for site care reviewed with patient _____
RN signature: _____
Follow-up visit no. 1 (date _____) Describe site and care instructions (attach photo): _____
_____

Follow-up visit no. 2 (date _____) Describe site and care instructions (attach photo): _____
_____

Follow-up visit no. 3 (date _____) Describe site and care instructions (attach photo): _____
_____

Source: Goodman M: Rush Cancer Institute, Chicago.

In cases involving flare at the site (redness or itching along the vein) and loss of blood return, the nurse should stop injecting the drug, switch to saline, and give 10–30 cc of saline through the line while observing for swelling and symptoms of discomfort. If the vein is determined to be patent, the vesicant is again connected and injected slowly. The blood return again may be evident as the drug is given. *The nurse should not try to reposition the needle or press down on the cannula to obtain a blood return.* This strategy may result in damage to the vein and seepage of the drug out of the vein (i.e., an extravasation).

11. If extravasation is suspected, what should the nurse do?

1. Stop the drug.
2. Aspirate and leave the needle in place.
3. Call the physician.
4. Give an antidote (when appropriate) through the needle or by subcutaneous injection if the needle is already removed.
5. Remove the needle, and avoid undue pressure.
6. Apply cold or heat (depending on the extravasated drug) for 15 minutes 4 times/day for 24 hours.
7. Arrange consultation with a plastic surgeon.
8. Document the incident (see form in question 10).

12. How often should a VAD be checked during continuous infusion of a chemotherapeutic agent or vesicant?

Extravasations with VADs are rare but may occur. Exit sites need to be inspected frequently for signs of edema, erythema, or fluid drainage. The site should be checked every 1–2 hours or more often according to the patient's condition. Many nurses focus on checking blood return to ascertain catheter tip and needle placement; however, there is no consensus about how often this should be done. It is probably reasonable to check blood return less frequently (every 4–8 hours) because of concerns about infection risk, catheter clotting, or needle dislodgements in implanted ports.

13. A patient with breast cancer needs only one more dose of doxorubicin. She has absolutely no usable veins in her good arm. Is it safe to use her other arm, even though she has had a node dissection?

After consultation with the physician about the risks of performing venipuncture on the operative side, the arm should be assessed thoroughly. If there is no evidence of swelling, if the patient is fully informed about the involved risks, and if an excellent vein is available, it is safe to proceed. If there is any question about the integrity of the vein or if the veins are small and frail, a temporary central line may be considered.

14. What can be done to minimize the pain of needlestick?

For many patients the pain of the needlestick (e.g., an implanted port, peripheral line, or Zoladex injection) is the most dreaded part of treatment. For some patients an ethyl chloride spray is adequate to partially numb the site. For others, more anesthesia (intradermal lidocaine) is needed. Placement of an ice cube over a port site for 2 minutes, followed by ethyl chloride spray, is a good option.

The most effective solution, however, is Emla cream, which is placed over the port site 1–2 hours prior to the needle puncture. The port is then covered with a transparent dressing. Emla cream also may be used over peripheral veins. Patients often can identify their best veins by running the hand or forearm under warm water and placing the Emla cream on the site before they come for treatment. An exception is the patient receiving a vesicant agent; Emla cream may numb the site sufficiently to mask the discomfort associated with extravasation.

15. What is the safest way to administer a vesicant through a peripheral vein?

The safest way to administer a vesicant agent via a peripheral vein is first to select the best vein, preferably one in the forearm, where soft tissue density is greater. However, a straight, supple, easily cannulated vein in the hand is preferable to a smaller, deeper vein that is more difficult to cannulate in any other location. Next, select a method of administration—either the two-syringe technique or infusion through the side-arm of a freely running IV line. The two-syringe technique is used most often when fluids are not needed to hydrate the patient. A 23-gauge butterfly needle is large enough to permit adequate dilution yet causes minimal trauma to the vein. Flushing with a minimum of 3–5 cc of saline before and after vesicant administration is mandatory to ensure venous access and safe vesicant administration. When the two-syringe technique is used, the nurse should aspirate immediately if extravasation is suspected.

Injecting a vesicant through the side-arm of a freely running IV line (angiocath) is preferred when hydration is also needed or when the drug is known to cause vein irritation (e.g., nitrogen mustard). The main problem with side-arming is that the nurse has less control over fluid flow in the event of an extravasation. Gravity propels the vesicant into the patient as the nurse clamps off the IV line and then attempts to aspirate the vesicant. The potential result is a greater amount of drug infiltration. Both methods are equally safe for peripheral administration of vesicant drugs.

16. Which needle size is best for administering chemotherapy?

This issue is controversial, and current research provides no definitive answer. In addition, it is not known whether it is best to use an angiocath, a butterfly needle, or a scalp vein needle for administration of vesicants. Many nurses believe that angiocaths should be used for vesicants because they offer more stability and reduce the risk for infiltration, whereas other nurses are more comfortable and proficient with insertion of butterfly needles. Butterfly needles are acceptable for infusions lasting only a few minutes, but angiocaths are recommended for longer infusions and for vesicant or irritant drugs. Many nurses prefer small 23- or 25-gauge butterfly needles because they are easier to insert, less likely to puncture the vein wall, and also may cause less pain or scar tissue formation. Angiocaths (gauges 19 and 21) are favored because they are large-bore and enable the drug to reach the circulation more quickly.

17. Why is the antecubital fossa avoided for chemotherapy administration?

The antecubital fossa is an extremely difficult site to heal in the event of infiltration or extravasation. Infiltrations are also more difficult to detect in the antecubital fossa. Many nurses reserve this area for drawing blood or emergency use. Chemotherapy may cause venous thrombosis or fibrosis, making the antecubital fossa unusable for other purposes.

18. What is a hypersensitivity reaction?

A hypersensitivity reaction (HSR) occurs when the immune system is overstimulated by a foreign substance (e.g., chemotherapy) or antigen and forms antibodies that cause an immune response. Sensitization results, and subsequent exposures to the antigen cause a type I allergic reaction. HSRs may occur during the initial or subsequent administration of a chemotherapeutic agent.

19. What are the symptoms of a hypersensitivity reaction?

Most HSRs occur within the first 15 minutes of infusion or injection, but they are not limited to this time frame. HSRs may present as one or more of the following signs and symptoms: dizziness, flushing, nausea, generalized itching, hives, rash, rhinitis, abdominal cramping, chills, hypotension, dyspnea, bronchospasm, cyanosis, and feelings of agitation, uneasiness, or impending doom.

20. Which drugs are most often associated with an HSR?

Paclitaxel (Taxol). The vehicle in which it is mixed (Cremophor EL) rather than the drug itself appears to cause allergic reactions. Most reactions occur with the first or second treatment. Patients are pretreated with glucocorticosteroids and antihistamines with each course of paclitaxel; diphenhydramine may be used if needed but is not given routinely after the third uneventful course.

Commonly Used Chemotherapeutic Agents That May Cause Hypersensitivity Reactions

AGENT	OVERALL INCIDENCE (%)	CLINICAL PRESENTATION	COMMENTS
L-Asparaginase	20–35	Fevers, aches, chills, urticaria, hypotension, diaphoresis, edema, asthma, laryngeal constriction, loss of consciousness	Incidence may increase with each subsequent administration Emergency medications and equipment should be readily available during administration. Consider substitution of a similar drug (e.g., *Erwinia* L-asparaginase instead of *Escherichia coli*).
Paclitaxel (Taxol)	3–28	Bronchospasm, dyspnea, stridor, facial flushing, edema, hypotension, urticaria, rash Generally occurs within first 10 min of infusion	Most patients are premedicated with dexamethasone, 20 mg orally 12 and 6 hr before infusion, as well as diphenhydramine, 25–30 mg IV, and cimetidine, 300 mg, famotidine, 20 mg IV, 30 min before infusion.
Docetaxel (Taxotere)	Undetermined	Flushing, rash, pruritus, dyspnea, chest discomfort, bronchospasm, angio-edema, hypotension	Currently patients receive Decadron, 8 mg orally 2 times/day on day before treatment and continuing for 5 days. Patients also may receive IV Benadryl, 25–50 mg, 30 min before infusion.
Etoposide (VP-16)	1–3	Rash, facial flushing, angio-edema, pruritus, urticaria, hypotension, diaphoresis, wheezing, and dyspnea Usually occurs with first dose	Etoposide is formulated in solution (Tween 80 and benzyl alcohol) that may contribute to HSR. Generic brands may be associated with higher incidence of HSR. Cross-hypersensitivity between pacli-taxel and etoposide appears to be more likely with repeated exposures.
Teniposide (Vumon)	5% overall 13% in cancers of central nervous system	Rash, facial flushing, angio-edema, pruritus, urticaria, hypotension, wheezing, dyspnea Usually occurs with first dose	Teniposide is formulated in Cremo-phor EL, which may contribute to HSR.
Cisplatin (Platinol)	5	Anxiety, pruritus, cough, dyspnea, diaphoresis, angio-edema, vomiting, rash, urticaria, hypotension	HSRs have been observed with intravenous and intravesicular administrations. HSRs have been reported with man-nitol, which can be used as a premedication for cisplatin.
Procarbazine (Matulane)	15	Maculopapular rash, urticaria, angioedema, toxic epidermal necrolysis Rare type II reactions of interstitial pneumonitis and eosinophilia	Rechallenge is usually unsuccessful, despite pretreatment with cortico-steroids or antihistamines.
Anthracycline antibiotics (doxorubicin, daunorubicin)	1–15	Urticaria, pruritus, angioedema, dyspnea, bronchospasm, hypotension Local flare reaction may mani-fest as erythema, pruritus, and urticaria around injection site.	Cross-reactivity among anthracyclines has been demonstrated.

Etoposide (VP-16). Administration over a minimum of 45–60 minutes prevents a hypotensive episode. Bronchospasm with severe wheezing and flushing also has been observed and generally responds to antihistamines and glucocorticosteroids. More HSRs occur with the generic formulation than with the brand-name drug. Pharmacists need to inform the nurse administering the drugs if this is the case.

Cisplatin. Cisplatin and its analogs may cause a type I allergic reaction. Although most clinicians expect HSRs to occur with the first or second use, many reported cases involving cisplatin required repeated exposure (4 or 5 times).

21. What additional steps should be taken to prevent an HSR?

Although any patient may experience a serious reaction, people who say that they are allergic to everything should give cause to pause. Take the extra time to elicit a medical/allergy history. Make note of the drugs to which the patient is allergic, and find out whether they have had previous exposure to the chemotherapeutic agent(s) that you are about to administer. Instruct the patient to report any symptoms to you immediately. Make sure that patients who are treated in a private room have a call light or bell.

22. How should an HSR be managed if it occurs?

A policy and procedure for management of an HSR should be readily available; emergency drugs and emergency equipment should be in good working condition and located in the immediate work area. Posting a quick reference list of medications commonly associated with HSRs, along with management guidelines (laminated) that include the doses and methods of emergency drug administration, is helpful. In the event of an HSR, the first step is to take a deep breath and call for help; then implement the following guidelines:

1. Stop the infusion immediately, stay with the patient, and have the physician notified. Reassure the patient and family.
2. Maintain the IV line with normal saline.
3. Obtain all emergency drugs that may be needed to treat the patient.
4. Monitor vital signs, and maximize rate of infusion of IV fluid if the patient is hypotensive.
5. Administer emergency drugs according to policy and procedure or physician order:
    - Epinephrine, 0.1–0.5 mg (1:10,000 solution) by IV push or subcutaneously every 10 minutes as needed.
    - Diphenhydramine HCL, 25–50 mg IV
    - Albuterol inhaler to promote bronchodilation.
    - Solu-Medrol, 30–60 mg IV, Solu-Cortef, 100–500 mg IV, or dexamethasone, 10–20 mg IV, to ease bronchoconstriction even more.
    - Aminophylline, 5 mg/kg (average dose: 300–500 mg) over 30 minutes if the patient has evidence of bronchospasm or wheezing.
    - Dopamine (Intropin), 2–20 µg/kg/min, to maintain blood pressure and organ perfusion.
6. Put the patient in supine position to promote adequate perfusion of vital organs.
7. Monitor vital signs every 2 minutes until the patient is stable, every 5 minutes for 30 minutes, and every 15 minutes until a determination of the patient's condition is made.
8. Document the incident and patient reaction in the chart.
9. Because pharmaceutical companies make note of incidents such as an HSR, it is important to provide information to the company about drug lot numbers, diluents, preservatives, and any other factor that may contribute to a better understanding of the cause of the reaction.

23. Can patients who have had an HSR receive the causative drug again?

In most cases, patients should not receive the remainder of the drug on the day of the reaction or at any future time, especially if the reaction was significant (bronchospasm, severe hypotension, or generalized urticaria). If the reaction is mild (rash that resolves with diphenhydramine), the physician may choose to continue the drug once the patient stabilizes. If the drug is absolutely necessary and no suitable substitute is available, rechallenge may be appropriate and safe. With subsequent dosing, the patient may require preparation with antihistamines and corticosteroids; emergency drugs and personnel should be in attendance during the rechallenge. The drug also may be further diluted during rechallenges to minimize an HSR.

24. What different types of drug interactions may occur in the oncology setting?

A true drug interaction occurs when the effects of one drug are altered by concomitant administration of other medications. Drug interactions may be advantageous by producing synergy between drugs or detrimental by causing antagonism, enhanced toxicity, or inhibition of effects. Pharmacokinetic drug interactions are characterized by alteration in the absorption, distribution, metabolism, bioavailability, and elimination of a particular medication. Such interactions may occur directly at the cellular level; for example, coadministration of aspirin and methotrexate causes displacement of methotrexate from its protein-binding site, which results in a higher blood level of methotrexate, decreased elimination of methotrexate, and increased toxicity.

Physical and chemical incompatibilities may occur when multiple drugs are mixed or administered together. A physical incompatibility occurs when the mixture of two or more agents results in a change in appearance of solution (e.g., color, precipitation, or turbidity). Chemical incompatibility results in drug degradation, thereby diminishing its effectiveness. Interactions are not always visibly detectable in an IV bag or tubing; thus, it is crucial to refer to compatibility data before administering IV chemotherapy (see table below).

Compatibility Guidelines for Drugs Commonly Used in an Ambulatory Oncology Clinic*

	LASIX	MANNITOL	K+	MG	HEPARIN	DECADRON	ZOFRAN	KYTRIL
Carboplatin							C	C
Carmustine							C	
Cisplatin	C	C	C	C for 48°	C	C	C	C
Cyclophosphamide	C	C in D5 ½ normal saline for 48°			C	C	C	C
Cytarabine	C		C		I	C	C	C
Dacarbazine					I		C	C
Doxorubicin	I				I	I	C	C
Etoposide			C				C	C
5-Fluorouracil	C		C	C	C		I	C
Ifosfamide							C	C
Methotrexate	C				C	C	C	C
Mitomycin	C				C		C	
Mitoxantrone			C		I		C	
Paclitaxel			C	C	C	C	C	C
Vinblastine	I				C		C	
Vincristine	I				C		C	C
Zofran	I	C	C	C	C	C		
Kytril	C		C	C				

• Compatibilities apply to Y site infusion or injection unless otherwise specified.
K = potassium, MG = magnesium, C = compatible, I = incompatible.

Other comments about drug compatibility and interactions include the following:

Carboplatin
- Dose should be adjusted for patients with decreased creatinine clearance.
- Aluminum equipment causes precipitant formation and reduces potency.
- Compatible with paclitaxel and ifosfamide.

Carmustine
- Incompatible with polyvinyl chloride or sodium bicarbonate.

Cisplatin
- Incompatible with sodium bicarbonate, 5-FU, metoclopramide, etoposide, and paclitaxel.
- Cytotoxic synergy with etoposide.
- Dose should be reduced for patients with decreased creatinine clearance.
- Antitumor activity enhanced with tamoxifen.
- Administration via aluminum needles decreases efficacy and causes black plating on needles or equipment.
- Compatible with etoposide and paclitaxel.

Cyclophosphamide
- Compatible with doxorubicin, cisplatin, metoclopramide, droperidol, 5-FU, and mesna.
- Co-administration with allopurinol increases myelosuppression.
- May block metabolism of barbiturates and sedatives.

Cytarabine
- Incompatible with penicillin and 5-FU.
- Compatible with methotrexate, idarubicin, daunorubicin, etoposide, sodium bicarbonate, and metoclopramide.
- Synergy with methotrexate.

Dacarbazine
- Compatible with cyclophosphamide, doxorubicin, dactinomycin, and methotrexate.

Doxorubicin
- Compatible with vincristine, cyclophosphamide, dacarbazine, and vinblastine.
- Incompatible with hydrocortisone, methotrexate, and 5-FU.

Etoposide
- Compatible with cisplatin, carboplatin, cytarabine, daunorubicin, 5-FU, paclitaxel, and ifosfamide.
- Incompatible with idarubicin.

5-Fluorouracil
- Compatible with leucovorin, methotrexate, and vincristine.
- Incompatible with cisplatin, cytarabine, daunorubicin, doxorubicin, and idarubicin.

Ifosfamide
- Compatible with Mesna in solution for 24°, carboplatin, cisplatin, and etoposide.

Methotrexate
- Compatible with cytarabine, dacarbazine, leucovorin, vincristine, 5-FU, hydrocortisone, and sodium bicarbonate.
- Incompatible with bleomycin, doxorubicin, prednisone, and metoclopramide.

Mitomycin
- Compatible with 5-FU and leucovorin.

Mitoxantrone
- Synergy with cytarabine.
- Compatible with hydrocortisone and sodium succinate.
- Incompatible with hydrocortisone and sodium phosphate.

Paclitaxel
- Incompatible with polyvinyl chloride bags and infusion sets.
- Should be given before platinum-based agents in combined chemotherapy.
- Compatible with carboplatin, cisplatin, etoposide, and famotidine.

Thiotepa
- May exaggerate effects of muscle relaxants when given in combination.

Vinblastine
- Compatible with 5-FU, dacarbazine, doxorubicin, and bleomycin.
- Incompatible with infusaid pumps.
- May increase cellular uptake of methotrexate by malignant cells.

Vincristine
- Compatible with bleomycin, cytarabine, doxorubicin, 5-FU, methotrexate, and metoclopramide.
- Additive neurotoxicity when given with other neurotoxic agents.

Zofran
- Incompatible with sodium bicarbonate and lorazepam.
- Compatible with diphenhydramine, droperidol, famotidine, hydrocortisone, hydromorphone, leucovorin, metoclopramide, and morphine sulfate.

Kytril
- Kytril is chemically stable and physically compatible when injected with diphenhydramine, morphine, and lorazepam.

25. What should be said to a patient who asks, "Can I drink alcohol while receiving chemotherapy?"

The ingestion of alcohol may be contraindicated in certain patients while receiving chemotherapy. For example, patients who drink alcohol while taking procarbazine may experience an Antabuse-like reaction with facial flushing, headache, nausea, and hypotension. Similarly, the incidence of methotrexate-induced hepatotoxicity is increased in patients who consume alcohol. However, patients may be reassured that with other chemotherapeutic agents, alcohol in moderation is safe.

26. What special precautions should a health care professional take to minimize exposure while mixing, administering, or handling chemotherapeutic agents?

All chemotherapeutic agents should be admixed in a biologic safety cabinet (BSC). Personnel should wear protective clothing, including surgical Latex gloves and a disposable, lint-free, nonabsorbent gown, while mixing chemotherapy. Careful hand washing is essential. Gloves should be replaced immediately if punctured. Spills should be cleaned up as expediently as possible, and exposed garments should be replaced. If a BSC is not available, protective eye gear and a respirator mask should be worn in addition to the gloves and gown. An absorbent, disposable pad should be placed under the arm or body part to which chemotherapy is given to catch any spills. For handling excreta, surgical Latex gloves should be worn; a disposable gown should be added if splashing is possible.

27. Can a nurse administer chemotherapy through an Ommaya reservoir?

Yes—if she or he has demonstrated competency. An Ommaya reservoir is a small plastic, domelike device placed beneath the scalp. An attached catheter is threaded into the lateral ventricle for administration of chemotherapy intrathecally in patients with central nervous system leukemia or into the spinal fluid in patients with metastatic disease and for obtaining samples of cerebrospinal fluid for examination. The following *sterile* procedure should be followed:

1. Wear a mask and sterile gloves.

2. Prepare the scalp area with Betadine or chlorhexidene scrub (parting the hair or shaving the area if necessary). Dry with sterile gauze.

3. Use a small-gauge or butterfly needle attached to a syringe, and insert gently into the Ommaya reservoir. (Local anesthetic is usually not needed before puncturing.)

4. Withdraw the spinal fluid (the amount should equal the volume of the infusate).

5. Inject preservative-free chemotherapeutic agent slowly into the reservoir.

6. Remove the needle, and gently pump the reservoir several times.

7. Place a Bandaid over the site, and ask the patient to lie supine for 15 minutes.

Patients should be instructed to notify the physician of signs and symptoms of infection, such as fever > 101° F, tenderness, erythema or swelling at the site, neck stiffness, or headache.

BIBLIOGRAPHY

1. Berg DT: New chemotherapy options and implications for nursing care. Oncol Nurs Forum 24(Suppl): 5–12, 1997.
2. Dorr RT, Von Hoff DD: Cancer Chemotherapy Handbook. Norwalk, CT, Appleton & Lange, 1994.
3. Erlichman C: Pharmacology of anticancer drugs. In Tannock IF, Hill RP (eds): The Basic Science of Oncology, 2nd ed. New York, McGraw-Hill, 1992, pp 317–337.
4. Finley R: Drug interactions in the oncology patient. Semin Oncol Nurs 8(2):95–101, 1992.
5. Ford JM: Modulators of multidrug resistance. Hematol Oncol Clin North Am 9:337–361, 1995.
6. Goodman M, Riley MB: Principles of chemotherapy administration. In Groenwald S, Frogge M, Goodman M, Yarbro C (eds): Cancer Nursing: Principles and Practice, 4th ed. Boston, Jones & Bartlett, 1997.
7. Perry MC (ed): The Chemotherapy Source Book, 2nd ed. Baltimore, Williams & Wilkins, 1996.
8. Powel LL, Fishman M, Mrozek-Orlowski M (eds): Cancer Chemotherapy Guidelines and Recommendations for Practice. Pittsburgh, Oncology Nursing Society, 1996.
9. Trissel LA: Handbook on Injectable Drugs, 8th ed. Bethesda, MD, American Society of Hospital Pharmacists, 1994.
10. Van Meerten E, Verweij J, Schellens JHM: Antineoplastic agents: Drug interactions of clinical significance. Drug Safety 12(3):168–182, 1995.
11. Wickham R, Purl S, Welker D: Long term central venous catheters: Issues for care. Semin Oncol Nurs 8(2):133–147, 1992.

9. BIOLOGIC THERAPY

Heidi Mahay, PharmD

GENERAL PRINCIPLES

1. What are biologic response modifiers?

A biologic response modifier is defined as any substance capable of altering (modifying) the immune system with either a stimulatory or a suppressive effect. This definition includes agents that restore, augment, or modulate the host's immunologic mechanisms. Biologic agents produce direct antitumor activities as well as other effects; they may interfere with the ability of tumor cells to survive, metastasize, or differentiate. Biologic therapy involves the use of the following agents: interferons, interleukins, hematopoietic growth factors, monoclonal antibodies, and tumor necrosis factor.

2. What are monoclonal antibodies?

Monoclonal antibodies are antibodies generated against a specific antigen. Hybridoma technology, developed in the mid 1970s, fuses an antibody-secreting cell with a malignant cell resulting in a single antibody that can recognize a single antigen. This technology allows the production of unlimited amounts of pure monoclonal antibody (MAB) that are highly specific for a single antigen. The use of antibodies as carriers to deliver drugs and toxins to tumor cells was proposed in the early 1900s and was given the name "magic bullets." Today, monoclonal antibodies tailored to recognize specific antigenic determinants on tumor cells can be used diagnostically to detect cancer cells or therapeutically to enhance or cause the destruction of cancer cells.

COLONY-STIMULATING FACTORS

3. What are colony-stimulating factors?

Colony-stimulating factors (CSFs) or hematopoietic growth factors (HGFs) are hormone-like proteins present endogenously in the human body. They are essential to the hematopoietic system for proliferation, differentiation, and maturation of blood cells. CSFs bind to receptors on the hematopoietic cell membrane and regulate the growth and maturation of the specific stem and precursor cells. Several growth factors have been identified; however, only granulocyte colony-stimulating factor (G-CSF), granulocyte-macrophage colony-stimulating factor (GM-CSF), and erythropoietin-alpha (EPO) are commercially available for clinical use.

Pharmaceutical Characteristics of Colony-Stimulating Factors

CYTOKINE	GENERIC NAMES	COMMERCIAL SOURCE	BRAND NAMES	NORMAL ENDOGENOUS SOURCES
G-CSF	Filgrastim Lenograstim	*E. coli*	Neupogen Neutrogin	Monocytes, macrophages, fibroblasts, endothelial cells, keratinocytes
GM-CSF	Sargramostim Molgramostim Regramostim	*E. coli* Yeast	Leukine Leucomax Prokine	T-lymphocytes, monocytes, macrophages, fibroblasts, endothelial cells, osteoblasts, epithelial cells
EPO	Epoetin-α		Epogen Procrit	Renal cells, hepatocytes

4. What is the difference between G-CSF and GM-CSF?

G-CSF: Commercially available G-CSF is derived from *Escherichia coli*. The main biologic and pharmacologic effect of G-CSF is to increase proliferation and differentiation (maturation) of neutrophils from their precursors, the committed progenitor cells. G-CSF enhances both function and endurance of neutrophils.

GM-CSF: Unlike G-CSF, GM-CSF affects multiple hematopoietic stem cells, including the precursors for granulocytes, macrophages, eosinophils, and megakaryocytes. The major effect of GM-CSF is to stimulate production of mature neutrophils and macrophages. GM-CSF potentiates the survival and function of mature neutrophils and also may increase microbial killing by enhanced phagocytosis and superoxide production.

5. What uses of G-CSF and GM-CSF are approved by the Food and Drug Administration (FDA)?

The FDA has approved the use of G-CSF and GM-CSF to decrease the incidence of infection in patients undergoing myelosuppressive chemotherapy and bone marrow transplant. Both agents are also approved for use in patients with HIV infection, myelodysplastic syndromes, aplastic anemia, and congenital, cyclic, and acquired neutropenia. However, only G-CSF is approved to treat neutropenia in selected adults with acute myelogenous leukemia, but this use is controversial because studies indicate that certain cell lines with receptors for G-CSFs may be stimulated by G-CSF.

6. Is timing crucial in drawing blood levels after G-CSF and GM-CSF are given?

An initial transient leukopenia occurs about 1 hour after injection of G-CSF because of the transient decrease in circulating neutrophils and monocytes. This effect occurs with every dose and is followed by an increase in neutrophils. Blood samples for monitoring the hematologic effects of G-CSF, therefore, should be drawn before rather than after the daily dose.

Transient leukopenia resulting in disappearance of circulating neutrophils, eosinophils, and monocytes also occurs with each dose of GM-CSF. The leukopenia may be accompanied by pulmonary sequestration of neutrophils. GM-CSF prolongs the half-life of circulating neutrophils from 8 to 48 hours. The proliferation of eosinophils is enhanced, and neutrophilia is seen in the blood.

7. What are the side effects of G-CSF or GM-CSF?

The most frequent adverse effect of G-CSF is bone pain characterized by a transient mild, dull ache; this effect occurs in approximately 20% of patients. Bone pain is usually managed with mild analgesics such as actaminophen or other nonsteroidal antiinflammatory drugs (NSAIDs). Other infrequent adverse effects include vasculitis after administration. Patients receiving G-CSF for longer than 1 year may experience hair thinning, splenomegaly, persistent bone pain, and, in rare cases, thrombocytopenia. Minor elevations of lactate dehydrogenase (LDH) and alkaline phosphatase have also been reported.

GM-CSF has been reported to cause a first-dose effect in certain patients within 3 hours of administration. This effect is characterized by flushing with hypotension, tachycardia, arterial oxygen desaturation, musculoskeletal pain, shortness of breath, and nausea; it is more common after intravenous than subcutaneous administration. Fortunately, intravenous administration of GM-CSF is relatively uncommon. GM-CSF can also induce fever and chills at doses ≥ 3 µg/kg. Doses ≥ 20 µg/kg/day are not well tolerated. The major dose-limiting side effects are weight gain with fluid retention, pleural and pericardial inflammation and effusions, and venous thrombosis.

8. What are the general guidelines for using CSFs in oncology practice?

CSFs are used primarily to decrease anticipated morbidity (infections) and possibly mortality from the severe neutropenia that accompanies myelosuppressive chemotherapy. CSFs are generally administered after subsequent cycles of chemotherapy to patients with documented occurrence of febrile neutropenia in an earlier cycle. This practice is termed secondary administration or prophylaxis. Other circumstances for secondary administration of CSFs include prolonged neutropenia that may delay chemotherapy or cause inappropriate dose reductions. CSFs are also recommended to stimulate hematopoietic progenitor cells and reconstitute bone marrow elements after high-dose chemotherapy.

9. Are there circumstances in which CSFs should not be used?

Since CSF therapy can be costly, about $100 to $200/day, guidelines have been suggested by expert panels. According to the guidelines by the American Society of Clinical Oncology for the use of CSFs, primary prophylaxis with CSFs is cost-saving only if the rate of hospitalization for febrile neutropenia is 40% or more; current standard regimens are not close to that figure. Further data are necessary for expanding the use of CSFs based on benefits of improved survival, decreased hospitalizations, and reduced supportive care.

10. Describe the dose and route of administration of CSFs.

The recommended dose is 5 µg/kg/day of G-CSF or 250 µg/m^2/day of GM-CSF. The effect of G-CSF is dose-related; doses of 5–10 µg/kg/day have little effect on cell lines other than neutrophils. However, higher doses of G-CSF are associated with a 25% decrease in platelets.

CSFs can be administered subcutaneously or intravenously. Subcutaneous self-administration is convenient and can be taught to most patients. If intravenous administration is preferred, infusions of approximately 15–20 minutes are suggested. Side effects are sometimes increased with intravenous administration. Neupogen is contraindicated in patients with hypersensitivity to *E. coli*–derived proteins. Dosage escalation of the CSFs is not recommended. Currently available data suggest that rounding the dose to the nearest vial size may improve patient convenience and decrease costs without affecting clinical efficacy.

11. When should the CSFs be initiated? For how long should they be continued?

CSFs should not be given within 24 hours prior to and no earlier than 24 hours after cytotoxic therapy, because they may enhance the myelotoxicity of chemotherapeutic agents by increasing cell turnover rate. Clinical data have shown that beginning G-CSF or GM-CSF 24–72 hours after the completion of chemotherapy provides optimal neutrophil recovery. The manufacturer recommends the continuation of G-CSF administration until the absolute neutrophil count (ANC) has reached 10,000/ml; however, a shorter duration can be recommended if patients achieve clinically adequate neutrophil counts (ANC = 5000). The appropriate ANC is still debated among physicians. CSF therapy should be monitored by obtaining blood counts at least once weekly.

ERYTHROPOIETIN

12. What is erythropoietin?

Erythropoietin (EPO) was the first hematopoietic growth factor approved for clinical use. EPO, a glycoprotein hormone produced by the kidney, stimulates the production of red blood cells. EPO primarily regulates the production of the red blood cell line with little effect on other cells. It is currently approved for the treatment of anemia associated with chronic renal failure, chemotherapy, and use of zidovudine. Recent studies have also shown that EPO may also be of benefit for other chronic anemias, including anemia associated with neoplastic infiltration of the bone marrow, and in the treatment of myelodysplastic syndromes. Side effects of EPO include flulike symptoms (Epogen), occasional headache, and bloodshot eyes (Procrit).

13. What is the role of erythropoietin in patients with cancer?

Many factors cause anemia in patients with cancer; however, the predominant causes are thought to be related to the cancer itself or to cytotoxic chemotherapy. The anemia results from both increased destruction and decreased production of red blood cells. Studies evaluating the effects of EPO levels in patients with cancer have shown substantial rises in hemoglobin, subjective improvement in anemia-related symptoms, improvement in performance status, and decreased transfusion requirements.

14. What is the dose of EPO? How is it given?

The dose for renal failure is 50–100 U/kg administered subcutaneously 3 times/week. The dose for the treatment of anemia due to cancer chemotherapy is 150 U/kg subcutaneously 3 times/week.

The dose can subsequently be titrated based on the rate of hematocrit rise and should be decreased when the hematocrit reaches the target range of 30–36% or increases by more than 4 points during 2 weeks.

Doses should be increased if the hematocrit does not increase by 5–6 points after 8 weeks of therapy and is still below the target range. The dose of EPO varies with individual patients. Maintenance doses of EPO range from 12.5–525 U/kg/dose 3 times/week.

INTERLEUKIN-2

15. What is interleukin-2?

Interleukin-2 (IL-2) is a glycoprotein produced by helper T-cells after stimulation by antigens and IL-1. The primary function of interleukins (between leukocytes) is immunomodulation and immunoregulation of leukocytes. IL-2 promotes proliferation and differentiation of B- and T-cells as well as monocytes and also has many immunologic effects. The IL-2 receptor is present mainly on activated T-cells. The effects of IL-2 include proliferation of various cytotoxic cells, including natural killer (NK) cells, lymphokine-activated killer (LAK) cells, and tumor-infiltrating lympho-cytes (TIL), which aid in the destruction of tumor cells without damaging normal cells. FDA-approved aldesleukin (Proleukin) or IL-2 is produced by recombinant DNA technology (placement of human genes inside bacteria or yeast cells to produce large quantities of highly purified protein).

16. What are the uses of IL-2?

IL-2 is used to cause tumor regression in metastatic renal cell cancer, malignant melanoma, and colorectal cancer resistant to conventional chemotherapy agents. Responses in patients with renal cell cancer have been ~ 20%. When used as a single agent in patients with malignant melanoma, IL-2 has shown response rates of ~ 15%. The overall response rate for colorectal cancer is 10%. Regimens using IL-2 in combination with other agents are currently under investigation.

17. How should IL-2 be administered?

IL-2 is administered most commonly by intravenous infusion; it also has been administered subcutaneously. The dosage of IL-2 should be adjusted carefully according to patient tolerance, response, and route of administration. The potency of aldesleukin usually is expressed in international units (IU). Other units have also been reported, including Cetus units (CU) and Roche units (RU), but they are not equivalent (1 RU = 3 IU; 1 CU = 6 IU).

18. Discuss the toxicities associated with IL-2.

Most IL-2–induced toxicities appear to be dose-related and are reversible or manageable with appropriate supportive care. IL-2 can potentially cause side effects in nearly every organ system. The most common dose-limiting toxicities of IL-2 are hypotension, fluid retention, and renal dysfunction. IL-2 causes a decrease in peripheral vascular resistance with peripheral va-sodilatation and tachycardia, thus producing hypotension. Most patients receiving intense ther-apy with IL-2 require blood pressure support with pressors such as dopamine.

A problematic side effect of therapy with IL-2 has been **vascular leak syndrome** (VLS), which presents as peripheral edema and weight gain (often > 10% of body weight). Ascites with or without pleural effusions and pulmonary edema may accompany VLS. Patients with underly-ing cardiovascular or renal abnormalities may be more susceptible to these side effects. VLS is managed with vasopressors (e.g., dopamine), fluid support, diuretics, and oxygen.

A major side effect is a flulike syndrome 4–6 hours after initiation of therapy. Another sig-nificant side effect is fatigue, which may be due to cytokine release. Other adverse effects associ-ated with IL-2 include nausea, vomiting, and diarrhea, which can be managed with adequate antiemetic therapy and antidiarrheals. Patients receiving IL-2 may also experience thrombocy-topenia, anemia, eosinophilia, and a skin erythema with burning and pruritus. Skin erythema can be managed with a moisturizing cream such as Eucerin. Neurologic changes, hypothyroidism, and bacterial infections are also common.

INTERFERONS

19. What are the interferons? How do they act as chemotherapeutic agents?

The interferons (IFNs) are proteins belonging to the cytokine family. Three types have been described in humans: alpha (IFN-α); beta (IFN-β); and gamma (IFN-γ). Each type originates from a distinct cell and has different biologic and chemical properties. The cellular activities of the IFNs consist of three types: antiviral, immunomodulatory, and antiproliferative.

The antiviral effects of the IFNs include inhibition of intracellular replication of viral DNA as well as protection of cells from viral attack. The immunomodulatory effects include stimulating T-lymphocytes and increasing the killing potential of natural killer (NK) cells. IFNs directly inhibit DNA and protein synthesis in tumor cells and increase tumor cell recognition by stimulating expression of human lymphocyte antigens (HLAs) and tumor-associated antigens on tumor cell surfaces. In addition, IFNs increase all cell phases, prolonging the overall generation time and thus inhibiting the rate of cell growth.

20. What are the therapeutic uses of the interferons?

Most of the trials to date have used recombinant IFN-α. Labeled indications in cancer include hairy cell leukemia and acquired immunodeficiency disease (AIDS)-associated Kaposi's sarcoma. Response rates in patients with hairy cell leukemia have been ~ 70%; however, most patients relapse after discontinuation of therapy. Patients with Kaposi's sarcoma have shown response rates of 30–40%. Other uses of IFN-α include some non-Hodgkin's lymphoma, multiple myeloma, and chronic myelogenous leukemia, all of which have shown response with IFN-α therapy. Solid tumors in which good responses have been seen include renal cell carcinoma and malignant melanoma. Nononcologic indications include the use of IFN-β for multiple sclerosis and IFN-γ for chronic granulomatous disease.

21. How are the interferons administered?

Recombinant IFN-α-2a and IFN-α-2b are administered by intramuscular or subcutaneous injection.

22. Discuss the adverse effects associated with interferon use. How can they be managed?

Pharmacologic doses of IFNs have been associated with various toxicities, including an acute flulike syndrome with fever, chills, malaise, myalgias, and headache that begins 2–8 hours after the first subcutaneous injection. Flulike symptoms may be prevented or at least alleviated with administration of acetaminophen before the IFN injection and every 4 hours thereafter for a total of 24 hours. Administration of IFN at bedtime enables the patient to sleep through the flulike symptoms of initial therapy. Tolerance to the flulike effects develops over several days to weeks.

Other side effects include fatigue, which is the most common dose-limiting and dose-related side effect of IFN-α. Bedtime administration may help to minimize the fatigue, along with strategies to reduce activities and conserve energy. Severe fatigue, however, may require dosage decreases or discontinuation of therapy. Gastrointestinal symptoms such as anorexia, nausea, vomiting, and diarrhea are rare at low doses but increase in frequency and severity as the dose increases. Antiemetics and antidiarrheals may help to control some of these symptoms. Patients should be encouraged to maintain adequate nutritional intake. Neurologic effects such as vertigo, decreased mental status, confusion, depression, and paresthesias are rare at low doses but may increase in severity and incidence at increased doses. Hematologic effects include mild leukopenia with a reduction in counts of 40–60%. This is followed by a rapid increase to normal 3–10 days after discontinuation of therapy.

INVESTIGATIONAL AGENTS

23. What is tumor necrosis factor?

Tumor necrosis factor (TNF) is a natural substance produced by activated macrophages, monocytes, and lymphocytes after exposure to endotoxin. It causes tumor and healthy tissue necrosis by decreasing or stopping blood flow. In vitro studies in mice and other animal models have shown that TNF has cytotoxic or cytostatic effects on tumor cells with virtually no effect on normal cells. TNF is released in the bloodstream and binds to receptors on tumor cell membranes where it produces cell arrest and cell lysis. TNF has been used for the treatment of melanoma, colorectal carcinoma, AIDS-related Kaposi's sarcoma, B-cell lymphoma, non-small-cell lung cancer, ovarian cancer, and glioma. To date, however, TNF has not shown significant palliative or curative therapy for any type of cancer. Phase II clinical trials are underway to investigate tumor response, immune system modulation, dose, route of administration, and toxicities.

24. What is PIXY321?

PIXY321 is an example of a fusion molecule made by combining interleukin-3 (IL-3) and GM-CSF. Fusion molecules should have greater bioactivity than either of the single agents used alone. Although current studies with PIXY321 have been disappointing, there is potential for future development of better fusion products.

25. Is there any biologic agent available to stimulate platelets?

Clinical trials in humans are under way for the use of c-mpl ligand for treatment of thrombocytopenia. Interleukin-11 is further along in trials and has shown a potent effect to elevate platelet counts after chemotherapy. Its clinical applicability may be limited by patient complaints of fatigue, arthralgias, and myalgias. The clinical benefit of these agents will be based on their efficacy in reducing the duration of severe thrombocytopenia and the need for platelet transfusions.

26. What are some resources for using biologic therapy?

The following pharmaceutical companies offer excellent instruction books, monographs, and videotapes for staff and patient education, as well as professional advice from Clinical Support Specialists:

Amgen, Inc.	800-77-AMGEN (Neupogen)
Chiron Therapeutics	800-244-7668 (IL-2)
Immunex Corporation	800-IMMUNEX (Leukine)
Ortho Biotech	800-2BIOTECH (Procrit)
Roche Laboratories	800-7ROFERON (Interferon)
Schering Corporation	800-526-4099 (Interferon)

BIBLIOGRAPHY

1. American Society of Clinical Oncology: Recommendations for the use of hematopoietic colony-stimulating factors: Evidence based, clinical practice guidelines. J Clin Oncol 12:2471–2508, 1994.
2. Bociek RG, Armitage JO: Hematopoietic growth factors. Cancer 46:165–187, 1996.
3. Chabner BA, Longo DL (eds): Cancer Chemotherapy and Biotherapy. Philadelphia, J.B. Lippincott, 1996.
4. Kaye JA: Clinical development of recombinant human interleukin-11 to treat chemotherapy-induced thrombocytopenia. Curr Opin Hematol 3:209–215, 1996.
5. Lieschke FJ, Bergess AW: Granulocyte colony-stimulating factor and granulocyte macrophage colony-stimulating factor. N Engl J Med 327:28–35, 1992.
6. Rieger PT (ed): Biotherapy: A Comprehensive Overview. Boston, Jones & Bartlett, 1995.
7. Rubin JT: Interleukin-2: Its biology and clinical application in patients with cancer. Cancer Invest 11:460–472, 1993.
8. Siegel JP, Puri RK: Interleukin—toxicity. J Clin Oncol 9:694–704, 1991.
9. Smith TJ: Economic analysis of the clinical uses of the colony-stimulating factors. Curr Opin Hematol 3:175–179, 1996.
10. Snead RB, Harker LA: Preclinical studies and potential clinical applications of c-mpl ligand. Curr Opin Hematol 3:197–202, 1996.
11. Vose JM, Armitage JO: Clinical applications of hematopoietic growth factors. J Clin Oncol 13:1023–1035, 1995.

10. BONE MARROW TRANSPLANTATION

Mary Roach, MS, RN, OCN, *and*
Marie B. Whedon, MS, RN, AOCN, FAAN

1. What is a bone marrow transplant?

A bone marrow transplant (BMT) is the intravenous administration of bone marrow–containing stem cells capable of reproducing and differentiating into mature red and white blood cells and platelets. The different types of transplants reflect the possible sources of stem cells. **Autologous** transplants use the patient's own bone marrow, which is harvested, processed, frozen, and then returned after the patient receives chemotherapy and/or radiotherapy. **Allogeneic** transplants use bone marrow from a donor who may be unrelated or related to the patient (sibling or other close relative). If the bone marrow donor is the patient's identical twin, the transplant is termed **syngeneic**.

2. What is a blood cell transplant?

Stem cells circulate in the peripheral bloodstream as well as the bone marrow. It is possible to collect peripheral blood stem cells (PBSCs) by circulating the patient's blood through a cell-separating machine. Transplants, mostly autologous, have been performed using PBSCs. Clinical experience over the past 10 years has shown that blood cell recovery can be reliably achieved with the use of PBSCs. The term **blood cell transplant** (BCT) refers to transplants using stem cells and other blood cells in different stages of differentiation and maturation collected from the peripheral blood.

3. How common are bone marrow and blood cell transplants?

Statistics from the International Bone Marrow Transplant Registry indicate continued annual growth in the numbers of autologous transplants at a rate of 20% per year. It is estimated that more than 8,000 allogeneic BMTs and 12,000 autologous (including blood cell and bone marrow) transplants are performed annually.

4. How is a bone marrow donor selected?

The immune system is designed to reject tissue seen as "foreign." When donor marrow is used, it is generally from a family member, preferably one with an identical tissue match to the patient. The match is determined by testing for the genes located within the major histocompatibility complex located on chromosome 6. These genes encode the human leukocyte antigens (HLA), which are proteins located on cell surfaces and involved in cell self-recognition. Three separate gene sites have been identified as important for transplantation: A, B, and D/DR. HLA typing is done by a simple blood test to determine how closely a potential donor matches the patient at these sites. An HLA-identical sibling is the ideal donor, but the donor also may be an HLA-nonidentical family member. The greater the mismatch between patient and donor, the greater the risk of complications. There is approximately a 30–35% chance that a suitable family donor can be found. In the late 1970s, transplants began to be performed using HLA-matched unrelated donors.

5. How does a patient find a compatible unrelated donor?

The National Marrow Donor Program (NMDP), established in 1986, maintains a registry of thousands of volunteer marrow donors. The NMDP also administers the various collection, transplant, and donor centers around the country and maintains stringent standards for these institutions. The potential unrelated marrow donor must be in good health and between 18 and 55 years old. The American Red Cross and National Marrow Donor Program occasionally conduct donor drives, similar to blood drives, to attract more potential donors into the pool. Special efforts are ongoing to recruit minority donors, particularly African Americans, Hispanics, and Asians, who are currently underrepresented in the registry. Interested donors should be instructed to contact the National Marrow Donor Program at 800-MARROW-2.

If a patient requires a transplant but has no family match, a computer search is initiated among volunteer donors on the NMDP registry. It takes weeks to months from the first request to locate an unrelated donor. If a matched donor is located, he or she is requested to undergo an information session and informed consent procedure. Additional blood testing may be done at that time to ensure a good match between donor and recipient. The marrow is harvested from the donor at an approved collection center. All expenses are paid by the NMDP and then billed to the patient and transplant center. The harvested marrow is transported by trained personnel (by ground or air) under strict conditions directly to the recipient and immediately infused. The donor harvest must be carefully timed with the recipient's treatment schedule.

6. When are BMTs indicated?

Hematologic disorders and malignancies in children and adults were the first diseases to be treated with BMT and remain the most common indication for allogeneic transplant. Certain rare genetic and immunologic disorders are also treated with BMT. The cancer most frequently treated with autologous BMT is breast cancer. Evidence is evolving that high-dose therapy can extend disease-free survival in some patients with metastatic disease and may reduce the risk of recurrence in women with high-risk primary breast cancer. BMTs are increasingly used to treat solid tumors that require high-dose chemotherapy as well as many malignant and nonmalignant diseases.

Diseases Treated with Bone Marrow Transplant

DISEASES	REASONS FOR BONE MARROW TRANSPLANT
Leukemias	
Chronic myelocytic leukemia	High-dose chemotherapy and/or radiation is needed to eradicate
Chronic lymphocytic leukemia	disease; disease does not respond to conventional treatment; or
Myelodysplastic syndrome	no conventional treatment is available. Diseased marrow is
Acute myelocytic leukemia	removed by preparative regimen (chemotherapy, radiation) and
Acute lymphocytic leukemia	replaced by disease-free marrow.
Anemias	
Thalassemia	Nonfunctioning bone marrow is replaced by functioning marrow.
Severe aplastic anemia	
Fanconi's anemia	
Sickle cell anemia	
Solid tumor cancers	
Neuroblastoma	High-dose chemotherapy and/or radiation is needed to eradicate
Ewing's sarcoma	tumor, but the therapy also eradicates bone marrow. Marrow
Brain cancer	transplant is needed as a rescue.
Testicular cancer	
Ovarian cancer	
Lung cancer	
Lymphomas	
Non-Hodgkin's lymphoma	Chemotherapy and radiation are needed to kill tumor but also kill
Hodgkin's disease	bone marrow. Marrow transplant is needed as a rescue.
Multiple myeloma	
Immune deficiencies	Deficient marrow and immune system are replaced by normally
Severe combined immune	functioning marrow.
deficiency syndrome	
Combined variable immune	
deficiency	
Wiskott-Aldrich syndrome	

Table continued on following page.

Diseases Treated with Bone Marrow Transplant (Continued)

DISEASES	REASONS FOR BONE MARROW TRANSPLANT
Inborn metabolic disorders	
Hurler's syndrome	Enzyme deficiency causes alterations in growth and development,
Hunter's syndrome	ultimately resulting in death. Transplanted marrow contains
Gaucher's disease	components to produce the missing enzymes.
Sanfilippo's disease	
Krabbe's disease	
Leukodystrophy	

From Oncology Nursing Society: Manual for Bone Marrow Transplant Nursing: Recommendations for Practice and Education. Oncology Nursing Press, 1994, with permission.

7. What criteria must be met for a disease to be treated by autologous BMT?

In addition to consideration of the patient's age and general physical condition, the disease being treated must meet four criteria for an effective transplant:

- Tumor is responsive to chemotherapy.
- The dose-limiting toxicity of chemotherapy is myelosuppression.
- BMT can be done early in the disease when tumor burden is low and drug resistance is minimal
- Source of stem cells is free of tumor cells.

8. Why are blood and bone marrow transplants performed for breast cancer and other solid tumors?

Research has shown that certain solid tumors cannot be cured by standard-dose chemotherapy and that high-dose chemotherapy is needed for potential cures. Blood and bone marrow transplants provide stem cell rescue to reconstitute the hematopoietic and immunologic systems, thereby permitting the administration of potentially curative high-dose chemotherapy that otherwise would be limited by myelosuppression. The stem cells are collected and stored before chemotherapy is administered and then returned to the patient after high-dose chemotherapy.

9. What is meant by harvesting bone marrow? How are bone marrow and peripherally derived stem cells obtained?

Stem cells, which have the ability to differentiate into all of the blood cells, are most numerous in the bone marrow, although some circulate in the peripheral blood. Stem cells are obtained in two ways. Traditionally, bone marrow has been harvested or collected in the operating room under general anesthesia. Marrow stem cells are collected by repeated bone marrow aspirations (1–2 L of marrow) from the posterior and/or anterior iliac crests and occasionally the sternum. The procedure takes an average of 1–3 hours. In the operating room, the marrow is filtered to remove bone particles and large fat globules and then poured into transfusion bags for further processing and freezing (autologous marrow) or immediate infusion into the recipient (allogeneic marrow).

A small percentage of stem cells also circulate in the peripheral blood. The number of these cells can be increased by administering chemotherapy and/or colony-stimulating factors (CSFs) before collection. Timing the collection of stem cells to coincide with blood cell recovery after chemotherapy decreases the number of hemaphereses required to collect adequate numbers of stem cells. Granulocyte CSF (G-CSF) or granulocyte-macrophage CSF (GM-CSF) is also used prior to hemapheresis to increase stem cell numbers in the peripheral blood. Protocols vary, but commonly G-CSF or GM-CSF is given by subcutaneous injection daily, with stem cell collections beginning on day 4 or 5 of injections. This procedure is termed **priming** or **mobilization**. Some institutions also prime bone marrow-derived stem cells. The cells can then be collected by a process of apheresis, in which a machine separates and collects the desired blood stem cells and returns the unneeded blood elements to the patient. Three to four collections, each lasting 2–4 hours, are usually required to collect adequate numbers of stem cells. The stem cells are then processed and frozen.

Various advantages have been identified with the use of peripheral stem cells. Most obviously, peripheral stem cell collection obviates the need for a bone marrow harvest with the attendant risks of anesthesia. A theoretical benefit is less tumor contamination of peripherally derived stem cells. In addition, marrow recovery is more rapid with the use of primed peripheral stem cells, probably because mobilization stimulates progenitor cells to maturity.

10. What does "purging" mean? How is it done?

The aim of "purging" bone marrow or stem cells used in autologous transplants is to remove any contaminating malignant cells while leaving the stem cells intact to reconstitute the hematopoietic system. In hematologic malignancies, bone marrow harvests and stem cell collections are usually done while the patient is in complete remission. In addition, methods of eliminating malignant cells include the use of chemical agents (cyclophosphamide, mafosfamide, etoposide, cisplatin), and antibody purging (monoclonal antibodies combined with complement, cytocidal agents, or magnetic microspheres). Positive selection also has been explored as a means of eliminating the potential of returning malignant cells in the stem cell product. Crude selection can be done on the basis of the physical characteristics of stem cells, but current efforts focus on selection using stem cell surface antigens such as CD34.

The contribution of contaminating tumor cells in stem cell products to relapse is not firmly established. No randomized studies and only a few controlled studies assessing the efficacy of purging have been done. Purging with antibodies and chemicals has the potential to damage stem cells and to delay engraftment and return of normal blood counts. Research continues to clarify the role of purging in transplantation.

11. What is the role of colony-stimulating factors in transplant?

CSFs, also known as hematopoietic growth factors, are cellular proteins (cytokines) that occur naturally in the body and are responsible for the proliferation, differentiation, and maturation of all hematopoietic cells. The discovery of CSFs and their availability clinically through recombinant DNA techniques have changed the transplant process by significantly decreasing neutropenia and its sequelae. Prior to growth factors, neutropenia-related fatal infections had thwarted attempts to improve survival and reduce toxicity of this potentially curative therapy.

Growth factor has been used before transplant to increase the number of stem cells harvested from the periphery and to stimulate posttransplant neutrophil recovery. Some concern existed about the use of growth factor in transplant for leukemia. The same receptors to growth factor that exist on normal white blood cells are also found on leukemic blast cells. The initial concern was that administration of growth factor might increase leukemia relapse rates by causing undesired stimulation or proliferation of residual leukemia cells. Therefore, growth factor was initially used only after transplantion for solid tumors. Studies using growth factor in patients with leukemia, however, showed no increase in relapse. Growth factor is now used for priming before harvest of stem cells from leukemia patients in remission as well as after induction therapy for selected elderly patients with leukemia. Growth factor is also used in an attempt to stimulate functional cells to repopulate the marrow in patients experiencing delayed engraftment or graft failure.

12. How are blood or marrow stem cells returned to the patient?

In allogeneic BMT the donor's marrow is harvested, filtered, and infused through a central line immediately into the recipient, much like a blood transfusion. If the recipient is not at the same center as the donor, the donor's marrow is transported immediately after collection to the transplant center by courier.

In autologous transplants, previously harvested marrow and/or blood stem cells are preserved with dimethyl sulfoxide (DMSO) and frozen in liquid nitrogen. At transplant, the frozen bags of blood and marrow stem cells are rapidly thawed in a water bath and infused directly by bag or syringe into a central venous catheter. This procedure is usually well tolerated by the patient. The DMSO preservative used in freezing the cells may cause nausea, vomiting, flushing, chest discomfort, and occasional hypotension. DMSO also has an unpleasant odor that can persist for up to 24 hours, and patients report an unpleasant taste as the cells are infused. Premedication with an antiemetic and an antihistamine helps to alleviate these side effects. Storage of the stem cell product may cause some red cell lysis, and patients may note hematuria for 24 hours after the infusion.

13. What is a conditioning regimen?

In allogeneic BMT for hematologic disorders, the transplant is preceded by a conditioning regimen of chemotherapy with or without total body irradiation (TBI). Conditioning regimens have three functions: (1) to create space in the marrow for the stem cell graft, (2) to immunosuppress the host to prevent graft rejection, and (3) to ablate residual malignant cells and thus prevent relapse. Furthermore, the conditioning regimen needs to accomplish these goals with tolerable morbidity and no mortality. The conditioning regimen results in a dangerous period of 1–3 weeks of marrow aplasia; morbidity from complications ranges between 5–25%.

Dose-intensive chemotherapy required for treatment of solid tumors is used in autologous BMT conditioning regimens primarily to kill residual malignant cells. Doses range from 4–10 times the standard-dose chemotherapy. Even with infusions of stem cells to protect against the myelosuppressive effects of chemotherapy, doses are still limited by other major organ toxicities caused by drugs such as cytosine arabinoside and cyclophosphamide. Multiple agents are often combined to achieve the dual goals of immunosuppression and adequate antineoplastic effect. However, the narrow therapeutic index of these drugs at high doses makes it difficult to deliver all drugs at maximum tolerated doses (MTDs).

Future developments are likely to target cytotoxic therapy more specifically to tumor cells. Such targeting may involve sensitizing tumor cells to the cytotoxic effects while simultaneously protecting normal tissue. Another approach may be to accept the limits of chemotherapy to eradicate all malignant disease and to combine transplantation with monoclonal antibodies or post-transplant immunotherapy to eradicate residual microscopic disease.

Chemotherapeutic Agents Used in Autologous Bone Marrow Transplants

AGENT	MTD	LIMITING TOXICITY
Thiotepa	1200 mg/m^2	Central nervous system, gastrointestinal
Etoposide	3600 mg/m^2	Stomatitis
Busulfan	15 mg/kg	Stomatitis
Total body irradiation	1500 cGy	Pulmonary
Amsacrine	960 mg/m^2	Gastrointestinal
Melphalan	240 mg/m^2	Gastrointestinal
Carmustine	1200 mg/m^2	Pulmonary, hepatic
Nitrogen mustard	2.4 mg/kg	Central nervous system
Carboplatin	2.0 gm/m^2	Hepatic, renal, central nervous system
Cyclophosphamide	200 mg/kg	Cardiac
Dacarbazine	3750 mg/m^2	Not reached
Mitomycin-C	40 mg/m^2	Hepatic, gastrointestinal
Ifosfamide	1.5 gm/m^2	Renal, central nervous system

From Crouch MA, Ross JA: Current concepts in autologous bone marrow transplantation. Semin Oncol Nurs 10:12–19, 1994, with permission.

14. What is the role of total body irradiation in transplantation?

TBI is the exposure of the entire body to gamma radiation and is an important component of many BMT conditioning regimens for leukemia. Radiation doses ranging from 1200–1575 cGy are usually used in combination with cyclophosphamide. One TBI regimen for allogeneic BMT in patients with acute myelogenous leukemia uses a total dose of 1200 cGy delivered in twice daily fractions of 100 cGy for 6 days. Experience has shown that patients treated with divided doses of

radiation (fractionated radiation) experience fewer acute and chronic side effects than patients treated with single doses of radiation. Radiation has a number of unique benefits, including:
- Lack of cross-resistance to chemotherapeutic drugs
- Ability to treat sanctuary sites (testes, central nervous system)
- Potent immunosuppression required for allogeneic BMT
- No detoxification or excretion required after radiation
- Dose distribution may be tailored by shielding (e.g., lungs) or "boosting" to areas of bulk disease

15. What are the side effects and complications of TBI?

Many normal tissues are affected by TBI. Potential acute side effects include nausea and vomiting, diarrhea, enlarged salivary glands, and dry mouth. The most critical areas affected are the lung (idiopathic interstitial pneumonia), gastrointestinal tract, reproductive system, central nervous system, and lens of the eye. As a result, some long-term side effects of TBI may include sterility, cataracts, chronic pulmonary disease, leukoencephalopathy, hormonal impairments, and secondary malignancy.

16. What are the major problems in the early posttransplant period?

The major effects of conditioning and marrow infusion for both autologous (marrow and blood cell) and allogeneic transplant are similar despite differences in preparative treatment and disease. Graft-vs.-host disease (GVHD) and interstitial pneumonia are the major causes of death after allogeneic BMTs. The chemotherapy and/or radiation conditioning regimen causes the following major side effects and complications in the immediate posttransplant period:
- Hematologic effects: neutropenia, thrombocytopenia, hemolytic uremic syndrome
- Infection due to neutropenia (major cause of death during the intensive chemotherapy phase). Bacterial and fungal infections and herpes virus reactivation are the most common examples immediately after BMT. Ninety percent of first fevers are caused by bacteria.
- Gastrointestinal effects: nausea, vomiting, oral mucositis, esophagitis, and severe diarrhea. Nausea and vomiting result from the conditioning therapy as well as from prophylactic and therapeutic antibiotics. The combination of mucosal damage and nausea and vomiting can make eating difficult or impossible, necessitating parenteral nutrition.
- Pulmonary effects: pulmonary congestion or infection and diffuse alveolar hemorrhage (generally fatal)
- Cardiac effects (less common): cardiac arrythmias, myocardial edema or fibrosis, and congestive failure
- Hemorrhagic cystitis (cyclophosphamide)
- Nephrotoxicity or renal failure related to radiation nephritis, amphotericin B, or DMSO
- Neurotoxicity (carmustine and busulfan): seizures, dementia, confusion, and diplopia
- Dermatologic toxicity, ranging from mild rashes to severe blisters and bullae (due to multitude of medications)
- Venoocclusive disease of the liver, an obstructive disease of the hepatic venules resulting in portal hypertension and liver failure, occurs in up to 50% of patients, more commonly among patients with preexisting liver abnormalities or previous abdominal radiation therapy.

17. What is graft-versus-host disease?

Acute GVHD, which is unique to allogeneic transplant, results when the infused donor marrow recognizes the recipient as foreign tissue. Symptoms include an immune T-cell mediated reaction in the skin (rash), gastrointestinal tract (enteritis), and liver (elevated liver function tests). The incidence ranges from 40–50%. The greater the degree of immunologic HLA mismatch between the donor and recipient, the more common and more severe the GVHD reaction. The severity of disease is identified by a grading system, as depicted in the table below.

Staging of Acute Graft-Versus-Host Disease

	CLINICAL STAGE			CLINICAL GRADE OF SEVERITY	
STAGE	SKIN	LIVER	GUT	GRADE	DEGREE OF ORGAN INVOLVEMENT
+	Maculopapular rash < 25% body surface	Bilirubin 2–3 mg/dl	Diarrhea 500–1000 ml/day	1	+ to ++ skin rash; no gut involvement; no decrease in clinical performance
++	Maculopapular rash 25–50% body surface	Bilirubin 3–6 mg/dl	Diarrhea 1000–1500 ml/day	2	+ to +++ skin rash; + gut or liver involvement (or both); mild decrease in clinical performance
+++	Generalized erythroderma	Bilirubin 6–15 mg/dl	Diarrhea > 1500 ml/day	3	++ to +++ skin rash; ++ to +++ gut or liver involvement (or both); decrease in clinical performance
++++	Desquamation and bullae	Bilirubin > 15 mg/dl	Pain or ileus	4	Similar to grade 3 but with ++ to ++++ organ involvement and extreme decrease in clinical performance

From Oncology Nursing Society: Manual for Bone Marrow Transplant Nursing: Recommendations for Practice and Education. Oncology Nursing Press, 1994, with permission.

18. What is the graft-versus-leukemia effect?

Graft-versus-leukemia effect refers to the potentially beneficial immunologic effect of mild GVHD in fighting off residual leukemia in the host. The lack of a GVHD reaction in autologous BMT is suspected to play a role in the higher relapse rate in autologous transplants, and some groups are attempting to induce GVHD in autologous marrow recipients.

19. How is GVHD prevented or treated?

The first and most important way to prevent GVHD is by finding an identically matched donor. Even in this case, however, prophylactic immunosuppressive drugs (cyclosporine, methotrexate, and steroids) are used singly or in combination to minimize the recipient's immunologic response to donor marrow. These drugs have their own side effects and toxicities. Another preventive method is called T-cell depletion. Because T cells are believed to be responsible for the recognition and immunologic reaction in GVHD, reducing their numbers in the donor marrow may reduce the incidence and severity of the problem. However, because T cells also seem to play a role in engraftment of the marrow, this procedure has potential risks.

Intensive nursing interventions are needed to manage skin (erythroderma, bullous formation, desquamation) and other organ toxicities (e.g., severe diarrhea, mucositis). In particular, patients are even more susceptible to infections than during the period of neutropenia from the immunosuppressive effects of both GVHD and the drugs used to treat it.

20. Are the infectious problems after BMT different from the infectious problems after standard chemotherapy?

The type of infectious problems after BMT differ from those normally encountered after standard chemotherapy because of the more severe and prolonged immunologic insult caused by the intensive chemotherapy and radiation treatment of transplant. Except for patients receiving growth factors, profound neutropenia (granulocyte counts near 0) may last for approximately 3 weeks. The white blood cell count slowly and gradually increases towards normal if engraftment of the infused marrow occurs on schedule. During the period of profound neutropenia, patients are extremely vulnerable to serious, potentially life-threatening infections and sepsis. This threat is further increased by the disruptions that chemotherapy, radiation therapy, and invasive procedures inflict on the body's first line of defense, the skin and mucous membranes. Immunologic defects are intensified and further prolonged in the allogeneic patient with GVHD.

Protective isolation procedures (private room, visitor restrictions, low microbial diet, and handwashing) are employed to minimize the transmission of microbes from the external environment to the defenseless patient. However, such procedures do not remove the threat from normally present body flora and latent viral invaders. These pathogens are able to reactivate or colonize and invade tissues unimpeded by the normal surveillance system of an intact immune system.

21. What isolation precautions are needed during BMT?

Different degrees of immunosuppression are associated with autologous and allogeneic transplants; suppression is less with autologous BMT. Isolation procedures vary from center to center, but patients who have undergone autologous BMT usually are treated in a private room. Ill visitors are restricted, and all visitors must wash their hands before coming in contact with the patient. Fresh flowers are not allowed in patient rooms, and patients are given a low microbial diet (no fresh fruits or vegetables). Some centers use special air-filtering systems called high-efficiency particulate air filters (HEPA). Because several studies examining the benefits of protective isolation in BMT centers have not supported the use of strict protective isolation, many centers have relaxed their restrictions and allow patients to leave their rooms without masks, relying on handwashing as the main protective technique. The advent of early-discharge and outpatient BMTs has contributed to the reexamination of protective isolation procedures.

For patients with allogeneic transplants, the same general guidelines apply. Laminar air flow isolation is used by some centers with HLA-matched unrelated donor transplants or partially matched transplants because of the greater risk of GVHD and its associated immunosuppression. This level of isolation is difficult for patients to cope with. Contact with caregivers and visitors is limited, and all persons must gown, glove, and mask before entering the patient's room.

22. Do patients need to be hospitalized for BMT?

Traditionally, patients have been hospitalized for both autologous and allogeneic BMT. With the use of peripheral stem cells and CSFs in autologous BMT, the duration of severe neutropenia has been shortened, thereby reducing morbidity and mortality. However, an emphasis on cost containment in health care has influenced a movement to provide more transplant care in outpatient clinics or through home care companies.

Currently there are three patterns of care for patients who have undergone autologous and blood cell transplants. In the traditional approach, the patient is hospitalized for the conditioning regimen and throughout the period of pancytopenia until blood counts have recovered. The early-discharge approach is to hospitalize the patient for the conditioning regimen and then to discharge the patient from the hospital with daily follow-up in the outpatient clinic. Care provided in the outpatient clinic includes physical assessment, bone marrow and progenitor cell infusion, parenteral antibiotics, electrolytes, and blood transfusions. In the outpatient model of BMT, the patient receives both conditioning therapy and post-chemotherapy care in the outpatient setting. In both the early-discharge and outpatient models, a caregiver must be present to care for the patient outside the hospital. Usually patients are housed in a "medical-motel" type of facility. With such changes, transplant centers are challenged to provide complex care in the outpatient setting. Ongoing teaching of the patient and caregiver is crucial.

Current data from the Duke University Transplant Program, which began a pilot program of early discharge after BMT in 1991, indicate that approximately 35% of patients are readmitted to the hospital. Reasons for readmission include new-onset fever, dehydration, or protracted nausea and vomiting. A number of patients receiving BMT in the outpatient setting report acceptance and increased independence.

Most patients with allogeneic BMT remain in the hospital from the initiation of conditioning therapy through recovery of blood counts. However, some centers that formerly required patients to receive care from the transplant center for the first 100 days now allow earlier return to the care of referring physicians.

23. Can BMTs be done at the community level or only at academic centers?

The first investigational procedures were performed only within large academic research centers. By 1996, more than 400 centers were listed worldwide with the International Bone Marrow Transplant Registry (IBMTR). A center must meet certain minimal standards to be listed with the IBMTR. Several professional groups have identified the criteria that are important to perform allogeneic and autologous transplants competently. These criteria require specifically trained personnel, performance of minimal numbers of BMTs to maintain expertise, and environmental specifications.

With the expanded indications for autologous marrow and blood cell transplants, many non-research-based community institutions have organized programs to serve this growing market of patients. Such institutions usually build on the expertise of already existing oncology units and programs and perform a limited type of transplants (usually autologous marrow or blood cell transplants rather than allogeneic transplants). Educated consumers should evaluate such programs carefully to ensure that they meet the minimal requirements of professional organizations.

24. How does a patient choose a transplant center? What questions should the patient ask?

Depending on the type of disease and treatment, nurses can advocate for patients to be knowledgeable consumers regarding the quality of the program in which they seek treatment. Patients should be encouraged to ask some or all of the following questions:

- What types of diseases are treated and what types of transplants are performed?
- Are nurses and doctors specially trained to perform transplants?
- How long has the program been in existence, and how many BMTs have been performed?
- What are the outcomes of other patients treated for the same disease?
- Does the center perform investigational treatments and report results to a national organization?
- Can the patient talk to previous patients at the center?
- What support resources and housing are available for the patient and family?

25. What type of follow-up care do BMT patients require?

Important aspects of follow-up care in the early recovery period are the prevention and management of complications from BMT. Blood counts may not have fully recovered, and patients may experience fatigue, fever, and bleeding. Close assessment and administration of antibiotics, blood products, and GVHD therapy may be required. The gastrointestinal tract may not be fully recovered, necessitating antiemetics, antidiarrheals, fluids, electrolytes, and nutritional support. The intensity of needs depends largely on how early the patient is discharged after the conditioning therapy and bone marrow/stem cell reinfusion. Initially, the patient may be seen in clinic 3–7 days per week for physical and laboratory assessment. An important aspect of BMT follow-up care is emotional support. Many patients experience anxiety along with excitement at hospital discharge. Consistent caregivers, ongoing contact with a social worker, and support groups are helpful. As the acute toxicities of BMT resolve, outpatient follow-up is less frequent.

26. What are the expected long-term effects of BMT?

Long-term effects of BMT are varied and involve the physical, social, psychological, and spiritual domains. Most physical effects occur within the first year and result from the transplant: GVHD, chemotherapy, radiation therapy, immunosuppressive drugs, or the original disease (relapse). Effects from chronic GVHD include skin changes, dry eyes and mouth, diarrhea, weight loss, anorexia, and pulmonary and liver involvement. The skin is involved in 95% of patients who develop chronic GVHD. Symptoms include dryness, itching, and absence of sweating; later, skin tightness and contractures may develop. The mouth and eyes are also frequently affected, with symptoms of dryness and pain. Extensive chronic GVHD can cause disability as a result of contractures, skin disfigurement, weight loss, and malaise. Late infectious complications include encapsulated bacteria, varicella zoster virus, and *Pneumocystis carinii*.

Cataracts, endocrine dysfunction, cognitive dysfunction, and sterility may result from TBI. In addition to sterility, problems with sexuality, both physiologic (vaginal dryness, and ejaculatory problems) and psychologic (related to body image) may occur. Other potential delayed complications after BMT include immunodeficiency, autoimmune disorders, dental problems, and aseptic necrosis. The rate of second malignancies appears to be no higher in BMT patients than in patients undergoing other curative cancer therapy.

27. How long does it take for patients to return to normal after BMT? How does a BMT affect a person's quality of life?

The trauma of undergoing transplant usually affects all aspects of well-being: physical, psychological, social, and spiritual. The first year after transplant often is characterized by great emotional intensity and fear as patients cope with continued treatment of transplant-related complications, including GVHD and infections. Many of the physical effects lessen over time, and most patients can resume a more normal function within 1 year after the procedure. A minority of patients (5–15%) experience lasting physical effects that may not improve and require permanent adaptation or significant rehabilitation. Chronic GVHD, pulmonary problems, reproductive effects, and second malignancies are among the most devastating complications.

Many patients do not experience a linear recovery from the psychological, social, and existential effects of transplant. Most BMT survivors report only mild-to-moderate psychological distress. Survivor guilt, changed relationships with family and friends, and changes in employability and insurability are unpredictable nonphysical effects. Some beneficial effects are also reported by patients, including renewed sense of purpose and meaning in life and reprioritizing what is important. Most report they are "glad to be alive" or to have a "second chance" at life. With regard to social functioning, the ability for patients to resume their pre-BMT role has a positive impact. The influence of these factors on recovery has been studied only recently. Early conclusions suggest that follow-up services and resources that allow patients an outlet to talk about their stories and to share long-term emotional challenges are important aspects of the nurse's tasks. Because some BMT patients encounter difficulties in returning to work, vocational retraining may be an important component to full recovery.

Long-term survivors may be reluctant to share seemingly "minor" issues with their health care providers because they do not want to appear ungrateful for a second chance at life. Informing patients of survivor groups and celebrations, networks, newsletters, and on-line computer resources is a first step to providing good follow-up care to the growing number of long-term survivors. Despite the physical, psychological, and social difficulties that BMT patients may face, the majority indicate that, given the same circumstances, they would still elect to undergo a BMT.

28. Is it difficult to get insurance coverage for BMT?

Obtaining insurance coverage for BMT is a complex and changing issue. The transplant procedure is quite costly (estimated at $50,000–150,000) because of intensive preevaluation testing, high-dose chemotherapy, antibiotics, colony-stimulating factors, blood products, and intensive inpatient, ambulatory and possibly home care needs. Some patients without insurance would not be eligible for the procedure unless they were able to pay out of pocket or raise adequate money to pay for the procedure upfront. Some policies are vague about coverage for transplant, whereas others specifically deny coverage for transplant or "experimental treatments" in general. As the number of patients with diseases eligible for transplant increased, so did the financial burden and risk for private insurance companies—and some declined payment. Patients won many lawsuits forcing insurance companies to pay, prompting insurance companies to look for other solutions to the increasing financial risk. Collaborations between insurance companies and specific institutions or "centers of excellence" have evolved in parallel with other changes in health care economics, such as managed care and capitated payment. In some cases, transplant centers compete with other centers in terms of which can offer an insurance company the lowest capitated fee. If patients' expenses for care exceed the agreed upon price for the procedure, the transplant center assumes the additional cost. The financial issues surrounding transplant can create significant ethical dilemmas for patients, providers, and insurance companies.

29. What educational and support resources are available to patients and their families to help cope with the stresses of BMT?

BMT programs often have extensive patient education and support resources. Books, monographs, and videos, for and by patients, are now available. The topics range from description of the procedure to specific care practices (e.g., Hickman catheter) and long-term effects and care. Active newsletters are sent out by some centers, and one patient-developed newsletter has a regular subscription list. Support and survivor groups can be contacted through the larger BMT programs as well as the Internet. Many programs offer formalized psychosocial consultations with social workers, nurses, or psychologists to all patients.

30. What are the likely new directions for BMT in the future?

One new direction in bone marrow transplantation is gene therapy, which is the introduction of genetic material into human cells. The focus of gene therapy has been on correcting or compensating for specific genetic defects or mutations that can cause or predispose to disease.

The hematopoietic stem cell is an ideal vehicle for gene therapy. Recent technical advances have improved the effectiveness of inserting genetic material into cells of interest. Among the approaches under investigation are blocking the expression of an oncogene, preventing the inactivation of tumor suppressor genes, or altering genes that affect the manner in which chemotherapy drugs are metabolized by tumor cells to increase drug effectiveness. Many obstacles remain, but gene therapy probably will be part of a multimodality approach to cancer treatment early in the next century.

ACKNOWLEDGMENT

The authors thank Pamela Ely, MD, BMT physician at Lahey Hitchcock Clinic and Professor at Dartmouth Medical School, for her thoughtful review of this manuscript.

BIBLIOGRAPHY

1. Appelbaum F, Fay J, Herzig G, et al: American Society for Blood and Marrow Transplantation Guidelines for Training. Biol Blood Marrow Transplant 1:56, 1995.
2. Crouch MA, Ross JA: Current concepts in autologous bone marrow transplantation. Semin Oncol Nurs 10:12–19, 1994.
3. Horowitz MM: New IBMTR/ABMTR slides summarize current use and outcome of allogeneic and autologous transplants. IBMTR Newslett 2:1–3, 1995.
4. Oncology Nursing Society: Manual for Bone Marrow Transplant Nursing: Recommendations for Practice and Education. Oncology Nursing Press, 1994.
5. Phillips G, Armitage, J Bearman S, et al: American Society for Blood and Marrow Transplantation Guidelines for Clinical Centers. Biol Blood Marrow Transplant 1:54–55, 1995.
6. Stewart S: Bone Marrow Transplants: A Book of Basics for Patients. BMT Newsletter, Highland Park, IL, 1992.
7. Whedon MB, Ferrell BR: Quality of life after bone marrow transplantation:Beyond the first year. Semin Oncol Nurs 10:42–57, 1994.
8. Whedon, MB, Wujcik D: Blood and Marrow Stem Cell Transplantation: Principles, Practice and Nursing Insights, 2nd ed. Boston, Jones & Bartlett, 1997.
9. Whedon MB, Stearns D, Mills L: Quality of life of long-term adult survivors of autologous bone marrow transplantation. Oncol Nurs Forum 22:1527–1537, 1995.

11. GENETIC ADVANCES

Constance Engelking, RN, MS, OCN

1. Why is the science of genetics significant to oncology nurses?

A growing scientific database relevant to molecular genetics has revealed a strong link between genetics and a wide range of multifactorial disorders, including cancer. An estimated 5–8% of the population has genetically induced disorders. Among the nonmalignant disorders associated with genetic abnormalities are Huntington's chorea, cystic fibrosis, Alzheimer's disease, sickle-cell anemia, familial hypercholesterolemia, and various birth defects. Genetic defects also are associated with a number of malignancies. For example, approximately 1 in 200 women are predisposed to the development of breast cancer by inheriting the oncogenes BRCA-1 and BRCA-2. Women who carry these abnormal genes have an 80–90% chance of developing breast cancer in their lifetime. The risk for ovarian cancer also appears to be higher in women with these genes. Cancer-specific genes have been implicated in the causation of up to 8% of colorectal cancers. Hereditary nonpolyposis colorectal cancer (HNPCC) and familial adenomatous polyposis (FAP) occur in carriers of certain genes (i.e., hMLH 1 and 2, hPMS 1 and 2; APC genes) and are known to produce susceptibility to development of colorectal cancers. Emerging data also indicate relationships between genetic mutations and malignancy in retinoblastoma, endocrine neoplasia, Wilms' tumor, and various other solid tumors, including lymphomas, melanoma, and lung, brain, and prostate cancers.

2. What benefits will advances in genetic science bring to oncology?

Understanding the genetic basis for cancer will open doors in both prevention and management. The elucidation of identifiable genetic characteristics known to produce high risk for particular malignancies will facilitate more accurate prediction of personal cancer risk and help to target preventive interventions at people with risk factors. In fact, this newfound understanding of genetic science will permit us to tailor programs of total cancer risk management to people with cancer-prone genetic profiles.

Novel diagnostic and treatment options also will become available. DNA-based diagnostic approaches that subcategorize various malignancies according to molecular prognostic indicators will make possible the customization of treatment recommendations based on more accurate probabilities of response and risk for recurrence. Therapeutic management strategies that involve repair or replacement of missing or malfunctioning genes and the use of various genetic techniques to eradicate existing tumor will be added to the armamentarium of anticancer therapies. Furthermore, exquisitely detailed descriptions of biochemical factors that dictate both the incidence and severity of drug-induced side effects will facilitate development of less toxic drugs.

3. What elements constitute the human genome?

The genome is composed of all genetic material necessary for the development and operation of a living organism. Analyzing the genome is analogous to dissecting the human body. Just as the anatomy can be separated into organs and organs into tissues, so the genome can be reduced to molecular components that are progressively less complex. The largest and most complex elements are chromosomes. Found within the nucleus of the cell, these rodlike structures are composed of proteins and DNA. DNA, the cornerstone of the genome, is organized at the molecular level as a double-stranded helical structure that is often described as having a twisted ladder appearance. Sugar and phosphate molecules compose the two side bars of the ladder. Four nitrogenous bases complete the structure: two purines, adenine (A) and guanine (G), and two pyrimidines, thymine (T) and cytosine (C). These four bases bind selectively to one another to form the four possible base pairs: AT, TA, GC, or CG. The pairs act as rungs that connect the two side bars of the ladder. Every three nitrogenous bases along the DNA molecule constitute a codon that holds either instructions for assembly of different amino acids (i.e., protein-building blocks) or cues to start or stop the protein assembly process. Collectively, the DNA protein-coding sequences and the sequences that regulate when and how much of a protein is made constitute the gene. The genome is defined as the full set of genes.

4. What is the relationship among genotype, phenotype, and karyotype?

All three terms describe various levels of genomic expression. **Genotype** encompasses the inheritable characteristics that distinguish one species from another (i.e., man or mouse). **Phenotype** refers to the physical, morphologic, and biochemical manifestations of an individual genotype, which result from the interaction between genetic characteristics and the environment. **Karyotype** refers to the identifiable pattern of an individual's specific complement of chromosomes.

5. What is the relationship of DNA to genes?

Genes are functional subsections of the DNA chain with an estimated length of 10,000–100,000 nucleotides. Genes are the smallest functional units of DNA; they hold the instructions or messages that guide cellular production of specific products (e.g., protein) necessary for an organism's replication and function. Each gene is an ordered sequence of nucleotides found at a certain location on a specific chromosome. For example, BRCA-1, the susceptibility gene for breast cancer, encodes a protein of 1863 amino acids and is found on the long arm of chromosome 17 in the interval 17q12-21. BRCA-2, another breast cancer susceptibility gene, has been localized to the long arm of chromosome 13. It is estimated that approximately 5000 genes are organized along the average human chromosome. Only a small percentage of the total human DNA (3 billion base pairs) is thought to constitute the protein-coding regions known as genes. The remainder is labeled "junk DNA" and has no known function.

6. Do certain genes play a role in the development of cancer?

Specialized classes of tumor susceptibility genes are known to play a key role in the development of cancer, including protooncogenes, oncogenes, and antioncogenes. Protooncogenes and oncogenes are important to the regulation, control, and differentiation of normal cells. Normal protooncogenes are altered to become oncogenes as a result of various mutational events. Oncogenes subsequently stimulate uncontrolled cellular reproduction by encoding for proteins that cause dysregulation of normal cell growth and differentiation. Thus, oncogenes can be thought of as accelerators of neoplastic cellular proliferation. Anti-oncogenes (tumor suppressor genes), on the other hand, encode for proteins that block cellular growth and neoplastic transformation; they are considered "watch-dog" genes that are activated by oncogenic activity. Cancer may result if this genetic regulatory function is lost because the responsible tumor suppressor gene (e.g., P53) is either damaged or absent.

Neoplastic transformation also may occur if the DNA repair process becomes dysfunctional. In this situation, DNA mismatches are not halted by the normal mechanisms, leading to an accumulation of genetic errors that ultimately result in the development of malignancy.

7. What genetic mutations may lead to the development of cancer?

Genomic mutations are reproducible changes in the DNA sequence. They can be spontaneous or result from physical, chemical, biologic, or genetic factors. Mutations are categorized as somatic or germ-cell. Somatic mutations affect genes in the cells of the body and are acquired through carcinogenic exposures. Germ-cell mutations affect genes in gametes and are inherited. A range of DNA changes has been associated with the development of cancer. The following are among the mutations known to play a role in cellular neoplastic transformation:

Deletions: loss or removal of a DNA sequence with subsequent joining of the regions on either side of the missing section.

Insertions: gain or addition of a sequence(s) of DNA not typically present.

Missense mutation: change in the DNA that produces a sequence of three base pairs that encodes for a different amino acid than the original code.

Nonsense mutation: change in the DNA that produces a sequence of three base pairs that does not encode for an amino acid, thus ending the protein sequence.

Point mutation: substitution of one nucleotide for another.

Chromosomal translocation: exchange of chromosomal material between at least two non-homologous chromosomes.

8. What are the concerns about DNA testing and the storage of genetic information in DNA databanks?

The genetic profile has been characterized as a person's "future diary." It is a blueprint describing the person's possible physiologic destiny. Genetic information is exceedingly unique in ways that raise concerns about whether such data should be shared publicly. First, genetic information is still a code that has been only partially deciphered and that is highly sensitive to external forces. The full implications of a person's genetic profile in relation to cancer are still to be defined. It is not yet known, for example, what percentage of people will actually experience malignant diseases for which genetic risk has been identified, when it may occur, and how it may manifest. Such gaps in knowledge place the value of personal genetic information about cancer risk in question and raise the psychosocial dilemma of revealing risks with no known management approaches. Presymptomatic screening for cancer may produce high levels of anxiety and a sense of fatalism that interferes with preventive health care.

Another concern is that public knowledge of a person's genetic profile may give others power over the person's life. For example, if an insurer or employer becomes aware of a genetic predisposition for cancer, the person may be offered reduced health benefits or eliminated as a candidate for promotion. At its worst, discrimination based on projections of bad health outcomes would result in denial of health insurance or employment despite the lack of data to support the idea that a genetic predisposition will be actualized.

In addition, genetic data reveal facts about the person's family members and have health implications for future generations. The disclosure of information about family members without their consent gives rise to ethical issues related to rights to privacy and choice. Moreover, family secrets (e.g., paternity issues) may be exposed as DNA testing is undertaken with far-reaching effects on interpersonal relationships and emotional well-being. Transmitter and survivor guilt as well as depression and overprotection or abandonment of a child also may result when people learn that they may have passed a genetic disorder to their offspring.

Because the availability of personal genetic information is a new phenomenon, uniform standards and guidelines regulating the privacy of information stored in DNA databanks have not yet been established, although various groups (e.g., National Advisory Council for Genomic Research, American Cancer Society) and ethicists are currently addressing such issues. Currently, the best efforts to maintain confidentiality are the "shadow charts," which are shared only with the geneticist or genetic team and the individual.

9. What is the position of key oncologic organizations in regard to commercially available genetic testing?

Considerable controversy surrounds the commercial availability of genetic testing. In 1996, several groups published position statements designed to protect the individual. The American Society of Clinical Oncology (ASCO) has recognized three categories of genetic testing indications: (1) families with well-defined hereditary syndromes for which either a positive or negative result will change medical care, (2) hereditary syndromes for which the medical benefit of identification of a carrier (heterozygote) is presumed but not proved, and (3) people with family histories of cancer or syndromes in which germline mutations have been identified. In general, ASCO recommends cancer predisposition testing only when: there is a strong family history of cancer (especially early age of onset); the test can be adequately interpreted; and the results will influence the medical management of test takers or their family members.

Similarly, the National Advisory Council for Human Genome Research has devised a list of crucial questions to be answered about DNA testing for presymptomatic identification of cancer risk. Examples include definition of the number and incidence of disease-causing gene mutations and actual risk of cancer, laboratory and technical issues relevant to testing for cancer genes, and methods of quality control. Other areas of study include what methods are most effective and feasible for educating large numbers of at-risk people and how to ensure informed consent, provide culturally sensitive genetic counseling, and avoid genetic discrimination.

Both the American Society of Human Genetics and the National Breast Cancer Coalition want to limit BRCA-1 testing to research protocols until more is known about the mutation. They have called for a written plan to manage potentially discriminatory consequences and to establish therapeutic options before widespread testing is permitted.

In contrast, commercial organizations that offer screening tests for various types of cancer (e.g., breast, ovarian, and colorectal cancers) argue that genetic testing is an individual choice and that availability will force the refinement of such testing and bring potentially life-saving diagnostic tests to the public.

10. What are the primary sources of genetic information?

The various data sources for collecting genetic information include family history, physical examination, and selected laboratory studies. Family history is particularly important as a case-finding tool. Historical data permit construction of a family tree or pedigree that may illuminate the existence of a trait or disorder across generations. At a minimum, data-gathering should encompass three generations of relatives and include copies of death certificates, medical records, pathology reports, and cancer registry data to ensure accuracy and comprehensiveness. Physical examination reveals characteristics associated with genetic disorders (e.g., polycystic kidneys, familial adenomatous polyposis) and thus provides another piece in the genetic puzzle. Laboratory testing completes the picture, although tests for cancer genes have two obvious shortcomings: (1) the imperfect association between a mutation isolated by laboratory testing and actual development of cancer and (2) the current inability to detect all mutations that may result in a malignant condition.

11. What is the Human Genome Project (HGP)?

Officially launched in 1990 under the aegis of the National Institutes of Health and the Department of Energy, the HGP is a federally funded, multibillion dollar international initiative designed to describe fully the genomes of humans and selected model organisms by the year 2005. This goal is to be accomplished systematically by mapping genetic and physical characteristics of the 23 chromosome pairs in human cells, isolating the 100,000 genes contained within, and sequencing the estimated three billion base pairs in human DNA. Adjunctive goals focus on defining the most critical ethical, legal, and social concerns likely to emerge as the genome is unveiled. To address such issues, funding has been dedicated to the development of a project component known as the Ethical, Legal, and Social Implications branch (ELSI). ELSI seeks to develop strategies that will ensure: (1) confidentiality and fair use of genetic information, (2) appropriate presentation of genetic information in clinical settings, and (3) effective education of providers and consumers of health care.

12. How do linkage, physical, and sequence maps differ?

Gene mapping consists of three interdependent map construction methods. The primary difference among the three types of genetic maps is the level of detail. In general, linkage mapping is a method of identifying specific genes, whereas physical and sequence maps describe the overall and specific DNA sequencing of the genome. Linkage maps contain representations of physical and disease traits known as "random polymorphisms" that can be located to particular chromosomes and then mapped in relation to one another. (Random polymorphisms are discrepancies in DNA among people that are considered useful clues for linkage analyses when they occur in more than 1% of the population.) The linkage map appears as a grid of evenly spaced genetic markers onto which the positions of identified genes are superimposed. In contrast, the physical map is constructed by "snipping" overlapping collections of DNA fragments with biochemical scissors known as restriction enzymes, copying, and then reassembling the DNA clones in the order in which they appear on the chromosome. The DNA fragments are analyzed by various methods to determine the base-by-base DNA sequence. The sequence map is the most detailed of the maps, providing the actual order of the base pairs in a specific gene. A laboratory technique known as polymerase chain reaction (PCR), in which DNA fragments can be amplified (i.e., duplicated without cloning) for analysis, has automated the mapping process significantly.

13. How will advances in genetic science be applied to the treatment of cancer?

Understanding the make-up of the human genome, coupled with advanced laboratory technology, permits manipulations to "normalize" an individual's genetic profile. Gene transfer is a relatively new intervention performed for the first time 6 years ago in a child with severe combined immunodeficiency (SCID). Using gene transfer techniques, a functional gene can be introduced into a patient's cells to replace a missing gene, to correct a genetic defect, or to endow the cells with new capability. The two primary clinical applications at this point are gene marking and gene therapy. The two strategies differ in that gene marking is diagnostic, entailing the insertion of an identifiable gene into patients' cells to label them for future recognition, whereas gene therapy has a therapeutic intent and involves the introduction of a functioning gene to replace a missing or malfunctioning gene responsible for a particular disease state. An application of gene marking under investigation is to ascertain whether reinfused marrow is the source of relapse after autologous blood cell transplant by inserting the marker gene responsible for conferring neomycin resistance (i.e., Noe$_R$) into the cells of transplant patients. Five different techniques for clinical application of gene therapy include:

1. Stimulation of immune responses via tumor cell vaccination with a cytokine gene (i.e., IL-2 or TNF in neuroblastoma, melanoma, renal cell carcinoma)

2. Injection of a foreign human leukocyte antigen (HLA) gene (e.g., HLA-B7 to heighten tumor immunogenicity in melanoma)

3. Insertion of a "suicide gene" into neoplastic cells (e.g., gene for herpes simplex thymidine kinase [TK] into brain tumor cells followed by a course of ganciclovir to destroy tumor cells that have taken up the TK gene)

4. Introduction of a multidrug resistance gene into bone marrow (e.g., to protect normal hematopoietic cells from myelosuppression induced by dose-intensive chemotherapy)

5. Introduction of tumor suppressor gene to "turn off" tumor cell proliferation (e.g., P53 gene into colorectal cancer cells)

Currently, all gene transfer is investigational and involves only somatic cell techniques, that is, genetic alterations are achieved in individual patients and cannot be passed along to their offspring. However, the technology for germ-line gene transfer does exist. Although currently considered unethical, in the future it may be used to prevent cancer in people at high risk.

14. By what methods is gene transfer carried out?

The cellular insertion of genes can be accomplished by one of two sophisticated delivery methods: (1) ex vivo insertion using a retroviral vector or (2) in vivo injection via physical or chemical transport mechanisms. Use of a viral vector is an indirect method of altering the target cells, whereas the in vivo method is direct.

In the ex vivo method, retroviral vectors are used as carriers to bring the desired genetic material to the host cell for insertion. Retroviruses are particularly well-suited for this task because cytoplasmic incorporation of genetic material is one of their natural functions. Sophisticated laboratory procedures are used to make the viral vector safe by removing the genes responsible for viral replication (i.e., specific segments of DNA that carry the instructions for self-replication of the virus). In the next step, the marker or therapeutic gene is introduced into the vector. The genetically modified viral vector is then combined in cell culture with the particular target cells (e.g., peripheral stem cells, lymphocytes) that have been removed from the patient. Various cytokines are added to stimulate cellular proliferation. The vector "infects" or enters the cell and inserts the gene into the chromosome of the host cell for subsequent replication. Within a week or two the desired number of cells are produced and processed for reinfusion into the patient. The actual administration procedure is similar to a blood transfusion.

In contrast, in vivo gene transfer is accomplished by injecting the desired genetic material directly into the target cell. Among the array of direct injection methods being studied, liposomal transport is the most clinically feasible at this point. The gene-containing liposome fuses to the cell membrane, after which the gene is transported across the membrane for chromosomal incorporation. In addition to being easy to prepare, liposomal delivery systems are nontoxic and biodegradable. Recently, the HLA-B7 gene has been studied in patients with advanced melanoma on the theory that it will act as an immune system stimulant, causing the release of cytokines locally to bring about a T cell attack response against tumor cells.

15. What safety considerations are associated with gene transfer therapy?

As with the development of other anticancer therapies, safety concerns are related to potential occupational hazards associated with the administration of gene therapies, especially with the use of retroviruses. However, specific regulations serve to protect the clinician. Specifically, FDA regulations do not permit clinical use of retroviral vectors until they have been modified to eliminate their replicating ability. Accordingly, protocols involving retroviral vectors cannot begin until confirmatory quality control testing has been conducted. In addition, compliance with universal precautions is considered adequate protection against any viral hazards that may exist, although none have been demonstrated to date.

16. How will advances in genetic science affect cancer nursing?

Although the implications of advances in genetic knowledge and technology are yet unknown, such advances certainly will contribute significantly to an already transforming paradigm of cancer nursing practice and care. Three areas in which change will be evident include professional perspective, practice focal points, and patient/client profiles. The current emphasis on disease management will be increasingly replaced by attention to cancer prevention and screening for indicators of high risk, transforming nursing practice and care from a short-term, episodic approach to a longer-term, continuous approach. The content of patient education will be altered. The current concentration on symptom management is likely to shift toward wellness promotion and preventive lifestyle behaviors. Patient profiles will change in relation to the point on the health/illness continuum at which patients present to the health team. Rather than presenting at or immediately after diagnosis, often because they are symptomatic, patients will enter the health care system as a result of risk for developing cancer. Outcomes will be less certain than in the past, because at this point it remains unclear who will actually develop cancer. As a result, anxiety may be significant and sustained in people at risk. Conversely, high-risk people may adopt a fatalistic attitude and not engage in prevention behaviors because they believe that cancer is inevitable. Both attitudes create the need for intensive and targeted counseling for people at risk and their families. In addition, the focus of clinical practice will move from the individual and physical care skills to the family network and interpersonal interactive skills. The team will expand to include geneticists and experts in genetic counseling techniques. Oncology nurses will be in a strategic position to pioneer new gene therapies and screening approaches and to define human responses to new strategies.

BIBLIOGRAPHY

1. American Society of Clinical Oncology: Statement on the genetic testing for cancer susceptibility. J Clin Oncol 14:1730–1736, 1996.
2. Engelking C: The human genome exposed: A glimpse of promise, predicament, and impact on practice. Oncol Nurs Forum 22(Suppl): 3–9, 1996.
3. Engelking C: Genetics in cancer care: Confronting a pandora's box of dilemmas. Oncol Nurs Forum 22 (Suppl):27–34, 1996.
4. Jenkins J, Wheeler V, Albright L: Gene therapy for cancer. Cancer Nurs 17(6):447–456, 1994.

5. Loescher L: Genetics in cancer prediction, screening, and counseling. Parts I & II Oncol Nurs Forum 22(Suppl):10–19, 1996.
6. National Advisory Council for Human Genome Research: Statement on the use of DNA testing for presymptomatic identification of cancer risk. JAMA 271:785, 1994.
7. Rothenberg KH: Genetic information and health insurance: State legislative approaches. J Law Med Ethics 23:312–319, 1995.
8. Scanlon C, Fibison W: Managing Genetic Information: Implications for Nursing Practice, Washington, D.C., American Nurses Association, 1995.
9. Wheeler VS: Gene therapy: Current strategies and future applications. Oncol Nurs Forum 22:20–26, 1995.

12. CLINICAL TRIALS

Pamela A. Rosse, RN, MS, CCRA, *and Mary T. Garcia,* RN, BSN, MPH, CCRA

1. Describe how a clinical trial differs from a protocol.

A **clinical trial** is a planned investigation involving patients. It is designed according to accepted scientific methods and is intended to determine the most efficacious treatment for future patients with a given medical condition.

A **protocol** is the written form of a clinical trial; it outlines the objectives of the study and summarizes research information currently available relative to the treatment under study. In addition, a protocol explicitly delineates criteria for inclusion and exclusion of participants. It also provides a detailed description of the treatment involved and specifies parameters for evaluating outcomes.

2. What types of studies is the oncology nurse likely to encounter?

Studies may be designed as therapeutic or preventive, or they may address biologic or genetic questions and involve tissue/specimen collection and testing. Therapeutic studies may include one or several modalities, e.g., chemotherapy, radiation therapy, surgery, hormonal therapy, immunotherapy, or alternative therapies for symptom management.

3. How does an institutional review board (IRB) function?

An IRB is entrusted with the task of protecting the rights and welfare of human participants in research by asking the following questions:
1. Do the benefits outweigh the risks?
2. Is there adequate protection for the participants, including informed consent?
3. Is the selection of participants equitable?

Membership requirements for IRBs in the United States are established by the Food and Drug Administration (FDA). A minimum of five members of varied backgrounds, gender, and racial and cultural perspectives is required. A typical IRB may include physicians, pharmacists, nurses, scientists, lawyers, clergy, and community representatives. One nonmedical person with no direct affiliation to the reviewing institution is mandated. All studies must be approved by the IRB before any patients may be enrolled. The IRB also must be kept abreast of changes and informed of adverse events related to the studies.

4. How can informed consent be ensured?

To inform potential participants adequately about the study, specific points must be covered:
- Reason for the study
- Specific procedures that will be utilized, both for diagnosis and treatment
- Alternative treatments
- Potential risks and benefits to participation (including the right to refuse without consequence)
- Assurance of confidentiality
- Clarification of compensation (or lack thereof)

The consent process involves discussion of all of the above points with the patient. Information about the study may be provided by the physician, research nurse/data manager, pharmacist, or others knowledgeable about the clinical trial. Researchers are strongly encouraged to provide consent forms written at a 6th-grade reading level; however, the abundance of medical terms is often confusing. Frequently patients have just learned of their diagnosis; although seemingly aware of what they have heard and agreed to do, they have many questions later that require further clarification of the study process.

5. Are there special circumstances when informed consent may not be available?

Yes. Sometimes the only access to a new therapy is through a clinical trial. In an emergency in which the patient may be not be capable of giving consent, the study treatment may be considered. In cases involving minors or legal guardianship, the patient may not be the person providing consent

In certain unique situations, eligibility criteria may be waived. On occasion, the IRB may approve participation in a study for a single patient on a compassionate basis, usually when no alternative treatment is available.

6. Are patients reimbursed for participation in a study?

Studies may be sponsored by government sources, pharmaceutical companies, or individual institutions and investigators, and funding varies accordingly. Usually, patients do not receive money for participation, although study costs or drugs may be provided. In special circumstances reimbursement for participation may be approved by the officiating IRB. Typically, if the patient is insured, routine health care costs are billed; remaining expenses are absorbed by the funding source. For-profit, not-for-profit and charitable organizations may wish to contribute financially and help to defray patients' costs.

7. Describe the three phases of therapeutic studies.

Every new chemotherapy drug is tested in three subsequent trials called phase I, phase II, and phase III before it is approved by the FDA for general use.

Phase I studies are dose-escalating clinical trials designed to determine the maximal tolerated dose (MTD) of a new drug, alone or in combination with another drug or modality. A phase I trial also helps to establish an optimal therapy schedule, to determine pharmacokinetic properties, and to identify toxicities associated with the therapy. It is not a primary goal of a phase I trial to determine the efficacy of the therapy. Frequently, phase I involves patients who have had extensive treatment, and different types of cancer may be included for study in a phase I trial. Because the study is concluded once the MTD is reached, the numbers are usually small (e.g., 20 patients).

Phase II studies evaluate antitumor activity in specific tumors and further define toxicities. The number of patients involved typically ranges from 20–80.

Phase III trials compare a promising new treatment to established therapy in clinical practice to determine whether one is superior in treating a specific disease. Large numbers of participants are required.

Adjuvant trials are designed to provide additional therapy to patients who have been deemed free of disease after treatment. The goal is to prevent recurrence.

8. Why is it important to understand the terms *eligibility* and *evaluability*?

Eligibility refers to meeting the qualifications stipulated in the protocol for participation in the study. **Evaluability** refers to how well the protocol was followed once the patient was enrolled; essentially, it determines how usable the patient's data are. Both concepts are crucial to the integrity of the study. For example, if a patient does not have the same type, grade, or stage of cancer as required in the protocol, the progress of disease may not be affected by the proposed therapy. Significant differences among patient characteristics make it difficult to include them in the same pool for analyses. Similarly, if patients are not treated for their disease in a standardized manner, it is difficult to generalize about the results. Of equal importance, if a patient does not meet one of the criteria (e.g., adequate renal or cardiac function), serious toxicities may occur.

9. In clinical trials with multiple treatment regimens, who decides which regimen a particular patient will receive?

In studies with multiple treatment regimens, each regimen is called an arm. Patients are often randomized to specific arms of a study or assigned to different treatments by a process similar to flipping a coin. Usually, the randomization schedule is generated by a computer. For some studies assignment may be blinded (that is, the patient does not know which treatment he or she is receiving) or double-blinded (neither the patient nor the healthcare team knows which drug is being administered). At times, failure to achieve a response to one treatment will result in crossover (switching) to another arm of treatment.

Example of Multiple Arms and Randomization

Randomize	
Arm I:	Drug X for 6 cycles
Arm II:	Drug X for 9 cycles
Arm III:	Drug Y for 12 cycles
Evaluate	
Arms I, II:	If equal to or greater than a partial response, randomize to drug Z or observation.
Arm III:	If less than a partial response, treat with drug Z and radiotherapy.

10. Define equipoise and its significance in clinical trials.

Equipoise means *even balance*. In relationship to clinical trials, it refers to approaching studies from an unbiased perspective. The concept of equipoise is fundamental in conducting clinical research and is particularly relevant during presentation of a clinical trial to patients. Because of the investigational nature of a study, it is important to impress on patients that no known benefits may occur directly to them. It is also paramount, in studies with more than one treatment option, to present all treatments with equal enthusiasm. Sometimes this is a difficult task for the health care team because, based on professional experience, they may believe one therapy to be more promising than others.

Studies that compare therapy with no therapy (observation) are particularly challenging. It is often difficult to do nothing when a patient is faced with the diagnosis of cancer. In such cases it may be beneficial to remember that many investigational cancer therapies ultimately have been deemed ineffective, and many are associated with numerous and significant toxicities.

11. What role do pharmacokinetics play in clinical trials?

Often the drug tested in a clinical trial is reviewed for its pharmacokinetic properties. To measure absorption rates, duration of action, distribution within the body, and excretion, blood or other types of samples are collected at specifically designated intervals before and after administration of therapy. Sometimes no samples or perhaps only one or two samples are required. In other cases, samples may be required only when a patient experiences significant untoward side effects.

Timing in obtaining samples is often critical to the validity and reliability of data. Every effort should be made to adhere to blood-draw or other sampling times. The study coordinator should be informed of instances in which the schedule cannot be maintained in case other arrangements are needed; special notation should be documented in the patient's clinical trial record.

12. In general, what kinds of information do investigators look for once a study has ended?

At the conclusion of a clinical trial the primary investigators pay particular attention to data that answer the following questions:

1. Were the original study questions (usually found in the objectives section of the protocol) answered? Most commonly these questions are related to the endpoints such as survival time, types of tumor responses, and time to recurrence.

2. What were the toxicities (in detail)? Do they outweigh the benefits?

3. Was each patient eligible and evaluable? If not, it may be difficult to generalize about the data.

13. What are the implications if the treatment schedule stipulated in the protocol is not followed?

Obviously, clinical trials are designed with specific scientific questions in mind. The schedules of treatments are typically based on previously conducted trials—animal, human, or both. Often the primary treatment schedules are discontinued as a result of significant toxicities. Many protocols provide a schedule for modification of therapy based on specific toxicities and their severity. When no modification schedule is provided or for unique patient situations, the primary investigator should be contacted to discuss whether the patient should remain in the study.

As a general rule, the protocol schedule should not be violated because it is inconvenient or because the treating physician does not agree with the way the protocol is written. Such issues should be taken into consideration before the patient enters a clinical trial. Deviation from the stipulated protocol may be dangerous, because the alternative treatment may not have been studied at great length. Furthermore, deviation may make the patient's data inevaluable. Compromise of treatment may jeopardize timely completion of select studies and even preclude some patients from participating in an innovative study. The following is an example:

> In a phase I study, drug X is tested on a limited sample size. Additional patients were hopeful of entering the study, but only 20 patients were accepted before the study was closed for analyses. During the analyses it is discovered that patient 18 did not receive drug X on days 1, 7, and 21 as stipulated in the protocol. Instead, the patient received the drug on days 1, 10, and 42 because she was out of town. If the investigators had known this information before beginning the analyses, they may have chosen to allow an additional patient to enter the study as a replacement for patient 18. The unfortunate patient who would have been number 21 was precluded from joining the study because the investigators believed that all previous patients were eligible and evaluable.

14. What if a patient decides to discontinue treatment earlier than the protocol stipulates?

Each patient has the right to discontinue participation in a clinical trial at any time, and this right should be clearly stated in the consent form. In such cases, the patient, family, and health care team should thoroughly discuss appropriate alternatives, including no treatment.

Even though the patient discontinues therapy, some of the early data may still be useful to the study. Examples include toxicities and perhaps tumor response. In the final analysis, the primary investigators and biostaticians decide whether the patient is evaluable.

Many clinical trials require follow-up of the patient's status until death. In such cases, even if the patient has discontinued active participation in a clinical trial, the study remains open at an institution until all patients have died.

15. How much information is shared with the patient whose condition precludes treatment at the full dose specified by the protocol?

The heart of this question is patients' right to know about their treatment. At the same time, the health care team must struggle with other fundamental questions: Will a modified investigational therapy be any better or worse than the originally proposed investigational therapy—or, for that matter, standard therapy? Do the benefits outweigh the risks? Because it is mandated that patients be adequately informed about participation in research studies, it seems logical that they be provided with the facts necessary to make a truly informed decision. Therein lies the difficulty—all of the facts are not typically known to the health care team. If they were, there would be no need for an investigational study. One of the most honest approaches is to provide the facts that are known and to discuss issues for which the answers remain unknown.

16. How can the oncology nurse contribute to the validity of clinical trials?

1. **Identification of potential study patients**

   Oncology nurses are in a critical position for fostering clinical trial research. They possess knowledge of cancer disease processes and understand the rationale for treatment. They frequently have unique insights into whether a patient is likely to be able to comply with a protocol.

2. **Protecting the integrity of the study**

   Most patients participate in an oncology clinical trial believing that in some way they are contributing to cancer research. If information about their case is compromised on the part of the heath care team, the patients' efforts have been undermined. Thus, adherence to a protocol is paramount. Because the nurse is frequently responsible for coordinating patient care, the nurse should be aware of protocol guidelines and remain in contact with the coordinators of the clinical trial. The treatment plan must be followed exactly, including drug administration, pre- and posthydration guidelines, anti-emetic therapy, specified antibiotics, and use of cell-stimulating factors. Various tests must be performed at specified times, and radiotherapy and/or surgery must be synchronized accordingly. The nurse may be able to provide suggestions that promote feasibility and ensure compliance.

3. **Documentation in the medical record**

   In addition to routine requirements, it is of great value to those who review the data for study purposes to find notations relative to (1) the patient's current performance status; (2) dose modifications or schedule changes and reasons for them; (3) specific symptoms of toxicity, including onset and duration; and supportive care, particularly as related to symptom management.

4. **Patient advocacy**

   Often the oncology nurse is in a position to support patients' decisions to begin, continue, or discontinue treatment. Similarly, in investigational studies the nurse may need to help patients verbalize their decision to participate or not participate to family or other health care team members. The nursing staff also can help patients to feel comfortable with their informed decision or even to change their decision, if circumstances permit.

BIBLIOGRAPHY

1. Berry DL, Dodd MJ, Hinds PS, Ferrell BR: Informed consent: Process and clinical issues. Oncol Nurs Forum 23:507–512, 1996.
2. Jassak P, Ryan MP: Ethical issues in clinical research. Semin Oncol Nurs 5(2):102–108, 1989.
3. Protection of Human Subjects and Institutional Review Board Requirements: Food and Drug Administration Regulatory Primer. Rockville, MD, Office of AIDS and Special Health Issues, U.S. Department of Health and Human Services, 1996.
4. Varricchio CG, Jassak, PF: Informed consent: an overview. Semin Oncol Nurs 5(2):95–98, 1989.
5. Wager E, Tooley PJH, Emanuel MB, Wood SF: Get patient consent to enter clinical trials. BMJ 311:27–30, 1995.
6. White-Hershey D, Nevidjon B: Fundamentals for oncology nurse/data managers—preparing for a new role. Oncol Nurs Forum 17:371–377, 1990.

13. ALTERNATIVE THERAPIES

Mary Jo Cleaveland, RN, MS

1. How are alternative therapies characterized?

Alternative therapies or alternative medicine is the umbrella term for unproven remedies and techniques prescribed or provided by a variety of licensed and unlicensed health care practitioners. Alternative therapies are used by millions of people in the United States. In other countries, they are called complementary therapies because they are used in conjunction with allopathic or mainstream medicine. Despite the lack of scientific research supported by acceptable methodologies, anecdotal evidence and case studies suggest the efficacy of many alternative therapies.

2. Which are the most common unproven therapies used by people with cancer?

Diet and nutrition are the most common unproven cancer treatments. The macrobiotic diet is the most popular anticancer diet therapy. Diet supplements with megavitamins and antioxidants also are widely used. Mind–body techniques used by people with cancer include relaxation and visualization, meditation, group support, individual psychotherapy, hypnosis, and biofeedback. These therapies often are sought to relieve symptoms of anxiety, insomnia, and depression or to lessen the side effects of cancer treatments. Intercessory prayer and the laying on of hands are often included in mind–body descriptions of alternative therapies. Less frequent remedies include touch therapies and herbal preparations. The most controversial alternative therapy is the use of alternative pharmacologic treatments, which include shark cartilage, immunoaugmentative therapy (IAT), antineoplastins, and Cancell. Some patients seek metabolic therapies, primarily available in Mexico. A number of practitioners prescribe these therapies.

Alternative Therapies for Cancer

TYPE OF THERAPY	PROVIDER
Psychological approaches (includes imagery, cancer support groups, group therapy, individual therapy)	MD, RN, psychotherapist
Nutritional-metabolic programs (includes macrobiotics, nutritional supplements)	MD, naturopath (ND), chiropractor
Acupuncture and herbs	Traditional Chinese medicine (OMD), ND, acupuncturist (DAc), MD
Alternative pharmacologics	PhD, MD
Prayer, laying on of hands	Religious and folk healers
Therapies with proven absence of effect, i.e., laetrile, hoxsey, hydrogen peroxide, coffee enemas (clinics in Mexico, Southern California)	MDs

3. How often do people with cancer seek alternative and complementary therapies?

In a 1990 survey of 5,047 people with cancer, Lerner and Kennedy[6] found that 9% had used at least one unproven therapy. Mind therapies were used most frequently, followed by diet therapies. The demographics revealed that younger women who were affluent and better educated used the therapies more often than other segments of the population. In a smaller Canadian study,[8] 75% of 300 patients with cancer reported using some form of alternative therapy in conjunction with biomedical treatments.

4. How does use of alternative therapies by patients with cancer compare with use by people with other life-threatening or chronic illnesses?

A 1990 Harvard survey found that 1 in 3 Americans used unconventional therapies, with visits to providers of alternative therapies exceeding visits to primary care medical doctors. In addition, 70% of reported consumers of alternative therapies did not tell their allopathic physician about their use of unconventional remedies or techniques. The therapies were used more often in conjunction with conventional therapies. An interesting finding was the relative lack of use of alternative therapies by persons with cancer. The demographics were similar to those in the survey of patients with cancer: women who were younger, well educated, and affluent. The most frequent consumers were people with acute or chronic conditions that were not life-threatening, i.e., back problems, allergies, asthma, arthritis, insomnia, anxiety, and depression.

5. At what stage in the course of cancer do patients seek information or use alternative therapies?

In the past, the majority of cancer patients turned to alternative therapies when response to conventional treatments had failed or no further therapies were available. Often patients were not ready to give up and searched for any treatment that might halt the course of the disease. Rarely did they chose alternatives in lieu of conventional treatments. Increased consumer interest and media promotion of alternative therapies are influencing patients to combine unproven therapies with conventional treatments, but it is still rare for patients to reject conventional treatments and follow alternative therapy programs exclusively. When conventional therapies fail or when cancer returns, some patients turn to unproven therapies in hope of curing the cancer. Because most of the therapies are costly and not reimbursable by conventional insurance, patients often lack financial resources for alternative therapies.

6. Are there research protocols or studies to determine the effects of alternative therapies?

Both basic research and clinical studies are under way to determine the activity and effectiveness of many alternative therapies. Some of the current studies focus on cancer prevention, the role of specific dietary factors, and the role of antioxidants. Others focus on the use of bio-electromagnetics and bovine cartilage. Chinese herbs are under investigation in animal models. Quality-of-life studies are under way to determine the effects of mind–body techniques on well-being as well as length of survival. Some nursing studies have documented the effects of mind–body interventions such as relaxation and imagery, therapeutic massage, and biofeedback for the control of pain and side effects of treatments.

7. What political and social factors affect the use of unproven therapies?

A person with cancer may receive information about alternative therapies from family members and friends. In an effort to be helpful and supportive, the community often presents the lay person's view of the many choices of therapies. It is often reported that someone who was given a grim prognosis was "saved" by an alternative therapy. The media, too, in news reports and magazine articles, provide another source of information, much of it misinformation. Proponents of alternative therapies use seductive advertising. Perusal of titles in popular bookstores, e.g. *Sharks Don't Get Cancer* and *The Cure for All Cancers*, demonstrates the allure of these therapies. Many people turn to pamphlets and workers in health food stores for information about "healthy" choices. Many health care practitioners promote themselves as having the cure for cancer. Such promotion is unethical and, in some cases, illegal.

8. Where can the person with cancer get information about alternative therapies?

In an attempt to facilitate the evaluation of alternative therapies, Congress mandated the formation of the Office of Alternative Medicine (OAM) within the National Institutes of Health. The organization resulted from the efforts of congressional leaders who had personal experience with alternative therapies and wanted to integrate them into mainstream medicine. In 1996, MD Anderson Cancer Center received OAM funding to research alternative therapies in the treatment of cancer. The OAM has an information line, 301-402-2466. At a conference on alternative therapies, Dr. Wayne Jonas, Director of OAM, reported that 80% of the 600 monthly calls were for information about alternative therapies for cancer. The American Cancer Society provides information on specific unproven therapies and organizations that advocate freedom of choice in unproven therapies. The Food and Drug Administration provides information about testing with various alternative therapies. The Cancer Information Service (1-800-4-Cancer) provides patients and health care professionals with resources and information about these therapies.

9. What is quackery?

Quackery in its purest sense is the deliberate prescription or administration of a therapy for personal gain of either notoriety or money. Often practitioners advertise their therapies as a cure for cancer. Opponents of unconventional, unproven, or alternative therapies have determined that practitioners prescribing such remedies are practicing quackery. Proof of quackery requires scientific, legal, and ethical documentation. A loose network of experts in these disciplines has succeeded in exposing some therapies as quackery. An example is the scientific proof of the ineffectiveness of Laetrile as a cancer therapy through studies conducted at the National Cancer Institute in the 1970s. Persons continuing to prescribe Laetrile either have labeled the drug as a nutritional supplement or integrated it into a nutritional-metabolic approach in clinics in Mexico and Southern California. The language now used to describe these therapies avoids the word *cure*.

10. Are any unproven therapies known to be dangerous?

The greatest danger in alternative therapies is that the patient may choose to use an unproven therapy *instead* of conventional therapies. This danger is minimized when the patient has widespread disease at the time of initial diagnosis. The three key considerations for use of unproven therapies are (1) the training and experience of the practitioner; (2) open disclosure of known effectiveness and potential side effects, and (3) quality of service delivery, including costs. The dangers of some unproven therapies used with conventional therapies include possible interactions between the therapies; for example, a pseudo-mushroom drink that contains large numbers of fungi was the source of opportunistic infections in some persons experiencing immunosuppression. Some herbal preparations have potential harmful and dangerous effects. The best scenario for the person wanting to combine therapies includes dialogue between the physician administering the conventional therapies and the alternative practitioner. Together they can design a plan that is not harmful and may be helpful to the patient.

11. What do people with cancer expect from their oncology physicians and nurses?

The primary wish of all persons with cancer is that their doctors and nurses listen to their struggles with the diagnosis and treatment choices. Often persons with cancer are confused by the language of biomedicine and turn to more understandable alternatives and lay information sources for guidance. Patients often fear that they will be judged foolish or hysterical if they consider choices other than conventional treatments. Many patients are well educated and are looking for guidance that makes them a full partner in designing their treatment for cancer. Patients may turn first to a nurse to explore his or her thoughts and to practice what to say with the physician. Being fully informed is the key to guiding choice. Often patients need multiple methods of receiving information: verbal, written, and visual. Often they need to review the information several times to absorb it fully. They may need a trusted person to help them put together their questions and assimilate and review the answers. A nonjudgmental approach is essential to the support of the patient's choices.

12. What is the major ethical consideration for nurses in facilitating choices?

The ethical dilemma facing nurses is to balance the patient's rights of free choice and personal control with the duty to protect the patient from harm—both from alternative therapies and from false hopes that result only in psychological distress. Often the provider of unproven therapies offers hope that is missing from conventional treatments, usually when a patient has recurrent disease and the next available treatments offer little hope of cure. The nurse can help the patient to consider whether he or she is getting full information from the alternative provider about risks, benefits, and costs.

13. What can a nurse say on discovering that a patient is using a harmful unproven therapy?

Some patients are reluctant to share their use of unproven and potentially harmful therapies with their physicians. The patient may choose the nurse as a confidant. The disclosure often reveals uncertainty about a choice of treatment. First, the nurse must honor the confidence of the patient, while acknowledging the uncertainty of all therapies. The nurse then should negotiate with the patient to share the information with the physician, including an offer to be present when the discussion occurs. If the patient refuses, the nurse must explain that the nursing code of ethics compels intervention, either to discontinue dangerous therapies or at least to document continued use so that the patient can be treated appropriately if dangerous effects occur. Finally, if the patient is a minor and the parent refuses to discontinue dangerous, unproven therapies, the situation demands intervention by ethical and legal professionals.

14. What are practice guidelines for the oncology nurse?

The nurse must know his or her own values yet practice neutrality in helping patients explore alternative therapies. By keeping current with the evolving field of unproven therapies, the nurse can give appropriate information to the patient and guide the patient toward sources of understandable information. Seeking support from colleagues while patients and families struggle with choices will help the nurse to remain supportive. Protecting the patient from harm while maintaining a relationship may challenge the nurse's personal and professional resources. Sharing this responsibility with colleagues helps.

15. What nursing interventions are complementary to medical treatments for cancer?

Mind–body therapies and use of touch are complementary nursing interventions that can be used throughout the patient's journey with cancer in different settings, from inpatient units and ambulatory clinics to the patient's home. They can be offered as interventions for various symptoms and side effects. Many interventions have self-help components and also can be taught to family members. In a recent study, children with cancer were asked what nurses did to help them. The children gave examples of the gentle, friendly, and available nurse as the "good" nurse. Although technical support such as the use of topical anesthetics to lessen procedural pain is important, gestures such as holding hands and using a soothing voice during difficult times were highly valued by the children. The therapeutic use of self is the primary "mind–body" intervention used by many nurses.

16. What is a specific mind–body therapy?

The most frequently used mind–body therapy is relaxation. Relaxation is an alert, hypometabolic state of decreased sympathetic nervous system arousal that can be achieved in various ways. The most common and simple method is to breathe slowly and deeply while tensing and relaxing various parts of the body. Verbal cues induce this state of relaxation. More complex systems of relaxation are hypnosis with suggestion and biofeedback.

17. Is there a simple technique for helping patients to relax?

The practice of relaxation taught by Benson[1] uses the following steps:
1. Sit in a comfortable position, either upright in a chair or lying down.
2. Close your eyes.
3. Deeply relax all of your muscles, beginning with your feet and progressing upward to your face. Alternately, take in a deep breath while tensing all the muscles in your body, and release the breath while relaxing all of your muscles.
4. For a few minutes, turn your attention to your breath. Watch your breath coming in and going out.
5. Now, as you breathe out, mentally say the word *one*. (Other words may be suggested, such as calm, peace, Amen, OM, whatever the patient is comfortable with.)

6. Continue breathing naturally, and mentally say the word or phrase.

7. Continue for 10–20 minutes. You may open your eyes to check the time or use a soft alarm. If thoughts come in, let them go and return to the word.

8. When you are finished, sit quietly for a few minutes, with eyes either closed or opened. Do not stand up immediately.

9. Practice once or twice each day, but not within 2 hours of eating. The relaxation response will come with less and less effort.

18. How does guided imagery work?

Guided imagery is more controversial than relaxation. In general, imagery is the use of the imagination to bring about an internal experience that can serve to connect body, mind, and spirit. It was pioneered with cancer patients in the 1970s by the Simontons. The therapist is the guide, but the person being guided decides what imagery works for him or her. One of the potential difficulties with imagery is that the person may identify completely with the image and experience a sense of failure if the imagery does not "cure" the cancer. Guided imagery should be provided by therapists trained and skilled in the art and science of imagery. Audio tapes often are used for continuing the experience after sessions with the therapist. Nurses can use guided imagery to enhance states of relaxation.

19. Are there any contraindications to massage therapy?

The major concern is that massage may aid the cancer in spreading because of increased circulation. Although this belief is taught in massage therapy schools, no research supports this theory. Deep tissue work around areas of metastasis to bones may cause fractures. The general rule is to use gentle massage and to avoid sites of lymphatic drainage around the tumor. An exception is the use of massage for treatment of lymphedema after mastectomy. No pressure massage should be used when platelets are low, i.e., in patients with leukemias and severe marrow depression secondary to therapies. In the nursing literature, gentle, slow-stroke massage enhances relaxation and increases feeling of well-being. Patients who have had tumors surgically removed can receive deep massage throughout adjuvant therapies.

20. What is therapeutic touch?

Therapeutic touch is a systematic method for promoting healing or comfort through the use of hands. It is derived from ancient practices of laying on of hands. This healing practice, originated by Krieger,[5] involves the intentional use of the hands to direct energy to the patient. The three steps in the therapy are (1) centering oneself, letting go of busy thoughts and activities, and intending to be with the person; (2) using the hands and scanning the person's body with the hands a few inches away from the body—this scanning or assessment of the person's energy identifies for the practitioner areas of heat or cold or other differences; and (3) moving the hands over the person, a process called "unruffling," and then directing energy with the hands to places within the body that feel tense or distressed. The entire process takes 15–20 minutes. Research has shown that therapeutic touch is effective in reducing pain, relieving anxiety, reducing behavioral distress in infants and toddlers, and decreasing headache pain. For patients with cancer, therapeutic touch may be used when massage is contraindicated for the general relief of anxiety and stress and for management of pain. Nurses throughout the United States can learn therapeutic touch in nursing schools, through continuing education offerings, or from a video produced by the National League for Nursing.

21. How does the oncology nurse identify practitioners who are trained in massage and other touch therapies?

One of the best sources of referral for touch therapies is patients who have used these practitioners. Asking patients for their sources acknowledges the value of their experiences with complementary practitioners. In addition, many nurses are trained in massage and therapeutic touch, and some have private practices. They are often listed in the directories of their professional organizations. To find nurses trained in massage therapy, contact the National Association of Nurse Massage Therapists (800-336-2668). Nurses experienced in therapeutic touch are often members of the Nurse Healers-Professional Associates (412-355-8476) or the American Holistic Nurses Association (919-787-5181).

22. Are there indications for the use of music and sound therapies?

Nursing studies using music as an intervention for nausea and vomiting, pain relief, and distraction for children undergoing procedures have been reported in the literature. The positive results demonstrate the usefulness of selected music as a complementary modality. The guidelines for individualizing a music listening program include patient preferences, an environment in which the patient is minimally disturbed, use of audio headphones, and allowing a minimum of 20 minutes for listening. Other sound therapies used by individual patients include toning and listening to rhythmic drumming. Creation of music therapies is best facilitated by a music therapist.

23. What other complementary therapies are nursing interventions?

Nurses have become certified or licensed in biofeedback, hypnosis, aromatherapy, and acupressure, all of which may be considered nursing interventions. Practice issues must be addressed through the Nurse Practice Act in each state. In some states the interventions may be practiced only under the supervision of a medical doctor or alternative practitioner. Each nurse must know the regulations in his or her state.

BIBLIOGRAPHY

1. Benson H, Klipper MZ: The Relaxation Response. New York, Avon Books, 1976.
2. Cassileth BR, Chapman CC: Alternative and complementary cancer therapies. Cancer 77:1026–1034, 1995.
3. Eisenberg DM, Kessler RC, Foster C, et al: Unconventional medicine in the United States. N Engl J Med 328:246–252, 1993.
4. Fletcher DM: Unconventional cancer treatments: Professional, legal, and ethical issues. Oncol Nurs Forum 19:1351–1355, 1992.
5. Krieger, D: Accepting Your Power to Heal: The Personal Practice of Therapeutic Touch. Santa Fe, NM, Bear and Company, 1993.
6. Lerner IS, Kennedy BJ: The prevalence of questionable methods of cancer treatment in the US. Cancer 42:181–191, 1992.
7. Lerner M: Choices in Healing: Integrating the Best of Conventional and Complementary Approaches to Cancer. Cambridge, MA, MIT Press, 1994.
8. Montbriand MJ: Freedom of choice: An issue concerning alternative therapies chosen by patients with cancer. Oncol Nurs Forum 20:1195–1200, 1993.
9. Spiegel D: Psychosocial intervention in cancer. J Natl Cancer Inst 85:1198–1204, 1993.

III. Hematologic Malignancies

14. HODGKIN'S DISEASE

Elder Granger, MD, FACP

Quick Facts—Hodgkin's Disease

Incidence	In the United States, Hodgkin's disease will be diagnosed in 7500 people in 1997; < 1% of all new cancers. Rare in children under 10 years of age. Bimodal age distribution: first peak at 25–30 years (5 cases per 100,000) and second peak at 75–80 years (7 per 100,000). Sex distribution nearly equal in adults (before age 10, more frequent in males.
Mortality	Estimated 1500 deaths in 1997.
Etiology	Unknown; possibly viral.
Risk factors	Increased parental education and small family size (delayed-infection); > 90% of cases in Caucasians

Rye's Histologic Classification

TYPE	INCIDENCE (%)	PRESENTATION	PROGNOSIS
Lymphocyte-predominant	5	Healthy young male, stage I–II	Excellent
Mixed cellularity	30	Any stage, often retroperitoneum, HIV cases	Fair
Nodular sclerosis	60	Female predominance; neck or mediastinum	Good
Lymphocyte-depleted	2	Wasting syndrome, febrile, liver +, marrow +	Poor

Signs and symptoms	Asymptomatic cervical, supraclavicular, and mediastinal nodes Enlarged superficial nodes (70%) Mediastinal adenopathy (50–60%) Involvement of spleen and paraaortic nodes (25–40%) Infradiaphragmatic presentations (about 15%) Unexplained weight loss Unexplained fever with temperatures above 38.5° C (101° F) Drenching night sweats Pruritus (10–15%) Lymph node pain with alcohol ingestion (1–10%)
Metastases	Liver and bone marrow (5–10%)
Ann Arbor staging system	Stage I Involvement of single lymph node region (I) or single extralymphatic organ or site (I_E) Stage II Involvement of 2 or more lymph node regions on same side of diaphragm (II) or localized involvement of extralymphatic organ or site (II_E) Stage III Involvement of lymph node regions on both side of diaphragm (III), possibly with an extralymphatic organ or site (III_E), involvement of spleen (III_S), or both (III_{SE}) Stage IV Disseminated involvement of 1 or more extralymphatic organs, with or without associated lymph node involvement, or isolated extralymphatic organ site with distant nodal involvement All stages are subclassified as A (asymptomatic) or B (fever, night sweats, loss of > 10% of body weight).

Table continued on following page.

91

Quick Facts—Hodgkin's Disease

Treatment	Stages I, IIA		Radiation therapy
	Stages IB, IIB, IIIA, IIIA$_1$		Radiation therapy or chemotherapy
	Stages IIIA$_2$, IIIB		Chemotherapy ± radiation therapy
	Stage IVA, IVB		Chemotherapy alone
	Bulky mediastinal disease		Chemotherapy + radiation therapy
5-year	Stages I, IIA	85–95%	Stages IIIA$_2$, IIIB 60–80%
disease-free	Stages IB, IIB	80–85%	Stages IVA, IVB 30–50%
survival rate	Stages IIIA, IIIA$_1$	60–85%	

1. What is Hodgkin's disease?

Hodgkin's disease (HD) is a malignancy of unknown etiology usually arising in lymph nodes. It often affects young adults and is one of the most curable cancers. The histologic pattern and anatomic distribution vary with age. HD is a histologic diagnosis based on the recognition of multinucleated Reed-Sternberg (RS) cells surrounded by a background of benign-appearing host inflammatory cells composed of lymphocytes, plasma cells, and fibroblasts.

2. Describe a Reed-Sternberg cell.

The RS cell is considered malignant. To be diagnostic of HD, it must have two or more nuclei or nuclear lobes and two or more large nucleoli. The origin of the RS cell is unknown. In rare instances, cells resembling RS cells are found in benign illnesses and other malignancies.

3. How is Hodgkin's disease related to a viral cause?

Although the cause of HD is unknown, a viral association is implicated by occasional case clusterings, immune defects, and the presence of Epstein-Barr genome in involved lymph nodes.

4. Compare the four histologic types of HD.

Lymphocyte-predominant (nodular and diffuse). Nodular lymphocyte-predominant HD is essentially B-cell lymphoma. Most patients present with early-stage disease; systemic symptoms are infrequent (10%). The 5-year survival rate is approximately 90%.

Mixed cellularity. RS cells are rare and may be mistaken for T-cell or diffuse large cell lymphomas. It often presents in older patients with more advanced-stage disease and is most common among patients with acquired immunodeficiency syndrome (AIDS). The 5-year survival rate for all stages is 50–60%.

Nodular sclerosis. The most common histopathologic type, nodular sclerosis, is found more often in women and young adults. It is associated with the lacunar cell variant of the RS cell. Patients often present with neck or mediastinal lymphadenopathy. The incidence of systemic symptoms is about 30%. Prognosis is good, with a high 5-year survival rate.

Lymphocyte-depleted. This rare form of HD was earlier mistaken for large-cell lymphoma. It presents primarily in older patients with advanced-stage disease and has the worst prognosis of the four types. The 5-year survival rate is < 50%.

5. What are the Cotswolds staging modifications?

In 1989 an international conference in Cotswolds, England recommended the following modifications of the Ann Arbor staging system:

- Suffix X should be added to patients with bulky disease (maximal dimension of nodal mass > 10 cm or mediastinal mass > $\frac{1}{3}$ of the chest wall diameter).
- The number of anatomic regions involved should be indicated by a subscript (e.g.,II$_3$).
- A new category of response to therapy, unconfirmed/uncertain complete remission (CRu), should be used to designate patients achieving > 90% partial response with stable adenopathy.

6. What signs and symptoms are associated with HD?

Cervical, supraclavicular, and mediastinal nodes are involved in 50–70% of cases. In contrast to non-Hodgkin's lymphoma, HD can be isolated and exhibits more orderly or contiguous lymph node spread. Generalized pruritus occurs in 10–15% of the cases and lymph node pain with alcohol ingestion in 1–10% of the cases. Patients also may be anergic (i.e., they do not react to normal skin antigens). B symptoms (indicative of larger tumor burden) consist of unexplained loss of > 10% of body weight in the previous 6 months, unexplained fever with temperatures above 38.5° C (101° F), and drenching night sweats. Common laboratory findings include elevated sedimentation rate and elevated levels of alkaline phosphatase.

7. What are the poor prognostic factors in HD?

The stage or extent of disease is the most important prognostic variable. Other factors indicative of a poorer prognosis include bone marrow, lung, or liver involvement; bulky disease (nodal diameter > 10 cm); B symptoms; high erythrocyte sedimentation rate; low hematocrit and high lactate dehydrogenase (higher rate of relapse); large mediastinal mass; and age over 65 years. Extensive splenic involvement has a poor prognosis if treated with primary irradiation. Elderly patients tend to present with more advanced stages, a worse prognostic histology, and other medical problems that cause difficulty in tolerating chemotherapy.

8. How is the diagnosis of HD usually established?

In addition to adequate surgical biopsy of involved tissue, the following procedures for staging are recommended:

- Detailed history recording duration and presence or absence of B symptoms and unexplained pruritus
- Detailed physical examination with special attention to all node-bearing areas
- Radiologic studies: chest radiograph; computed tomography (CT) of thorax, abdomen, and pelvis; bipedal lymphangiogram optional.
- Hematologic studies: complete blood count (CBC); erythrocyte sedimentation rate; bilateral bone marrow biopsy
- Biochemistry: liver function tests; renal function test; serum lactate dehydrogenase (LDH), albumin, calcium, and alkaline phosphatase
- Other procedures: gallium and technetium isotope scanning; multiple-gated acquisition blood-pool scan (MUGA); magnetic resonance imaging (MRI); laparotomy

9. How does stage affect treatment choice?

Radiation therapy is highly effective for early-stage disease, whereas chemotherapy is more effective for late-stage disease.

10. When is staging laparotomy indicated?

Diagnostic staging laparotomy is indicated only if the findings will significantly alter therapy. Staging laparotomy is generally indicated for stage I and stage II patients who are candidates for radiotherapy alone. Laparotomy alters clinical staging in about one-fourth to one-third of patients, of whom two-thirds will be upstaged and one-third downstaged.

The risk of abdominal involvement is < 10% in (1) women with clinical stage I disease, (2) patients with clinical stage I disease and mediastinal disease only, (3) men with clinical stage I disease and lymphocyte-predominant histology, and (4) women with clinical stage II disease younger than 27 years with 2–3 sites of involvement. High risk factors for below-the-diaphragm disease include involvement of four or more nodal sites above the diaphragm, hilar or extramediastinal extension, large mediastinal mass (> $\frac{1}{3}$ of the diameter of the chest), or B symptoms. At surgery the spleen is removed; needle and wedge biopsies of the right and left lobes of the liver, and samples of multiple lymph groups are obtained. If not already done, a bilateral bone marrow biopsy is obtained.

11. How is HD treated?

More than 75% of cases are curable, and more than 50% of recurrent disease after primary therapy can be cured. HD responds to radiation therapy alone, combination chemotherapy, or combined treatment with radiation and chemotherapy.

12. What chemotherapy regimens are effective in treating HD?

The most common regimens are MOPP and ABVD (see table). Each regimen is given over 28 days, and most patients receive 6 cycles. If tumor burden is reduced between the fourth and sixth cycles, two more cycles are given. Patients are treated over 6–12 months (2 months after complete remission). Both regimens have similar therapeutic results. Variations of these regimens include MOPP/ABV hybrid and alternating MOPP/ABVD.

Chemotherapy for Hodgkin's Disease

DRUGS	DOSE (MG/M^2)	ROUTE	DAYS
MOPP			
Mechlorethamine (nitrogen mustard)	6	IV	1, 8
Oncovin (vincristine)	1.4	IV	1, 8
Procarbazine	100	PO	1–14
Prednisone	40	PO	1–14
ABVD			
Adriamycin (doxorubicin)	25	IV	1, 15
Bleomycin	10	IV	1, 15
Vinblastine	6	IV	1, 15
Dacarbazine	375	IV	1, 15

IV = intravenously, PO = orally.

13. Discuss the common complications of chemotherapy.

Complications and side effects include nausea, vomiting, alopecia, sterility in men and women, myelosuppression, neuropathy, cardiomyopathy, and aseptic necrosis of femoral heads (related to prednisone). Although secondary malignancies (acute nonlymphocytic leukemia and non-Hodgkin's lymphoma) are associated with chemotherapy alone, they are more common after radiation plus chemotherapy. ABVD causes leukemia less frequently and is better for preserving fertility than MOPP; however, it is associated with more cardiac and pulmonary toxicity.

14. What is the most common complication of radiation therapy?

Hypothyroidism is the most common complication as a consequence of mantle radiation therapy. It can be treated with replacement therapy. Other complications include myelosuppression, pericarditis, pneumonitis, myelopathy, and transient aspermia. Secondary cancers related to radiation therapy include solid tumors (e.g., breast, thyroid cancer), sarcomas, and salivary and skin cancers.

15. What is Lhermitte's syndrome?

From 6–12 weeks after mantle radiation therapy, approximately 15% of patients develop a shocklike sensation radiating down the back of the extremities when the head is flexed. This is due to radiation causing temporary demyelinization of the spinal cord. The symptoms resolve spontaneously and do not cause any permanent neurologic damage.

16. What is the role of bone marrow transplantation in the present and future treatment of HD?

The results of clinical studies of autologous bone marrow transplantation vary because of its uses as salvage therapy for diverse patient populations. Multiple studies have shown complete remission rates of 40–70%, with a 5-year relapse-free survival rate of 20–40%. Further studies are currently being conducted to identify high-risk patients who may benefit from bone marrow transplantation after their first remission. Peripheral blood stem cells can be used instead of autologous bone marrow for patients with inadequate marrow.

17. Discuss the most important nursing considerations in caring for patients with HD.

In addition to providing patient education and coping support through a long and highly toxic regimen of primary therapy, nurses need to pay particular attention to providing information about potential long-term effects and development of secondary cancers and to explaining the prolonged period of appropriate follow-up for possible recurrence after therapy. The patient must understand that a small foci of Hodgkin's disease may cause no symptoms but still lead to relapse or recurrence. All members of the multidisciplinary team should be sensitive to the patient's fear of recurrence. The patient may interpret every word or facial expression of the treatment team as a likely clue that the Hodgkin's disease has recurred. The risk of relapse is greatest within the first 2 years and decreases with time. Follow-up should include physical examinations, chest radiographs, and appropriate blood work (e.g. LDH, CBC, alkaline phosphatase) every 2–3 months for the first two years, every 4–6 months for the third and fourth years, and then annually. Generally, patients are considered cured if they remain in remission for 10 years.

18. What is the effect of pregnancy on HD? Of HD on pregnancy?

Pregnancy has no documented adverse effect on the natural history of HD, and HD has no effect on the course of gestation, delivery, or incidence of prematurity or spontaneous abortions. The management of HD during pregnancy must be individualized. Therapeutic abortion is not mandatory, and many patients have been successfully treated while pregnant with no adverse effect on the fetus. A therapeutic abortion may be medically indicated if treatment with chemotherapy or irradiation is required because of evidence of rapid disease progression, visceral involvement, or systemic symptoms. If treatment cannot be delayed, modified supradiaphragmatic irradiation or chemotherapy with vinblastine can be used safely.

19. Are patients with AIDS at increased risk of developing HD?

HIV-positive patients are at increased risk of developing HD and usually present with aggressive, advanced-stage disease and B symptoms. Treatment with standard chemotherapy may produce long-term remissions. The overall survival rate is decreased by AIDS-related complications and refractory disease.

20. Discuss future directions for HD.

Investigations are being conducted for administration of less toxic regimens, use of biologic response modifiers, and administration of high-dose chemotherapy with bone marrow transplantation.

The views expressed in this chapter are those of the author and do not necessarily reflect the views of the Department of Defense or any of its agencies.

BIBLIOGRAPHY

1. Beahrs OH, Henson DE, Hutter RVP, Kennedy BJ: American Joint Committee on Cancer: Manual for Staging of Cancer, 4th ed. 1992, pp 253–255.
2. Brain MC, Carbone PP (eds): Current Therapy in Hematology-Oncology, 5th ed. St. Louis, Mosby, 1995.
3. Canellos G, Anderson JR, Propert KJ, et al: Chemotherapy of advanced Hodgkin's disease with MOPP, ABVD, or MOPP alternating with ABVD. N Engl J Med 327:1478–1484, 1992.
4. DeVita VT, Hellman S, Rosenberg SA (eds): Cancer: Principles and Practice of Oncology, 5th ed. Philadelphia, J.B. Lippincott, 1997.
5. Kennedy BJ: Hodgkin's disease. Cancer 43:325–346, 1993.
6. Murphy GP, Lawrence W, Lenhard RE: Hodgkin's disease and non-Hodgkin's lymphomas. In American Cancer Society Textbook of Clinical Oncology, 2nd ed. 1995, pp 451–469.
7. Parker SL, Tong T, Bolden S, Wingo PA: Cancer Statistics, 1997. CA Cancer J Clin 47:5–27, 1997.
8. Prior E, Goldberg AF, Conjalka MS, et al: Hodgkin's disease in homosexual men: An AIDS-related phenomenon? Am J Med 81:1085–1088, 1986.
9. Rubin P, McDonald S, Qazi R: Clinical Oncology: A Multidisciplinary Approach for Physicians and Students, 7th ed. 1993, pp 217–239.
10. Vose JM, Bierman PJ, Armitage JO: Hodgkin's disease: The role of bone marrow transplantation. Semin Oncol 8:749–757, 1990.
11. Ward FT, Weiss RB: Lymphoma and pregnancy. Semin Oncol 16:397–409, 1989.
12. Williams SF, Farah R, Golomb HM: Hodgkin's disease. Hematol Oncol Clin North Am 3, 1989.

15. LEUKEMIA

Libby Tracey, RN, PhD(c), OCN, and Scott Kruger, MD

ACUTE LEUKEMIA

Quick Facts

Incidence	Hematopoietic malignancies account for 6–8% of all new cancers diagnosed annually. An estimated 35,500 new cases of all leukemias will be reported in the United States in 1997; of these, 9200 are **acute myelocytic leukemia (AML)** (2.3/100,000 people). and 3000 are **acute lymphocytic leukemia (ALL)** (1.5/100,000 people).
Mortality	In 1997 there will be an estimated 34,000 deaths from all forms of leukemia—6300 from AML and 1410 from ALL.
Etiology and risk factors	• Ionizing radiation exposure (atomic bomb survivors) • Prolonged exposure to benzene (workers in rubber and shoe leather industries) and petroleum products with a 10–30-year interval between exposure and onset of disease • Chromosomal abnormalities • Cigarette smoking • Prior chemotherapy with alkylating agents and prolonged therapy with epipodophyllotoxins • Genetic disorders such as Down's syndrome, autosomal recessive syndromes such as Bloom's and Fanconi's anemia, and ataxia-telangiectasia • Diseases of the bone marrow—polycythemia vera, paroxysmal nocturnal hemoglobinuria, myelodysplastic diseases, aplastic anemia • Retroviruses (adult T-cell leukemia and hairy cell leukemia)
Survival	**AML:** fatal within months if untreated; with aggressive therapy, 70–80% achieve remission and 25–30% are cured. **ALL:** fatal within months if untreated; with aggressive therapy, 80–90% achieve remission and 70–80% are cured.
Signs and symptoms	• Life-threatening panctyopenia manifested as fatigue, pallor, dyspnea, fevers, infection, petechiae, bruising, and mucosal bleeding • Mental status changes as a result of leukocytosis • Cranial nerve palsies, priapism, dyspnea, and chest pain from tumor emboli • Soft tissue tumors consisting of collections of leukemic cells (granulocytic sarcomas or chloromas) • Monocytic leukemia: 50% of patients have gingival hypertrophy or skin infiltration (leukemia cutis) • Increased risk of central nervous system disease presenting with headache, diplopia, cranial nerve palsies, and mental status changes • Hyperuricemia with kidney obstruction • Coagulopathy and disseminated intravascular coagulation (DIC) presenting with bleeding and thrombocytopenia • Common symptoms in children: bone pain, hepatomegaly, splenomegaly, lymphadenopathy, and testicular swelling (ALL)
Classification	**French-American-British (FAB) Classification** of acute leukemias

	AML	M0	Undifferentiated
		M1	Myeloblastic without differentiation
		M2	Myeloblastic with differentiation
		M3	Acute hypergranular promyelocytic leukemia
		M3v	Micro or hypogranular promyelocytic leukemia

Table continued on following page.

	M4	Myelomonocytic leukemia
	M4Eo	Myelomonocytic with abnormal eosinophilia
	M5	Acute monocytic, poorly differentiated
	M5a	Monocytic with > 80% monoblasts
	M5b	Monocytic with > 20% promonocytes and monocytes
	M6	Erythroblastic leukemia
	M7	Megakaryoblastic leukemia
ALL	L1	Lymphoblastic leukemia (homogeneous common childhood variant)
	L2	Lymphoblastic leukemia (heterogeneous common adult variant)
	L3	B-cell lymphoblastic (rare; similar to Burkitt's leukemia)

1. What is leukemia?

Leukemia was first described in 1889 as a disease with too many white blood cells in the blood. It is now defined as a cancer of the blood-forming elements and is identified by the type and stage of maturity of the affected blood cell. The diseased cells can be either white blood cells (lymphocytes or granular cells of myeloid origin, which mature and make neutrophils, eosinophils, or basophils), red blood cells, or megakaryocytes (which make platelets). The FAB cooperative group classifies AML into three main groups according to the predominant cell type: granulocytic (M1, M2, M3), monocytic (M4, M5), and erythroid (M6). The abnormal clones of cells interfere with the ability of the normal bone marrow to make healthy cells, resulting in depression of normal cellular elements of bone marrow. This puts the patient at risk for fatigue, bleeding, and infections.

2. What is the difference between acute and chronic leukemia?

Acute leukemia is a disease of early precursors or immature cells (blasts), whereas **chronic leukemia** is a disease of more mature (differentiated) and functioning cells. Before effective therapy was available, patients with acute leukemia died within several weeks, whereas patients with chronic leukemia lived for many years.

3. Is leukemia hereditary?

Although the direct cause of leukemia is unknown, there are several genetic links. There is recognized risk for cancer development in families with two or three cases in two or more generations and increased incidence of leukemia in twins and siblings. This increased risk does not necessarily mean that leukemia will occur in subsequent generations. Other hereditary or congenital disorders associated with leukemia include Down's syndrome (alterations of chromosome 21), Fanconi's anemia, and Bloom's syndrome.

4. What age groups are most commonly associated with leukemia?

AML, also referred to as acute nonlymphocytic leukemia (ANNL), is usually an adult disease representing 80% of the adult leukemias, presenting after age 40. It is also the predominant form of leukemia in the neonatal period. Fifteen percent of acute leukemias in children are ANLL.

ALL represents 85% of acute leukemias in children and is the most common malignancy of childhood. A specific incidence peak is observed between the ages of 2–4 years, with a second peak in mid-life in adults.

In contrast with acute leukemias, chronic leukemia usually occurs after the age of 30. Juvenile chronic myelocytic leukemia (CML) is an exception, occurring predominantly in white males.

5. Discuss the common presenting symptoms of leukemia.

Symptoms result from effects on the hematopoietic system. Patients complain of fatigue, weakness, bruising, bleeding from gums, or nosebleeds. Frequently patients present with an infection and fever. The diagnosis is not suspected until a complete blood count (CBC) is done. Common constitutional symptoms include generalized malaise, dyspnea, bone pain, and weight loss. Infiltration of the leukemic cells sometimes results in swollen gums, testicular swelling, hepatosplenomegaly, and lymphadenopathy (ALL). Mental status changes, cranial nerve palsies, seizures, priapism, and respiratory failure are associated with leukostasis.

6. What are the common abnormal laboratory findings in acute leukemia?
- Varying degrees of anemia, thrombocytopenia, and neutropenia (< 1000/μl in half of patients at presentation) or pancytopenia
- Hyperuricemia and elevated lactic dehydrogenase (LDH) due to rapid cell turnover
- Abnormal coagulation profiles indicative of DIC
- Abnormal cerebrospinal fluid in patients with leptomeningeal disease (elevated protein with abnormal cytology)

7. How is leukemia diagnosed?
Patients usually present with an abnormal blood count. Review of the peripheral smear may show immature cells called blasts. Microscopic cytochemical stains and immunophenotypic markers help to determine whether the blasts are of myeloid or lymphoid origin. This distinction is important because the treatment is different for ANLL and ALL. Sometimes one can see specific abnormal cells in the blood, which help to establish the diagnosis (cells with Auer rods are seen in AML).

Bone marrow aspiration and biopsy are performed to make the definitive diagnosis. Bone marrow with 30% or more blasts establishes the diagnosis of leukemia. The aspirate reveals cell morphology, and the biopsy is examined for marrow cellularity. The diagnosis of AML (M1–M5) is identified by at least 30% blasts (> 30% of all nucleated red blood cells) in the bone marrow. Erythroleukemia (M6) is diagnosed if erythroblasts make up > 50% of the nucleated bone marrow cells. Cytochemical stains and immunologic marker studies help to determine the type of leukemia. Chromosome analysis is also useful; for example, ALL with hyperdiploidy (extra chromosomes) and CALLA antigen (common acute lymphoblastic leukemia antigen) is a favorable prognostic sign, whereas multiple translocations or deletions are unfavorable.

8. What are the staining characteristics of acute nonlymphoblastic leukemia?
Leukemia may be characterized by flow cytometry and cytochemical staining methods. In AML (M1–M4) the myeloid blasts stain positive with myeloperoxidase and Sudan black, monocytic cells (M5–M6) stain with nonspecific esterase, while tdt is a fluorescent stain that marks lymphoblasts.

9. How do flow cytometry and immunophenotyping help in establishing a diagnosis of leukemia?
Flow cytometry is a machine that uses laser light to identify cell surface markers. Cells are labeled with antibodies directed at different antigens (monoclonal antibodies) specific for leukemia. A panel of CD (designated cluster groups of differentiation) antigens is mixed with the cells. When a laser light hits the cells with bound antigen, a fluorescent color is produced. The fluorescent cells are counted, and their percentage relative to the total number of cells is calculated. This information is useful to refine rather than to make the diagnosis. As depicted in the chart, AML is characterized by MABs directed at CD13, CD33, and CD15 (monoclonal myeloid markers); C14 (monoclonal monocytic marker); CD34 (monoclonal marker for precursor cells); and human leukocyte antigen (HLA-DR). CD41 is a monoclonal marker for megakaryocytes.

	M0	M1	M2	M3	M4	M5	M6	M7
HLA DR	0	+	+	0	+	+	+	+
CD34	+	+	0	0	0	0	0	+
CD13	+	+	+	+	+	+	0	0
CD33	+	+	+	+	+	+	0	0
CD15	0	0	+	+/0	+	+	0	0
CD14	0	0	0	0	+	+	0	0
CD41	0	0	0	0	0	0	0	+

10. Discuss the common cytogenetic abnormalities and their implications for prognosis.

Cytogenetics (analysis of a cell's chromosomal pattern) helps to confirm a diagnosis, to evaluate prognosis, to identify chemotherapy resistance, and to detect minimal residual disease. Abnormalities may be expressed as losses (–), gains (+), deletions (del), or translocations (t). Deletion refers to partial chromatin loss from a single chromosome. Translocation refers to chromatin exchange between different chromosomes. Approximately 60–90% of patients with AML have cytogenetic abnormalities that may have prognostic significance. For example, M4Eo with inv(16) and M2 with t(8;21) are associated with good prognosis and higher cure rate. Trisomy of chromosome 8 or deletions or losses of chromosomes 5 or 7 are related to poorer prognosis.

11. What factors are related to the prognosis of acute leukemia?

- Older patients and patients with comorbid illness do worse.
- Cytogenetic abnormalities, especially deletions and translocations, are usually a poor prognostic variable; e.g., presence of Philadelphia chromosome t(9;22).
- Hyperdiploidy and CALLA antigen are favorable variables in ALL; in AML t(15,17), t(8,21) and inv (16) are good prognostic variables
- Elevated white blood cell counts are a poor prognostic variable, especially counts > 50,000.
- Sepsis at the time of presentation is a negative variable.
- CNS involvement is a negative variable.
- Leukemia arising from a myelodysplastic syndrome is difficult to treat; most patients die even with aggressive therapy.

12. What is myelodysplasia?

Myelodysplasia is a group of bone marrow diseases also involving the stem cells. They are sometimes referred to as "preleukemias" because eventually many patients progress to acute leukemia. Varying amounts of bone marrow abnormalities result in progressive anemia, thrombocytopenia, and leukopenia. Some patients may have pancytopenia, resulting in the regular need for transfusion of blood products. Many patients benefit from growth factors such as erythropoietin and granulocyte colony-stimulating factor (G-CSF), which help to raise blood counts and to decrease transfusion requirements. When using growth factors, one must be careful that the blast count does not rise and cause the disease to progress to acute leukemia. Usually stopping the growth factor reverts the disease into the preleukemic state. Acute leukemia has 30% or more blasts in the marrow; myelodysplasia has 5–29%; and normal bone marrow has 5% or less blasts.

13. How are myelodysplastic diseases treated?

Patients with myelodysplastic diseases may live for several months or even years with supportive care, including transfusion therapy and antibiotics. Platelet infusions are used to treat clinical bleeding. Androgens (Danazol) sometimes are useful for treatment of anemia and thrombocytopenia. Corticosteroids such as prednisone may improve cell counts in some patients but also increase the risk of infection. Conventional antileukemic chemotherapy may induce short remissions, but treatment complications are high, including a death rate of 25–40%. Because most patients are elderly, one must weigh the risk:benefit ratio before considering aggressive chemotherapy. Bone marrow transplantation is considered for younger patients with suitable donors. A new agent that shows promise in refractory anemia with excessive blasts and CMML is topotecan. Some patients also benefit from growth factors (erythropoietin, G-CSF), which may decrease transfusion requirements.

14. Define secondary leukemia and therapy-related leukemia.

Secondary leukemia results from a preexisting condition such as myelodysplasia or Down's syndrome. Therapy-related leukemia is a special kind of secondary leukemia, associated with the following:

Alkylating agents used to treat cancer or immunologic diseases
- Melphalan (most leukemogenic), followed by cyclophosphamide and nitrogen mustard
- Long-term daily drug exposure (greatest risk)
- Concurrent radiation exposure

Topoisomerase II inhibitors
- Etoposide, teniposide, doxorubicin, daunorubicin, and mitoxantrone
- Cytogenetic abnormalities of 11p23 or 21q22
- Absence of myelodysplasia before onset of leukemia

15. Why is acute promyelocytic leukemia (APL) distinct from other subtypes of AML?

M3 promyelocytic leukemia is frequently associated with disseminated intravascular co-agulopathy (DIC). The granules of the promyelocytes release procoagulants, which consume clotting factor and platelets. Low-dose heparin is sometimes used to control DIC by stopping the consumption of coagulation factors. Patients who are bleeding are given platelets and fresh frozen plasma. Chemotherapy to kill the promyelocytes is necessary because heparin and transfusion support only buy time until the disease can be controlled.

16. How is APL treated? When is transretinoic acid used?

The characteristic 15;17 gene translocation in M3 APL has led to a unique treatment option for APL. The translocation of genes fuses the retinoic acid receptor alpha gene on chromosome 17 with the promyelocytic leukemia gene on chromosome 15. Transretinoic acid has been shown to cause the tumor cells to differentiate, which offers the advantage of a shorter period of neu-tropenia with normalization of the marrow and cytogenetics in 30–60 days.

17. What is retinoic acid syndrome?

About 25% of patients develop a syndrome of fever, pulmonary infiltrates and severe dysp-nea, pleural effusions, and cardiovascular collapse associated with transretinoic acid treatment. Many patients develop leukocytosis with white blood cell counts > 100,000. Treatment involves temporary discontinuation of the drug, corticosteroids, and initiation of a cytoreductive agent, such as hydroxyurea or conventional chemotherapy, to control the leukocytosis.

18. What does remission mean in acute leukemia?

Remission means that bone marrow function returns to normal with no evidence of the leukemic clone (blast cells < 5%), normal myeloid-to-erythroid ratio, adequate platelets, and peripheral blood counts with hemoglobin concentration >12 gm/dl, granulocyte count > 2000/μl, and platelet count > 100,000/μl. Any chromosomal abnormalities should no longer be present.

19. Explain induction treatment for AML.

Cytarabine (Ara-C) and an anthracycline (idarubicin or daunorubicin) are used to induce re-mission. The rate of complete remission is 55–70%. Many physicians do weekly bone marrow examination from day 14 to evaluate the response to chemotherapy. If on day 14 the marrow is not clear, patients may receive another dose of therapy.

Example of induction therapy:
Ara-C 100 mg/m^2 by continuous infusion for 7 days
and
Idarubicin, 12 mg/m^2 by slow intravenous push on days 1,2, and 3*
If a second cycle is needed on day 14:
Ara-C 100 mg/m2 by continuous infusion for 5 days
and
Idarubicin 12 mg/m^2 by slow intravenous push for 2 days*
* Some physicians substitute daunorubicin, 45 mg/m^2, and reduce dose to 30 mg/m^2 in elderly patients.

20. How is the CNS treated in AML?

CNS treatment is recommended for patients with disease or patients at high risk for disease (white blood cell count > 50,000 or M4 and M5 disease). Choices for treatment include high-dose cytarabine (3 gm/m^2), which crosses the blood-brain barrier, or intrathecal methotrexate or cytarabine.

21. What is consolidation therapy of AML?

Once remission of AML is achieved, consolidation therapy is required. Use of a higher dose of chemotherapy than during induction is sometimes called intensification therapy. Usually at least 2 cycles are given after remission therapy. Maintenance therapy (many months to years of chronic chemotherapy) is not needed. In adults 5-year survival rates range from 15–30%.

Example of consolidation therapy:

Ara-C 3 gm/m^2 every 12 hours intravenously as a 3-hour infusion for 6 doses

or

Ara-C 200 mg/m^2 by continuous infusion for 5 days

and

Idarubicin 12 mg/m^2 by slow intravenous push for 2 doses

Each cycle is repeated every 28 days.

22. What is the treatment for relapsed AML?

Treatment of relapsed or refractory AML involves drugs such as mitoxantrone, etoposide, carboplatin, and amsacrine. Newer approaches include cyclosporin to block multiple-drug resistance (MDR) gene expression and to prevent efflux of the therapeutic agent from the cell. Antibody-targeted therapy and toxins such as ricin are under study. Bone marrow transplant also may be used for salvage therapy. In general, each subsequent remission is shorter in duration than the previous one.

Example of relapse therapy for AML:

Ara-C 3 gm/m^2 every 12 hours as a 3-hour infusion for 8 doses

and

Mitoxantrone 12 mg/m^2 by slow intravenous push for 3 days

or

Etoposide 100 mg/m^2 by intravenous infusion over 2 hours for 5 days

23. Can induction therapy be administered in the outpatient setting?

Most patients are hospitalized for several weeks during induction therapy; consolidation and maintenance therapy are given in the outpatient setting. However, patients with uncomplicated acute leukemia or uncomplicated neutropenic sepsis may be treated completely on an outpatient basis for induction, consolidation, and maintenance therapy. Patients need to live close to the hospital and must be seen daily (including weekends) for physical assessment, blood counts, and antibiotic and transfusion needs. The major criterion for admission is severe neutropenia and complicated sepsis characterized by extremely high fevers, hypotension, and cardiovascular compromise.

24. What is the role of hematopoietic growth factors in leukemia?

Growth factor support in the treatment of leukemia is controversial. The concern is that growth factors may stimulate the growth of the leukemic clone. Growth factors are sometimes used in patients with sepsis or prolonged bone marrow aplasia.

25. What is a blast crisis?

Peripheral blast counts > 50,000–100,000/μl may result in impaired blood flow and leukostasis because large and "sticky" blasts plug arterioles and infiltrate local perivascular tissue. Brain or lung leukostasis may be fatal. Leukostasis occurs most commonly in patients with ALL. A medical emergency requiring immediate treatment is indicated by the following symptoms: headache (increased intracranial pressure), altered mental status, dyspnea, and priapism.

26. What is the treatment for blast crisis?

Treatment options depend on the type of leukemia and the severity of the illness. Hydrea in large doses destroys myeloblasts. Corticosteroids in high doses destroy lymphoblasts. Immediate treatment consists of leukopheresis to remove the abnormal white blood cells from the blood and radiation therapy to treat brain or severe pulmonary compromise. High doses of chemotherapy are used to decrease the blast cell burden.

27. What is the treatment for ALL?

Patients undergo induction therapy to place them in clinical remission. After remission is obtained, patients receive consolidation treatment consisting of 3–8 cycles of chemotherapy with non–cross-resistant drugs. Patients also receive CNS prophylaxis with radiation and/or intrathecal chemotherapy. They are then placed on a maintenance regimen for 2–3 years.

Treatment for ALL: Linker Regimen

1. Induction
   Vincristine 2 mg intravenously on days 1, 8, 15, and 22
   Daunorubicin 50 mg/m^2 on days 1, 2, and 3
   Prednisone 60 mg/m^2 on days 1–28
   L-Asparginase 6000 U/m^2 intramuscularly on days 17 and 28
2. In patients with residual leukemia on day 28:
   Vincristine 2 mg intravenously on days 29 and 36
   Daunorubicin 50 mg/m^2 on days 29 and 30
   Prednisone 60 mg/m^2 days 29–42
   L-Asparginase 6000 U/m^2 intramuscularly on days 29–35
3. Consolidation
   A (cycles 1, 3, 5, and 7)
   Vincristine 2 mg intravenously on days 1 and 8
   Daunorubicin 50 mg/m^2 on days 1 and 2
   Prednisone 60 mg/m^2 on days 1–14
   L-Asparginase 12,000 U/m^2 intramuscularly on days 2, 4, 7, 9, 11, 12, 13, and 14
   B (cycles 2, 4, 6, and 8)
   Ara-C 300 mg/m^2 by intravenous piggyback on days 1, 4, 8, and 11
   Teniposide 165 mg/m^2 on days 1, 4, 8, and 11
   C (cycle 9)
   Methotrexate 690 mg/m^2 by continuous infusion for 42 hours
   Leucovorin 15 mg/m^2 intravenously every 6 hours for 12 doses after methotrexate, beginning at hour 42
4. Central nervous system prophylaxis (weeks 5–7)
   Radiation therapy, 1800 Gy
   Methotrexate 12 mg intrathecally each week for 6 weeks
5. Maintenance (begin after cycle C until week 130)
   6-Mercaptopurine 75 mg/m^2/day orally
   Methotrexate 20 mg orally each week

28. What is the most useful index of infection risk in patients with leukemia?

Infection is the leading cause of death in patients with leukemia and lymphoma. The risk rises as the granulocyte count drops below 1000/mm^3, and the incidence of infection increases dramatically as the count drops below 500/mm^3. A rapidly declining granulocyte count, compared with a more gradual decline, is associated with a higher risk of infection. Because of the low granulocyte count, patients may not have the usual signs of infection such as fever, erythema, or pus. A careful physical examination with particular attention to catheter exit sites, surgical wounds, and the perineal region is necessary. A high index of clinical suspicion warrants cultures and empiric antibiotic therapy.

29. What are the sources of infecting organisms?

Endogenous organisms colonize sites inside the body, such as the nose, alimentary tract, and upper respiratory tract. Gram-positive infection has become more common because of the insertion of indwelling catheters such as Hickman or Broviac catheters. **Exogenous organisms** may come from the five F's: food, fingers, feces, flies, and fomites (inanimate transmission). Flowers, including water in vases, and plants harbor *Pseudomonas aeruginosa*.

30. What precautions are appropriate in neutropenic patients?

Patients with absolute granulocyte counts < 1000 are at increased risk of developing infection. All people who come in contact with the patient must wash their hands, and anyone who is sick should wear a mask or not be allowed contact with the patient. Most institutions do not require visitors to wear masks. Patients should avoid all fresh fruits and vegetables, and all foods should be cooked to avoid bacterial contamination. Patients should practice exceptionally careful personal hygiene to decrease the risk of infections.

31. What are the common causative organisms and sites of infection in neutropenic patients?

Myelosuppressed patients are most prone to gram-negative sepsis from organisms such as *Escherichia coli*, *Pseudomonas* sp., and *Klebsiella* sp., which are normal body flora. Meticulous body hygiene is important because infections may be self-induced.

Site	Organisms
Skin	*Staphylococcus aureus, Pseudomonas aeruginosa, Klebsiella pneumoniae, Escherichia coli,* herpes zoster
Pharynx	*S. aureus,* gram-negative bacilli, *Candida albicans*
Mouth and esophagus	*C. albicans,* herpes simplex, cytomegalovirus, gram-negative bacilli
Lungs	*P. aeruginosa, E. coli, S. aureus, Aspergillus flavus, A. fumigatus, Pneumocystis carinii*
Urinary tract	*E. coli, K. pneumoniae, P. aeruginosa*
Perianal region	*Bacteroides* sp., *K. pneumoniae, E. coli, P. aeruginosa*

32. What precautions are appropriate in thrombocytopenic patients?

Patients with platelet counts of < 10,000 to 20,000 are at risk for spontaneous bleeding (e.g., CNS bleed). The risk is greatest for counts < 5,000 or with a rapid fall in platelet count. Prophylactic platelet transfusions may be given for counts between 10,000 and 20,000. During induction therapy in adult acute leukemic patients, prophylactic platelet transfusions given for a platelet count threshold of ≤ 10,000 compared with ≤ 20,000 reduce total platelet utilization with only a minor adverse effect on bleeding with no statistically significant effect on morbidity. (The ≤ 10,000 platelet count threshold may be applied to other patient groups so long as they do not have bleeding predispositions related to coagulation or anatomic abnormalities.) Treatments to decrease the risk for bleeding include H_2 blockers such as Zantac, stool softeners, aggressive control of nausea/vomiting, and hormonal manipulation in women to stop menses. Drugs that impair platelet function and invasive procedures or treatments should be avoided (e.g., intramuscular injections, rectal medications/enemas, rectal temperatures).

33. What sexual modifications should be considered by patients undergoing treatment for leukemia?

Sexual contact is not dangerous for the patient. Certain modifications need to be made during intercourse based on blood count. For example, if the white cell count is below normal, sexual intercourse should be avoided until the granulocyte count is > 1,000. Both partners should carefully cleanse the genital area (e.g., with bacteriostatic soap) to avoid infection even when the blood count is acceptable. Proper lubrication and avoidance of excessive friction decrease the possibility of bleeding if the platelet count is low. If the partner has any evidence of genital infection, it is best to check with the doctor first to discuss ways of reducing chances of transmission.

Birth control is essential to prevent pregnancy. Birth control pills and condoms should be used at all times. Pregnancy should be avoided until 1 year after all treatment has stopped to decrease the risk of teratogenesis to the fetus.

34. Discuss important nursing interventions for patients with leukemia.

Leukemic patients require the complete range of supportive oncology nursing care interventions. Assessment and early detection of complications or side effects of the disease and therapy are particularly critical, as is administration of chemotherapy, blood components, antibiotics, antifungals, and symptom control therapy. The nurse must also offer creating coping strategies and address the many psychosocial concerns faced by patients with a potentially fatal disease. Patients may be referred to the Leukemia Society of America (800-955-4LSA), a national voluntary health agency that offers patient support groups, financial assistance, professional educational programs, and research grants. Common symptoms and nursing care are listed below:

Symptoms	*Nursing Care*
General health Leukemic patients often complain of weakness, poor appetite and weight loss. Myelosuppression results in persistent infection, low-grade or high fever, chills, bleeding tendencies, and fatigue. Psychosocial concerns include fear and anxiety, body image and self-esteem changes, sensory/perceptual alterations during reverse isolation, disruption of relationships, etc.	1. Instruct patient and significant others about chemotherapy and potential side effects, complications of myelosuppression and how to prevent infections and bleeding, venous access device care, body image changes (e.g., alopecia), sexual concerns, anticipated length of treatment and hospitalization, and ways to cope.
Head and neck Mouth sores and bleeding from gums, mouth, and nose are common problems. As a result of bleeding into the sclera of the eyes, the whites of the eyes may be pink or red. This condition is normally not painful. Infections and swollen lymph glands may cause neck discomfort.	2. Institute neutropenic precautions. *Good handwashing is the single most effective way to prevent infection.* 3. Examine patient daily from head to toe, with particular attention to skin and venous access sites for signs of infection and bleeding.
Cardiopulmonary system Blood in sputum may result from infection or platelet reduction. Respiratory distress and shortness of breath may result from infection (e.g., pneumonia) or anemia with decreased oxygenation. Rapid heartbeat may result from infection.	4. Encourage or assist patient to shower daily. Instruct and assist patient to practice meticulous oral and personal hygiene. Administer antibiotics, antivirals, and antifungals as needed. 5. Help patients to conserve energy and ensure adequate sleep and rest. Recommend sleeping aids as needed. Administer red blood cells as needed.
Gastrointestinal tract GI bleeding may be visible or hidden, in vomitus or from the rectum. Perirectal lesions may give rise to discomfort, with delayed healing and possible infection. Diarrhea, a side effect of chemotherapy, may cause irritation or excoriation of the rectal area.	6. Assess for bleeding and petechiae, particularly in mouth, sclera, rectum, and vagina. Institute thrombocytopenic precautions. Give stool softeners, sitz baths, platelets (as ordered). Apply topical thrombin to bleeding sites as indicated. 7. Assess for changes in mental status or complaints of headache.
Genitourinary tract Signs of bleeding may develop (e.g., vaginal bleeding or blood in urine). Urinary tract infection may be seen.	8. Monitor vital signs for sepsis and changes in cardiopulmonary status. 9. Monitor urine output, serum electrolytes, blood urea nitrogen, creatinine, complete blood counts, prothrombin time, partial thromboplastin time, and fibrinogen.
Musculoskeletal system Patients may present with symptoms of arthralgia and/or sternal pain caused by excessive numbers of white cells packing the bone marrow. Uric acid levels may be elevated, resulting in goutlike pain, especially in the joints.	10. Ensure adequate caloric intake. Give antiemetics as needed. 11. Provide adequate pain control. 12. Administer chemotherapy and monitor for side effects.

CHRONIC MYELOGENOUS LEUKEMIA

Quick Facts

Incidence	Accounts for 20% of all the cases of leukemia. In the U.S. there will be 4300 estimated new cases of CML in 1997. The disease usually occurs in middle-aged adults, although 10% of all cases occur in the 5–20 year-old-age group. CML represents 3% of all childhood leukemia.
Mortality	The 1997 estimated number of deaths from CML is 2400 (approximately 1.5 per 100,000/year). Eventually all patients with CML die unless a successful bone marrow transplant is performed. The average time from diagnosis to blast crisis is 5 years.
Risk factors	Ionizing radiation from the atomic bomb, radiation for treatment of cervical carcinoma, and therapeutic radiation for ankylosing spondylitis
Signs and symptoms	Early disease is usually asymptomatic and discovered during an incidental CBC. Symptoms are vague and gradually progressive. Fatigue, anorexia, early satiety (from splenomegaly), weight loss, excessive sweating, and other constitutional symptoms. Occasionally a patient will present with a dramatic hypermetabolic state with drenching sweats, weight loss, heat intolerance, priapism, gout, severe abdominal pain and mental status changes. Fever should raise the suspicion of a splenic infarction or infection.

35. How is CML staged?

Chronic phase. Patients may be asymptomatic or have a white blood cell count > 25,000 and often > 100,000. The blood smear reveals granulocytes in all stages of maturation. The bone marrow is hypercellular; the predominant cell type is a myelocyte. Leukocyte alkaline phosphatase (LAP) is low, whereas levels of LDH, B12, and uric acid are elevated. The Philadelphia chromosome is present T(9,22)(q34;Q11). Median survival: 3.5–5 years.

Accelerated phase. This transition phase occurs when the blood becomes more abnormal with > 15% blasts, > 30% blasts and myelocytes, > 20% basophils, and < 100,000 platelets. Patients have progressive cytogenetic abnormalities. Drug requirement may increase with worsening symptoms. Median survival: 18 months.

Blast phase. This phase resembles acute leukemia with > 30% blasts in the bone marrow or blood. Patients have increased symptoms such as weight loss, fevers, sweats, bone pain, and progressive abnormalities of the blood. Extramedullary disease with tumor in the skin or other organs may be found. Median survival: 3–6 months.

36. What is the treatment for CML?

Chronic phase disease is treated with drugs (hydroxyurea or busulfan) to lower blood counts and shrink the spleen. Decreasing the number of cells helps to control the symptoms. Interferon has the advantage of decreasing the number of copies of the Philadelphia chromosome and may place patients in cytologic remission, which has shown a survival advantage in some studies. Interferon also has more side effects (flulike illness, myalgias, fever). In accelerated and blast phases the prognosis is poor. Patients with myeloid blast crisis are treated with cytarabine drug combinations. Lymphoid blast crisis has a better prognosis and responds to conventional ALL treatment.

37. What is the Philadelphia chromosome?

The Philadelphia chromosome is formed when the long arm of chromosome 22 is translocated to chromosome 9, t(9,22). This creates an abnormal piece of DNA by attaching the *bcr* (breakpoint cluster region) area of chromosome 22 to the *c-abl* oncogene on chromosome 9. The abnormal protein produced has increased tyrosine kinase activity, resulting in the overproduction of cells.

38. Review the role of bone marrow transplant and peripheral stem cell rescue.

Allogeneic transplant is the only cure. Transplant is best scheduled within 1 year of diagnosis. Transplant during accelerated or blast phases is associated with 4-year survival rates of only 10–30%.

Autologous transplantation has been used to place a patient from the accelerated or blast phase back into the chronic phase. This treatment is sometimes used when an allogeneic donor is not available. Patients may achieve a short-lived remission, but early relapse is common. The stem cells for the transplant can be obtained from the bone marrow or peripheral blood. Stem cells are immature cells that have the potential to develop into any kind of blood cell (pluripotential cell). Normal stem cells look similar to lymphocytes. They are stimulated by growth factors such as granulocyte-stimulating factor, granulocyte-monocyte stimulating factor, erythropoietin, interleukins, and thrombopoietin to mature into granulocytes, monocytes, eosinophils, basophils, erythrocytes, and platelets. Stem cells are normally dormant and are not harmed by standard doses of chemotherapy or radiation therapy.

B-CELL CHRONIC LYMPHOCYTIC LEUKEMIA

Quick Facts

Incidence	CLL is the most common leukemia in the U.S., representing 30% of all types of leukemia. The incidence of CLL is 3 per 100,000 people. In the U.S. there will be an estimated 7400 new cases of CLL in 1997. CLL is usually diagnosed in elderly patients (median age: 65–70 years). It is rare in patients under 30.
Mortality	Median survival is excellent, averaging over 6 years. There will be an estimated 4900 deaths in 1997.
Etiology	Unknown. No documented association with radiation, chemotherapy, or chemicals except some chemicals used in agriculture. Genetic factors: trisomy 12, abnormalities of chromosomes 12, 14 and 18 (BCL-2)
Signs and symptoms	Approximately 20% of patients are asymptomatic and the diagnosis is made on a routine CBC. Patients may present with constitutional symptoms of fatigue, malaise, weakness, and symptoms related to lymphadenopathy; e.g. early satiety, abdominal pain or a lump from an enlarged lymph node. Infections may result from suppressed immune status due to hypogammaglobulinemia.
Staging (Rai)	Stage 0 Blood and marrow lymphocytosis (median survival: > 10 yr)
	Stage I Lymphocytosis and enlarged nodes (median survival: 6 yr)
	Stage II Lymphocytosis and enlarged liver or spleen (median survival: 6 yr)
	Stage III Lymphocytosis and anemia (< 11) (median survival: 2 yr)
	Stage IV Lymphocytosis and thrombocytopenia (< 100,000) (median survival: 2 yr)

39. What are the diagnostic criteria for CLL?
• Peripheral blood lymphocytes > 10,000 for at least 4 weeks and bone marrow infiltration with at least 30% mature lymphocytes or clonality of peripheral blood lymphocytes.
• Peripheral blood lymphocytes > 5,000 for at least 4 weeks and bone marrow infiltration with at least 30% mature lymphocytes and clonality of peripheral blood lymphocytes.

40. What are the indications for treating CLL?
• Symptomatic anemia   • Enlarged painful liver or spleen
• Thrombocytopenia   • Symptomatic adenopathy
• Disease-related symptoms   • Rapidly increasing lymphocytosis

41. What are the major signs or symptoms of advanced CLL?
In advanced disease any organ may be infiltrated with the malignant clone of cells. Hepatosplenomegaly is a common example. When the bone marrow is packed with malignant cells, the patient may be pancytopenic and require transfusion support. Autoimmune anemia and thrombocytopenia are late findings.

42. How is CLL treated?
Early-stage asymptomatic disease may not require therapy for several years. Alkylating agents (chlorambucil or cyclophosphamide) with or without prednisone are usually the first treatments.

Prednisone may be particularly useful to treat autoimmune anemia and thrombocytopenia. Fludarabine and other nucleoside analogs such as cladribine are also highly effective; they are used for patients who have failed alkylating therapy. On occasion, combination chemotherapy with cyclophosphamide, vincristine, and prednisone, with or without doxorubicin, is used for severe disease that has failed other therapies. Radiation therapy and splenectomy may be used to palliate symptoms. Intravenous immunoglobulin is sometimes used to treat hypogammaglobulinemia in patients with frequent life-threatening infections.

43. What is the role of bone marrow transplant in CLL?

Transplant is an investigational treatment for CLL.

44. What is prolymphocytic leukemia?

Prolymphocytic leukemia is a variant of CLL in which over one-half of the leukemic cells are large lymphocytes called prolymphocytes. Patients commonly present with advanced disease. The disease has a median survival of 3 years and is more resistant to chemotherapy.

45. What is T-cell CLL?

T-cell CLL is rare in the United States but represents the dominant form of leukemia in Asia. Patients present with pancytopenia and splenomegaly without lymphadenopathy. Median survival is 2–3 years.

46. What is T-gamma lymphoproliferative disorder?

T-gamma lymphoproliferative disorder is a disease of the large granular lymphocyte. The clinical course is variable, ranging from indolent to severe (as with acute leukemia). Usually the disease is indolent with a 4-year survival rate of 75%. Patients present with fevers, infections, cytopenias, and abnormal CBC. T-gamma lymphoproliferative disorder is associated with autoimmune diseases and hepatitis.

BIBLIOGRAPHY

1. Beutler E, Lichtman M, Coller B, Kipps T (eds): Williams' Hematology, 5th ed. New York, McGraw-Hill, 1995.
2. Devine SM, Larson RA: Acute leukemia in adults: Recent developments in diagnosis and treatment. Cancer J Clin 44(6):326–352, 1994.
3. DeVita V, Hellman S, Rosenberg S: Cancer: Principles and Practice of Oncology, 5th ed. Philadelphia, J.B. Lippincott, 1997.
4. Faguet GB: CLL: An updated review. J Clin Oncol 12:1974–1990, 1994.
5. Haskell C: Cancer Treatment, 4th ed. Philadelphia, W.B. Saunders, 1995.
6. Heckman KD, Weiner GJ, Davis CS, et al: Randomized study of prophylactic platelet transfusion threshold during induction therapy for adult acute leukemia: 10,000/µL versus 20,000/µL. J Clin Oncol 15:1143–1149, 1997.
7. Kantarjian HM, Deisseroth A, Kurzrock R: Chronic myelogenous leukemia: A concise update. Blood 82:691–703, 1993.
8. Lessin LT (ed): Medical Knowledge Self Assessment Program in the Specialty of Hematology. Philadelphia, American College of Physicians, 1994.
9. O'Brien S, Del Giglio A, Keating M: Advances in the biology and treatment of B cell chronic lymphocytic leukemia. Blood 85:307–318, 1995.
10. Parker SL, Tong T, Bolden S, Wingo PA: Cancer Statistics, 1997. CA Cancer J Clin 47:5–27, 1997.
11. Pazdur R (ed): Medical Oncology—A Comprehensive Review, 2nd ed. Huntington, NY, PRR, 1996.
12. Pazdur R, Cola L, Hoskins W, Warman L (eds): Cancer Management: A Multidisciplinary Approach—Medical, Surgical and Radiation Oncology. Huntington, NY, PRR, 1996.
13. Viele CS: Chronic myelogenous leukemia and acute promyelocytic leukemia: New bone marrow transplantation options. Oncol Nurs Forum 23:488–502, 1996.
14. Wujcik D: Update on the diagnosis of and therapy of acute promyelocytic leukemia and chronic myelogenous leukemia. Oncol Nursing Forum 23:478–487, 1996.
15. Yeager KA, Miaskowski C: Advances in understanding the mechanisms and management of acute myelogenous leukemia. Oncol Nurs Forum 21:541–548, 1994.

16. MULTIPLE MYELOMA

Cathy E. Pickett, RN, BSN, and Paul Seligman, MD

Quick Facts—Multiple Myeloma

Incidence	1% of all malignancies; in 1997, approximately 13,800 new cases will be diagnosed in the United States.
Mortality	In 1997, 10,900 estimated deaths
Etiologic factors	No single predisposing factor; suggested factors include chronic exposure to various types of low-level radiation, occupational exposures (agriculture, chemicals, rubber plant, leather tanners) and chemical exposure to benzene formaldehyde, hair dyes, paint sprays.
Risk factors	Increasing age (median age: 50–70 yr); increased risk in men; more common among African Americans than Caucasians (2:1)
Signs and symptoms	Many patients present with complications because the disease is a slow-growing neoplasm, typified by a long prodromal or asymptomatic period. Most patients present with systemic involvement indicated by bony disease (many present with back pain), renal disease, increased calcium, anemia, and/or infections.
Diagnostic studies	**Urinary and serum protein electrophoresis** (UPEP/SPEP) to assess for presence of monoclonal protein
	Quantitative immunoglobulins to evaluate specific amounts of immunoglobulin
	Skeletal survey to evaluate degree of bone marrow involvement as indicated by percentage of plasma cells
	Complete blood count to evaluate for anemia, neutropenia, and thrombocytopenia
	Serum chemistries to evaluate renal function and hypercalcemia
	β2 microglobulin (prognostic indicator) increases with advancing disease

Staging*	Stage I	< 0.5 myeloma cells $\times 10^{12}/m^2$
		All of the following:
		1. Hemoglobin value > 10 gm/100 ml
		2. Serum calcium value normal (< 12 mg/100 ml)
		3. On radiographs, normal bone structure (scale 0) or solitary bone plasmacytoma only
		4. Low M-component production rates
		a. IgG value < 5gm/100 ml
		b. IgA value < 3 gm/100 ml
		c. Urine light-chain M-component on electrophoresis: < 4 gm/24 hr
	Stage II	> 0.6–1.20 myeloma cells $\times 10^{12}/m^2$ (intermediate)
		Fitting neither stage I nor stage III
	Stage III	> 1.20 myeloma cells $\times 10^{12}/m^2$ (high)
		One or more of the following:
		1. Hemoglobin value of 8.5 gm/100 ml
		2. Serum calcium value > 12 mg/100 ml
		3. Advanced lytic bone lesions (scale 3)
		4. High M-component production rate
		a. IgG value > 7 gm/100 ml
		b. IgA value > 5 gm/100 ml
		c. Urine light-chain M-component on electrophoresis: > 12 gm/24 hr
	Subclassification	
		A = Relatively normal renal function (serum creatinine value < 2.0 mg/100 ml)
		B = Abnormal renal function (serum creatinine value > 2.0 mg/100 ml)

---

* Criteria vary, and standard definitions are lacking. Some clinicians monitor serum levels of B2 microglobulin, which correlate with renal function and myeloma cell tumor burden. Although good indicators of prognosis and survival, current staging systems do not indicate treatment. The staging system presented above was developed by Durie GB, Salmon SE: A clinical staging system for multiple myeloma. Cancer 36, 852, 1975. © 1975 American Cancer Society. Reprinted by permission of Wiley-Liss, Inc., a subsidiary of John Wiley & Sons, Inc.

1. What is multiple myeloma?

Multiple myeloma is a malignant proliferation of plasma cells that results in an overproduction of a specific immunoglobulin, generally detected in the blood or urine. M-protein is the abnormal immunoglobulin produced by the malignant plasma cell. It is produced excessively and is not able to make effective antibodies. Plasma cells are responsible for production of immunoglobulin (the basic unit of antibodies) and arise from stem cells in the bone marrow. Myeloma cells are present in bone marrow and in the outer part of bones.

2. How is multiple myeloma diagnosed?

A few patients are diagnosed by chance with the identification of abnormal protein in the blood or urine. Most present with a common complication of myeloma and are further evaluated using diagnostic studies (see Quick Facts).

Diagnostic Criteria for Various Forms of Monoclonal Gammopathies

Multiple myeloma
1. Plasmacytoma on tissue biopsy
2. > 30% marrow plasmacytosis
3. Monoclonal spike
   a. IgG > 3.5 gm/dl
   b. IgA > 2.0 gm/dl
   c. Urinary light chain > 1.0 gm/24 hr
4. Additional features
   a. Lytic bone lesions
   b. Low residual immunoglobulins

Diagnosis requires 1, 2, or 3 plus either 4a or 4b if plasmacytosis and monoclonal spike are present but lower than above. Diagnosis can be made if 4a or 4b present.

Indolent myeloma
Same as for myeloma except
1. 0–3 bones lesions, no fractures
2. Monoclonal spike < 7 gm/dl IgG; < 5 gm/dl IgA
3. No associated features: anemia, hypercalcemia, renal dysfunction, infection; good performance

Smoldering myeloma
Same as indolent myeloma except
1. No bone lesions
2. Marrow plasmacytosis < 30%

Monoclonal gammopathy of unknown significance (MGUS)
1. Monoclonal gammopathy
   a. IgG < 3.5 gm/dl
   b. IgA < 2.0 gm/dl
   c. Urinary light chain < 1.0 gm/dl
2. Marrow plasmacytosis < 10%
3. No bone lesions
4. No symptoms

From Gautier M, Cohen H: Multiple myeloma in the elderly. J Am Geriatr Soc 42:653–664, 1994, with permission.

3. What is monoclonal gammopathy of unknown significance (MGUS)?

The diagnosis of MGUS is made when patients have no symptoms, no skeletal involvement, a marrow plasmacytosis of < 10%, and M protein levels lower than described. Because 20–25% of these patients eventually develop multiple myeloma, frequent and ongoing evaluation is necessary.

4. What is a plasmacytoma?

A plasmacytoma is a single isolated collection of malignant plasma cells in the bone that can be treated with local therapy such as surgery and/or radiation. Because some of these patients eventually develop multiple myeloma, close monitoring is necessary.

5. What is the significance of Bence-Jones protein in the urine?

Some malignant plasma cells produce only the light-chain part of the immunoglobulin. These low-molecular-weight proteins are excreted in the urine; they allow the diagnosis of light-chain myeloma and may contribute to the development of renal failure (referred to as **myeloma kidney**).

6. Why are patients with multiple myeloma so prone to the development of renal failure?

Renal failure in patients with multiple myeloma is multifactorial. The causes generally include an accumulation of Bence-Jones proteins, hypercalcemia, hyperuricemia, and dehydration. It is important that patients with multiple myeloma receive adequate hydration before receiving diagnostic dyes or contrast media. The degree of hydration depends on the patient's creatinine value and stage of disease, but treatment generally involves the administration of at least 1 liter of normal saline and reevaluation of the patient's renal function and fluid status.

7. What are lytic lesions?

Many patients present with skeletal involvement and bony destruction caused by the accumulation of plasma cells. Plasma cells also increase bone resorption, resulting in further bony destruction that may present as "punched-out" lesions on radiographs. A lytic lesion is a destructive loss of bone in an isolated area secondary to metastatic cancer infiltration. Diffuse osteoporosis also may result. Skeletal involvement may lead to pathologic fractures, increased serum calcium, and severe pain. The administration of intravenous biphosphonates, such as pamidronate, which inhibit osteoclastic activity and decrease bone resorption, is currently recommended every 3–4 weeks to minimize bony destruction.

8. If patients with multiple myeloma have an increase in a specific immunoglobulin, why are they at increased risk for infection?

The elevated monoclonal protein is impaired and does not function normally to provide protection. Because it is produced in large quantities, it also results in a decrease in the levels of other normal and functional immunoglobulins. As the percentage of bone marrow infiltration by plasma cells increases, neutropenia further predisposes patients to infection.

9. What medical emergencies are patients with multiple myeloma prone to develop?

The common oncologic emergencies in patients with multiple myeloma are hypercalcemia, spinal cord compression, and hyperviscosity.

10. Define hyperviscosity. How is it exhibited?

The presence of high concentrations of M protein in the blood may lead to occlusion of blood vessels and circulatory problems. The patient may develop claudication, visual disturbances, and neurologic symptoms such as headache, drowsiness, and confusion.

11. How is multiple myeloma treated?

Systemic treatment begins when symptoms appear. Because multiple myeloma has a long prodromal phase in which patients are asymptomatic, treatment is generally reserved for patients who have developed complications. Radiation may be used effectively to treat a solitary lesion or palliatively to treat bony lesions and control pain.

12. What chemotherapy is used for the treatment of multiple myeloma?

The combination of melphalan and prednisone (MP), which has been a primary treatment modality since the 1960s, induces a temporary (duration of 2 years) remission in 40% of previously untreated patients. There is a low frequency of complete response. (Response is defined as a 75% reduction in the rate of myeloma protein production, a 95% decrease in the rate of Bence-Jones protein excretion, and < 5% marrow plasma cells, as determined by bone marrow biopsy). A continuous infusion of vincristine and doxorubicin combined with oral dexamethasone (VAD) is primarily used as a treatment for relapses or for patients who fail MP therapy. VAD has response rates of 55% and quicker remission but no improvement in long-term survival. Younger patients may initially receive VAD or other combinations at higher doses with some evidence of longer remissions.

13. What are the major complications of treatment?
    Side effects of all treatments include drug resistance, infection in an already immunocompromised patient, and leukemia as a result of long-term use of alkylating agents.

14. What is the prognosis for patients with multiple myeloma?
    Multiple myeloma is normally treated with chemotherapy, and initially patients respond well. It is considered an incurable disease, because most patients relapse and fail to respond to chemotherapy as the disease progresses. Once symptoms develop, the median survival time without treatment is 7 months. Standard treatment can extend survival to 2–3 years. The 5-year survival rate increased from 12% in the 1960s to 27% in the 1980s. Although this increase represents progress, the lack of a cure has led to ongoing investigation of other treatment modalities.

15. What current studies are under way in the management of multiple myeloma?
    Studies investigating the use of interferon after chemotherapy have produced conflicting results. Although trials are still in progress, little evidence indicates that interferon improves survival. The use of interferon as maintenance therapy (after chemotherapy) may, however, prolong response to initial treatment. Bone marrow transplantation (generally autologous transplants after high-dose chemotherapy) is also under investigation; results indicate prolonged remission and increased survival but increased morbidity.

16. If bone marrow transplantation can increase survival and achieve a complete response in some patients, why is it not a standard treatment?
    Many patients with multiple myeloma are elderly and, thus, more susceptible to the major side effects of the regimen. They may choose to enjoy a period of symptom-free survival with standard chemotherapy. Younger patients in early stages of the disease may be the best candidates for bone marrow transplantation, but they must accept the increased risk of morbidity. Until morbidity is decreased, many patients may be hesitant to accept bone marrow transplantation as a treatment option. Trials are under way to determine the most effective chemotherapy regimen, the best source of stem cells (peripheral or bone marrow), and the best time for transplantation.

17. How can nurses promote safety and improve the quality of life in patients with multiple myeloma?
    The nurse's role involves facilitating diagnosis and managing disease-related complications or treatment-induced side effects.
    Nurses can help patients with skeletal involvement to achieve optimal pain control while avoiding side effects of medication. Education about positioning and ambulation also may help to prevent further pathologic fractures and continued bone destruction.
    Nurses also can educate patients about the importance of hydration and avoidance of renal toxic drugs and hypercalcemia to promote optimal renal function and prevent further damage. Because infection is the leading cause of death, patient education about prevention, recognition, and treatment of infection is critical.

18. What resources are available to provide patients and families with more information?
    Patients and families should contact their local American Cancer Society for resources and support group information. The Physician Data Query is a valuable resource for patients and

families looking for current information and investigational trials in progress. The Leukemia Society of America (800-955-4LSA) can be accessed by computer and also has pamphlets and resources for patients with multiple myeloma. "Surfing the net" is recommended to explore a variety of resources. The International Myeloma Foundation (800-452-CURE; e-mail: TheIMF@aol.com) offers patient seminars, a newsletter, resources, publications, and a patient-to-patient directory.

BIBLIOGRAPHY

1. Alexanian R, Dimopoulos M: The treatment of multiple myeloma. N Engl J Med 330:484–489, 1994.
2. Bensinger W, Rowley S, Demirer T, et al: High-dose therapy followed by autologous hematopoietic stem-cell infusion for patients with multiple myeloma. J Clin Oncol 14:1447–1456, 1996.
3. Berenson J, Lichtenstein A, Porter L, et al: Efficacy of pamidronate in reducing skeletal events in patients with advanced multiple myeloma. N Engl J Med 334:488–493, 1996.
4. Bubley G, Schnippe L: Multiple myeloma. In Holleb A, Fink D, Murphy G (eds): American Cancer Textbook of Clinical Oncology. Atlanta, American Cancer Society, 1991, pp 397–409.
5. Gautier M, Cohen H: Multiple myeloma in the elderly. J Am Geriatr Soc 42:653–664, 1994.
6. Hjorth M, Westin J, Dahl I, et al: Interferon-α2b added to melphalan–prednisone for initial and maintenance therapy in multiple myeloma. Ann Intern Med 124:212–222, 1996.
7. Lawrence J: Critical care issues in the patient with hematologic malignancy. Semin Oncol Nurs 10:198–207, 1994.
8. Parker SL, Tong T, Bolden S, Wingo PA: Cancer Statistics 1997. CA Cancer J Clin 47:5–27, 1997.
9. Sheridan C: Multiple myeloma. In Groenwald S, Frogge M, Goodman M, Yarbro C (eds): Cancer Nursing: Principles and Practice. Boston, Jones & Bartlett, 1993, pp 1229–1237.

17. NON-HODGKIN'S LYMPHOMA

Scott Kruger, MD, and Libby Tracey, RN, PhD(c), OCN

Quick Facts—Non-Hodgkin's Lymphoma	
Incidence	4% of all cancers in the United States, with an estimated 53,600 new cases in 1997 (increase associated with AIDS and elderly). In adults, the median age at diagnosis is over 50 years.
Mortality	Overall survival has improved with newer treatments. It is estimated that in the United States, 23,800 people will die from the disease in 1997.
Etiology	The exact causes of non-Hodgkin's lymphoma (NHL) are unknown.
Risk Factors	**Infections** • Human immunodeficiency virus (HIV) • Epstein-Barr virus (African Burkitt's lymphoma) • Human T-cell lymphoma virus (HTLV-1) (T-cell lymphoma) • *Helicobacter pylori* associated with gastric mucosa-associated lymphoid tissue lymphomas (MALT) **Environmental factors:** pesticides and fertilizers, wood and cotton dust, early and prolonged use of hair dyes, and possibly smoking **Therapy-related factors** • Chemotherapy (alkylating agents) and radiation therapy with latency period of about 5–6 years • Immunosuppressants (azathioprine or cyclosporine) **Congenital immune deficiencies:** Bloom's and Wiskott-Aldrich syndromes **Autoimmune disorders:** Sjögren's syndrome, systemic lupus erythematosus, rheumatoid arthritis, celiac disease
Signs and symptoms	B symptoms of fevers, weight loss, and drenching sweats may be present. **Low-grade lymphomas** present with painless, slowly progressive lymphadenopathy that at times may spontaneously regress in size and then grow at a later time. Extranodal involvement and B symptoms may be found in advanced disease. Patients often present with higher-stage disease than intermediate and high-grade types (III and IV). **Intermediate- and high-grade lymphomas** sometimes present with rapidly growing adenopathy. One-third present with extralymphatic disease in the GI tract, skin, sinuses, and central nervous system (CNS). B symptoms are common. Patients often present with lower-stage disease (I and II). Lymphoblastic lymphoma may present with a large mediastinal mass, superior vena cava syndrome, or cranial nerve involvement due to leptomeningeal disease. American Burkitt's lymphoma often starts with a large abdominal mass and obstructive symptoms.
Staging	NHL is staged according to the Ann Arbor Staging System.
	Stage I Involvement of a single lymph node region or lymphoid structure (spleen, thymus, or Waldeyer's ring)
	Stage II Involvement of 2 or more lymph node regions on same side of diaphragm (the mediastinum is a single site, hilar nodes are lateralized). The number of anatomic sites should be indicated by a suffix (e.g., stage II$_3$).
	Stage III Involvement of lymph node regions or structures on both sides of diaphragm
	Stage III$_1$ Splenic, celiac, or portal nodes
	Stage III$_2$ Paraaortic, iliac or mesenteric nodes

Table continued on following page.

1. What are the non-Hodgkin's lymphomas (NHLs)? How are they diagnosed?

The NHLs are a diverse group of seemingly unrelated diseases arising from lymphoid tissues. NHL is caused by a malignant clonal expansion of one of the elements of a lymph node. Because lymphatic tissue is present throughout the entire body, the disease may develop anywhere. It may begin in a lymph node, spleen, liver, or bone marrow as well in extralymphatic sites such as skin, gastrointestinal tract, pharynx, and central nervous system. The diagnosis is established by biopsy of abnormal tissue and evaluation with histologic and immunophenotypic examination.

2. What are the most common cytogenetic abnormalities? How do they correlate with histology?

Chromosomal abnormalities are associated with oncogene expressions involved in lymphogenesis, as depicted below:

Cytogenetic Abnormality	Oncogene Expression	Histology
t(14;18)	bcl-2	Follicular and diffuse large cell
t(11;14)	bcl-1	Mantle zone
t(14;19)	bcl-3	B-cell chronic lymphocytic lymphoma (CLL)
t(8;14), t(2;8), t(8;22)	c-myc	Burkitt's and non-Burkitt's lymphoma
Trisomy 12		B-cell CLL
14q11 abnormalities	tcl-1, tcl-2	T-cell acute lymphocytic lymphoma (ALL)
7q35 abnormalities	tcl-4	T-cell ALL and lymphoblastic lymphoma
t(2;5)	npm; alk	Anaplastic large cell

3. What characteristics of an enlarged node raise the suspicion of lymphoma?

A painless, enlarging lymph node that feels rubbery is suspicious for lymphoma. Infectious nodal enlargement is usually tender. Supraclavicular nodes are always suspicious for malignancy.

4. Why is the classification of NHL so confusing?

The classification is confusing because the NHLs are a heterogeneous group of diseases that seem to have little relationship to each other. They are named according to growth pattern (follicular vs. diffuse) within the lymph node, cell size (large vs. small), and appearance (cleaved or noncleaved). Until the mid 1980s, the Rappaport classification was widely used in the United States, but it has been replaced by the Working Formulation, which attempts to simplify classification into risk categories of low, intermediate, and high grade. However, the Working

Formulation does not include all lymphomas. The REAL (Revised European American Lymphoma) classification was recently proposed by the International Study Group in an effort to accommodate newly described lymphomas not included in the Working Formulation.

Classification of Non-Hodgkin's Lymphomas

WORKING FORMULATION	RAPPAPORT
Low grade	**Low grade**
A Small lymphocytic	Diffuse, well differentiated lymphocytic
B Follicular, small cleaved cell	Nodular, poorly differentiated lymphocytic
C Follicular, mixed, small cleaved and large cell	Nodular, mixed
Intermediate grade	**Intermediate grade**
D Follicular, large cell	Nodular, histiocytic
E Diffuse, small cleaved cell	Diffuse, poorly differentiated lymphocytic
F Diffuse, mixed, small cleaved and large cell	Diffuse mixed
G Diffuse, large cell	Diffuse, histiocytic
High grade	**High grade**
H Immunoblastic	Diffuse, histiocytic
I Lymphoblastic	Lymphoblastic
J Diffuse, small noncleaved cell	Burkitt's and non-Burkitt's types

5. Which lymphomas are not classified by the Working Formulation?

Disease	Description
Mantle zone	Resembles follicular small cleaved cell but is derived from a cell in mantle zone surrounding B-cell follicles. Aggressive disease with high risk for extranodal spread. Low potential for cure.
Monocytoid B-cell lymphoma	Low-grade indolent disease. Predominant lymph node involvement.
Mucosa-associated lymphoid tissue (MALT)	Low-grade indolent disease. Affects GI tract, lung, breast, thyroid, and salivary glands.
Anaplastic large cell Ki-1 lymphoma	Skin is often involved. Cells infiltrate the sinusoids of nodes. Often confused with Hodgkin's disease or carcinoma. Most cases are of T-cell origin. Behaves as an intermediate-grade lymphoma.
Mycosis fungoides	Indolent cutaneous T-cell lymphoma that may later spread to lymph nodes and invade other organs. More advanced forms with peripheral blood involvement and diffuse erythema are called Sezary syndrome. Involvement of organs results in poor prognosis.
Angiocentric lymphoma	T-cell disease that invades and destroys blood vessels.
T-cell–rich B-cell lymphoma	Usually aggressive and behaves like large cell lymphomas.
Angiotropic large cell	Diffuse intravascular proliferation, usually of B-cell lineage.
Angioimmunoblastic lymphadenopathy (AILD)	Diffuse adenopathy, hepatosplenomegaly, skin rash, cytopenias, systemic symptoms, polyclonal hypergammaglobulinemia. Often evolves into T-cell lymphoma.
Divergent or discordant composite lymphoma	Large cell histology in lymph node but low grade in marrow. The low-grade component usually turns into high-grade disease.Two histologic subtypes in the same node; sometimes coexists with Hodgkin's disease.
Castleman's disease	Benign lymphoproliferative disorder, sometimes related to HIV. Increased rate of evolving into malignancy.
Adult T-cell leukemia lymphoma	Aggressive malignancy associated with skin infiltration, hypercalcemia, and lytic bone lesions.

6. What are favorable and nonfavorable lymphomas? Are favorable lymphomas more curable?

Favorable lymphomas are low-grade lymphomas. Unfavorable lymphomas are intermediate- and high-grade lymphomas. Low-grade lymphomas are considered "favorable" because of their relatively long natural course without treatment. Unfortunately, they are not considered curable. Most patients with low-grade lymphoma require treatment for a few years, but it is generally for palliation rather than cure. The 5-year survival rate for patients with low-grade lymphomas ranges from 50–70%. In contrast, the unfavorable lymphomas are potentially curable with combination chemotherapy regimens. The higher-grade lymphomas are considered "unfavorable" because without active treatment the natural prognosis is poor. The 5-year survival rate for intermediate-grade lymphoma ranges from 33–45%; for high-grade lymphomas, from 23–32%. Treatment may achieve complete remission in 60–80% of patients with diffuse, aggressive NHL.

7. What is the International Index?

The International Index consists of five factors used by the major cooperative groups to predict overall survival in patients with unfavorable lymphomas. Two or more of the following risk factors signify a less than 50% chance of relapse-free and overall survival at 5 years.
- Age (> 60 years)
- Elevated levels of serum lactate dehydrogenase (LDH)
- Performance status (levels ≥ 2)
- Stage III or IV disease
- Two or more sites of extranodal involvement

8. What other prognostic factors are useful in unfavorable lymphomas?

- Tumor biology: Ki-67 (marker for cellular proliferation), abnormal cytogenetics, T-cell lymphoma
- Presence of B symptoms
- Tumor burden: bulky sites (diameter > 7 cm), elevated B2 microglobulin
- Drug resistance

9. What is the significance of immunophenotyping in NHLs?

NHLs are typed for T and B cells; however, whether this distinction influences patient outcome is still debated. Some studies indicate a shorter disease-free survival time in patients with T-cell, diffuse large cell lymphoma than in patients with B-cell lymphomas of similar histology.

10. How does Hodgkin's lymphoma differ from non-Hodgkin's lymphomas?

Pathologically the characteristic Reed-Sternberg cell is not found in NHLs. NHLs spread by skipping lymph node areas, whereas Hodgkin's disease is orderly and does not skip lymph node groups. NHLs are usually seen in older adults, whereas Hodgkin's disease has a bimodal incidence with the first peak in young adults.

11. What is the treatment of low-grade lymphomas?

Low-grade lymphomas are characterized by indolent behavior and median survival times of 6–10 years. Most patients are elderly and have advanced disease at presentation. Only 10–20% have stage I or II disease.

Stage I or II disease. Radiation alone is rarely used because NHLs do not spread contiguously and often skip to other lymph node areas. It has been used for localized tumors of the head and neck, orbit, and other single sites of disease. Many oncologists use a combination of radiation and chemotherapy for localized disease with the hope that it will produce long-term disease-free survival and even cure. For patients with comorbid illnesses, a watch-and-wait approach is a reasonable alternative. Chemotherapy is used when patients become symptomatic. Total nodal irradiation is not generally used because of its relapse rate (> 50%).

Stage III and IV. Treatment options include watching and waiting. Various systemic chemotherapy regimens are begun when patients become symptomatic. Chemotherapy is usually started early in patients with unfavorable prognostic features such as marrow involvement, bulky disease, high levels of serum LDH, many extralymphatic sites of disease, and decreased performance status.

12. What is the treatment of intermediate-grade lymphomas?

Intermediate-grade lymphoma is frequently diagnosed in early stages. High-grade immunoblastic lymphoma is treated like intermediate-grade diseases.

Stage I and II. A combination of chemotherapy and radiation is the treatment of choice. The 5-year disease-free survival rate ranges from 78–95% for stage I disease and from 70–75% for stage II disease. Patients usually receive 3–4 cycles of chemotherapy followed by involved-field radiation therapy. For patients who do not receive radiation, 6–8 cycles of chemotherapy are used.

Stage III and IV. Most patients are treated with 6–8 cycles of systemic chemotherapy. Radiation is sometimes added to sites of bulky disease to decrease the risk of local recurrence. Despite the availability of multiple chemotherapy regimens, the 5-year disease-free survival rate is approximately 40%.

13. What chemotherapy regimens are commonly used for treating NHL?

Palliation of low-grade disease
    Oral chlorambucil with or without prednisone
    Oral cyclophosphamide with or without prednisone

Intermediate and high-grade disease
    CVP (cyclophosphamide, vincristine, prednisone)
    CHOP (cyclophosphamide, doxorubicin, vincristine, prednisone)
    MACOP-B (methotrexate, doxorubicin, cyclophosphamide, vincristine, bleomycin, prednisone
    ProMACE-CytaBOM (cyclophosphamide, etoposide, doxorubicin, cytarabine, bleomycin, vincristine, methotrexate, leucovorin, prednisone)
    m-BACOD (methotrexate, leucovorin, bleomycin, doxorubicin, cyclophosphamide, vincristine, dexamethasone)

Salvage chemotherapy
    DHAP (dexamethasone, cytarabine, cisplatin)
    IMVP (ifosfamide with mesna, methotrexate, etoposide)
    ESHAP (etoposide, methyl prednisone, cisplatin, cytarabine)
    MIME (mesna, ifosfamide, mitoxantrone, etoposide)
    CEPP (cyclophosphamide, etoposide, procarbazine, prednisone)

14. Which of the above regimens is the best treatment for intermediate- or high-grade NHL?

Many researchers believe that CHOP, one of the first combination regimens to be used, is the gold standard for treatment of intermediate- or high-grade NHL. Clinical trials to date have not determined that the newer regimens are superior to CHOP in terms of survival or cure rates.

15. What is tumor lysis syndrome?

While undergoing therapy for leukemia and high-grade lymphomas, patients develop multiple electrolyte abnormalities due to the release of chemicals in the blood from the dying blast cells. All patients should be adequately hydrated and receive allopurinol to decrease the production of uric acid. Alkalinization of the urine is sometimes performed to increase the solubility of uric acid. Hyperkalemia, hypocalcemia, and hyperphosphatemia may be life-threatening. Despite prevention, in some patients dialysis is needed to treat metabolic abnormalities. Risks for the patient include renal failure, cardiovascular collapse, and death.

16. What paraneoplastic syndromes are associated with NHL?
- Non–parathyroid hormone-induced hypercalcemia
- Subacute motor neuropathy
- Polymyositis

17. How is lymphoblastic lymphoma treated?
Lymphoblastic lymphoma is uncommon in adults, but in children it is the most common type of NHL. Treatment is the same as for acute lymphoblastic leukemia: high-dose chemotherapy, intrathecal chemotherapy for CNS involvement, and/or radiation to the brain.

18. Which patients should receive CNS prophylaxis with radiation or intrathecal therapy?
All patients with Burkitt's, non-Burkitt's, and lymphoblastic lymphoma receive treatment to the CNS. Other patients with involvement of bone marrow, testes, nasopharynx, or sinuses should be evaluated for CNS disease. Epidural and brain disease is treated with intrathecal therapy using methotrexate or cytarabine (Ara-C) or with radiation therapy.

19. What is the treatment for mycosis fungoides?
Topical chemotherapy with nitrogen mustard or carmustine (BCNU) and ultraviolet light A activation of skin with psoralen (PUVA) are usually the initial therapies. Extracorporeal photopheresis and total skin electron beam therapy are used for more advanced disease. Systemic chemotherapy may be used to palliate symptoms.

20. What is the role of bone marrow transplant and stem cell rescue in NHLs?
The role in initial presentations is unclear. In relapsed disease, high-dose therapy with autologous bone marrow transplant or stem cell support may be used; initial results are encouraging.

21. What is Richter's transformation?
Evolution of a low-grade lymphoma into a diffuse large cell lymphoma is called Richter's transformation. The term was first used in 1928 to describe a case of CLL that developed into aggressive lymphoma.

22. What public resources are available for patients with lymphoma?
- Cure for Lymphoma Foundation
  Telephone: 212-319-5857; E-mail: InfoCFL@aol.com
  Raises funds for research and provides patient educational materials. Patient support is available through a patient-to-patient telephone network, library, and newsletter.
- Leukemia Society of America
  Telephone: 800-955-4LSA; 212-573-8484
  National voluntary health agency that offers support groups and financial assistance.
- Lymphoma Research Foundation of America
  Telephone: 310-204-7040; E-mail: lrfa@aol.com
  Nonprofit agency that provides research grants and educational information. It offers a support group (Los Angeles) and a national "buddy system."
- Lymphoma Foundation of America
  Telephone: 202-223-6181
  Nonprofit agency that provides educational materials, patient support groups, treatment updates, and patient advocacy.

BIBLIOGRAPHY

1. Armitage JO: Treatment of non-Hodgkin's lymphoma. N Engl J Med 328:1023–1030, 1993.
2. Beutler E, Lichtman M, Coller B, Kipps T (eds): Williams' Hematology. 5th ed. New York, McGraw-Hill, 1995.
3. Devine SM, Larson RA: Acute leukemia in adults: Recent developments in diagnosis and treatment. Cancer J Clin 44(6):326–352, 1994.

4. DeVita V, Hellman S, Rosenberg S: Cancer: Principles and Practice of Oncology, 5th ed. Philadelphia, J.B. Lippincott, 1997.
5. Engelking C, Hubbard SM: Current Issues and Controversies in the Management of Non-Hodgkin's Lymphoma. New York, Triclinica Communications, 1996.
6. Haskell C: Cancer Treatment, 4th ed. Philadelphia, W.B. Saunders, 1995.
7. Lessin LI (ed): Medical Knowledge: Self Assessment Program In the Specialty of Hematology. Philadelphia, American College of Physicians, 1994.
8. Parker SL, Tong T, Bolden S, Wingo PA: Cancer Statistics, 1997. CA Cancer J Clin 47:5–27, 1997.
9. Melynk A, Rodriquez A: Intermediate-and high-grade non-Hodgkin's lymphomas. In Pazdur R (ed): Medical Oncology—A Comprehensive Review, 2nd ed. Huntington NY, PRR, 1995.
10. Pazdur R, Cola L, Hoskins W, Wagman L (eds): Cancer Management: A Multidisciplinary Approach— Medical, Surgical and Radiation Oncology. Huntington, NY, PRR, 1996.

IV. Solid Tumors

18. AIDS-RELATED MALIGNANCIES

David C. Faragher, MD

1. What are the AIDS-defining malignancies?

Kaposi's sarcoma (KS), non-Hodgkin's lymphoma (NHL), and invasive cervical cancer.

2. Does Kaposi's sarcoma occur with equal frequency in all groups of patients with acquired immunodeficiency syndrome (AIDS)?

KS is much more frequent in gay and bisexual men with human immunodeficiency virus (HIV) than in other risk groups. Studies from the early 1980s revealed that up to 50% of gay/bisexual men presented with KS as the initial manifestation of AIDS. In 1991 this percentage had decreased to 11%. Over 90% of all AIDS-related KS occurs in gay/bisexual men. KS has also been described in non-HIV infected gay men. KS is quite uncommon in intravenous drug users, heterosexual men, and women. However, KS is more common in women who have bisexual male sexual partners than in women who are intravenous drug users.

3. Does KS occur only in patients with AIDS?

KS was initially described by Moricz Kaposi in 1872 in elderly men of eastern European or Mediterranean descent. It was primarily limited to skin involvement of the legs and was rarely life-threatening (classic type). Cases of lymph node involvement or visceral disease were rare. An endemic form has also been described in younger men and women of sub-Saharan Africa. The endemic form is more aggressive with visceral and lymph node involvement as well as cutaneous disease. A third category of non-HIV KS involves patients who are immunocompromised from organ transplantation or autoimmune diseases. In patients with organ transplants, the incidence of KS is 200–400 times greater than the incidence in the general population. KS found in patients with AIDS is the epidemic form of the disease.

4. Why are malignancies included in the Centers for Disease Control (CDC) list of AIDS-defining conditions?

Malignancies are a relatively common complication of a broad range of immunodeficiency states. There have been many reports of malignancies in patients with organ-transplants as well as various congenital immunodeficiency conditions. Immunosuppression predisposes to malignancies for several possible reasons: (1) absence of protective immune surveillance to eliminate abnormal clones; (2) dysregulation of cell proliferation and differentiation; and (3) chronic antigenic bombardment of the immune system by various infections. The marked rise in incidence of lymphoma and KS in HIV-infected individuals has been noted since 1982. KS was one of the first recognized conditions in AIDS. Epidemiologic studies subsequently showed that non-Hodgkin's lymphoma and, most recently, invasive cervical cancer in women are much more common in patients with AIDS than in age-matched controls. It is the greater than expected frequency of finding these malignancies that leads to their inclusion as AIDS-defining conditions.

5. Have any other malignancies been associated with AIDS?

Several non–AIDS-defining malignancies have been described in patients with AIDS, including Hodgkin's disease (HD), squamous cell carcinomas (SCC) of the head and neck, SCC of the anus, germ cell cancer, lung cancer, melanoma, basal cell carcinomas of the skin, colon cancer, and plasmacytoma. There are also several reports of myelodysplastic syndrome (pre-leukemia) and acute leukemia in patients with AIDS. Some of these malignancies, such as HD and germ cell cancers, are more common in 30–45-year-olds, which is the age group most often afflicted with AIDS. The results of epidemiologic studies to determine whether these cancers have a higher incidence in patients with AIDS than in age-matched controls are conflicting. There is also some controversy about different biologic behavior of malignancies in patients with AIDS compared with immune-competent patients. There are many examples of malignancies that are significantly more aggressive and more advanced in patients with AIDS.

6. Is HTLV-1 associated with AIDS-related malignancies?

The human T-cell leukemia/lymphoma virus (HTLV-1) is not the AIDS virus. It is a retro-virus endemic to southwest Japan, the Caribbean basin, Melanesia, and parts of Africa. There have been some reports of HTLV-1 in urban areas of the United States, such as New York City and Miami. Transmission routes are the same as for HIV— transplacental, blood transfusions, sexual contact, and sharing contaminated intravenous needles. In 1988, the Food and Drug Adminstration (FDA) formally recommended screening all whole blood and blood component donations for HTLV-1. In the United States, seroprevalence rates are approximately 0.016%. HTLV-1 is associated with adult T-cell leukemia/lymphoma as well as HTLV-1-associated myelopathy and tropical spastic paresis, a neurologic disease.

7. What causes KS?

There have been multiple theories about the cause of KS in AIDS. Some of the original the-ories even involved induction of KS by inhalation of amyl nitrates. Because KS was seen primar-ily in gay and bisexual men, it was hypothesized that KS was caused by an infectious agent such as cytomegalovirus (CMV), Epstein-Barr virus (EBV), or human papillomavirus (HPV). These viral DNA sequences were reported in some, but not all, samples of KS tumors. It is known that various soluble factors (cytokines) stimulate growth of KS in tissue culture systems as well as in the human body. These cytokines include interleukin-1 (IL-1), IL-6, tumor necrosis factor-beta (TNF-β), platelet-derived growth factor (PDGF), and Oncostatin-M. Cytokine production is also stimulated by opportunistic infections and some medications (e.g., steroids). In addition to cyto-kines, KS production and growth are stimulated by a protein product of the HIV virus. The HIV-tat protein has been found to induce and stimulate KS in animal systems. Recently, however, a new virus has been identified—KS-associated herpes virus (KSHV), also known as human herpes virus-8 (HHV-8). KSHV has been isolated from most AIDS-KS tumor cells, but it is not found in normal cells from the same patients. It is thought that KSHV may be the agent that transforms normal mesenchymal cells into "pre-KS" cells; further activation by cytokines (e.g., IL-1, HIV-tat, TNF) may trigger a true monoclonal malignant condition.

8. What types of NHL occur in AIDS?

The predominant types of NHL in AIDS are high-grade B-cell NHLs, such as immunoblas-tic, Burkitt's, non-Burkitt's small noncleaved (70%) lymphoma, and intermediate-grade large cell lymphomas (30%). Epidemiologic studies have shown a sharp rise in incidence of NHL since 1983, occurring predominantly in men aged 20–54 years. In a study of 100,000 patients with AIDS from 1981–1989, 3% had NHL. This is a 60-fold increase in incidence compared with the general population. NHL also may be clinically undetected before death. In an autopsy study of 101 patients with AIDS, 20 were found to have NHL.

9. Does HIV-related NHL follow the same natural history as in non-immunocompromised patients?

AIDS-associated NHL is significantly more aggressive than NHL in immunocompetent pa-tients. Typically it is more extensive and frequently involves extranodal sites (central nervous system, bone marrow, gastrointestinal tract); it is therefore diagnosed as stage IV disease. Patients also frequently have B symptoms (fevers, night sweats, and weight loss). Lymphomas of the central nervous system may occur as mass lesions or with leptomeningeal involvement only. The risk for NHL rises significantly as immunosuppression worsens. The incidence of NHL is much greater in patients with CD4 lymphocyte counts < 50. (A healthy person normally has a CD4 count of 500–1000). Opportunistic infections (infections that occur only because of the host's immunosuppression) are likely in individuals with CD4 counts < 200. Another unique finding in AIDS-associated NHL is the presence of polyclonal malignant cells. Monoclonality generally is considered a hallmark of malignancy. However, the patient with AIDS is exposed to repeated infections and subsequent polyclonal B-lymphocyte activation and transformation to a polyclonal malignancy.

10. How is KS staged?

Most malignancies are staged by parameters developed and standardized by the American Joint Committee on Cancer (AJCC). This system uses the tumor-node-metastasis (TNM) classification. However, KS has a unique presentation, prognosis, and natural history. Many staging systems modeled after the TNM classification have been proposed. However, they do not accurately predict the prognosis of AIDS-associated KS. Recently, the Oncology Subcommittee of the NIH-sponsored AIDS Clinical Treatment Group (ACTG) proposed a new staging scheme based on factors that more accurately predict the natural history and prognosis of KS.

Good risk—all of the following:	Poor risk—any of the following:
Tumor confined to skin and/or lymph nodes	Extensive oral, gastrointestinal, or other visceral disease, tumor associated with edema or ulceration
CD4 ≥ 200	CD4 < 200
No opportunistic infection, thrush, or B symptoms	History of opportunistic infection, or B symptoms
Karnofsky performance status ≥ 70%	Karnofsky performance status < 70

11. What is the treatment for HIV-associated NHL?

Because AIDS-associated NHL is an aggressive disease that usually presents with multiorgan involvement, chemotherapy is generally the standard of care. However, patients most likely to develop AIDS-associated NHL are severely immunocompromised and frequently have active opportunistic infections. A complete evaluation must be done to determine whether any treatment is appropriate. If treatment is chosen, multiagent chemotherapy is necessary. In immunocompetent patients, multiagent chemotherapy yields response rates as high as 80% and long-term survival rates of approximately 40%. However, in AIDS-associated NHL, response rates are 50% and median survival is approximately 5–6 months. Subgroups of patients have significantly better survival. Patients with CD4 > 100, Karnofsky performance status >70%, no opportunistic infections, and absence of extranodal disease have significantly improved survival with aggressive chemotherapy.

12. What special precautions are needed in giving chemotherapy for AIDS-associated NHL?

Completing full courses of chemotherapy may be more difficult because of frequent dose reductions and delays due to prolonged bone marrow suppression and opportunistic infections. Recent studies confirm improved outcomes with use of modified chemotherapy regimens and the generous use of hematopoetic growth factors (granulocyte colony-stimulating factor [G-CSF], granulocyte-macrophage colony-stimulating factor [GM-CSF]). Original studies, using full-dose chemotherapy, revealed excessive morbidity and mortality as a result of infections. The likelihood of morbidity increases as the degree of immunosuppression increases. Current recommendations include use of attenuated doses and/or use of hematopoetic growth factors if CD4 < 100, and standard chemotherapy doses (with or without G-CSF or GM-CSF) if CD4 > 200. Because the risk of leptomeningeal relapse is extremely high, use of meningeal prophylaxis is encouraged for all patients with AIDS-associated NHL. Such patients also should be treated with aggressive antiviral therapy and prophylaxis against *Pneumocystis carinii* pneumonia (PCP).

13. What are the indications for treatment of AIDS-associated KS?

The first factor to consider in the treatment of KS is the indications for treatment. KS often presents as limited skin involvement, which may not require immediate treatment. Some patients request immediate treatment for body image and cosmetic reasons. But if KS is asymptomatic, treatment may be postponed until there is further indication. The primary indications for treatment include (1) cosmetic control; (2) painful, bulky lesions; (3) oral lesions interfering with eating or swallowing; (4) lymphedema from lymph node or lymph vessel infiltration; (5) pulmonary involvement; (6) extensive gastrointestinal involvement causing GI obstruction; and (7) rapidly progressive disease.

14. Which treatment modalities are used for AIDS-associated KS?

The many options for treatment of KS include local or systemic therapy. Local treatments include radiation therapy, intralesional therapy, and cryotherapy (liquid nitrogen). Intralesional therapy usually involves dilute solutions of vincristine, but other agents also have been used. Systemic treatment includes single-agent chemotherapy, multiagent chemotherapy, and alpha-interferon (with or without concomitant antiretroviral therapy). Life-threatening disease, usually pulmonary disease, requires aggressive treatment with multiagent chemotherapy. Response rates have ranged from 70–100% with these regimens. Alpha-interferon has had response rates up to 65% in a select subset of patients with good prognosis (CD4 > 200, no opportunistic infection or B symptoms). The combination of antiretroviral therapy with alpha-interferon has allowed continued high response rates with lower doses of interferon. There has been no significant antitumor activity from antiretroviral therapy alone. A treatment recently approved by the Food and Drug Administration for KS is liposomal Adriamycin. The liposomal coating allows long circulation time, higher intralesion drug levels, and high response rates (up to 70%) with lower toxicity. A side effect common to nearly all of these treatments is neutropenia. Use of hematopoetic growth factors has helped to minimize cytopenia and infections and maximizes tolerated doses of therapy. All treatment for KS is palliative; therefore, risks and benefits must be weighed before initiating therapy.

15. Can treatment of HIV with antiretroviral therapy increase the risk of NHL?

This is a controversial question. Several reports have investigated this possibility. An autopsy study in 1992 found an association of increasing incidence of NHL with cumulative doses of zidovudine (AZT). An animal study also found a higher incidence of NHL in mice treated with Didanosine. However, a study in 1991 revealed no increase in the incidence of NHL with increased cumulative doses of AZT. The authors reported a risk of approximately 0.8% for each 6 months of AZT treatment, with an incidence up to 3.2% after 24 months of AZT treatment. This study suggests that an increased incidence of NHL correlates with increased survival due to antiretroviral therapy. If patients treated with antiretrovirals live longer, they have more time to become immunosuppressed, leading to increased exposure to lymphomagenic stimuli (e.g., viruses, oncogenes).

16. Why has invasive cervical SCCA been included as a AIDS-defining malignancy?

The incidence of women infected with HIV has risen significantly. HIV infection in women now accounts for 40% of all infections worldwide, and for up to 12% in the United States. In selected regions in the U.S., such as New York City, up to 25% of HIV cases are female. Most HIV infections in American women are from heterosexual transmission. It is also known that the incidence of cervical neoplasia is significantly higher in congenital immunodeficiencies, autoimmune diseases and acquired immunodeficiency states, such as organ transplantation. Reported rates of cervical neoplasia in such patients reach as high as 40%; the risk of anogenital neoplasia is 9–14-fold compared with matched controls. Immunosuppressed women with HIV have a much higher incidence of monilia vaginitis, sexually transmitted diseases, genital ulcers, and pelvic in-flammatory disease. Vaginal candidal infection may occur much earlier than oral thrush and be more resistant to conventional therapies. The association of human papillomavirus (HPV) and cervical neoplasia is well known. The oncogenic HPVs have been identified in 80–90% of inva-sive cervical cancer as well as high-grade cervical intraepithelial neoplasia (CIN). Several studies have reported a high incidence of HIV in women under 50 years of age with invasive cervical cancer. Furthermore, cervical cancer in the setting of HIV appears to be much more biologically aggressive, less responsive to conventional therapies, and associated with a poorer prognosis. Because of these findings, CDC revised the AIDS-defining criteria in 1993 to include invasive cervical cancer.

17. Is preinvasive neoplasia of the cervix included in the revised AIDS-defining CDC list?

The term *cervical intraepithelial neoplasia* (CIN) generally refers to cervical dysplasia, car-cinoma in situ, and preinvasive neoplasia. The incidence of HIV infection in women with CIN varies by risk group and geographic region. In high-risk areas, such as New York City, up to 13% of women in screening clinics were found to be HIV-positive. HIV-positive women have up to 10-fold increased risk of abnormal cervical cytology; some studies report abnormal cervical cy-tology in 30–60% of HIV-positive women. However, a high degree of discordance between cy-tology and biopsy have been found in HIV-positive women with negative cytology and abnormal cervical biopsies. Although preinvasive cervical neoplasia is not included in the AIDS definition, cervical dysplasia and CIA are considered AIDS-related conditions. The degree of cervical neo-plasia is correlated with the degree of immune suppression. Women with CIN tend to have lower CD4 counts than HIV-positive women without CIN.

18. What is the proper screening for cervical neoplasia in HIV-positive women?

Papanicolaou smears should be done every 6 months as well as baseline colposcopy or cer-vicography. It should also be remembered that there is an extremely high association between HPV and anal neoplasia. All HIV-positive women with HPV or cervical dysplasia should have a thorough anal examination, including visual and digital exam, anal cytology smear, and anoscopy, to rule out anal neoplasia.

19. What is the appropriate treatment for invasive malignancy of the cervix in women with AIDS?

Patients with AIDS-associated cervical cancer present with more advanced disease than age-matched controls. Incidence of high-grade tumors, lymph node involvement, and aggressive bio-logic behavior is more common in women with AIDS. In addition, risk of recurrence is higher and survival times are shorter for patients with AIDS. Therapy for invasive disease should be based on the patient's condition and stage of malignancy. Patients with relatively good immune function tolerate surgery quite well. Patients with advanced inoperable disease should be consid-ered for chemotherapy or radiation therapy. Patients with poor immune function do not tolerate pelvic radiation treatment or chemotherapy because of depressed hematologic reserve.

20. Are any nursing considerations different in patients with AIDS-related malignancies from those in other oncology patients?

Nursing care and symptom control are similar in patients with AIDS-related malignancies and other oncology patients, except that even more vigilance may be required for early identifica-tion of life-threatening infectious complications and assessment of neurologic abnormalities. Patients need to be well educated about prevention of infection and signs and symptoms of op-portunistic infections, particularly PCP (symptoms include shortness of breath with or without exertion and dry, nonproductive cough). In addition to other neutropenic precautions, HIV-in-fected patients should be instructed not to handle or eat raw meat, to avoid eating raw shellfish due to risk of vibrio, and to wear gloves when handling litter boxes because of the potential for contacting toxoplasmosis. Assessment of neurologic abnormalites can be complicated because mental status changes may be associated with HIV-related dementia, central nervous system involvement, drug side effects, viral or opportunistic infections, or depression.

Psychosocial issues and stresses may differ and be more complicated than in the oncology patient without AIDS. Even in communities who are accepting of AIDS, the patient with AIDS and cancer may experience more social isolation, particularly as the illness progresses,

A particularly difficult nursing challenge in patients with AIDS-related malignancies is keeping track of various drug interactions and incompatibilities in patients who are on multiple drug regimens to treat malignancy, underlying HIV disease, and opportunistic infections. Patients need to be encouraged to inform health care providers if they are taking any other drugs, remedies, or alternative care substances that also may interact with prescribed therapies. There is a large potential for drug interactions that may be synergistic or antagonistic and result in increased effect, decreased effect, or enhanced toxicity.

21. Are there any "red flags" to alert the health care provider about potential drug interactions in HIV-infected patients?

Red flags that should alert nurses to potential drug interactions include the following: treatment or prophylaxis for mycobacterial infections with rifamycins (e.g., rifampin, rifabutin) or macrolides (e.g., erythromycin); therapy with azole antifungal drugs (e.g., ketoconazole) or protease inhibitors (e.g., ritonavir); and any multidrug regimen. Although most interactions do not require changes in drug selection, nurses should be aware of clinically significant interactions. For example, patients with advanced HIV disease and cancer frequently receive palliative care drugs such as opioids, antidepressants, sedatives, and/or hypnotics. Serious clinical consequences may result from increased concentrations due to altered clearances when these drugs are taken along with ritonavir (an antiretroviral, protease inhibitor drug).[7]

BIBLIOGRAPHY

1. Emmanoulides C, Miles SA, Mitsuyasu RT: Pathogenesis of AIDS-related KS. Oncology 10:335–341, 1996.
2. Kaplan LD, Northfelt DS: Malignancies associated with AIDS. In Kaplan LD, Northfelt DS (eds): The Medical Management of AIDS, 4th Ed. Philadelphia. W.B. Saunders, 1995.
3. Levine AM: Acquired immunodeficiency syndrome-related lymphoma. Blood 80:8–20, 1992.
4. Levine AM, Bernstein L, Sullivan-Halley J, et al: Role of zidovudine antiretroviral therapy in the pathogenesis of AIDS-related lymphoma. Blood 86:4612–4616, 1995.
5. Moore PS, Chang Y: Detection of herpesvirus-like DNA sequences in KS in patients with and those without HIV infection. N Engl J Med 332:1181–1185, 1995.
6. Northfelt DW: Cervical and anal neoplasia and HPV infections in persons with HIV infection. Oncology 8:33–37, 1994.
7. Piscitelli SC, Flexner C, Minor JR, et al: AIDS commentary: Drug interactions in patients infected with human immunodeficiency virus. Clin Infect Dis 23:685–693, 1996.

19. BLADDER CANCER

Patrick Judson, MD, and Mark Nishiya, MD

1. How many new cases of bladder cancer will be reported in the United States in 1997? How many deaths will be due to bladder cancer?

In 1997, there will be an estimated 54,500 new cases and 11,700 deaths.

2. Is bladder cancer more common in men than in women?

Almost three times as many men as women are affected by bladder cancer.

3. What are the risk factors for bladder cancer?
- Exposure to aromatic amines and smoking cigarettes (contains aromatic amines)
- Schistosomal haemotobium infections (squamous cell carcinoma of the bladder)
- Chronic irritation from bladder stones or chronic indwelling Foley catheter

4. Which chromosome is most commonly affected in bladder cancer?

Although others may be affected, chromosome 9 is commonly altered.

5. What are the histologic types of bladder cancer?

Transitional cell carcinomas (90%) may be solid or papillary. They are low-grade, noninvasive, and most commonly found in the United States. In the Middle East, where schistosomal haemotobium infections are common, squamous cell carcinomas are the most common histologic type of bladder cancer. Chronic bladder irritation is also a predisposing factor. Primary adenocarcinoma of the bladder may occur but is rare.

6. What are the signs and symptoms of bladder cancer?

The most frequent signs and symptoms are gross and microscopic hematuria (80%) and irritative symptoms (urgency, frequency, dysuria) in approximately 20% of all patients.

7. What are the most common sites of metastases?

The most common metastatic sites are bones, lungs, lymph nodes, and liver. Of interest, in patients who have been successfully treated with combination chemotherapy, the central nervous system is a common site of metastases.

8. What are the most appropriate tests for the staging of bladder cancer?
- History and physical examination (including bimanual examination at the time of transurethral resection)
- Complete blood count, chemistry profile, urinalysis, chest radiograph, urine cytology
- Intravenous pyelography (IVP)
- Cystoscopy and transurethral resection of bladder tumor (TURBT) + bladder mapping and sampling of the floor of the prostatic urethra in men with high-grade bladder cancer
- In patients with muscle invasion, an abdominal computed tomography (CT) scan and bone scan should be considered.
- CT scan of the chest should be considered in high-grade, muscle-invading tumors.

9. What prognostic features are important?
- Tumor grade
- Muscle invasion
- Blood vessel or lymphatic invasion

10. Describe the tumor, node, metastasis (TNM) system for staging bladder cancer.

T0	No evidence of primary tumor
TA	Noninvasive papillary tumor
TIS	Carcinoma in situ
T1	Invasion of lamina propria
T2	Invasion of superficial muscle
T3a	Invasion of deep muscle
T3b	Invasion of perivesical fat
T4a	Invasion of prostate, uterus, vagina
T4b	Invasion of pelvic or abdominal wall
N0	No nodal metastases
N1	One lymph mode metastasis < 2 cm in size
N2	Metastases in one node, 2–5 cm, or multiple nodes with none > 5 cm
N3	Nodal metastases > 5 cm
M0	No distant metastases
M1	Distant metastases

11. Do grade and stage have a bearing on rate of progression?

The progression of grade I tumors is about 2%; of grade II tumors, about 11%; and of grade III tumors, about 45%. About 4% of stage TA tumors and 30% of stage T1 tumors progress. In general, one may think of bladder cancer as superficial or invasive. Superficial cancers are stages TA, TIS, and T1; invasive cancers are stages T2–T4. Superficial cancers tend to recur throughout the patient's life but remain superficial; they require continued monitoring and local treatment. Invasive cancers usually require radical surgery and are worrisome for metastatic spread.

12. What is the treatment of superficial tumors after cystoscopy?

Stage TIS tumors should be treated with intravesical agents, such as BCG (bacillus Calmette-Guérin—an attenuated strain of *Mycobacterium bovis*), doxorubicin, mitomycin, and thiotepa. The agent with the best response rate is BCG. In controlled trials, BCG has been shown to be superior to most available intravesical agents. It decreases both the risk of recurrence and the risk of progression. TA and T1 lesions can be managed with surveillance, cystoscopy, and cytology every three months if they are low grade. Recurrent and high-grade superficial tumors may be treated with intravesical agents after resection of the tumor.

13. What is the standard regimen for intravesical BCG?

The standard regimen is weekly treatment for 6 weeks with repeat cystoscopy 6 weeks after the last treatment. Some evidence suggests that maintenance BCG improves results.

14. What systemic reaction occurs in some patients treated with BCG?

Fever > 103° F is seen in approximately 3% of patients receiving BCG. Patients are hospitalized and treated with cycloserine, isoniazid (INH), and rifampin. BCG therapy should not be reinstituted. Some patients experience low-grade fevers, which usually resolve within 24 hours. No INH or rifampin is necessary, and BCG may be continued with close monitoring. Patients with low-grade fevers that last longer than 24 hours can be pretreated with INH, and BCG therapy can be safely continued.

BCG sepsis occurs in 0.4% of patients. Traumatic catheterization with bleeding is the most common cause of intravascular absorption of BCG and development of sepsis syndrome. Treatment includes INH, rifampin, and cycloserine. The use of prednisone is controversial. Patients definitely should not receive BCG again.

15. Which patients should not be treated with BCG?

BCG should be avoided in patients who are immunosuppressed, who have active urinary tract infections, or who have exhibited previous sensitivity to BCG.

16. What is the treatment for muscle-invading transitional cell carcinoma?

In the United States radical cystectomy is the treatment of choice. This procedure involves removal of the local pelvic lymph nodes and radical cystoprostatectomy in men and anterior exenteration in women. Patients have urinary diversions (e.g., ileal-conduit with external bag or continent urinary diversions that do not involve external drainage).

17. What morbidities are associated with cystectomy? How can they be decreased?

- **Impotence.** Potency can be maintained by surgical techniques that spare the nerves traveling posteriorly to the prostate gland. However, most patients become impotent if classic surgical techniques are used.
- **Need for urinary stoma.** Neobladders such as Indiana and Koch pouches prevent continuous loss of urine. A neobladder is formed from the bowel and may enable a patient to achieve urinary continence.

18. What is an ileal conduit?

Compared with continent diversions, an ileal conduit may have less morbidity. However, it is an incontinent type of diversion and requires an external drainage bag. The ureters are not brought to the skin directly after removal of the bladder because of the high rate of stoma stenosis, which may lead to renal obstruction and failure. By interspersing a segment of ileum between the ureters and skin, this complication is virtually eliminated. The ileal conduit maintains its blood and nerve supply and continues to peristalse and eliminate urine.

19. What is an Indiana pouch? How is it formed?

An Indiana pouch is a continent, catherizable neobladder. It is made from the terminal ileum and proximal colon. The colon portion is opened, then folded back on itself to decrease the pressure within the pouch as well as to increase the volume. The terminal ileum is left attached to the colon and brought to the skin. The ileal-cecal valve keeps the urine from leaking out of the colon and can be catheterized through the stoma to drain the pouch. No bag is required over the stoma because it should not leak. The pouch should be catheterized every 4–6 hours using a clean technique. A 4×4 gauze pad is all that is needed to cover the stoma.

20. What is a Studer pouch? How is it formed?

A Studer pouch is a neobladder made entirely from ileum. In men, it can be connected to the urethra so that they can void through the urethra and maintain continence. More of these pouches will be seen in the future for men with bladder cancer.

21. Does neoadjuvant or adjuvant therapy have a role in bladder cancer?

Evidence suggests that in high-risk patients combination cisplatin-based therapy before or after surgery decreases the risk of recurrence and increases cure rates.

22. Is there an effective treatment for metastatic transitional cell carcinoma?

Cisplatin-based chemotherapy is effective in metastatic transitional cell carcinoma. Methotrexate, vinblastine, Adriamycin, and cisplatin (M-VAC) is a commonly used regimen. The patient should have a good performance status, adequate myocardial reserve, and adequate renal function. Growth factors may be useful in conjunction with M-VAC. An alternative regimen is taxol and cisplatin. Adequate hydration should be ensured with vigorous use of antiemetics. Carboplatin may be substituted for cisplatin.

23. What types of alteration should nurses expect after cystectomy?

- Because the bowels normally make mucous, neobladders and ileal conduits will continue to make mucous. Mucous freely passes out of ileal conduits but may need to be irrigated from continent neobladders.
- Infections are managed with antibiotics. Urine cultures are always positive because of intestinal colonization by bacteria. True infections are manifested by fever and possible flank pain.

- Reflux of urine to the kidneys may contribute to pyelonephritis and late renal deterioration.
- Stones may develop in the kidney or pouch if urinary stasis is present.

24. What metabolic alterations may patients experience after surgery for bladder cancer?

Patients may develop metabolic disturbances depending on the type of urinary diversion and segment of intestine used. The intestine is responsible for absorption; therefore, if urine is in prolonged contact with the intestine, metabolic disturbances may result. Ileal conduits probably have the least amount of metabolic abnormalities because of the short time of urine contact. Continent diversions using ileum and colon may cause hyperchloremic metabolic acidosis, which in turn may cause osteoporosis over the long term. Patients may have frequent loose bowel movements after an intestinal urinary diversion. This symptom may resolve over a 3-month period. A few patients have persistent change in bowel habits, especially if the ileal-cecal valve is removed.

Patients with presurgical renal dysfunction (creatinine > 2.0) may have a problem compensating for this metabolic alteration and probably are candidates for ileal conduits only.

Patients with neobladders and patients with resection of large amounts of terminal ileum are at risk for vitamin B12 deficiency, possibly leading to megaloblastic anemia. Blood levels should be monitored.

BIBLIOGRAPHY

1. Kelly LP, Miaskowski C: An overview of bladder cancer: Treatment and nursing implications. Oncol Nurs Forum 23:460–468, 1996.
2. Parker SL, Tong T, Bolden S, Wingo PA: Cancer Statistics 1997. CA Cancer J Clin 47:5–27, 1997.
3. Wilding G: Genitourinary cancer chemotherapy. In Brain MC, Carbone PP (eds.): Current Therapy in Hematology/Oncology, 5th ed. St. Louis, Mosby, 1995, pp 444–450.

20. BONE AND SOFT TISSUE SARCOMAS

Kyle M. Fink, MD, and Ioana Hinshaw, MD

Quick Facts—Sarcomas

Incidence	**Rare tumors**, <1% of all cancers; 6,000 new cases of soft tissue sarcomas, 2,000 new cases of bone sarcomas annually
Mortality	<1% of all cancer deaths; 3,100 deaths from soft tissue sarcomas, 1,200 deaths from bone sarcomas annually
Risk factors	Most patients have no known risk factors; rarely: genetically inherited diseases (von Recklinghausen's disease), prior radiation therapy, Paget's disease (osteosarcoma)
Histology	**Soft tissue sarcomas** have at least 70 histologic subtypes (liposarcoma, rhabdomyosarcoma, leiomyosarcoma, malignant fibrous histiocytoma) **Bone sarcomas** (osteosarcoma, Ewing's sarcoma, chondrosarcoma, malignant fibrous histiocytoma of bone)
Symptoms	Local pain, soft tissue swelling, palpable mass

Staging	**Soft tissue sarcomas** (tumor, node, metastasis [TNM])
	    Stage I: well differentiated, no nodes, no metastases
	    Stage II: moderately differentiated, no nodes, no metastases
	    Stage III: poorly differentiated, no nodes, no metastases
	    Stage I, II, III: subclassified into A (< 5cm) and B (> 5 cm)
	    Stage IV: any differentiation, with nodes and/or metastases
	Bone sarcomas (surgical staging more often used)
	    Stage I: low grade
	    Stage II: high grade
	    Stage I, II: subclassified into A (intracompartmental) and B (extracompartmental)
	    Stage III: any grade, with regional and/or distant metastasis

Treatment	**Soft tissue sarcomas**

Treatment		
	Small, well differentiated tumors	Surgery alone
	Large, poorly differentiated tumors	Multimodality treatment, including chemotherapy, surgery, and, rarely, radiation therapy
	Osteosarcoma, Ewing sarcoma	Chemotherapy followed by surgery followed by chemotherapy

1. What are sarcomas?

Sarcoma is derived from the Greek *sarkoma*, meaning fleshy growth; it refers to a group of malignant tumors that originate from a common embryologic ancestry, the primitive mesoderm. The mesoderm gives rise during embryogenesis to soft tissues (e.g., muscles, tendons, fibrous tissue) as well as bone and cartilage. Sarcomas are tumors derived from any of these structures.

2. Are any risk factors associated with the development of sarcomas?

The majority of sarcomas appear in patients with no known predisposing factors. Some genetically transmitted diseases, however, are associated with an increased incidence of sarcomas. For example, von Recklinghausen's disease (neurofibromatosis) carries a 7–10% chance of developing neurofibrosarcoma, an otherwise rare sarcoma. There are also a few reported cases of sarcomas arising in damaged tissues after radiation therapy. Radiation therapy-related sarcomas, more common after high doses of radiation, tend to be high grade and occur after a latency of more than 10 years. Their distribution involves the sternum, sternoclavicular joint, cervical/thoracic spine, and soft tissue areas in the radiation fields used for treatment of lymphomas, seminomas, and Hodgkin's disease. Paget's disease carries an increased risk for developing osteosarcoma in the affected bones (estimated to be 1000 times higher than that of the normal population).

3. How are sarcomas classified?

Sarcomas are divided into soft tissue sarcomas and bone sarcomas. There are at least 70 different histologic subtypes of soft tissue sarcomas, which are classified according to the appearance of the tissue it has formed (e.g., fibrosarcoma, liposarcoma). Bone sarcomas include osteosarcoma, Ewing's sarcoma, and malignant fibrous histiocytoma (MFH) of bone.

4. What are the most common sarcomas in adults? In children?

In adults the most common sarcomas are malignant fibrous histiosarcoma, liposarcoma, leiomyosarcoma, and osteosarcoma. Children most often have rhabdomyosarcoma, osteosarcoma, or Ewing's sarcoma.

5. Describe the importance of histologic grade in sarcomas.

Histologic grade is of paramount importance in evaluating the aggressiveness of sarcomas and is included in the pathology report along with the exact histopathologic type. The grade may be low, intermediate, or high; high-grade sarcomas are the most aggressive. High-grade tumors more often have distant metastasis and are associated with a lower survival rate. Low-grade tumors in general have a better prognosis. The histopathologic grade is based on the degree of differentiation, cellularity, number of mitoses, pleomorphism, and amount of necrosis.

6. What is the clinical presentation of patients with sarcomas?

The early symptoms of sarcomas are nonspecific and include mild pain and mild soft tissue swelling; they are often attributed to local trauma, which leads to frequent delay in diagnosis. Eventually they grow to form palpable masses. Of interest, in osteosarcoma the pain precedes the soft tissue swelling and is caused by stretching of the periosteum by the tumor.

7. What steps are necessary in the diagnosis and staging of sarcomas?

The steps needed in diagnosing sarcomas include computed tomography (CT) and magnetic resonance imaging (MRI) of the affected area and open biopsy. MRI is the most sensitive imaging modality because of high resolution and accurate distinctions between normal and abnormal tissues. After MRI confirmation an open incisional biopsy is done. Although fine-needle aspiration (FNA) and core biopsy can give a diagnosis of malignancy, they rarely provide the exact histopathologic type and grade of the tumor. The incision should be made in a direction that allows incorporation into the subsequent excision, which prevents local recurrence. Therefore, it is recommended that the biopsy be done by the surgeon who will ultimately excise the tumor. Once the diagnosis is made, the next step is complete staging to define the extent of disease. This includes a CT of the chest and a bone scan to exclude metastasis in these two most frequent sites of distant spread.

8. How does staging differ between soft-tissue and bone sarcomas?

Bone sarcomas are staged using the TNM system with the additional factor of intra- vs. extracompartmental location. The staging of soft tissue sarcomas is unique in the use of histophysiologic grade to identify the stage of disease. The grade of malignancy has greater bearing on treatment planning and prognosis than apparent cell origin. The grade determines the stage.

9. What are the most important prognostic factors in sarcomas?

The TNM stage has direct influence on survival: stage I patients have a 5-year survival rate of 90%; stage II, 70%; stage III, 20–50%; and stage IV, < 20%. High-grade tumors > 5 cm have a more than 50% chance of recurrence, whereas tumors < 2 cm have an excellent prognosis with a cure rate of approximately 90%. It is important to emphasize the poor prognosis of local recurrence, which almost always correlates with the presence of systemic disease.

10. Describe the prognosis and management of pulmonary metastasis from sarcomas.

The lung represents the most common site of distant spread of sarcomas. It is important to recognize a subset of patients that benefits from surgical resection of pulmonary metastasis. This subset includes patients whose primary tumors have been controlled, who lack extrapulmonary disease, and who have adequate cardiac and pulmonary function. Important prognostic factors are number of pulmonary nodules (preferably < five), disease-free interval (> 1 year), and completeness of resection. Resection of up to 5 nodules or aggressive repeated metastectomies result in a long-term disease-free survival rate of 20–35%. The prognosis of patients who present with pulmonary metastases at diagnosis is uniformly fatal.

11. Where do soft tissue sarcomas most commonly arise?

Soft tissue sarcomas most often arise in the extremities with more frequent involvement of the lower (38%) than upper extremities (11%); rarely they are seen in other parts of the body, such as the retroperitoneal area (15%), trunk (13%), viscera (5%), and head and neck region (5%).

12. To what sites do soft tissue sarcomas metastasize?

The lungs are the most frequent site of metastasis (33%), followed by bones (23%) and the liver (15%).

13. What is the current therapy for soft tissue sarcomas of the extremities?

For low-grade sarcomas the treatment is complete surgical excision with negative margins, a prerequisite for local control and cure. Low-grade sarcomas are relatively chemo- and radio-resistant; therefore, chemotherapy and radiation therapy play no role in their management. High-grade sarcomas show higher response rates to chemotherapy and radiation. For small high-grade tumors the preferred modality is still surgery; however, for larger tumors (> 5 cm) a multi-modality approach that involves both chemotherapy and surgery is preferred. In this setting, some centers have used intraarterial neoadjuvant chemotherapy followed by limb-sparing surgery.

14. Which chemotherapy agents are most effective against soft tissue sarcomas?

The most effective drugs in this setting are Adriamycin and ifosfamide, which have response rates of 15–25% when used as single agents. The preferred approach is combination regimens such as MAID (mesna, Adriamycin, ifosfamide, and dimethyltriazenyl imidazole carboxamide [DTIC]), which show response rates as high as 40–50%.

15. What are osteosarcomas?

Osteosarcomas are malignant tumors usually arising in the bone that are characterized by bone or osteoid production.

16. Which age group and gender are most affected by osteosarcoma?

Osteosarcoma usually affects young patients, 10–20 years of age, with a peak incidence around the adolescent growth spurt. The second peak occurs during the sixth decade of life. Osteosarcoma affects men more than women (male-to-female ratio = 1.5:1).

17. Which sites are most often involved by osteosarcoma?

The knee is most often affected, with the distal femur being the most frequent primary site. The proximal tibia is second in frequency, followed by the proximal humerus.

18. What is the recommended management of osteosarcomas?

In the past osteosarcomas were treated by amputations one joint above the location of the primary tumor. Despite this mutilating surgery, survival was poor (in the range of 20%), with patients succumbing to metastatic disease. The modern approach involves preoperative (neoadjuvant) chemotherapy followed by limb-sparing surgery and more adjuvant chemotherapy. Preoperative chemotherapy decreases the size of the tumor and permits limb-sparing surgery; most importantly, however, response to chemotherapy is an important prognostic factor and correlates with survival. Limb salvage surgery is now possible in close to 90% of cases. Some institutions use preoperative intraarterial cisplatin with great success.

19. What is considered a good histologic response to chemotherapy in osteosarcoma? What are the clinical implications?

The response to preoperative chemotherapy as assessed by the pathologist through examination of the surgical specimen is an important piece of information and correlates with long-term survival. A good pathologic response is defined by more than 90% necrosis of the specimen. In general, patients with good response to chemotherapy have a 10-year survival rate approaching 90%, whereas the rate is much lower in patients without such a response.

20. What are the most effective drugs for treatment of osteosarcoma?

The most active drugs are high-dose methotrexate, cisplatin, Adriamycin, cyclophosphamide, and ifosfamide.

21. What is the long-term prognosis for osteosarcomas?

With modern therapy the long-term survival rate is approximately 80%. Almost 90% of patients are able to undergo limb-sparing surgeries. The local recurrence rate is approximately 5–10%.

22. What is Ewing's sarcoma? How does it differ from osteosarcoma?

Ewing's sarcoma is a rare tumor of the bone that affects mainly adolescents. It differs from osteosarcoma morphologically because of the presence of small, round, blue cells as opposed to the typical spindle cells of osteosarcomas. It also has a preference for the midshaft of the bone rather than the diaphysis and tends to involve the pelvic bones, scapula, and spine in addition to the femurs. Bone metastases are more common than in osteosarcoma.

23. Describe the usual plan of therapy and prognosis in Ewing sarcoma.

Therapy should involve a multimodality approach; the initial step is preoperative chemotherapy followed by radiation therapy to the primary lesion. The next step is limb-sparing surgery with adjuvant chemotherapy. The usual treatment program involves extended periods of chemotherapy (9–12 months). With this approach the long-term disease-free survival rate is approximately 80%.

24. How do you choose between limb-sparing surgery and amputation in the surgical treatment of sarcomas?

In experienced hands, limb-sparing surgery is considered safe and routine for a large number of carefully selected patients. Use of neoadjuvant chemotherapy increases the number of patients who undergo this procedure. Because limb-sparing surgery offers similar local control rates as amputation and provides better quality of life, it is the procedure of choice. However, in large and poorly differentiated tumors, the risks and benefits must be carefully weighed by the surgeon, keeping in mind that local recurrence is almost a death warrant.

25. What are contraindications for limb-salvage surgery?

Bone tumors with major neurovascular involvement	Pathologic fracture with hematoma at tumor site
Infection	Muscle involvement (extensive)
Inappropriate biopsy site	Immature skeletal age (< 10 years of age—rare).

26. What are the major issues facing nurses caring for patients with osteosarcoma?

Patients facing limb surgery with or without amputation have reduced mobility, which affects self care in dressing, personal care, and activities of daily living. Some restrictions affect employment, relationships, house, adaptation, and body image.

27. What are the toxicities associated with ifosfamide, a treatment for osteosarcoma?

Many patients undergo aggressive chemotherapy with high-dose ifosfamide. In the immediate period of drug administration, nausea and vomiting may be moderate to severe, requiring combinations of antiemetics. Central nervous system toxicity has also been reported and usually is manifested by a decrease in mental alertness, confusion, hallucinations, cerebellar signs, and seizures. These symptoms most commonly start within 2 hours after a bolus is administered and appear to be dose-related. The condition resolves with discontinuation of the drug. Toxicities to be expected later include hemorrhagic cystitis and myelosuppression. Hemorrhagic cystitis is prevented by aggressive hydration, frequent voiding, and administration of Mesna, which protects against ototoxicity. Mesna should be given along with ifosfamide, and patients may need to take Mesna in divided doses 4 hours and 8 hours after ifosfamide in the home setting.

BIBLIOGRAPHY

1. Daliani D, Patel SR: Soft-tissue and bone sarcomas. In Padzur R (ed): Medical Oncology: A Comprehensive Review. Huntington, NY, PRR, 1995, pp 511–529.
2. De Vita VT Jr, Hellman S, Rosenberg SA: Cancer: Principles and Practice of Oncology, 5th ed. Philadelphia, J.B. Lippincott, 1997.
3. Dorr RT, Von Hoff DD: Cancer Chemotherapy Handbook. Norwalk, CT, Appleton-Lange, 1994.
4. Fink K, Wilkins R: Intra-arterial chemotherapy and limb preservation in osteosarcoma in children [abstract]. ASCO 1001:1126, 1991.
5. Fletcher BD: Response of osteosarcoma and Ewing's sarcoma to chemotherapy: Imaging evaluation. AJR 157:825–833, 1991.
6. Haskell C: Cancer Treatment, 4th ed. 1995.
7. Jaffe N: Chemotherapy for malignant bone tumors. Orthop Clin North Am 30:487–499, 1989.
8. Lenhard RE, Lawrence W Jr, McKenna RJ: General approach to the patient. In Textbook of Clinical Oncology, 2nd ed. 1995.
9. Seeger LL, Gold RH, Chandnani VP: Diagnostic imaging of osteosarcoma. Clin Orthop Rel Res 270: 254–263, 1991.
10. Sim FH, Bowman WE, Wilkins RM, Choa EYS: Limb salvage in primary malignant bone tumors. Orthopedics 8:574–581, 1985.
11. Storm FK: Sarcoma: Surgery in brain MC. In Carbone PP (ed): Current Therapy in Hematology-Oncology, 5th ed. St. Louis, Mosby, 1995, pp 487–492.
12. Wilkins RM, Sim FH: Evaluation of bone and soft tissue tumors. In D'Ambrosia (ed): Musculoskeletal Disorders: Regional Examination and Differential Diagnosis, 2nd ed. Philadelphia, J.B. Lippincott, 1986.

21. BRAIN TUMORS

Betty Owens, RN, MS, and Kevin Lillehei, MD

1. Do cellular phones really cause brain tumors?

Why people develop brain tumors is unknown, with a few exceptions. The results of various studies do not support the hypothesis that cellular phones play a role in the development of brain tumors. In addition, no evidence suggests that electromagnetic fields or power lines contribute to brain tumor development. Exposure to certain chemicals is loosely associated with a higher incidence of brain tumors; however, the only clear association is with radiation therapy. The most common tumor, astrocytoma, has not been associated with a causal factor. Although familial clustering is rare, some families have a predisposition to develop brain tumors; these families are being studied. It is not helpful for patients with brain tumor to expend energy considering the cause. Instead, the patient's energy should be redirected to treatment and recovery.

2. Who gets brain tumors?
- Brain tumors develop in persons of all ages, but the two peak age ranges are 3–8 and 40–60 years.
- The overall incidence is slightly higher in males than females. The incidence of brain tumors is thought to be increasing, but only time will prove this hypothesis true or false.
- Patients with von Hippel-Lindau disease develop multiple benign vascular tumors called hemangioblastomas.
- Patients with neurofibromatosis develop multiple benign tumors called neurofibromas and have a higher risk of developing meningioma or astrocytoma.

3. What are the incidence and mortality rate of brain tumors?

In 1997, it is estimated that there will be 17,600 new cases of primary brain tumors and central nervous system neoplasms—10,100 in men and 7,500 in women; 13,200 deaths will be attributed to brain tumors. The U.S. Central Brain Tumor Registry reports an even higher incidence of primary brain tumors: > 28,500 new cases in 1996.

4. What is the difference between benign and malignant brain tumors?

The major difference between benign and malignant brain tumors is the aggressiveness of tumor histology. For example, meningioma is usually considered a benign tumor because it grows very slowly, does not invade normal brain, and has distinct borders. Thus, tumor removal can be accomplished with minimal risk of damage to surrounding brain. The most aggressive and malignant primary brain tumors, gliomas, start within the brain itself—not within the neurons but within the glials cells that carry nourishment to and waste from the neurons. Gliomas infiltrate normal brain and do not have distinct borders. This infiltrating border makes total surgical resection virtually impossible. Most gliomas have a relatively high growth rate. Even those that are initially low grade have the potential to degenerate into a more aggressive lesion.

In determining whether a tumor is benign or malignant, its location in the brain also needs to be considered. Histologically benign tumors may be located near critical structures and, therefore, cannot be surgically removed. Such tumors eventually cause neurologic deficits and possibly death. Thus a tumor may be benign by histology but cause severe problems because of its location within the brain.

The term benign should be used cautiously in describing brain tumors. Perhaps the best approach is to describe the nature of the tumor as it is now and what it may become, leaving the patient with hope but indicating that no one knows when and if the tumor will recur.

5. Which type of brain tumor is considered the most aggressive? Why?

Astrocytoma grade IV, or glioblastoma multiforme, strikes the greatest fear in health professionals and eventually in patients and family members as they learn the prognosis. These tumors grow at a phenomenal rate, quickly leading to significant neurologic problems. Prognosis without treatment is death within a few weeks. With surgery, radiation, and chemotherapy, survival can be extended to 12–18 months. Even within this classification, the growth rate of individual tumors varies. Glioblastoma behaves just as aggressively in children.

6. Describe the common problems experienced by patients with brain tumor.

All symptoms of a brain tumor are caused by tumor infiltration, pressure on normal brain, or treatment of the tumor. Headaches are common but usually can be managed by adjusting the doses of corticosteroids. Seizures occur frequently and, if not controlled, can be quite disturbing for the patient and family. Focal deficits involving motor or sensory loss, vision, or speech are common and relate to the location of the tumor within the brain. Fatigue is often a complaint and is managed by frequent rest periods. With conventional radiotherapy, hair loss is usually temporary but may be permanent, depending on the skin surface dose. Weight gain is caused by steroids, fluid retention, and ravenous appetite. Nausea and vomiting may be late signs of increased intracranial pressure from tumor growth or result from radiation and/or chemotherapy. Diarrhea, stomatitis, anorexia, and dyspnea are rarely experienced.

7. What is the most difficult problem to manage?

For short periods, living with a brain tumor is tolerable, but long illness becomes trying for patient and family. Family members who find it difficult to believe that the patient cannot control his or her behavior need repeated explanations and support. The most difficult problem for patients, family, and health care professionals is cognitive impairment, which may include the following:

1. **Reasoning and judgment** may decline before patients are diagnosed. For example, a business owner may make poor decisions, not follow through with plans, or fail to meet deadlines. If there are no other overt symptoms of the brain tumor, the business may become bankrupt before someone challenges the owner's judgment or recognizes the problem.

2. **Lack of initiative** is particularly common in patients with frontal lobe tumors. For example, the patient is aware that he or she needs to do something but cannot get started. The family may think that the patient is lazy or obstinate, and the supervisor at work knows only that the job is not getting done. Often relationships at work and home suffer, and the patient may be fired or divorced before the brain tumor is diagnosed.

3. **Lack of awareness** of neurologic deficits is also common. If a family member tries to point out such deficits, the patient may refuse to believe that anything is wrong. Athough the patient does not intend to be obstinate, this situation becomes exasperating for both patient and family member.

4. **Short-term memory deficit** may complicate the lack of awareness. The patient asks the same question over and over again and cannot follow through on tasks because he or she does not remember. Many of these symptoms are similar to those of patients with Alzheimer's disease.

5. **Personality change** is particularly difficult for the family. Roles usually change because the patient cannot perform normal physical tasks or offer the usual emotional support and companionship.

8. When is surgery indicated? Why are some brain tumors removed, whereas others are not?

After a brain tumor is diagnosed by computed tomography (CT) or magnetic resonance imaging (MRI), the physician, patient, and family determine which treatment approach is best. If at all possible, a tissue diagnosis is made. Tissue may be obtained from an open or needle biopsy; the method is determined by the location of the tumor, its proximity to critical structures, and the damage that may result from an open craniotomy or needle biopsy. Another factor in this decision is the predicted diagnosis—whether the tumor is thought to be benign or malignant by histology.

In most situations, the goal is to remove as much of the tumor as safely possible. If neurologic risk is minimal, gross total resection may be attempted. If neurologic risk is great, partial resection or biopsy may be the procedure of choice. For example, a brain scan may demonstrate that a meningioma is attached to a dural surface and has clear, distinct borders. If totally removed, a meningioma may not recur; even if only partially removed, it will probably grow back very slowly. The surgeon may choose to perform an open craniotomy and to remove as much tumor as is safe. On the other hand, if the tumor is thought to be an astrocytoma and is in a critical area, biopsy alone may be performed, followed by radiotherapy. Total or partial removal of an aggressive tumor may not be warranted if deficits result; in most cases, even with gross total removal, microscopic cells remain. The goal of surgery is to extend survival without sacrificing quality of life.

9. When is radiation therapy given?

After optimal tumor removal, radiotherapy is the treatment of choice for malignant lesions. Conventional radiotherapy is generally preferred; however, other modalities, such as hyperfractionated radiotherapy, stereotactic radiosurgery, and brachytherapy, are under investigation.

10. How are stereotactic biopsy and stereotactically guided craniotomy accomplished?

Stereotactic technology has greatly improved the quality and safety of neurosurgical procedures for patients with brain tumors. Stereotaxis is based on the concept that the location of a lesion can be determined more precisely by a fixed frame of reference in relation to the brain.

A spherical open frame (similar to a halo) is pinned to the skull, and the patient is taken for a CT or MRI scan. The subsequent films show not only the tumor but also points of reference on the frame. With the aid of a computer program, the surgeon can determine the x, y, and z coordinates of the lesion. During surgery, a special frame with degree markings is placed over the head and attached to the stereotactic halo. A needle is attached to the frame at a precise degree and trajectory and then passed to the target. If a biopsy is indicated, the target is usually the center of the lesion. Multiple samples are taken to ensure that representative tissue is obtained. If a craniotomy is indicated, the periphery of the lesion is targeted. During the craniotomy, the needle points to the edges of the lesion. A stereotactically guided craniotomy is indicated when the tumor is close to critical areas and its consistency makes it difficult for the surgeon to differentiate between tumor and normal brain.

A computerized robotic microscope also may be used to target the tumor more precisely. Instead of a stereotactic frame, small markers are glued to the skin of the head. An MRI is obtained immediately before surgery. The markers (rather than a frame) are the fixed reference points. In the operating room, the MRI images are inserted into a special computer, using a magnetic data tape attached to the robotic microscope. The MRI images are displayed on the computer screen, and the surgeon outlines the tumor on each image. Critical structures, such as a major artery or the central sulcus, also can be outlined. With these data, the computer can create a three-dimensional image of the tumor, showing the tumor's proximity to critical structures. Looking through the microscope, the surgeon registers the location of the fixed reference markers on the patient's head into the computer. With this information, the computer superimposes an image of the tumor through the microscope lens onto the operative surface. As the surgeon is operating, he can see where the edges of the lesion should be. As the microscope is moved during surgery, laterally or by depth, the computer adjusts the outline to accommodate the move. Such technology allows better resection with less risk to nearby critical areas, particularly when it is difficult to differentiate visually between normal brain and tumor.

11. What is stereotactic radiosurgery?

Stereotactic radiosurgery is effective treatment for small, well-defined lesions of the brain. The same stereotactic principle is used: a frame provides fixed reference points when an MRI or CT scan is obtained. The location of the lesion is determined, and a treatment plan is developed. Radiosurgery can be delivered by the linear accelerator with adaptive equipment for the stereotactic frame or Gamma Knife®. In both cases, treatment is delivered by narrow beams of radiation so that all beams come together at an isocenter, delivering a high dose to the isocenter with little radiation to surrounding tissues. The goal of radiosurgery is to deliver a dose of radiation that destroys everything in the target area. A full day is required to plan and prepare for the treatment, which takes approximately 10 minutes.

12. Is chemotherapy effective for brain tumors?

The answer depends on whom you ask. Optimists reply, "Yes, definitely," whereas pessimists ask, "Why bother?" The truth probably lies somewhere between the two responses. After radiotherapy, chemotherapy may be given immediately or when the tumor recurs. Chemotherapy is potentially effective only for aggressive tumors. Statistically, chemotherapy extends survival in patients with high-grade lesions only for a few weeks. On the other hand, a few patients may benefit significantly. The most commonly used regimens are 1,3-bis-(2-chloroethyl)-1-nitrosourea (BCNU) alone or PCV (procarbazine, lomustine, and vincristine). Because high doses of radiation therapy are toxic to the developing brain, more extensive chemotherapy regimens with multiple drugs are used in children. New drugs and new combinations of drugs are under investigation.

13. What long-term problems do children with a brain tumor face?

The long-term toxicity caused by multimodal therapy is a major concern in children because of the critical stage of brain development. Radiotherapy is delayed until after 2 years of age to decrease the risk and severity of long-term problems. Long-term toxicities are related to cognition (intelligence) and growth and development. Degrees of cognitive deficits range from mild to severe. Throughout the school life of the child it is imperative to assess cognitive function periodically and to adjust classroom work to fit specific deficits. Annual evaluation of the child should include input from teachers and other appropriate school personnel. Growth and development need to be assessed at least annually. Radiotherapy to the pituitary area may impair production of growth hormone. Sexual development, which is controlled by the pituitary, should be assessed, with appropriate hormone replacement as the child nears puberty.

Such physical and cognitive changes affect social development. Problems continue as the young adult pursues an independent life away from parents and considers marriage and fertility issues. Evaluations and interventions may be required throughout life.

14. Why are corticosteroids given to patients with brain tumors?

Patients with brain tumors most commonly present with neurologic deficits or symptoms of increased intracranial pressure (headache, nausea, vomiting) caused by mass effect of the tumor plus surrounding edema. The edema is caused by abnormal blood vessels within the tumor, which allow fluid to leak from the intravascular space into surrounding brain tissue. It was discovered many years ago that corticosteroids (most commonly dexamethasone) decrease the area of edema and improve symptoms, often dramatically. Corticosteroids are believed to improve the cell-to-cell adherence of endothelial cells within the tumor blood vessels, thereby lessening leakage of fluid into the surrounding brain. This in turn decreases the abnormal mass effect responsible for the symptoms.

15. What do patients and their families need to know about taking corticosteroids?

Because of their significant toxicity, the smallest effective dose of corticosteroids should be prescribed for the least amount of time. A patient should not discontinue treatment abruptly without instructions from a physician, because the body adjusts to the artificial steroids and stops producing natural steroids. Steroids taken for longer than 7–14 days must be gradually tapered. The longer a patient has taken steroids and the higher the dose, the longer and slower the taper must be. Patients also should be instructed about the following side effects:

• Alterations in body image caused by fluid retention and weight gain in varying degrees. Patients often complain about a ravenous appetite. The patient should be reassured that the weight can be lost after stopping the steroids. Other effects on body image include flushed face, abdominal striae, and growth of facial or body hair.

- Increased susceptibility to infection
- Stomach irritation, which can be relieved with an antacid
- Mood changes and irritability
- Muscle weakness in the proximal extremities, degenerative bone disease, and cataracts (caused by long-term use)

16. Which corticosteroid is used? How is it dosed?

Dexamethasone is commonly prescribed in oral doses ranging from 0.25–40 mg/day. Patients are often given an average dose of 2–4 mg every 6 hours. The maximal effective dose is often considered to be 40 mg/day. The patient should be cautioned not to discard unused medication because it may be prescribed intermittently throughout the course of their illness.

17. Are anticonvulsants prescribed for most patients? Do patients have to remain on anticonvulsants for life?

Anticonvulsants are often prescribed, depending on the physician's judgment and whether the patient has had a seizure. Seizures are caused by irritation to the brain. The brain tumor functions as an irritant, as does craniotomy. Even if anticonvulsants are not prescribed for long-term use, most patients receive a bolus before surgery; the drug may be continued for a few days postoperatively. Patients who experience a seizure are likely to remain on anticonvulsants for a longer period. If a patient remains seizure-free, anticonvulsants may be stopped after 6 months or 1 year. Although anticonvulsants may be stopped abruptly, often they are tapered to reduce the risk of severe seizure. In patients with brain tumors, attention should be paid to all minor complaints, which in fact may represent unrecognized seizure activity. Seizures occur in various forms and degrees and often are not identified as seizures by the patient or family.

18. What should patients be told about taking anticonvulsants?

The most commonly used anticonvulsant is phenytoin (Dilantin), followed by carbamazepine (Tegretol). Both drugs must be taken for 7–10 days to reach a therapeutic blood level. The patient should take a missed dose if it is remembered on the same day. If a day has passed, the patient should not try to make up the dose. Do not double dose!

19. What are the side effects of anticonvulsants?

If a patient is allergic to phenytoin and develops a skin rash, the drug should be stopped immediately. Because the rash may become severe, even life-threatening, it is imperative to instruct the patient to call the physician if a rash develops. Many patients feel sleepy and drowsy from the anticonvulsants. Major toxicities include nystagmus, slurred speech, dysarthria, hypotension, and coma (rare). Because anticonvulsants are metabolized by the liver, liver function should be evaluated at least annually. Often combinations of drugs are used if a single agent is not effective. Many new drugs are also available, including felbamate (Felbatol), clonazepam (Klonopin), gabapentin (Neurontin), and valproic acid (Depakote).

20. Should patients with brain tumors be allowed to drive?

Patients and families often ask when it is safe for the patient to drive. Reasons for restriction of driving privileges include seizures and cognitive deficits that affect processing of information and judgment. If a patient has had a seizure, many states have laws that restrict driving for 6–12 months. Although each state differs, most require a physician's approval. Rehabilitation programs often offer a safe driving evaluation. The patient who is not fit to drive but lacks awareness of deficits may resist the judgment of family and physician.

21. How does a patient or family know that the tumor is recurring? How does a patient with a brain tumor die?

In 90% of cases, the tumor recurs in the same general location, and the symptoms are similar to those at initial presentaion. As the tumor continues to grow, intracranial pressure increases, neurologic problems worsen, and the patient tends to sleep more hours each day. Eventually the patient can be awakened only with difficulty, usually for meals, and then quickly falls asleep again. As the patient spends more and more time in bed and ingests less fluid and nutrition, he or she is more prone to infections, thrombophlebitis, and other problems related to extended bedrest. In fact, an infection such as pneumonia may be the cause of death. Headaches are rarely a problem for patients with brain tumors. As the patient becomes more lethargic, he or she becomes less aware of deficits. Although watching neurologic deterioration is extremely difficult, families find comfort in the fact that the patient does not experience pain and is usually not aware of changes in mental status. Sudden death is possible but rare. Death usually occurs over days to weeks, depending on the growth rate of the tumor.

22. What factors influence survival? How do they affect treatment decisions?

Age, neurologic status at diagnosis, histology of the tumor, and extent of surgical resection are the primary factors that influence survival in adults. Younger patients with a good neurologic status at diagnosis statistically have a better chance of survival. If corticosteroids improve the neurologic deficit, it is likely that surgery will help as well. Tumor histology is a major factor influencing survival. The more aggressive the lesion, the poorer the prognosis. Complete (as opposed to partial) resection favors longer survival. Patients with multiple aggressive tumors have a poor prognosis and often are biopsied only and then treated with radiation. During craniotomy, as much tumor as possible is removed to relieve pressure and to reduce the tumor burden for subsequent therapies. Location is also a factor; the extent of tumor resection is often limited by its location. Tumors near or in the brainstem or adjacent to areas of motor or speech function are more difficult to treat.

Age alone does not usually affect treatment decisions; however, an aggressive surgical approach may not be recommended for elderly patients with an aggressive lesion, poor neurologic status, and other health problems that increase surgical risk. For such patients, diagnostic biopsy and radiotherapy may be the best treatment options. Intrinsic brainstem lesions often cannot be biopsied because the operative risks of neurologic deficit and death are too great.

23. What is the prognosis for common tumor types?

Survival is poorest for high-grade gliomas. The most common primary brain tumor is astrocytoma. Survival for glioblastoma (grade IV astrocytoma) treated with surgery, radiation, and chemotherapy is 12–18 months; for anaplastic (grade III) astrocytoma, 18–24 months; and for grade II astrocytoma, 6–7 years.

24. Describe new treatment options.

Progress in the treatment of brain tumors has been slow; however, in the past decade, neuro-oncology has gained the attention of the health care community. New efforts focus on basic science as well as clinical research, and both local and systemic approaches are under evaluation:

- Localized approaches for high-grade gliomas, including radiosurgery, radiosensitizers, brachytherapy, hyperthermia, and hyperfractionization
- Localized chemotherapy approaches, including direct delivery to the tumor via drug-impregnated, biodegradable wafers placed in the operative cavity and intraarterial delivery of chemotherapeutic agents
- Tumor vaccines that augment or manipulate the immune system. Because gliomas infiltrate normal brain, systemic treatment must include a way to search out the infiltrated cells
- Temporary interruption of the blood-brain barrier, which allows passage of chemotherapy agents to the tumor
- High-dose chemotherapy with bone marrow rescue
- Gene therapy

25. What resources are available to patients and families for education and support?

The foundations listed below provide free information about brain tumors and treatment to the public and health professionals. Related associations, often affiliated with rehabilitation medicine, provide education and support for patients with physical and mental disabilities related to traumatic brain injury. Such information also may be helpful to patients with brain tumor. A brain tumor support group is located on the Internet; however, patients should be cautioned to validate information with a trusted nurse or physician.

American Brain Tumor Association (ABTA)

2720 River Road, Suite 146

Des Plaines, IL 60018

(800) 886-2282, (847) 827-9910)

E-mail: ABTA@aol.com

Services include a listing of support groups, pen-pal program, newsletter, and information about treatment facilities and research funding.

National Brain Tumor Foundation (NBTF)

785 Market Street, Suite 1600

San Francisco, CA 94103

(800) 934-CURE, (415) 284-0208

E-mail:sstf39f@prodigy.com

Free information and counseling and support services to patients with brain tumor, survivors, and families. Also provides a newsletter, patient-to-patient telephone support line, free resource guide, and list of support groups.

BIBLIOGRAPHY

1. Broderson JM: Surgical options for brain tumor treatment. Crit Care Nurs Clin North Am 7:91–102, 1995.
2. Bronstein KS: Epidemiology and classification of brain tumors. Crit Care Nurs Clin North Am 7:79–89, 1995.
3. Lamb SA: Radiation therapy options for management of the brain tumor patient. Crit Care Nurs Clin North Am 7:103–114, 1995.
4. Laperriere NL, Bernstein M: Radiotherapy for brain tumors. Cancer J Clin 44(2):96–108, 1994.
5. Moore IM: Central nervous system toxicity of cancer therapy in children. J Pediatr Oncol Nurs 12(4):203–210, 1995.
6. Parker SL, Tong T, Bolden S, Wingo PA: Cancer Statistics 1997. CA Cancer J Clin 45:5–27, 1997.
7. Perry GF Jr: What occupations have been associated with brain cancer, and, more specifically, what is the connection between brain cancer and electric utility work? J Occup Environ Med 37:1067–1069, 1995.
8. Roman DD, Sperdoto PW: Neuropsychological effects of cranial radiation: Current knowledge and future directions. Int J Radiat Oncol, Biol Physics 31:983–998, 1995.
9. Shiminski-Maher T, Wisoff JH: Pediatric brain tumors. Crit Care Nurs Clin North Am 7:143–149, 1995.

22. BREAST CANCER

Patrice Y. Neese, MSN, RN, CS, ANP

Quick Facts—Breast Cancer

Incidence	30% of new cancers in women annually; in 1997, approximately 181,600 new cases will be diagnosed
Mortality	In 1997, 44,190 estimated deaths
Risk factors	**Increased age**
	History of breast cancer
	Early menarche, nulliparity
	Increased age at birth of first child
	Late menopause
	Use of exogenous hormones
	History of atypical hyperplasia
	Family history, radiation exposure
Histology	Adenocarcinoma most common; rare nonadenocarcinomas include squamous cell, cystosarcoma phyllodes, and angiosarcoma
Symptoms	**Painless mass more common than painful mass**
	Nipple discharge, nipple erosion
	Diffuse erythema of the breast
	Axillary adenopathy
Staging	Tumor, node, metastasis (TNM)
	Stage I — Tumor < 2 cm, no nodes, no metastases
	Stage II — Tumor 2–5 cm, with or without ipsilateral nodes, no metastases
	Stage III — Tumor > 5 cm, positive nodes, no metastases, and/or any of the following: peau d'orange, inflammatory skin changes, breast skin or nipple ulceration
	Stage IV — Tumor of any size, with or without nodes, positive distant metastases
Treatment	Stage I — Lumpectomy + radiation therapy or mastectomy
	If < 1 cm, no adjuvant treatment
	If > 1 cm and
	Premenopausal, ER+: physcian judgment, no adjuvant or tamoxifen (Nolvadex) for 5 yr
	Premenopausal, ER–: physician judgment, no adjuvant chemotherapy
	Postmenopausal, ER+ : tamoxifen for 5 yr
	Postmenopausal, ER–: physician judgment, no adjuvant or tamoxifen for 5 yr
	Stage II — Lumpectomy + radiation therapy or mastectomy
	If premenopausal, ER+: adjuvant chemotherapy with or without tamoxifen
	If premenopausal, ER–: adjuvant chemotherapy
	If postmenopausal, ER+: adjuvant chemotherapy with or without tamoxifen
	Stage III — May use neoadjuvant chemotherapy to shrink tumor; size may dictate mastectomy over lumpectomy; additional postoperative chemotherapy with or without radiation therapy; tamoxifen with increased estrogen receptors; stem cell or bone marrow transplants for > 10 positive nodes
	Stage IV — Extensive therapy may be of limited use; radiation therapy for palliation; if no visceral disease, premenopausal, ER+: consider oophorectomy or tamoxifen; with above criteria and postmenopausal: tamoxifen; if pre- or postmenopausal, ER–: chemotherapy until maximal response or bone marrow transplant

ER+ = increased estrogen receptors, ER– = decreased estrogen receptors.

1. What is the incidence of breast cancer among American women?

It is estimated that 181,600 new cases of breast cancer will be reported in the United States during 1997. With a life expectancy of 85 years, about 1 in 9 women will develop breast cancer at some time during their lives. Although the incidence has increased over the years, the mortality rate has been fairly stable for the past 60 years at about 27 per 100,000 patients. Breast cancer is the most common cancer diagnosis in women and the second major cause of cancer-related death. In addition, 1,400 cases of breast cancer in men are expected to be diagnosed during 1997.

2. What are some of the signs and symptoms of breast cancer? Is there one area of the breast in which more cancers are found?

Breast masses that are firm, nontender, irregular without distinct borders, nonmovable, and fixed to skin or deep fascia are often suspicious for cancer. Skin dimpling and nipple retraction are sometimes present. Erythema and peau d'orange (orange peel) are worrisome signs of inflammatory breast cancer. Unilateral nipple discharge, especially serous or bloody, is suspicious in older women. Enlarged axillary or supraclavicular lymph nodes are less common.

The primary site of breast cancer is described by the quadrant of the breast in which it is detected. The most common area is the upper outer quadrant, where approximately 50% of tumors are found. The upper inner quadrant is associated with a 15% incidence, the lower outer quadrant with 11%, the lower inner quadrant with 6%, and the central region (near the areola) with approximately 17%.

3. What are the diagnostic methods for breast cancer?

Before biopsy of a dominant mass, a patient should have a mammogram to define the extent of the lesion and to identify other suspicious areas. Because mammograms are not sensitive to approximately 15% of cancers, a negative test should not dissuade a physician from performing a biopsy on a dominant mass. Fine-needle aspiration (FNA) is often performed on palpable nodules because it is quick, relatively painless, and inexpensive. FNA cannot distinguish between ductal carcinoma in situ (DCIS) and invasive cancers, however, and its use is somewhat limited. Core-cutting needle biopsy has advantages similar to those of FNA, and a larger sample is usually obtained, giving a higher degree of accuracy. Both techniques depend on experienced persons performing the test and cytopathologic interpretation (such persons may not be present in small medical centers).

If a suspicious, nonpalpable nodule is seen on mammogram, it may be localized with needles guided by mammography. The needle-localized lesion is then excised for biopsy. Excisional biopsies are performed on any palpable nodule to provide the greatest diagnostic information, including size, receptor status, and margins. Most are performed in outpatient settings under local anesthesia.

4. What is the most common histologic type of breast cancer?

Approximately 80% of invasive or infiltrating cancers originate in the ductal system and are called ductal cancer. About 5–10% of infiltrating (invasive) cancers arise from the lobules; thus, they are called lobular cancers. The remaining invasive breast cancers are medullary, tubular, mucinous, comedo, and Paget's disease. Noninvasive cancer, or cancer that is confined within the lumen of the ducts or lobules (carcinoma in situ), is classified as either ductal (DCIS) or lobular (LCIS). Lobular carcinoma is not considered a true cancer. It is a marker for increased risk of future cancers of any kind in either breast. It requires only a simple local excision. It is usually found in younger women and is mammogram-negative. Inflammatory breast cancer is not a histologic type but is a clinical or pathologic diagnosis with skin or lymphatic invasion.

5. Do all breast cancers grow at a steady rate or is there variability in the rate of growth?

The majority of breast cancers have a doubling time of approximately 60–90 days. However, a small percentage will double as fast as 15 days and some every 600 days. The latter are associated with late recurrences > 10 years and sometimes 20 years after the original diagnosis.

6. What is the probability of lymph node metastasis of breast cancer?

Lymph node metastases are present at the time of diagnosis in 40–60% of cases. Lymph node metastasis is a prognostic aspect of staging; it represents the probability that the cancer has spread from the breast. In general, lateral lesions in the breast metastasize to axillary or supraclavicular nodes. Medial tumors are more likely to metastasize to internal mammary and mediastinal lymph nodes as well as supraclavicular nodes.

7. What are the cardinal prognostic factors in breast cancer staging?

The tumor-nodes-metastasis (TNM) staging system is used to predict the outcome of disease by analysis of prognostic factors and survival rates. Tumor size, extent of lymph node involvement, and presence of metastasis are graded and grouped according to the extent of disease. Approximately 96% of patients with stage I disease are alive at 5 years after diagnosis. The survival rates at 5 years for patients with stages II and III cancers are approximately 55% and 35%, respectively. Less than 15% of patients with metastatic disease or stage IV breast cancer are alive 5 years after diagnosis.

8. Define estrogen receptor status. Is it a prognostic factor?

Receptor levels are measured in the primary tumor, providing valuable information that is helpful in determining treatment. In general, tumors that are sensitive (i.e., have receptors) to estrogen and/or progesterone are slightly slower growing and have a better prognosis than tumors that are not. Postmenopausal women are more likely to be receptor-positive, whereas premenopausal women are more likely to be receptor-negative. Receptor-positive tumors are generally responsive to endocrine therapies such as tamoxifen, which is considered first-line therapy. Megestrol acetate and aminoglutethimide are reserved for treatment after tamoxifen has succeeded, then failed. Second-line therapy usually does not work if the patient does not initially respond to tamoxifen.

9. Are any other staging criteria used?

Because it takes years to establish scientifically the relationship between cutoff values of a new test and recurrence or survival data, several factors are used across the United States with variable justification. Flow cytometry measures the amount and type of DNA. A high amount of DNA found in aneuploid tumors is associated with a more aggressive form of breast cancer. Likewise, an elevated S-phase corresponds to a tumor that is dividing more rapidly and thought to be more aggressive. Angiogenesis (increased blood vessel/capillary development in primary tumors) has been linked to more aggressive tumors and may predict distant metastatic disease. Biomarkers, such as cathepsin-D, p53, and Her-2-neu, are currently available, but testing is expensive and results have varying abilities to prognosticate tumor growth or ability to respond to treatment.

10. What are some of the surgical options for treatment of breast cancer?

The most common surgical interventions for breast cancer are lumpectomy (breast conservation) with axillary node dissection or modified radical mastectomy (removal of breast and lymph nodes). Multiple randomized trials have demonstrated that the 10–20-year survival rate of patients with stage I or II breast cancer treated with lumpectomy and radiation therapy is equivalent to that of patients treated with mastectomy alone. Lumpectomy must be combined with radiation therapy for equivalent local control. Immediate or delayed reconstructive surgery is also an option for women who choose mastectomy. The decision is often difficult for women to make; it is based on personal preference, values, feelings about the body, priorities, and perceptions of risk.

11. The preoperative plan for patient education should include what basic points?

Because short-stay and outpatient procedures are becoming more standard for both lumpectomy and mastectomy, preoperative patient education from the nurse is imperative. The nurse should remind patients to stop taking aspirin and nonsteroidal antinflammatory agents, which may decrease platelet function. Hormonal therapy (birth control or replacement) should be stopped as soon as a diagnosis of breast cancer is made. The nurse also should teach the signs and symptoms of infection, wound care, Jackson-Pratt drain management, prevention and management of lymphedema, pain control, and comfort measures at home; recommend purchase of a postoperative bra (see question 13); and initiate referral to the Reach to Recovery Program of the American Cancer Society. Reach to Recovery is a one-on-one visitation program designed to help women meet the physical, emotional, and cosmetic needs related to breast cancer. Trained volunteers who have had breast cancer are available to visit women postoperatively. Information about exercises, temporary prosthetic devices, bras, and available support services is part of the program. In addition, it may be necessary to discuss appropriate birth control methods.

12. What additional information should be covered in the postoperative phase of patient education?

In addition to reinforcement of preoperative teaching, the postoperative phase of patient education should remind patients that individual coping is affected by exhaustion, from surgery, anesthesia, change in body image, and emotional aspects of dealing with a new diagnosis. The nurse should recommend moderation of habits related to eating, drinking, resting, socializing, and exercise (the patient should avoid lifting weights above 5 pounds for a few weeks). If the patient is a candidate for adjuvant chemotherapy, there is usually a period of several weeks between surgery and start of chemotherapy. This is an ideal time to have a dental examination and cleaning, which should be avoided during chemotherapy treatments when blood counts are low.

13. What kind of bra, if any, should be worn in the postoperative period?

Women are most comfortable after biopsy or lumpectomy if the breast is well supported. A sports bra is ideal, especially if one can be found with frontal closure (it is easier to put on than the overhead type). For example, a national discount chain carries an all-cotton, front-closing sports bra for less than 10 dollars. Wearing a bra to bed for the first few nights helps some women, as does lying on the opposite side with a towel rolled under the breast for support. Women should avoid underwire support postoperatively and during radiation therapy when the breast is tender and edematous.

14. What should be emphasized when teaching the patient about radiation therapy to the breast?

In general, 4500–5000 cGy are administered 5 days/week for 5–6 weeks after lumpectomy. Because the majority of radiation exposure is via tangential beam (through the breast instead of the body to avoid the heart and lungs), most women can expect few systemic effects. The most common side effects include local skin irritation similar to a bad sunburn. This symptom varies among women and may cause pruritus, edema, and occasionally moist desquamation in severe cases. Women should be encouraged to avoid ointments or oil-based products on the skin as well as all deodorant soaps and deodorants, most of which which have a high aluminum content that may interact with the radiation. A dusting of cornstarch may be used as a deodorant. Radiation to the axilla may increase the incidence of lymphedema (see chapter 36). Fatigue is another often reported side effect of therapy (see chapter 35). Less common is neutropenia.

15. Why do some women who have had a modified radical mastectomy receive radiation therapy?

Postmastectomy radiation therapy is recommended for women with a tumor larger than 5 cm, skin or chest wall involvement, positive surgical margin, or more than four positive lymph nodes. Depending on institutional protocols, radiation therapy is administered at different times during treatment. Most commonly it is administered after completion of chemotherapy. Occasionally, it is administered halfway through chemotherapy (sandwich). Less frequently, it is administered concomitantly with chemotherapy (i.e., cyclophosphamide, methotrexate, and fluorouracil). Patients tend to have more severe side effects with concomitant therapy and usually need dose reduction of either chemotherapy or radiation. Radiation therapy given concomitantly with doxorubicin has been associated with a worse cosmetic result and is rarely given. Radiation therapy is also used to treat some spot bone or brain metastases.

16. What is the role of neoadjuvant chemotherapy in breast cancer?

Neoadjuvant therapy is chemotherapy administered before surgery. Patients who present with locally advanced or inflammatory breast cancers (stage III), which generally are large tumors with skin and/or nipple involvement, usually respond with dramatic tumor shrinkage preoperatively. The same patients also may receive adjuvant chemotherapy.

17. Why do some women receive adjuvant chemotherapy whereas others do not?

Adjuvant chemotherapy is recommended in addition to primary treatment (surgery with or without radiation therapy) of breast cancer. According to the consensus statement of the National Cancer Institute, chemotherapy is recommended for all women with positive nodes unless contraindicated because of age or medical instability. Women who are estrogen receptor-positive and postmenopausal usually receive tamoxifen with or without chemotherpy, depending on age and general health. Women who do not receive adjuvant chemotherapy are node-negative and have tumors smaller than 1 cm.

18. What are the most common chemotherapy drug combinations?

Several hundred chemotherapy trials for breast cancer have provided data for the efficacious use of the following regimens:

The combination of cyclophosphamide (Cytoxan), methotrexate, and fluorouracil (CMF) is administered on days 1 and 8 every 28 days or on day 1 every 21 days for 6 cycles.

The combination of 5-fluorouracil, Adriamycin, and cyclophosphamide (FAC) is administered on day 1 every 21 days. Alternatively, fluorouracil may be administered on days 1 and 8 of a 28-day cycle for 6 courses. Adriamycin with cyclophosphamide (AC) is another option, administered in slightly higher doses every 21 days for 4 cycles.

Taxol or Taxotere is used with and without Adriamycin for metastatic or recurrent cancer; it is usually administered every 21 days.

19. When is bone marrow transplant recommended for women with breast cancer?

Stage IV breast cancer or high-risk primary disease (> 10 positive lymph nodes) is considered not curable by most oncologists with conventional therapy. This has led to the use of higher-dose regimens, which provide greater cell kill but also greater toxicity. Some clinical trials have demonstrated prolonged survival rates with a combination of high-dose chemotherapy and transplant of autologous stem cells harvested from bone marrow or peripheral blood before chemotherapy and administered after chemotherapy to prevent bone marrow suppression. Studies continue to evaluate the sequencing, dosing, and cost-effectiveness of such expensive therapy. Insurance companies contest the dollar value of survival periods, and coverage for patients who desire this treatment is inconsistent.

20. How does tamoxifen work? How long does treatment last?

Tamoxifen has been considered a standard adjuvant therapy for postmenopausal women with estrogen receptor-positive breast cancer. The role of tamoxifen alone in receptor-negative or premenopausal patients is controversial; the rate of response to tamoxifen in receptor-negative patients is about 5%. Tamoxifen acts by essentially blocking estrogen from breast cancer cells. It does not stop estrogen production in the body; in fact some studies have revealed estrogen-like effects on the uterus, bones, and liver. Women taking tamoxifen generally have increased bone uptake of calcium and less osteoporosis. They usually have lower serum cholesterol levels and less heart disease. However, tamoxifen also may increase the chance of uterine tumors, a finding that has prompted some women to stop treatment and oncologists to evaluate the length of treatment. Specialists prescribe treatment for 2–7 years; 5 years is the current recommendation in the adjuvant setting. However, patients with responsive metastatic disease or patients without a uterus may take tamoxifen indefinitely.

21. How often does breast cancer spread from one breast to the other?

It is rare for cancer to spread from one breast to the other. A woman who has had cancer in one breast, however, is 1–2 times more likely to develop cancer in the other breast. Therefore, most malignancies of the other breast are new cancers. It is also possible for one person to have one estrogen/progesterone-sensitive tumor and a second tumor that is receptor-negative.

22. What are the most common sites of metastases?

Metastatic spread from breast cancer may involve various organs. Lung, liver, bone, brain, and skin are reported most frequently. Breast cancer in the ovaries, spleen, peritoneum, adrenal glands, stomach, leptomeninges and retina of the eye is rare but documented in the literature. Although metastatic disease is considered incurable, it does not always mean that death is imminent. In fact, one-half of patients will live more than 2 years, and 10% will live a decade or more. Women with bone metastases only may live for a considerable length of time with the use of radiation, hormonal therapy, and chemotherapy. More recently strontium (metastron), a radioactive isotope, has been added because of its palliative effect in end-stage treatment of bone metastasis.

23. Should multiple regular screening tests be performed to monitor for metastatic disease or recurrence in women who have been diagnosed with breast cancer?

A European follow-up trial in 13,000 women with breast cancer demonstrated that numerous radiologic screenings give no survival advantage. Periodic physical examination, mammogram, and routine serum liver function studies, with bone scans, chest radiographs, and other radiologic studies performed only as needed, provide a simpler and more cost-effective approach. Serum circulating tumor markers (CEA and/or CA15-3) are evaluable in approximately 20% of patients with stage I or II breast cancer (nonmetastatic disease). Because of expense and challenges to their specificity, tumor marker tests are usually reserved for follow-up in women with metastatic disease.

24. What are some of the options for breast reconstruction?

No standard period of time between mastectomy and reconstruction can be considered ideal for all patients. Most mastectomy patients are medically appropriate candidates for reconstruction, which often may be performed at the same time that the breast is removed, especially if it is determined that cancer is not widespread. Some women are simply not comfortable with presentation of all of the options while they are struggling to cope with a new diagnosis of cancer, and delayed reconstruction may be best. Women who are obese, hypertensive, or diabetic, or who use tobacco should delay reconstruction until the condition is under control.

The goals of reconstruction are to enhance body image and to provide symmetry of the breasts when the woman is wearing a bra. The options, which are discussed with a plastic surgeon, depend on body type and breast size. Breast reconstruction may be accomplished as a prosthetic implant, tissue expansion, or flap procedure. After mastectomy, a balloon expander is inserted beneath the skin and chest muscle. Through a port mechanism, saline is injected periodically, stretching the skin until a more permanent saline implant may be inserted. Some patients do not require expansion before receiving an implant. An alternative approach involves creation of a skin flap using tissue from other parts of the body, such as the transverse rectus abdominis myocutaneous (TRAM) or the latissimus dorsi (LD). Although these alternatives do not require the use of implants and generally result in a more natural contour, they involve more extensive surgical procedures and scarring. Additional surgical procedures are available to reconstruct the areola and nipple.

25. What are some of the critical psychological issues facing families of patients with breast cancer?

Breast cancer is a crisis for the entire family. It may result in depression among family members, impaired marital relationships, lowered self-esteem, developmental delays in children, and behavioral problems with adolescents. Functional patterns of families are influenced by their structure and organization in both traditional and nontraditional modes; history of coping styles; and cultural, ethnic, and religious or spiritual influences. The oncology nurse is often the first observer of family dynamics in response to cancer. Identification of problems, provision of clear information, and referral to appropriate resources may assist the family to a successful coping style. This approach hopefully will enable family members to use the experience as an opportunity for growth and to avoid destructive outcomes as well as to assist the patient with her emotional response.

26. How can the oncology nurse support a couple coping with cancer?

Changes as a result of breast cancer in the quality of a couple's intimate relationship, communication problems, and fear of recurrence are issues that have been documented in the literature. The oncology nurse can support the partner during this time by being available to answer questions about procedures and treatments. Providing anticipatory guidance and education regarding possible challenges they may face as a couple can facilitate their sense of control and reduce feelings of uncertainty. Active listening is a valuable intervention, as is validation of their concerns.

27. What care interventions should guide nurses working with women who have a family history of breast cancer?

Approximately 5–10% of breast cancers can be attributed to inheritance of an altered gene. Mutations of genes BRCA1 and BRCA2 account for approximately 45% of hereditary breast cancer and the majority of heritable breast/ovarian cancer. The implications of a family history of breast cancer affect individuals differently, depending on various psychosocial issues and family dynamics. As assays are developed and validated, genetic screening may be appropriate for members of high-risk families. Nurses should recognize and discuss why some women exhibit high-risk behaviors or seem reluctant to comply with screening; they also should provide information about the benefits of early detection. By emphasizing and facilitating breast cancer screening and detection through monthly breast self-examination, periodic clinical examination, and screening mammography, the oncology nurse may reduce the fear of breast cancer.

28. What is the relationship between dietary fat intake and incidence of breast cancer?

Epidemiologists have long pondered whether a low-fat diet can prevent breast cancer. The incidence of breast cancer is clearly lower in countries where intake of animal fat is lower. Theoretically, added body weight is usually an increase in adipose or fat. Adipose tissue may be a tumor promoter, either through the production of estrogen or through the excessive calories that it represents. Animal fat also may be affected by growth hormones used to increase production and pesticide residues (dichlorodiphenyltrichloroethane [DDT]) that act like estrogen in the human body. There has been difficulty in designing a study to examine the relationship between a low-fat diet and rates of breast cancer. The ongoing Nurses' Health Study has not demonstrated an association between the two.

29. What issues related to breast cancer should we expect to hear about in the coming years?

Research is ongoing for chemoprevention of breast cancer. The National Surgical Adjuvant Breast Project (NSABP) is currently examing the role of tamoxifen in women at high risk for development of breast cancer. Identification of oncogenes and genetic predisposition has scientific interest as well as ethical and legal implications. Advances in surgical management of breast cancer also are under study. The use of lymphoscintography or lymph node mapping may reduce the morbidity of lymph node dissections. New and improved treatments with less systemic toxicity are always of interest. Taxol and the campothecins are not currently used as standard adjuvant chemotherapy, but phase II–III trials are currently under way. Survivorship (e.g., quality of life, fatigue, exercise, diet, hormone use, pregnancy, financial impact, and body image) is an area of increased interest. Alternative and complementary therapies are of interest to many practitioners and women with breast cancer; randomized trials rather than anecdotal recommendations may change breast cancer management.

30. What resources offer support, counseling, education, and information for patients with breast cancer?
- American Cancer Society
  800-ACS-2345
  Reach to Recovery Program
- Susan G. Komen Breast Cancer Foundation
  800-IM-AWARE (800-462-9273)
  Services include research and program grants, helpline.
- ENCORE–YWCA of USA
  e-mail: hn2202@handsnet.org
  Exercise program for women with breast cancer available through most local YWCA branches
- Mothers Supporting Daughters with Breast Cancer (MSDBC)
  (410) 778-1982
  e-mail: lillie@ix.netcom.com
  MSDBC helps women whose daughters have breast cancer so that they can better help their daughters cope with the disease and treatment.
- National Alliance of Breast Cancer Organization (NABCO)
  9 East 37th Street, 10th Floor
  New York, NY 10016
  (212) 709-0154 or 800-719-9154
  e-mail: nabcoinfo@aol.com
  Nonprofit agency representing over 300 organizations concerned about breast cancer; services range from physician referrals to job discrimination and professional education.
- Women's Healthcare Network
  800-991-8877
  Organization made up of independent businesses that specialize in serving women who have had breast surgery.
- Y-ME National Breast Cancer Organization
  800-221-2141

BIBLIOGRAPHY

1. Daly MB: New perspectives in breast cancer: The genetic revolution. Oncol Nurs 1:1–9, 1994.
2. Harris JR, Lippman ME, et al: Breast cancer (3 parts). N Engl J Med 327:319–328, 390–397, 473–480, 1992.
3. Henderson C: Breast cancer. In Murphy GP, Lawrence W, et al (eds): American Cancer Society Textbook of Clinical Oncology. Atlanta, American Cancer Society, 1995.
4. Hilton BA: Issues, problems, and challenges for families coping with breast cancer. Semin Oncol Nurs 9:88–100, 1993.
5. Ellis C: Breast reconstruction after mastectomy. Innov Oncol Nurs 10:2–26, 1994.
6. Love SM, Parker B, et al: Practice guidelines for breast cancer. Cancer J Sci Am 2:S7–S15, 1996.
7. Love SM: Dr. Susan Love's Breast Book. Reading, MA, Addison-Wesley, 1995.
8. Parker SL, Tong T, Bolden S, Wingo PA: Cancer Statistics 1997. CA Cancer J Clin 47:5–27, 1997.
9. Zahlis EH, Shands ME: The impact of breast cancer on the partner 18 months after diagnosis. Semin Oncol Nurs 9:83–87, 1993.

23. COLORECTAL CANCER

Diane K. Nakagaki, RN, BSN, ET, and
Brenda M. Hiromoto, RN, MS, CETN, OCN

Quick Facts—Colorectal Carcinoma

Incidence	15% of all new cancer cases in the United States. In 1997: 131,200 estimated new cases (94,100 colon and 37,100 rectal cancers). Colon cancer affects 1 in 20 people. Incidence is < 1 per 100,000 in persons under age 30 and 500 per 100,000 in persons over age 80.
Mortality	In 1997, 54,900 deaths will be due to colorectal cancer; 46,600 will be related to colon cancer and 8300 to rectal cancer; 11% of total cancer deaths annually. Mortality unchanged for three decades.
Etiology	Unknown; diet may be an influencing factor.
Risk factors	Adenomatous polyps are the most common risk factor. The larger the polyps, the greater the likelihood of malignancy (up to 40% in polyps > 2 cm) Family history and genetic syndromes: familial adenomatous polyposis (FAP), Gardner syndrome, Oldfield syndrome, Turcot syndrome, Peutz-Jeghers syndrome, hereditary non-polyposis colorectal carcinoma (HNPCC; originally named "cancer family syndrome") Inflammatory bowel disease; ulcerative colitis, especially > 10 years' duration Crohn's disease Diets rich in fat and cholesterol (high in red meat) Increased risk begins at 40 years and increases with age
Histology	**Adenocarcinomas** account for 98% of colon cancers and 95% of rectal cancers. **Anal carcinomas:** 65% squamous cell carcinomas, 25% transitional (cloacogenic or basaloid), < 10% adenocarcinoma, and < 5% miscellaneous.
Symptoms	Early: no symptoms; vague abdominal pain or flatulence Vary according to location of tumor, but usually a change in bowel movements is first symptom Other signs and symptoms include weakness due to anemia, pain, blood in stool, and bowel obstruction.
Diagnosis and staging tests	Digital rectal exam and fecal occult blood test (FOBT) Colonoscopy with biopsy of any lesions and/or air contrast barium enema Endoscopic ultrasound Chest radiograph, CT scan of abdomen and pelvis Complete blood count, liver and renal function tests, urinalysis, preoperative test for carcinoembryonic antigen (CEA) Immunoscintigraphy (antibody scan) to detect extrahepatic disease and radiolabeled monoclonal antibodies are currently under investigation to improve detection rates
Staging	**Astler-Coller modification of Dukes' classification**

	Stage A	Tumor confined to mucosa (2% of cases)
	Stage B1	Tumor penetrates into muscularis layer (11%)
	Stage B2	Tumor penetrates through muscularis into serosa or perirectal fat (30%)
	Stage C1	B1 tumor with positive regional lymph nodes (2%)
	Stage C2	B2 with positive regional lymph nodes (22%)
	Stage D	Distant metastases to other organs (33%)

Tumor, nodes, metastasis (TNM) system

Tumor stage

	TX	Primary tumor cannot be assessed
	T0	No evidence of tumor
	Tis	Carcinoma in situ

Table continued on following page.

Quick Facts—Colorectal Carcinoma (Continued)

Tl	Tumor invades submucosa
T2	Tumor invades muscularis propria
T3	Tumor invades through muscularis propria into submucosa
T4	Tumor perforates visceral peritoneum or invades other organs or structures

Lymph node stage

NX	Regional lymph nodes cannot be assessed
N0	No regional lymph nodes involved
N1	One to three pericolic lymph nodes involved
N2	Four or more pericolic lymph nodes involved
N3	Regional nodes along major named vascular trunk

Metastatic stage

MX	Distant metastasis cannot be assessed
M0	No distant metastasis
M1	Distant metastasis

Stage groupings

Stage 0	Tis, N0, M0
Stage I	Tl or T2, N0, M0 (Dukes' A)
Stage II	T3 or T4, N0, M0 (Dukes' B)
Stage III	Any T, Nl, N2, or N3, M0 (Dukes' C)
Stage IV	Any T, any N, Ml (Dukes' D)

1. What are the epidemiologic differences between colon cancer and rectal cancer?

The prevalence of colon cancer is nearly equal in males and females. Rectal cancer has a slight male predominance. Colorectal cancer is the third most common cancer for both genders and the second leading cause of death.

2. What other factors are related to the incidence of colorectal cancers?

The incidence of colorectal cancers is higher after the age of 40. The mean age of patients at presentation is 60–65 years. The incidence of colon cancer is higher in African Americans; the incidence for Native Americans is less than half the incidence for white Americans. The risk of colorectal cancer is much lower among Mormons and Seventh Day Adventists, who avoid alcohol and tobacco and eat mainly vegetables, fruits, and whole-grain cereals.

Other predisposing factors include history of colorectal or other cancer (e.g., breast, endometrial, or ovarian cancer); sedentary employment; and women with no or low parity or history of pelvic irradiation for gynecologic cancer. Alcohol consumption, especially beer, has been associated with a higher incidence of colorectal cancer. Charcoal or smoked meats and irradiated foods have no conclusive correlation to the risk of colorectal cancer. Irritation of the anal canal related to condylomata, rectal intercourse, fistulas, fissures, abscesses, and hemorrhoids may increase the risk for colorectal cancer. HIV-positive patients have a higher incidence of anal canal carcinomas.

3. Do other countries have a similar incidence of colorectal cancer as the United States?

There is wide variability among cultures and countries. Countries in which people consume large amounts of fruits and vegetables and low amounts of fat have a lower incidence of colorectal cancer. For example, the incidence is 3 per 100,000 in Nigeria and 7 per 100,000 in Japan vs. 40 per 100,000 people in the United States.

4. What is the survival rate for colorectal cancer?

The 1-year survival rate is 83%, and the 5-year survival rate is 61%. In general, the 5-year survival rate is based on the stage of disease (Astler-Coller modified Dukes' classification):

Stage A	75–100%	Stage C1	40%
Stage B1	65%	Stage C2	15%
Stage B2	50%	Stage D	< 5%

For anal cancer the 5-year survival rate is 48–66%.

5. **What are the most common signs and symptoms of colorectal cancer?**

Right colon: vague, achy abdominal pain; bleeding (dark or mahogany red); weakness due to anemia (common); obstruction (infrequent); palpable abdominal mass.

Transverse colon: blood in stool; change in bowel pattern; potential bowel obstruction.

Left colon: colicky pain; bleeding (red, mixed with stool); obstruction (common); weakness due to anemia (infrequent); nausea, vomiting; constipation alternating with diarrhea; decreased caliber of stool (pencil stools).

Rectum: steady gnawing pain; bleeding (bright red, coating stool); change in bowel movements (constipation or diarrhea); pencil stools; rectal urgency or fecal incontinence; spasmodic contractions with pain; perineal and buttock pain.

Anal: bleeding; pain; sensation of a mass; severe anal itching.

6. **What percentage of cancer is accounted for by the different segments of the colon?**

Descending and sigmoid colon: 52%

Ascending colon: 32%

Transverse colon: 16%

7. **What is the value of CEA in monitoring patients with colorectal cancer?**

Carcinoembryonic antigen (CEA) is a glycoprotein present in gastrointestinal mucosa. It is useful as a tumor marker for patients who have CEA-producing adenocarcinomas. CEA is most useful as a marker for tumor recurrence and in monitoring response to chemotherapy. An elevated, sustained postoperative CEA is related to tumor recurrence in most patients. Rising CEA levels (serial changes > 35% of baseline) may indicate progressive disease. Elevations in CEA are found in gastrointestinal, breast, and lung cancers and in smokers and patients with liver disease or cirrhosis, pancreatitis, inflammatory bowel disease, or rectal polyps.

8. **What are common sites of colon and rectal metastases?**

Common sites of metastasis for colon cancer are the liver, lungs, and peritoneum (with carcinomatosis). Colon cancer has a tendency to metastasize to the liver because most of the colon's venous drainage is through the portal system. Uncommon sites are brain, bone, ovaries, and adrenal glands. Rectal cancer has a tendency to metastasize to the lungs because its venous drainage is via the hemorrhoidal veins. Anal cancer may metastasize to the lung, liver, and inguinal nodes.

9. **How is colorectal cancer detected if no symptoms are present?**

Screening guidelines are controversial; however, the American Cancer Society recommends the following tests to screen for colorectal cancer in asymptomatic patients with no risk factors:

- Digital rectal examination: annually after age 40
- Fecal occult blood test (FOBT) × 3 specimens: annually after age 50
- Flexible sigmoidoscopy: every 3–5 years starting at age 50
- Barium enema if above tests reveal possible problem
- Colonoscopy: after age 50; every 3–5 years in high-risk patients and periodically (interval unknown) in patients with history of colorectal cancer; also if above tests reveal problems.

10. **What may cause false-positive or false-negative occult blood results?**

False positives: red meat, poultry, fish, turnips, horseradish, iron, aspirin, skin of cherries and tomatoes. Avoid for 72 hours before and during test.

False negatives: low-fiber diet 72 hours before test and vitamin C

11. **What foods are thought to reduce the risk of colorectal cancer?**

A diet low in fat and animal protein may reduce the formation of carcinogenic metabolites produced from the enzymatic activity of bacterial flora. The consumption of a diet high in vegetables, fruits, whole grains, and beans is associated with a decreased incidence of colorectal cancer. Additional studies have shown that cruciferous vegetables (e.g., cabbage, broccoli, cauliflower, brussels sprouts) reduce the risk for colorectal cancer. The recommendation is to eat 5 or more servings of fruits and vegetables daily.

12. How does a high-fiber diet protect against colon cancer?

Fiber in the diet may act as a protective agent against colon cancer by reducing the contact of possible carcinogens with bowel mucosa in five ways:

- Decreasing transit time within intestine
- Diluting carcinogens in stool
- Altering pH in colon
- Binding of possible carcinogens
- Decreasing ammonia concentration in intestine

13. Have any studies proved that the consumption of vitamins or other nutrients will prevent colorectal cancer?

The following products have not been shown to reduce the risk of colon cancer: vitamins, beta carotene, antioxidants, calcium, coffee, fish oils, fluorides, folic acid, food additives, garlic, olestra, olive oil, soybeans, salt, selenium, and tea.

14. Can nonsteroidal antiinflammatory drugs (NSAIDs) prevent colorectal cancer?

Recent clinical studies showed that sulindac (Clinoril) decreased the formation of colonic polyps and regression of rectal polyps in FAP. Indomethacin and aspirin have demonstrated a protective effect against bladder and colon cancer. Tumors may produce large amounts of prostaglandins, which can promote carcinogenesis. The role of prostaglandins in cancer initiation or promotion may be related to their activation of procarcinogens. Several studies have shown that after reaction with cyclooxygenase, certain substances in food may become mutagenic. By inhibiting cyclooxygenase, antiinflammatory agents may be able to block this activation. In addition to the inhibition of prostaglandin H synthetase (cyclooxygenase) and other enzymes important in carcinogenesis, NSAIDs may have important anticancer effects through modulation of the immune system, antiangiogenic effects, induction of apoptosis, and reduction of certain growth factor synthesis.

15. What is the treatment of choice for colorectal cancer?

Surgical resection is the primary treatment of choice in colorectal cancer. More than one-half of all patients can be cured by surgical resection of the involved intestinal segment and reanastomosis. Even if distant metastases are present, surgery is often performed to avoid problems related to bleeding or obstruction. Abdominal-perineal resections may be indicated for low rectal lesions, and newer sphincter-sparing procedures are under study. Clinical trials are ongoing to compare laparoscopic surgery with traditional open surgery. For anal canal carcinomas, a combination of radiation and chemotherapy is the treatment of choice. Surgery is reserved for patients who fail this combination.

Treatments for Colorectal Cancer

SITE	PROCEDURE	PHYSICAL ALTERATIONS
Appendix, cecum, ascending colon, hepatic flexure	Right hemicolectomy	Possible temporary or permanent cecostomy or ascending colostomy
Transverse colon	Transverse colectomy	Possible temporary or permanent transverse colostomy
Distal transverse colon	Left hemicolectomy	Possible temporary or permanent colostomy
Splenic flexure, descending colon	Left partial colectomy	Possible temporary or permanent descending colostomy
Sigmoid colon	Sigmoid colectomy	Possible temporary or permanent sigmoid colostomy

Table continued on following page.

Treatments for Colorectal Cancer (Continued)

SITE	PROCEDURE	PHYSICAL ALTERATIONS
Rectum	Low anterior resection for tumors > 10 cm from anal verge (upper third of rectum)	Possible temporary or permanent sigmoid colostomy
	Abdominal perineal resection (APR)	Permanent sigmoid colostomy (APR) in distal 6 cm of rectum
	Low anterior resection or APR controversial (cancer in mid-rectum 7–11 cm from anal verge)	Permanent sigmoid colostomy with APR

16. When is radiation therapy indicated?
- Preoperatively to reduce bulky rectal cancers, improve the rate of surgical resectability, and eradicate microscopic disease.
- Postoperatively in stage B or C rectal cancers to prevent local recurrence. Postoperative radiation is given to patients to eliminate remaining disease if surgical margins are positive, or for Dukes' stage B or C cancer of the rectum.
- Postoperatively in colon cancer if disease invades other organs (i.e., bladder, abdominal wall)
- Palliatively to decrease painful metastases or control bleeding for inoperable patients.

17. What is the role of chemotherapy in colorectal cancer?
- Adjuvant treatment after surgery
- Radiation sensitizer
- Palliation of advanced disease

18. What chemotherapeutic agents are given for cancer of the colon, rectum, and anus?
Chemotherapy is often used for patients with colorectal cancer, either as an adjuvant or for advanced disease. Adjuvant therapy is important because almost 50% of patients with colorectal cancer die of metastases primarily due to residual disease at surgery.
- Fluorouracil (5-FU) is the most widely used chemotherapy agent, with an overall response rate of 17–30%. Gastrointestinal effects (diarrhea and mucositis) or myelosuppression related to 5-FU vary according to the total dose, timing, combinations of drugs used, and method of administration. For example, continuous infusions commonly cause more gastrointestinal toxicity or hand-foot syndrome, whereas bolus dosing causes more myelosuppression.
- For patients with Dukes' stage B and C colon cancer, 5-FU is given along with levamisole (an oral immunorestorative drug) and/or leucovorin postoperatively as adjuvant therapy.
- Irinotecan (Camptosar) was approved in 1996 for patients with advanced disease refractory to 5-FU; it has a response rate of 23%.
- For metastatic disease, 5-FU with leucovorin (a vitamin that enhances the effectiveness of 5-FU) is usually given.
- For anal canal cancer, 5-FU and mitomycin C are frequently given concurrently with radiation therapy. In addition, 5-FU has radiosensitizing effects and is frequently given to improve the efficacy of radiation therapy.
- New agents under investigation include topoisomerase I inhibitors (Topotecan) and folate-based specific inhibitors of thymidylate synthases (D1694).

19. Are other treatments available for metastatic disease?
Treatment depends on the symptoms and extent of metastatic disease. Metastatic disease in the liver can be treated with radiation, hepatic artery chemoinfusion, or surgical resection if disease is limited to one area of the liver.

20. How is a colostomy managed?

The care of a colostomy is ideally taught by a nurse trained in enterostomal therapy (ET). Patients should be taught to:

- Clean the peristomal skin with soap and water.
- Apply disposable pouch over the stoma.
- Empty the pouch when it is one third full of stool and/or flatus.
- Change the pouch every 4–7 days if there is no leakage. Because pouches are now odor-proof and water-proof, they should not be punctured with holes, as recommended in the past.

21. What lifestyle changes occur with a colostomy?

Patients should be instructed about the following lifestyle changes:

Diet. No restrictions; continue to eat well-balanced meals with fluid intake of 6–8 glasses/day. Avoid or eat in moderation foods that may cause odor or gas.

Activity. Avoid heavy lifting, pushing, and pulling during the first three postoperative months. Continue participation in sports, including swimming, but avoid contact sports.

Traveling. No restrictions; always hand-carry supplies and take along extras.

Social issues. Be aware of initial reactions, including feelings of despair, invalidism, fear of accidents, feeling mutilated, loss of control, and fear of death and dying. Body image disturbance is greatest during the first year after surgery. As recovery from ostomy surgery progresses, patients become increasingly comfortable with their bodies, the ability to care for their pouch, and the desire to return to a normal lifestyle, including sexual activity. Ask to see an enterostomal therapist and/or trained ostomy visitor from the local ostomy association.

Hygiene. Bathe with or without pouch (be aware that stool can pass while bathing). Hot tubs should be avoided or used with caution.

Sexuality. Expect anxiety about initial sexual activity; suggestions to lower anxiety with an ostomy include:

- Empty the pouch before sexual activity.
- Deodorize the pouch 6-12 hours before sexual activity; avoid foods that can cause gas, urinary odor, or loose stools.
- Wear opaque pouch covers to conceal fecal material, or use lingerie or underwear made with pockets on the inside to hold the pouch.
- Experiment with sexual positions other than the missionary position.
- For women, consider vaginal lubricants for dyspareunia.
- For men, consider prostheses or reconstructive surgery (high incidence of impotence in men after abdominal perineal resection).

22. Should colostomies be irrigated?

Irrigations are generally taught for bowel regularity and may be necessary to cleanse the bowel for procedures. Colostomy irrigations can be done to regulate bowel activity in descending or sigmoid colostomies with formed stool. Irrigations are not recommended for the ascending or transverse colon because of the loose consistency of stool.

23. What resources are available to patients with colorectal cancer?

The American Cancer Society (800-ACS-2345) offers many educational and support services to all patients with cancer. The United Ostomy Association (800-826-0826) consists of local chapters that offer complete rehabilitative services and support groups to patients with ostomies. The Johns Hopkins Colorectal Cancer Registry (410-955-3875) provides information about genetic screening and counseling. The Wound, Ostomy, Continence Nurses Society provides educational and support services for patients with ostomies, incontinence, and wounds.

ACKNOWLEDGMENT

The authors thank John Mueh, MD, and Norman Levy, MD, Kaiser Foundation Medical Center, for their thoughtful review of this manuscript.

BIBLIOGRAPHY

1. American Cancer Society 1996 Advisory Committee: Guidelines on diet, nutrition, and cancer prevention: Reducing the risk of cancer with healthy food choices and physical activity. Cancer J Clin 46(6):325–341,1996.
2. Beahrs OH, Henson DE, Hutter RVP, Kennedy BJ (eds): American Joint Committee on Cancer: Manual for Staging of Cancer, 4th ed. Philadelphia, J.B. Lippincott,1992.
3. Bryant RA, Buls JG: Pathophysiology and diagnostic studies of gastrointestinal tract disorders. In Hampton BG, Bryant RA (eds): Ostomies and Continent Diversions: Nursing Management. St. Louis, Mosby, 1992, pp 299–348.
4. Cameron RB (ed): Practical Oncology. Norwalk, CT, Appleton & Lange, 1994.
5. Diaz-Canton EA, Padzur R: Colorectal cancer: Diagnosis and management. In Padzur R (ed): Medical Oncology: A Comprehensive Review, 2nd ed. New York, PRR, 1995, pp 263–284.
6. Giardiello FM: Clinical trials of non-aspirin NSAIDs to prevent colorectal neoplasia. In American Society of Clinical Oncology: Educational Book, 32nd Annual Meeting (May 18–21), Philadelphia, 1996, p 425.
7. Morra ME: Staging of cancer. In Gross B, Johnson BL (eds): Handbook of Oncology Nursing, 2nd ed. Sudbury, MA, Jones & Bartlett, 1994, pp 770–779.
8. Parker SL, Tong T, Bolden S, Wingo PA: Cancer statistics, 1997. CA Cancer J Clin 47:5–27, 1997.
9. Rothenberg ML, et al: Phase II trial of irinotecan in patients with progressive or rapidly recurrent colorectal cancer. J Clin Oncol 14:1128–1135, 1996.
10. Shell JA: The psychosexual impact of ostomy surgery. Progr Develop Ostomy Wound Care 4:3–15, 1992.
11. Steele GD Jr: Colorectal cancer. In Murphy GP, Lawrence W Jr, Lenhard RE Jr (eds): American Cancer Society Textbook of Clinical Oncology. Atlanta, American Cancer Society, 1995, pp 236–250.
12. Steele GD Jr: The national cancer data base report on colorectal cancer. Cancer 74:1979–1989, 1994.
13. UKCCCR Mal Cancer Trial Working Party: Epidermoid anal cancer results from the UKCCCR randomized trial of radiotherapy alone versus radiotherapy, 5-fluorouracil, and mitomycin. Lancet 348:1049–1054, 1996.

24. ENDOCRINE CANCERS

Michael T. McDermott, MD

1. What are endocrine neoplasms?

The endocrine glands secrete hormones directly into the bloodstream for transport throughout the body. Benign or malignant tumors may develop in these glands and cause clinical disease by secreting excessive amounts of hormones, by compressing or invading surrounding structures, or by metastasizing to distant sites. The most common endocrine neoplasms arise in the pituitary, thyroid, parathyroid, and adrenal glands and in the pancreatic islet cells. Although not strictly arising from an endocrine gland, carcinoid tumors are sometimes classified in this group because of their propensity to secrete large amounts of various substances into the circulation.

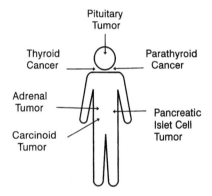

Location of endocrine neoplasms. Endocrine neoplasms arise from the hormone-secreting glands. The most common are tumors of the pituitary, thyroid, parathyoid, and adrenal glands and pancreatic islet cells. Carcinoid tumors, which may secrete large amounts of physiologic substances, are also often classified with the endocrine tumors, although they do not arise from an endocrine gland.

2. Name the different types of pituitary tumors.

The pituitary gland is the master gland that controls most of the other endocrine glands. It consists of five distinct cell types, each with a specific function. Any cell type may become neoplastic and produce excessive amounts of its specific hormone. Thus, pituitary tumors may secrete growth hormone (GH), prolactin (PRL), adrenocorticotropic hormone (ACTH), thyrotropin (TSH), or gonadotropins (luteinizing hormone [LH] and follicle-stimulating hormone [FSH]). Some tumors produce combinations of hormones, and others are nonsecretors.

Regulation and Function of the Pituitary Gland

CELL TYPE	HORMONE	TARGET	ACTION
Somatotroph	Growth hormone (GH)	All tissues	Tissue growth
Lactotroph	Prolactin (PRL)	Breast	Milk production
Corticotroph	Corticotropin (ACTH)	Adrenal	Cortisol production
Thyrotroph	Thyrotropin (TSH)	Thyroid	Thyroxine production
Gonadotroph	Follicle-stimulating hormone (FSH)	Ovary	Ovum development
		Testes	Sperm development
	Luteinizing hormone (LH)	Ovary	Ovulation induction
		Testes	Androgen production

3. What syndromes are associated with pituitary tumors?

GH-secreting tumors produce gigantism in children and acromegaly in adults. Prolactinomas cause galactorrhea (abnormal milk discharge from the breast) and amenorrhea (cessation of

menstruation) in women and impotence in men. ACTH-producing tumors cause the many manifestations of Cushing's disease. TSH-producing tumors result in hyperthyroidism, whereas go-
nadotropin-producing tumors paradoxically cause hypogonadism because of loss of pulsatile
hormone secretion.

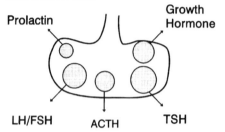

Functioning pituitary tumors. Pituitary tumors often
secrete excessive amounts of one or more of the pituitary hormones: growth hormone, prolactin, thyrotropin, corticotropin, or gonadotropins (LH and FSH).
Although the tumors are usually histologically benign,
significant morbidity and mortality may result from
the syndromes of hormone oversecretion or tumor
mass compression of surrounding vascular or neural
structures.

Clinical Features of Acromegaly

Enlargement of acral parts and multiple organs		Other features
Hands	Ears	Skin tags
Feet	Nose	Sleep apnea
Skull	Tongue	Osteoarthritis
Jaws	Heart	Hypertension
Sinuses	Liver	Diabetes mellitus

Clinical Features of Cushing's Syndrome

Central obesity	Purple striae	Emotional lability
Facial plethora	Easy bruising	Hypertension
Moon face	Muscle weakness	Diabetes mellitus
Buffalo hump		

4. Are pituitary tumors usually benign or malignant?
Pituitary tumors are almost always benign histologically and rarely metastasize to distant
sites. However, they often undergo progressive growth and frequently compress or invade local
structures such as the optic nerves and cavernous sinuses. Invasion may result in severe
headaches, significant visual defects, vascular thrombosis, and, occasionally, hydrocephalus.

5. How are pituitary tumors treated?
Prolactinomas are most often treated with medications such as bromocriptine and cabergo-
line, which produce significant reductions in tumor size and prolactin secretion. The treatment of
choice for other pituitary tumors is surgical resection; the tumor is usually removed through an
incision inside the nose (transsphenoidal hypophysectomy). Because many large and invasive
tumors cannot be completely removed, radiation therapy is often given postoperatively.

6. Name the most common types of thyroid cancer.
The thyroid gland is composed of follicular cells, which synthesize thyroid hormones, and
parafollicular c-cells, which produce calcitonin. Three main histologic types of cancer arise from
the follicular cells: papillary, follicular, and anaplastic carcinomas. Medullary carcinoma, on the
other hand, develops from the parafollicular c-cells.

7. How do thyroid cancers present clinically?
In 1997, there will be an estimated 16,100 new cases of thyroid cancer and 1,230 estimated
cancer deaths. Thyroid cancer usually presents as a painless thyroid mass, much like a benign thyroid nodule. Features suggesting that such a mass is malignant include size greater than 3 cm,
rock-hard consistency, lymphadenopathy, and hoarseness due to vocal cord paralysis. The diagnosis is most reliably made by fine-needle aspiration biopsy.

8. What is the prognosis for patients with thyroid cancers?

The prognosis for papillary carcinoma is excellent. The cure rate exceeds 90%, and the 10-year mortality rate is only 5%. Similarly, follicular carcinoma has a cure rate of over 80% and a 10-year mortality rate of 10%. Medullary carcinoma, however, results in a 10-year mortality rate of approximately 30%, and most patients with anaplastic carcinoma die within 8 months of diagnosis.

9. How are thyroid cancers treated?

Papillary and follicular carcinomas should be treated by a near-total thyroidectomy and daily suppression therapy with oral levothyroxine (LT4). Suppressive doses of LT4 are given to suppress pituitary secretion of TSH, which normally stimulates thyroid growth and function, and thus maintain the serum level of TSH below the normal range. Many patients also receive radioiodine (I-131) therapy, which involves discontinuation of LT4 for 4–6 weeks (allowing the serum TSH level to become elevated) followed by oral administration of a solution containing I-131. The patient is monitored in a radiation protection room for 3–5 days. Medullary carcinoma requires a total thyroidectomy and levothyroxine replacement therapy, which maintains the serum TSH level in the normal range. The treatment of anaplastic carcinoma is total thyroidectomy, levothyroxine suppression, and, in some cases, doxorubicin chemotherapy.

10. What are the features of parathyroid carcinoma?

Parathyroid carcinoma may present as a neck mass with associated lymphadenopathy or as hypercalcemia discovered on serum testing. The most strongly suggestive finding is extremely elevated serum levels of parathyroid hormone (PTH) out of proportion to the moderate degree of calcium elevation. The diagnosis ultimately depends on tissue examination.

11. Is there an effective treatment for parathyroid carcinoma?

The treatment of choice is aggressive neck dissection by an experienced surgeon. Chemotherapy and radiation therapy are rarely beneficial. The 5-year survival rate is less than 50%.

12. What are the most common tumors of the adrenal glands?

The adrenal glands consist of an outer cortex, in which steroid hormones are produced, and an inner medulla, in which catecholamines are made. Benign and malignant tumors may arise in either site. Adrenal cortical tumors may produce excessive cortisol, aldosterone, or androgens. Adrenal medullary tumors, called pheochromocytomas, often secrete norepinephrine and epinephrine.

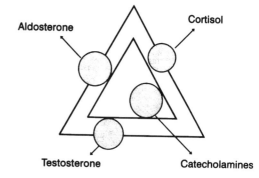

Functioning adrenal tumors. Adrenal tumors may arise from the outer zone (cortex) or the inner zone (medulla) of the adrenal glands. Tumors of the cortex often secrete excessive amounts of cortisol, aldosterone, or testosterone. Tumors of the medulla, known as pheochromocytomas, secrete catecholamines (epinephrine and norepinephrine). Symptoms result from hormone overproduction or, when tumors are malignant, from local invasion and distant metastases.

13. Describe the clinical manifestations of adrenal tumors.

Cushing's syndrome results when tumors secrete cortisol. An excess of aldosterone causes hypertension and hypokalemia. Androgen-producing tumors bring about virilization in women but may be asymptomatic in men. Pheochromocytomas often induce severe hypertension, sweating, and palpitations. Nonsecreting tumors, when large or malignant, present with pain and weight loss.

14. How are adrenal tumors treated?

Surgery is the treatment of choice for nearly all hormone-secreting adrenal tumors and for any nonsecreting tumors over 6 cm in diameter. When tumors prove to be malignant on pathologic examination, chemotherapy with mitotane may produce complete or partial remission. Other chemotherapeutic agents and radiation have not been shown to be effective.

15. What is the prognosis for patients with adrenal tumors?

The prognosis for patients with benign adrenal tumors is usually excellent. However, patients with adrenal carcinomas have a mean survival of 15 months and a 5-year survival rate of 20%.

16. Name the most common types of pancreatic islet cell tumors.

The pancreatic islets normally secrete three major hormones: insulin, glucagon, and somatostatin. Nonetheless, the most common islet cell tumor is gastrinoma, a neoplasm that secretes gastrin, which is normally made only in the stomach. Insulinoma is the second most common islet tumor; glucagonomas and somatostatinomas are rare.

17. What syndromes do pancreatic islet cell tumors produce?

Gastrinomas hypersecrete gastrin, which stimulates prolific acid overproduction by the stomach, resulting in the development of multiple, recurrent peptic ulcers and chronic watery diarrhea. This complex is also known as the Zollinger-Ellison syndrome. Excessive insulin secretion by insulinomas causes episodes of severe hypoglycemia, manifested by confusion, convulsions, and coma.

18. Are most islet cell tumors benign or malignant?

Approximately 80% of gastrinomas are malignant and 20% are benign. In contrast, only about 20% of insulinomas are malignant and 80% are benign.

19. Is there an effective treatment for islet cell tumors?

The treatment of choice for islet cell tumors is surgical resection. When gastrinomas are unresectable, symptomatic relief can be achieved by reducing gastric acid production with medications such as omeprazole or octreotide. Hypoglycemia from a persistent insulinoma may be prevented by frequent ingestion of small meals and administration of diazoxide, verapamil, or octreotide. Malignant tumors of either type also may respond favorably to streptozotocin given with doxorubicin or 5-fluorouracil.

20. What is the difference between carcinoid tumors and carcinoid syndrome?

Carcinoid tumors are neoplasms that arise from cells called enterochromaffin cells because of their peculiar histologic staining characteristics. They may occur in the lungs or gonads and throughout the digestive tract; the most common site is the appendix. Carcinoid syndrome is a symptom complex consisting of cutaneous flushing, diarrhea, and wheezing; it is associated with a tendency to develop progressive fibrosis of the right heart valves, endocardium, pleura, peritoneum, and retroperitoneum.

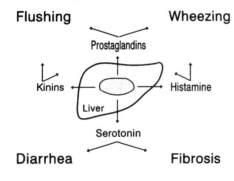

Carcinoid syndrome consists of a constellation of symptoms and signs that include flushing, wheezing, diarrhea, and growth of scar tissue in internal organs and body cavities. This syndrome most often occurs when an intestinal carcinoid tumor metastasizes to the liver and secretes into the systemic circulation active substances such as serotonin, prostaglandins, kinins, and histamine.

21. Describe the pathophysiology of carcinoid syndrome.

Many carcinoid tumors produce substances such as serotonin, bradykinin, tachykinin, histamine, prostaglandins, neurotensin, and substance P, all of which are readily metabolized by the liver. When carcinoid tumors metastasize to the liver, these humoral mediators gain access to the systemic circulation and cause manifestations of carcinoid syndrome.

22. Can carcinoid syndrome be treated or controlled?

Almost all patients who develop carcinoid syndrome have metastatic disease and cannot be cured; chemotherapy and radiation therapy are usually ineffective. However, because of the relatively slow growth rate of most carcinoid tumors, prolonged survival is common and control of the symptoms becomes necessary. Flushing may be alleviated with antihistamines (H_1 and H_2 antagonists) or steroids, whereas diarrhea frequently responds to codeine, diphenoxylate (Lomotil), loperamide (Immodium), or octreotide.

23. What are the endocrine paraneoplastic syndromes?

Endocrine paraneoplastic syndromes occur in association with some tumors but are not due to tissue invasion or metastases. They result from secretion by the tumor of hormones into the circulation. The three best known examples are the syndrome of inappropriate antidiuretic hormone (SIADH), hypercalcemia of malignancy, and ectopic ACTH syndrome.

24. Explain the pathophysiology of SIADH.

Antidiuretic hormone (ADH) is normally secreted by the posterior pituitary gland and acts on the kidney to promote water retention. In doing so, it protects the body against dehydration. Tumors, particularly those of the lung and brain, sometimes secrete large amounts of ADH that result in excessive water retention and dilutional hyponatremia. Dilutional hyponatremia may result in confusion, convulsions, and coma due to edema of the brain.

25. What are the mediators of the hypercalcemia of malignancy?

Most cases of hypercalcemia of malignancy result from tumor elaboration of a hormone known as parathyroid hormone-related peptide (PTHrp). Similar in some ways to PTH, this hormone normally functions to concentrate calcium in breast milk. When secreted in excessive quantities by tumors, such as those of the lung, it stimulates bone resorption and renal calcium retention, which combine to raise the serum calcium level.

26. Describe the pathophysiology of ectopic ACTH syndrome.

ACTH is normally secreted by the anterior pituitary gland and stimulates the adrenal glands to produce cortisol. Tumors of various organs, especially the lung, occasionally produce ACTH in quantities sufficient to stimulate excessive secretion of adrenal cortisol. This results in development of Cushing's syndrome, the manifestations of which are partly masked by tumor cachexia.

BIBLIOGRAPHY

1. Feldman JM: The carcinoid syndrome. Endocrinologist 3:129–135, 1993.
2. Friesen SR: Tumors of the endocrine pancreas. N Engl J Med 306:580–590, 1982.
3. Gagel RF, Robinson MF, Donovan DT, Alford BR: Medullary thyroid carcinoma: Recent progress. J Clin Endocrinol Metab 76:809–814, 1993.
4. Klibanski A, Zervas NT: Diagnosis and management of hormone-secreting pituitary adenomas. N Engl J Med 324:822–831, 1991.
5. Luton J-P, Cerdas S, Billaud L, et al: Clinical features of adrenocortical carcinoma, prognostic factors, and the effect of mitotane therapy. N Engl J Med 322:1195–1201, 1990.
6. Mazzaferri EL, Samaan NA (eds): Endocrine Tumors. Boston, Blackwell Scientific Publications, 1993.
7. Parker SL, Tong T, Bolden S, Wingo PA: Cancer statistics, 1997. CA Cancer J Clin 47:5–27, 1997.
8. Robbins J (moderator): Thyroid cancer: A lethal endocrine neoplasm. Ann Intern Med 115:133–147, 1991.
9. Wynne AG, Heerden JV, Carney JA, et al: Parathyoid carcinoma: Clinical and pathologic features in 43 patients. Medicine 71:197–205, 1992.

25. GASTRIC, PANCREATIC, HEPATOCELLULAR, AND GALLBLADDER CANCERS

Susan Morgan, MD

GASTRIC CANCER

Quick Facts

Incidence	In the United States the incidence is 10/100,000 persons compared with 78/100,000 persons in Japan. The number of new cases in the United States in 1997 is estimated at 22,400. Emigrants from high-incidence to low-incidence countries often have a decreased risk of developing gastric cancer. For unknown reasons, both incidence and mortality rates have decreased in all regions of the world.
Mortality	Highest in East Asia (Hong Kong, Japan, Singapore) and lowest in the United States. In 1997, 14,000 deaths in the United States due to gastric cancer are estimated.
Risk factors	**Environment:** lower socioeconomic status, diets low in fruits and vegetables, ingestion of salt-preserved or smoked foods, and smoking.
	Precursor conditions: previous partial gastrectomy for benign disease, chronic atrophic gastritis, pernicious anemia, achlorhydria, mucosal dysplasia, history of Barrett's esophagus, *Helicobacter pylori* infection, gastric adenomatous polyps.
	Heredity: blood group A, hereditary nonpolyposis colorectal cancer (Lynch syndrome 2)
Histology	Approximately 95% of gastric cancers are **adenocarcinomas.** The remainder are predominantly lymphomas or leiomyosarcomas. Other rare histologies include carcinoid tumors and squamous cell carcinomas.
Symptoms	Gastric cancer often progresses to an advanced stage before symptoms develop. Symptoms and signs of advanced disease include anorexia, early satiety, weight loss, palpable abdominal mass, dysphagia, severe anemia, and weakness.
Staging	American Joint Committee on Cancer (AJCC) tumor, node, metastasis (TNM) system based on postgastrectomy pathologic specimen:

Primary tumor (T)

TX	Primary tumor cannot be assessed
T0	No evidence of primary tumor
Tis	Carcinoma in situ
T1	Tumor invades lamina propria or submucosa
T2	Tumor invades muscularis propria or submucosa (classified as T3 with perforation of visceral peritoneum over gastric ligaments or omenta)
T3	Tumor penetrates serosa without invasion of adjacent structures
T4	Tumor invades adjacent structures

Regional lymph nodes (N)

NX	Regional lymph node(s) cannot be assessed
N0	No regional lymph node metastasis
N1	Metastasis in perigastric lymph node(s) within 3 cm of edge of primary tumor
N2	Metastasis in perigastric lymph node(s) more than 3 cm from edge of primary tumor or in lymph nodes along left gastric, common hepatic, splenic, or celiac arteries

Distant metastasis (M)

MX	Presence of distant metastasis cancer cannot be assessed
M0	No distant metastasis
M1	Distant metastasis

Table continued on following page.

Quick Facts (Continued)

Stage groupings:

Stage 0	Tis, N0, M0	Stage IIIA	T2, N2, M0
Stage IA	T1, N0, M0		T3, N1, M0
Stage IB	T1, N1, M0		T4, N0, M0
	T2, N0, M0	Stage IIIB	T3, N2, M0
Stage II	T1, N2 M0		T4, N1, M0
	T2, N1, M0	Stage IV	T4, N2, M0
	T3, N0, M0		Any T, Any N, M1

Treatment	• **Complete surgical resection of the tumor and adjacent lymph nodes** is the only chance for cure. Survival rates are best improved in patients with stage I disease. Patients with T3, T4, or any nodal involvement have a significant risk for relapse after surgical resection.
	• Currently postoperative radiation therapy and chemotherapy confer no benefit after complete surgical resection. For patients with locally advanced tumors that are unresectable, external beam radiation therapy may be palliative in reducing pain and relieving obstruction.
	• When chemotherapy is combined with radiation therapy in patients with locally advanced gastric carcinoma, survival is prolonged compared with either radiation therapy or chemotherapy alone.
	• For patients with metastatic gastric carcinoma, chemotherapy is the treatment of choice.

1. List the names associated with specific metastatic deposits in gastric cancer.

Virchow's node: left supraclavicular lymph node enlargement
Irish's node: left axillary lymph node enlargement
Sister Mary Joseph nodule: periumbilical nodule
Krukenberg's tumor: metastatic disease to ovaries
Blumer's shelf: mass in the cul-de-sac or rectal shelf

2. What paraneoplastic syndromes occasionally are seen in gastric cancer?

Acanthosis nigricans: a black or brownish wart-like eruption in intertriginous areas (axilla, groin, under breast); also may appear on palms of hands and soles of feet.
Trousseau's syndrome: recurrent, idiopathic deep vein thrombosis
Polymyositis/dermatomyositis: symmetrical proximal muscle weakness with or without skin rash.

3. What are the clinical manifestations of the "dumping syndrome"? What is its probable cause?

The dumping syndrome is a postoperative complication of gastric resection. Clinical manifestations include nausea, vomiting, diarrhea, epigastric fullness, tachycardia, diaphoresis, and weakness. Dumping syndrome most likely is due to removal of the reservoir function (antrum) of the stomach. Hypertonic foodstuffs empty directly into the small bowel, resulting in a major fluid shift out of the intravascular space and into the bowel. To improve symptoms, the patient needs to decrease the osmotic load presented to the small bowel by eating small, frequent meals that are low in carbohydrate and high in protein.

4. Monthly injections of which vitamin are necessary after subtotal or total gastrectomy? Why?

After gastric resection, vitamin B12 deficiency occurs within 6–10 years. The several-year delay in clinical evidence of vitamin B12 deficiency is due to adequate liver stores. Once these stores are exhausted, the deficiency becomes evident because the parietal cells of the stomach are responsible for producing intrinsic factor, which is necessary for absorption of vitamin B12 (distal ileum). Monthly administration of vitamin B12 prevents deficiency.

5. Is there a role for adjuvant (postoperative) chemotherapy or radiation therapy after curative resection for gastric cancer?

No. The only curative approach to gastric cancer is subtotal gastrectomy with resection of adjacent lymph nodes. Patients with stage I disease are the best candidates for curative resection. However, even when curative resection is attempted, cancer recurs in most patients within the first 2 years. The 5-year survival rate for stage I disease is 50–60%; for stage II disease, 29%; and for stage III disease, 13%. Despite the poor outcome, no adjuvant regimen has improved results.

6. Does radiation therapy in conjunction with chemotherapy confer a survival benefit on patients with locally advanced (nonmetastatic) gastric cancer?

Yes. Patients with locally advanced disease are unable to undergo resection for cure. Radiation alone may be palliative in reducing pain or relieving obstruction but does not improve survival. Nor does chemotherapy alone appear to improve survival. However, when radiation therapy (4000 cGy) is combined with chemotherapy (5-fluorouracil [5-FU]), survival appears to be prolonged. In one study comparing 5FU plus radiation therapy with radiation therapy alone, median survival was 12 months vs. 5.9 months, respectively.

7. What treatment options are available for patients with advanced (metastatic) gastric cancer?

Patients with advanced gastric cancer have incurable disease. Most die within a few months of diagnosis. Treatment options include investigational protocols; single-agent chemotherapy with 5-FU; multiagent chemotherapy such as 5-FU, Adriamycin, high-dose methotrexate, and leucovorin rescue (FAMTX); and etoposide, leucovorin, 5-FU (ELF); or comfort-directed supportive care. Depending on the patient's performance status (debilitated vs. good activity level), any one of the above options is acceptable.

Single-agent 5-FU has a response rate of about 20%. Complete responses are rare, and partial responses are of brief duration. FAMTX has a higher response rate (40–50%) and is associated with survival times of 6–10 months.

PANCREATIC CANCER

Quick Facts

Incidence	In the United States, the incidence of pancreatic cancer is 9/100,000 people; the estimated number of new cases for 1997 is 27,600. Incidence has been stable for the past 20 years. Males are 1.5–2.0 times more likely to develop pancreatic cancer than females. African-Americans are more frequently affected, with an incidence of 15/100,000 people.
Mortality	The median survival of patients with pancreatic cancer is 3–4 months, and the 5-year survival rate is only 3%. In the U.S., the number of estimated deaths in 1997 is 28,100. The prognosis is so dismal because most patients have advanced disease at the time of diagnosis.
Risk factors	Cause remains unknown but several factors are associated with its occurrence: • Cigarette smoking: most prominent risk factor for pancreatic cancer • Diet: high fat, low intake of fruits and vegetables, excessive alcohol • Previous partial gastrectomy for benign conditions • Diabetes mellitus • Occupational exposure: solvents, petroleum compounds, beta-naphthylamine, and benzidine • Lower socioeconomic status • Hereditary pancreatitis
Histology	Pancreatic cancer arises from both exocrine parenchyma and endocrine islet cells. Approximately 95% of pancreatic cancers occur within the exocrine portion of the pancreas. Among the exocrine malignancies, 80-90% are **adenocarcinomas**. The

Table continued on following page.

Quick Facts (Continued)

	majority arise in the proximal portion of the pancreas, which includes the head, neck, and uncinate process. Other less common malignant tumors of the pancreas include pancreatic islet cell tumors, lymphomas, and cystadenocarcinomas.
Symptoms	Most patients are symptomatic at the time of diagnosis. Symptoms include abdominal pain, anorexia, weight loss, early satiety, jaundice, nausea, vomiting, and diarrhea.
Staging	American Joint Committee on Cancer TNM staging system

Primary tumor (T)

TX	Primary tumor cannot be assessed
T0	No evidence of primary tumor
T1	Tumor limited to pancreas
T1a	Tumor ≤ 2 cm in greatest dimension
T1b	Tumor > 2 cm in greatest dimension
T2	Tumor extends directly to duodenum, bile duct, or peripancreatic tissues
T3	Tumor extends directly to stomach, spleen, colon, or adjacent large vessels

Regional lymph nodes (N)

NX	Regional lymph nodes cannot be assessed
N0	No regional lymph node metastasis
N1	Regional lymph node metastasis

Distant metastasis (M)

MX	Presence of distant metastasis cannot be assessed
M0	No distant metastasis
M1	Distant metastasis

Stage groupings

Stage I	T1, N0, M0
	T2, N0, M0
Stage II	T3, N0, M0
Stage III	Any T, N1, M0
Stage IV	Any T, Any N, M1

Treatment

- The approach to therapy differs according to stage of disease at presentation. Complete surgical resection remains the only effective treatment (possible in only 5–15% of patients). Procedures include pancreatoduodenectomy (Whipple procedure) for tumors in the head of the pancreas, distal pancreatectomy for lesions in the tail, and total pancreatectomy for large or diffuse lesions.
- Survival is improved with adjuvant chemotherapy plus radiation therapy after curative resection and no evidence of lymph node metastases.
- For patients with inoperable, locally advanced disease, radiation therapy plus chemotherapy improves survival compared with radiation therapy alone.
- For patients with metastatic disease, chemotherapy and supportive care are the treatment options.

8. What is the name of the standard operation for pancreatic tumors located in the head of the pancreas? What is removed?

The Whipple procedure (pancreatoduodenectomy) is the only potentially curative approach to pancreatic cancer located in the head of the pancreas. This procedure includes removal of the distal stomach, common bile duct, gallbladder, duodenum, pancreatic head to the midbody en bloc, and vagotomy. Unfortunately, resection is feasible in only 5–15% of cases because most patients have advanced disease (liver metastases, tumor extension into spleen, colon or stomach, vascular invasion, or nerve invasion) at presentation. Resection is also typically limited to patients with cancer located in the head of the pancreas because patients with tumors in the body or tail invariably have advanced disease (asymptomatic until well advanced). Patients with stage I tumors (T1–T2, N0, M0) are the best candidates for curative resection. However, even with resection, 90% of patients die from tumor recurrence within 1–2 years. The expected median survival is only 12–18 months.

9. Is there a role for adjuvant therapy after curative resection for pancreatic cancer?

Yes. Adjuvant therapy appears to be a reasonable approach for the few patients who are able to undergo curative resection and have no lymph node metastases identified on pathologic review. Only one prospective randomized trial (Gastrointestinal Tumor Study Group trial) has shown a survival benefit with the addition of postoperative 5FU and radiation therapy. Patients who received this combination showed significant improvement in median survival (20 months vs. 11 months), 2-year survival (43% vs. 18%), and 5-year survival (14% vs. 5%).

10. What is the newest chemotherapeutic agent for unresectable (locally advanced or metastatic) pancreatic cancer?

Gemcitabine is the newest drug for advanced pancreatic cancer. A randomized study demonstrated an advantage with gemcitabine over 5-FU in survival time and symptom control (pain, weight, performance status). Gemcitabine was given at 1000 mg/m^2 weekly for 7 doses, followed by a week of rest, and then weekly for 3 doses every 4 weeks thereafter. Approximately 24% of the gemcitabine-treated patients experienced improved symptom control compared with only 4.8% of the 5-FU-treated patients. The median survival for gemcitabine-treated patients was 5.65 months compared with 4.41 months for 5-FU-treated patients. Common side effects included nausea, vomiting, diarrhea, and neutropenia. At present, gemcitabine should be considered as first-line management of symptomatic patients with advanced pancreatic adenocarcinoma.

11. Which ganglion plexus is commonly involved in pancreatic cancer?

Pancreatic cancers may invade the celiac plexus, causing significant neuropathic pain. This pain is the worst symptom experienced by patients with advanced pancreatic cancer. Treatment to improve the pain includes opioid analgesics, surgical neurotomy, chemical neurolysis (celiac block), and radiation therapy. Medical management alone often is not enough to relieve the pain. Chemical neurolysis involves the injection of 50% alcohol directly into the region of the celiac plexus either intraoperatively or percutaneously and is associated with pain relief in 90% of cases. External beam radiation therapy is also effective in relieving neuropathic pain in approximately 50–70% of patients with advanced pancreatic cancer.

12. When Courvoisier's sign is present, what organ of the body can be palpated?

Gallbladder. Carcinoma of the head of the pancreas may cause biliary obstruction, resulting in a distended gallbladder. The distended gallbladder is typically nontender.

HEPATOCELLULAR CARCINOMA

Quick Facts

Incidence	The incidence of hepatocellular carcinoma is greatest in Southeast Asia, sub-Saharan Africa, and the Orient. The incidence in the United States, Canada, Britain, Australia, and South America is low. In 1997 in the United States, 13,600 new cases of liver and biliary passage cancers are estimated.
Mortality	High fatality rate. Among all patients the 5-year survival rate is approximately 3–5%. In 1997 in the United States, 12,400 deaths from liver and biliary passage cancers are estimated.
Risk factors	Chronic infection with either hepatitis B or hepatitis C, with or without underlying cirrhosis Preexisting cirrhosis: approximately 10% of patients with cirrhosis develop hepatocellular carcinoma. Aflatoxin: proved to be a potent hepatocarcinogen; appears to cause a specific mutation in the p53 tumor suppressor gene, leading to hepatocellular carcinoma. Hormones: the risk of liver cell adenomas and hepatocellular carcinoma is increased in women who have used oral contraceptives for 8 or more years; hepatocellular carcinoma has also been observed in patients with long histories of androgen administration.

Table continued on following page.

Quick Facts (Continued)

Histology	80–90% of primary liver cancers are hepatocellular, other less common tumors include hepatoblastomas, sarcomas, and primary lymphomas
Symptoms	Usual presenting symptoms are right upper quadrant pain, fatigue, abdominal swelling, and weight loss
Staging	American Joint Committee on Cancer TNM System

Primary tumor (T)

TX	Primary tumor cannot be assessed
T0	No evidence of primary tumor
T1	Solitary tumor < 2 cm in greatest dimension without vascular invasion
T2	Solitary tumor < 2 cm in greatest dimension with vascular invasion, or multiple tumors limited to one lobe, none > 2 cm in greatest dimension without vascular invasion, or a solitary tumor > 2 cm in greatest dimension without vascular invasion
T3	Solitary tumor > 2 cm in greatest dimension with vascular invasion, or multiple tumors limited to one lobe, none > 2 cm in greatest dimension, with vascular invasion, or multiple tumors limited to one lobe, any > 2 cm in greatest dimension, with or without vascular invasion
T4	Multiple tumors in more than one lobe or tumor(s) involving a major branch of portal or hepatic vein(s)

Lymph node (N)

NX	Regional lymph nodes cannot be assessed
N0	No regional lymph-node metastasis
N1	Regional lymph-node metastasis

Distant metastasis

MX	Presence of distant metastasis cannot be assessed
M0	No distant metastasis
M1	Distant metastasis

Stage groupings

Stage 1	T1, N0, M0
Stage II	T2, N0, M0
Stage III	T1, N1, M0
	T2, N1, M0
	T3, N0, M0
	T3, N1, M0
Stage IVA	T4, Any N, M0
Stage IVB	Any T, Any N, M1

Treatment	Surgery is the only curative modality for hepatocellular carcinoma, but its use depends on tumor size, location, and condition of the uninvolved liver. Only 10% of hepatocellular carcinomas are resectable with solitary or unilobar hepatic lesions at the time of diagnosis. There is no role for adjuvant chemotherapy or radiotherapy after curative resection. Other treatment options include hepatic intraarterial infusion of chemotherapy, chemoembolization, liver transplantation, radiation therapy, and single-agent chemotherapy (doxorubicin).

13. What tumor marker is commonly ordered for evaluating hepatocellular carcinoma?

Alpha-fetoprotein (AFP) is elevated in approximately 70% of patients diagnosed with hepatocellular carcinoma. Unfortunately, AFP is not specific for hepatocellular carcinoma and may be elevated in benign liver disease, germ cell tumor, gastric cancer, and pancreatic cancer. A normal level of AFP does not exclude the diagnosis of hepatocellular carcinoma.

14. List several paraneoplastic syndromes associated with hepatocellular carcinoma.

Fever	Gynecomastia
Hypercalcemia	Erythrocytosis
Hypoglycemia	Dysfibrinogenemia

15. What is the survival rate for patients with hepatocellular carcinoma?

The 5-year survival rate is approximately 40–45% for patients with small tumors (2–5 cm) and 10% for patients with tumors larger than 5 cm. Disease recurs in most patients undergoing resection.

Unfortunately, curative resection is appropriate for only 10% or fewer cases because of advanced disease (bilobar involvement), underlying cirrhosis (poor hepatic reserve), portal/vena caval thrombus, or other comorbid diseases. Survival for patients with unresectable disease is about 2–6 months.

GALLBLADDER CANCER

16. What risk factors are possibly associated with the development of gallbladder cancer?

The cause of gallbladder cancer is unknown. Chronic cholecystitis and cholelithiasis have been associated with the development of gallbladder cancer in 50% and 75% of cases, respectively. A calcified gallbladder ("porcelain gallbladder") has about a 15–20% chance of harboring cancer. Ulcerative colitis increases the risk for development of gallbladder cancer. The incidence of gallbladder cancer increases with age and peaks in the 6th–7th decades of life; it is rare before the age of 40. In 1997, 6,900 new cases and 3,500 deaths are estimated. Females are affected more commonly than males with a female-to-male ratio of 3:1–4:1. The incidence of gallbladder cancer is considerably higher in Mexicans, American Indians, and Alaskan natives. Employees of rubber industries have a higher incidence and earlier onset of gallbladder cancer.

17. Why is the prognosis for gallbladder cancer so dismal?

Gallbladder cancer is typically asymptomatic in its early resectable stages; by the time symptoms occur, the disease is advanced and unresectable. The cancer usually grows into the liver, stomach, and duodenum by direct extension, making resection impossible. The median survival period is approximately 6 months, and the 5-year survival rate is less than 5%.

Patients who are incidentally found to have stage I or II tumors at cholecystectomy for presumed symptomatic benign disease have an improved survival rate and are potentially cured.

18. Klatskin tumor refers to a cancer in what location?

A Klatskin tumor, named after a physician, is a primary extrahepatic bile duct cancer (cholangiocarcinoma) located near the bifurcation of the left and right hepatic bile ducts.

The views contained in this manuscript are solely those of the author and do not reflect the views or policies of Tripler Army Medical Command, the Department of Defense, or the U.S. Government.

BIBLIOGRAPHY

1. Brain MC, Carbone PP (eds): Current Therapy in Hematology-Oncology, 5th ed. St. Louis, Mosby, 1995.
2. Casciato DA, Lowitz BB (eds): Manual of Clinical Oncology, 3rd ed. Boston, Little, Brown, 1995.
3. DeVita VT, Hellman S, Rosenberg SA (eds): Cancer: Principles and Practice of Oncology, 5th ed. Philadelphia, Lippincott-Raven, 1997.
4. Macdonald JS, Haller DG, Mayer RJ (eds): Manual of Oncologic Therapeutics, 3rd ed. Philadelphia, J.B. Lippincott, 1995.
5. Padzur R (ed): Medical Oncology: A Comprehensive Review, 2nd ed. New York, PRR, 1995.
6. Parker SL, Tong T, Bolden S, Wingo PA: Cancer statistics, 1997. CA Cancer J Clin 47:5–27, 1997.

26. GYNECOLOGIC CANCERS

Patricia Novak-Smith, RN, MS, OCN,
and Susan A. Davidson, MD

1. What are the primary sites of gynecologic cancer?

Gynecologic cancers are associated with the female reproductive organs. The principal sites include the ovaries, fallopian tubes, uterus, cervix, vagina, and vulva. Additional rare cancers that are classified as gynecologic include gestational trophoblastic neoplasias (GTN), a group of pregnancy-related tumors that may persist and metastasize (such as hydatidiform mole and chorio-carcinoma), and primary peritoneal carcinoma, a tumor that originates on the peritoneal surfaces but demonstrates behavior similar to the epithelial ovarian cancers. The three most commonly diagnosed gynecologic cancers are the focus of this chapter: endometrial (epithelial surface of the uterus), ovarian, and cervical.

2. How are gynecologic cancers staged?

Gynecologic cancers are staged according to guidelines established by the International Federation of Gynaecology and Obstetrics (FIGO). FIGO adapted the traditional primary tumor-regional lymph nodes-distant metastasis (TNM) system to ensure consistency on the international level in the staging of gynecologic cancers. The primary features that distinguish this system from other staging systems are (1) reliance on clinical staging for cervical and vaginal cancer, which includes but is not limited to physical examination, chest radiograph, and intravenous pyelogram; (2) use of specific surgical staging for all other gynecologic cancers; and (3) adherence to the original staging designation for all disease sites despite later findings of persistence, metastasis, or recurrence.

3. Why is cervical cancer considered preventable?

Cervical cancer is considered a preventable cancer because it is characterized by a lengthy premalignant, preinvasive state that is amenable to early detection through routine Papanicolaou (Pap) smear sampling. These premalignant conditions may be completely eradicated with currently available treatment. Abnormalities of the cervix may be invisible to the naked eye. Exfoliative cytologic sampling of the cervix permits microscopic examination to detect the presence of cells with either atypical appearance or abnormal development. All premalignant lesions have the potential to regress, persist, or become invasive. It is believed that it may take as long as 7 years for early changes to progress to an invasive cancer. Cervical cancer is thus prevented when premalignant lesions are detected and treated before they undergo this transformation.

Quick Facts—Cervical Cancer

Incidence	2% of new cancer cases in women annually. In 1997: 14,500 estimated new cases.
Mortality	2% of cancer deaths in women annually. In 1997: 4,800 estimated deaths.
Risk factors	**Early coitus**
	Human papillomavirus (HPV), especially types 16 and 18
	Human immunodeficiency virus (HIV)
	Low socioeconomic status—decreased access to routine Pap smear screening
	Smoking (nicotine byproducts, measured in cervical secretions, are thought to favor development of precancerous changes of the cervix)
Histology	Squamous carcinomas are most common; other cell types include adenocarcinoma, adenosquamous carcinoma, small cell, and glassy cell.

Table continued on following page.

Symptoms	**Thin, watery vaginal discharge, heavier menses,** and **postcoital spotting** are most common; other symptoms include spontaneous, intermittent, painless uterine bleeding (metrorrhagia); back, flank, or leg pain; lower extremity edema; dysuria; hematuria or rectal bleeding; and cough.	
Staging	Stage I	Confined to cervix
	IA	Microscopic lesion < 7.0 mm wide, 5.0 mm deep
	IB	Microscopic lesion > IA or macroscopic lesion confined to cervix
	Stage II	Extension beyond cervix and/or upper two-thirds of vagina
	IIA	No parametrial involvement
	IIB	Parametrial involvement
	Stage III	Extension to lower third of vagina
	IIIA	No extension to pelvic side-wall
	IIIB	Extends to pelvic side wall and/or hydronephrosis
	Stage IV	Extension beyond true pelvis
	IVA	Involves adjacent organs (bladder, rectum)
	IVB	Distant metastasis
Treatment	Stage I	Total abdominal or modified radical hysterectomy
	Stages IB, IIA	Radical hysterectomy with lymph node dissection or radiation has equivalent prognosis **except** for bulky IB tumors (treated initially with radiation, may be followed with extra-fascial hysterectomy)
	Stages IIB, III, IVA	Radiation therapy (chemotherapy used as radiation sensitizer)
	Stage IVB	Palliative radiation and/or chemotherapy

4. What terms should the nurse be familiar with when explaining an abnormal Pap smear?

Terms used to identify abnormal Pap smears include atypia, dysplasia, cervical intraepithelial neoplasia (CIN), and squamous intraepithelial lesions (SIL). **Atypia** refers to cells with abnormal features that are not diagnostic and are considered to be of undetermined significance. **Dysplasia** indicates a distinct abnormality of cellular development and is associated with premalignant disease of the cervix. It is reported as mild, moderate, or severe, depending on the degree of deviation from the normal cells found on the cervix. The designation of **CIN** correlates with three dysplastic categories: (1) mild dysplasia/CIN 1; (2) moderate dysplasia/CIN 2; and (3) severe dysplasia/carcinoma in situ (CIS)/CIN 3. With the emergence of the human papillomavirus (HPV) as a deviation from normal cervical cytology and its association as a risk factor in the development of cervical cancer, it became necessary to include this category in the Pap smear reporting process. The term **SIL** was introduced in the current Bethesda classification system. Low-grade SIL (LSIL) encompasses changes due to HPV as well as CIN 1 or mild dysplasia. High-grade SIL (HSIL) includes CIN 2 or moderate dysplasia, CIN 3 or severe dysplasia, and CIS. In reporting these findings to the patient, it is important to stress that the classification is used to identify degrees of abnormality that are universally understood. This classification directs the practitioner to appropriate treatment and follow-up.

5. How should a nurse explain the evaluation and treatment of an abnormal Pap smear to a patient?

Patients should be reminded that the Pap smear is only a screening test; the actual cervical abnormality may be better or worse than the screening test indicates. To determine the extent of any abnormal Pap smear, the cervix must be examined with a colposcope, and diagnostic biopsies may be required. The treatment recommendations for an abnormal Pap smear depend on the colposcopy findings and, if necessary, the biopsy results. Colposcopy allows the health care provider to examine thoroughly the surface of the cervix using a colposcope for magnification. The colposcope is similar to using a pair of binoculars or a microscope to enhance visual inspection. Patients should be informed that the procedure is comparable to the process of obtaining a Pap smear, although it takes longer to complete. After insertion of the speculum, the cervix is thoroughly examined through the magnification of the colposcope. A 3–5% acetic acid (household vinegar) or other staining solution, such as Lugols' (strong iodine), may be used to demarcate cervical abnormalities. These solutions may cause a stinging or burning sensation, but they are not harmful to the cervical mucosa. Biopsies of abnormal areas, as well as curettage (scraping) of the endocervical canal above the external opening of the cervix, are then performed. These procedures are associated with mild discomfort, such as pinching or cramping sensations, and light vaginal bleeding or spotting. If precancerous changes are detected, further treatment is necessary. Treatment options that may be discussed with the patient include laser ablation, cryotherapy (freezing of abnormal tissue), loop excision, cold knife cone biopsy, and hysterectomy.

6. What should a nurse tell a patient who asks about the use of Pap smear screening for gynecologic cancers?

Patients often believe that Pap smears are used as screening tests for all gynecologic cancers. In reality, the Pap smear is specifically intended to detect abnormalities in the cells on the surface of the cervix, particularly preinvasive CIN (see question 4). On occasion, cellular abnormality of vaginal, endometrial, or ovarian origin may be detected. In these situations, additional work-up is required to determine the exact origin and significance of the abnormality. Overall, patients should be informed that the Pap smear is not intended to screen for either invasive cervical cancer or other gynecologic malignancies. Despite this limited application, the process of obtaining the Pap smear provides valuable information to the practitioner. Before insertion of the speculum, inspection of the external genitalia under bright light facilitates identification of abnormal or suspicious lesions on the vulva. Direct visualization of the cervix and vaginal tissue may reveal the presence of a gross lesion in an asymptomatic individual. After the speculum examination, palpation during bimanual examination assesses the ovaries for enlargement, a possible symptom of ovarian pathology. For these reasons, women should be encouraged to begin annual Pap smear screening and pelvic examination with the initiation of sexual activity or by age 18. After three or more consecutive normal annual screening tests and examinations, the Pap smear may be done less frequently as suggested by the health care provider. Establishing a life-long habit of annual testing as part of a well-woman examination offers the most consistent method of detecting abnormalities early. Both the American Cancer Society and the American College of Obstetricians and Gynecologists recommend annual examinations. After hysterectomy, Pap smear recommendations vary according to patient history.

7. Why would an examination under anesthesia be performed in a patient with cervical cancer?

Cervical cancer spreads primarily by direct extension to surrounding tissues and organs and involvement of regional lymph node chains. In the presence of visible, measurable tumor, it is important to assess the surrounding parametrial tissue for evidence of tumor infiltration. Although a pelvic examination is performed in the office, full assessment is not possible because of patient discomfort during the examination, presence of stool in the bowel, and anxiety about the findings. Patients, therefore, are frequently examined under anesthesia so that a thorough pelvic examination may be performed with the benefit of complete relaxation. This promotes a more accurate assessment of the clinical stage of disease. In addition, cystoscopic and sigmoidoscopic examinations may be carried out at the same time to rule out bladder and bowel involvement. Computerized axial tomographic (CAT) examination, although helpful in the determination of lymph node involvement, may be inconclusive in the determination of tissue invasion.

8. What is meant by parametrial spread in cervical cancer?

The parametrium is the space between the lateral portion of the cervix and the bony structure of the pelvic sidewall. It contains the supporting structures, such as the uterosacral and transverse cervical ligaments, that maintain the cervix in its relatively immobile position. The ureters pass through this area in rather close proximity to the uterus before insertion into the urinary bladder. Invasion of this space is common when a cervical tumor expands laterally. It may extend and become adherent to the bony structure of the pelvic sidewall. Patients with parametrial spread have an increased incidence of hydronephrosis, which requires ureteral stent placement because of compression by tumor growth. In addition, such patients may commonly complain of radiating hip or back pain secondary to mass effect, nerve infiltration, and possible bony metastasis. Spread of tumor to this location is an indication for primary treatment with radiation therapy. Chemotherapy may be used as a radiation sensitizer. Surgical excision after radiation therapy is generally not undertaken because of the poor healing properties of radiated tissue and the subsequent propensity for fistula formation. Nurses should understand that when parametrial spread is documented on bimanual pelvic examination, the patient has a more advanced stage of disease, which, as described above, affects the treatment recommendations.

9. When is hysterectomy indicated in cervical cancer?
The use of hysterectomy in the treatment of cervical cancer varies. Proper treatment of cervical cancer and potential sites of spread with surgery alone requires a radical hysterectomy with lymph node dissection. Patients with early cancers, characterized by tumors confined to the cervix that are smaller than 4 cm, may be the most appropriate candidates for this procedure if surgery does not expose them to increased morbidity. Patients with tumors that are larger than 4 cm but still confined to the cervix receive radiation therapy first to sterilize the regional lymph nodes and to shrink the tumor. This is followed by a simple hysterectomy to remove only the residual cervical tumor.

When the cancer extends beyond the cervix to the parametria and other surrounding tissue, radiation therapy without hysterectomy is the most effective treatment. It should be emphasized that cervical cancer may be effectively treated with radiation therapy. In the event that the patient has an early cervical cancer in the presence of comorbid factors that significantly increase operative risks, treatment with definitive radiation therapy offers individual survival rates that are comparable to those of the surgical procedure. The decision, therefore, to perform a hysterectomy is based on the stage of the cancer, age and health status of the patient, treatment plan, and preference of the patient.

10. Distinguish among an extrafascial, modified radical, and radical hysterectomy.
The nurse caring for a patient with gynecologic cancer should be aware that several classes of hysterectomies are routinely used in treatment. The differences among them have significance for recovery and potential postoperative complications.

An **extrafascial hysterectomy** is essentially synonymous with a simple hysterectomy in which the entire uterus and cervix are removed vaginally or abdominally. The adjacent supporting ligaments and vagina remain intact. This procedure may be used for benign conditions, such as fibroids. Extrafascial hysterectomy is also the procedure of choice following the administration of pelvic radiation because it allows removal of the uterus and cervix with minimal cutting damage to radiated tissue. The associated complications are low and include common surgical risks such as bleeding and infection.

In a **modified radical hysterectomy**, a small portion of the upper vagina and the inner third of the parametria (the space containing the uterosacral and cardinal ligaments) are removed along with the entire uterus and cervix. The ureters are partially dissected out of the uterosacral ligaments along with the bladder and the rectum. The higher complication rate is due to the increased potential for blood loss, ureteral injury, and postoperative bladder dysfunction. Patients commonly experience a more lengthy postoperative recovery period characterized by the need for either an indwelling Foley or suprapubic catheter until normal voiding patterns are reestablished. Some patients may be required to perform self-catheterization as a result of continued bladder dysfunction.

In a **radical hysterectomy**, the upper 3 cm of the vagina and most of the parametria are removed along with the entire uterus and cervix. The ureters are completely dissected out of the uterosacral ligaments. The bladder and rectum must be dissected further from the supporting tissue than for the modified radical hysterectomy. The complication rate is approximately 5%. Possible complications include infection, blood loss, ureteral injury, chronic bladder or rectal dysfunction, fistula formation (from ureter, bladder, or rectum), small bowel obstruction, and nerve injury. As with the modified radical hysterectomy, patients should expect the need for an indwelling Foley or suprapubic catheter for 1–4 weeks after surgery. In addition, chronic problems such as urinary frequency or incontinence, change in bowel elimination patterns, and pain or hypersensation associated with femoral-genital nerve disruption may be encountered.

Lymph node dissection during hysterectomy is the removal of the regional pelvic lymph nodes. This procedure is performed in patients with a diagnosis of cancer as a method of checking for cancer spread. It is frequently combined with the more radical hysterectomy procedures. Increased complications may be seen with lymph node dissection becauase the procedure lengthens operative time. Potential postoperative complications include lymphocyst formation and lower extremity edema.

Salpingo-oophorectomy (removal of the Fallopian tubes and ovaries) at the time of hysterectomy depends on the age of the patient and prior treatments. Women over the age of 45, who are approaching menopause, may choose to have the ovaries removed at the time of hysterectomy. For women with nonfunctioning ovaries, such as those who are postmenopausal or have received prior pelvic radiation therapy, removal of the ovaries is often recommended as a means of reducing future risk of ovarian cancer. The induction of surgical menopause in the pre- or perimenopausal patient results in an abrupt reduction of circulating estrogen, causing an acute vasomotor response. Depending on the diagnosis, initiation of estrogen replacement may be recommended for such patients.

11. What is a pelvic exenteration? When is it used?

Pelvic exenteration is a radical surgical procedure that involves the removal of the uterus (if it is still present), vagina, parametria, bladder (in a total or anterior exenteration), and rectum (in a total or posterior exenteration). The type of exenterative procedure—anterior, posterior, or total—is determined by the location of the cancer in the pelvis. The exenteration is followed by reconstructive procedures that include formation of a neovagina (with skin grafts or flaps), a urinary drainage system (either a conduit or continent pouch) fashioned from bowel, and either a colostomy or reanastomosis of the lower rectum to the sigmoid colon.

The most common use of pelvic exenteration is for cervical cancer that recurs in the central pelvis after radiation therapy. It also may be used for recurrent vaginal or endometrial cancer as well as for primary treatment of some extensive pelvic cancers. The rationale for complete and radical removal of tissues and organs in the pelvis after radiation therapy, as opposed to simple local excision, is based on the circulatory compromise and poor healing properties of radiated tissue, and to achieve free margins around the tumor. Once tissue has been radiated, it is less likely to heal normally. This compromise further increases the risk of infection, abscess, and fistula formation requiring ongoing intervention and corrective procedures. The intent of an exenterative procedure is curative. It should not be performed for palliation because of the high morbidity rate. For this reason, evidence of disease outside the central pelvis is a contraindication for exenteration.

Patients undergoing pelvic exenteration require intensive nursing care in the postoperative period. Patients may be hemodynamically unstable because of the length of the surgical procedure, blood loss, and fluid shifts. Infection and possible sepsis are concurrent concerns, along with early signs of failure of reconstructive procedures. Once the patient has stabilized, the process of patient teaching and adjustment to variations in elimination becomes the focus of nursing intervention. Overall, such patients represent a challenge to the nurse's technical, rehabilitative, supportive, and caring skills.

12. Why are radiation implants used in the treatment of cervical cancer?

The successful use of radiation therapy for the treatment of cancer depends, in part, on the ability to deliver an adequate dose of radiation to the source of the cancer. Tissue tolerance of the effects of radiation varies throughout the body. Continued administration of radiation beyond the known level of tolerance may result in permanent damage to the tissue. The vagina and cervix are relatively radiation-resistant compared with the surrounding bowel and bladder. Higher doses of radiation therapy, therefore, may be used to deliver a curative dose to the cervix. The usual radiation treatment plan for cervical cancer is biphasic. Approximately 5 weeks of external beam radiation therapy is administered to the pelvis to shrink the tumor and treat the regional lymph nodes. This is followed by brachytherapy, which is the placement of an intracavitary radiation source kept in place by a holder, such as a tandem and ovoid device, vaginal cylinder, or interstitial template. When loaded with the radioactive source, these devices deliver additional high doses of radiation to the vagina, cervix, and adjacent parametrial tissue. During the time that the implanted radiation source is in place, the uterus insulates the small bowel from the higher doses of radiation. In addition, packing placed into the vagina pushes the bladder and the rectum further away from the implanted radiation source. Thus, the cervix and vagina receive at least twice the dose of radiation that could be delivered if only external radiation were used.

13. What nursing care should be provided to a patient receiving a radiation implant?

The nursing care of patients receiving intracavitary radiation therapy, or brachytherapy, for gynecologic malignancies should focus on the safe delivery of the treatment and the recognition and prevention of complications. The most common devices used to deliver intracavitary radiation in gynecologic cancer are tandem and ovoids, vaginal cylinder, and interstitial afterload needles (see question 12). After placement of one of these hardware devices in the operating room, adequate recovery from anesthesia, and final planning in the radiation oncology department, the patient returns to her assigned room. Before loading the radioactive sources in the hardware, the nurse should have adequate time to perform a thorough postoperative assessment of the patient, review the postoperative orders, inform the patient of restrictions on activity, and prepare the patient for the loading procedure. The nurse should expect the patient to be on strict bedrest with minimal side-to-side turning to prevent dislodging the hardware. The head of the bed may be elevated no more than 30° to prevent perforation from the tandem or interstitial afterload needles. A Foley catheter to gravity drainage is used to eliminate use of the bedpan for urination. Complete bowel rest is desired to prevent hardware dislodgement. Patients are given a low residue diet along with Lomotil and/or opioid pain medications around the clock to promote constipation and discourage defecation.

Intravenous fluids may be administered until the patient has recovered from nausea due to anesthesia. Prophylaxis for deep vein thrombosis is initiated through the use of antiembolism or intermittent inflation stockings. Subcutaneous heparin may be used. Patients should be encouraged to use an incentive spirometer hourly during the day to promote adequate lung expansion and to prevent atelectasis. A patient-controlled analgesia (PCA) pump or epidural analgesia catheter may be used to prevent discomfort from the hardware placement. Vital signs should be assessed every 4 hours, and intake and output should be measured during every shift to monitor subtle changes in the patient's status. Assessment of the patient every shift is a key nursing function. Specific attention should be given to signs and symptoms of: (1) embolic episodes secondary to a diagnosis of pelvic malignancy, bedrest, and postoperative state; (2) perforation of the uterus by the tandem or bowel by the interstitial needles; (3) sepsis from the introduction of a foreign object (tandem or interstitial needle) through the necrotic tumor mass; and (4) dislodgement of the hardware through activity, bowel function, or inadvertent shifting of the device.

In performing these activities, the nurse must be organized and efficient so that minimal time is spent at the bedside after the radiation source has been placed. As a result, routine care activities, such as bathing, oral hygiene, and changing linen, are severely restricted. Whenever possible, the nurse should increase the distance from the source of radiation. Increasing the distance from the source of radiation decreases the amount or concentration of radiation that reaches a specific area. Lead shields may be placed around the patient's bed and/or just inside the entrance to the room as a protective device intended to absorb emitted radiation. Staff are expected to position themselves behind a shield when inside the room to minimize their exposure to radiation.

Shields may be impractical, however, when the patient requires direct care. Lead aprons do not afford additional protection from the gamma rays of this type of radiation; therefore, their use is not advocated. The nursing care of patients with radiation implants represents a challenge to all staff members. A coordinated team effort is required to ensure that the principles of time, distance, and shielding are followed without compromising the patient's physical and emotional care needs.

14. Are any screening studies useful in detecting ovarian cancer or monitoring response to treatment?

Unfortunately, no reliable tests are available for screening asymptomatic women for ovarian cancer. Although a combination of bimanual pelvic examination, transvaginal ultrasound, and CA-125 assay has been suggested by some, little evidence supports the effectiveness of this triad in an asymptomatic population. Bimanual pelvic examination may not alert the practitioner to the presence of an abnormality, particularly if the cancer is in an early stage or if the body habitus of the patient prevents optimal examination. Transvaginal ultrasound is helpful in defining the characteristics of an enlarged ovary but, like many radiographic studies, has limited predictive value.

Although serum tumor marker CA-125 is useful for monitoring treatment response, it lacks specificity for distinguishing ovarian cancer from various benign and malignant conditions. CA-125 tumor marker is elevated in approximately 80% of patients with ovarian cancer. The degree of elevation varies, and the actual CA-125 level may not be a direct reflection of the amount of tumor present. If the CA-125 is elevated when ovarian cancer is diagnosed, it is considered useful as a monitor of response to treatment and as an early indicator of cancer recurrence. Under these circumstances, the CA-125 level may be obtained monthly during treatment and every few months during follow-up after remission is achieved. Although the return of the CA-125 to normal levels early in the course of chemotherapy treatment may be considered a favorable prognostic indicator, it is not an indication of cure. Approximately one-half of the women with ovarian cancer who have a normal CA-125 after initial debulking surgery and chemotherapy have residual cancer if a second-look operation is performed. Residual cancer is frequently microscopic or of small volume; it may not be visible on radiographic studies or palpable on bimanual pelvic examination.

Quick Facts—Ovarian Cancer

Incidence	4% of new cancers in women annually. In 1997: 26,800 estimated new cases.
Mortality	5% of cancer deaths in women annually. In 1997: 14,200 estimated deaths.
Risk factors	**Age**—risk increases with age until age 70
	Family history of ovarian cancer, breast-ovarian cancer, or breast-ovarian-endometrial-colon cancer
	Incessant ovulation—conditions of uninterrupted ovulation such as nulliparity or infertility
	Northern European ancestry
	Industrialization/higher socioeconomic class
	Associations with perineal talc use, high dietary fat, and excessive coffee and alcohol consumption have been suggested but are considered weak
Histology	Adenocarcinoma of mucinous or serous papillary origin most common; other types include endometrioid, clear cell, Brenner, undifferentiated, and sarcomas.
Symptoms	**Abdominal distention and bloating** are most common; other symptoms include increased abdominal girth, nonspecific changes in GI function, increased flatus, weight gain, and pain.
Staging	Stage I — Limited to ovaries
	IA — One ovary
	IB — Two ovaries
	IC — Ruptured capsule, surface tumor, positive cytology

Table continued on following page.

Quick Facts—Ovarian Cancer (Continued)

Staging	Stage II	Pelvic extension
(cont.)	IIA	Uterus or tubes
	IIB	Other tissues
	IIC	Ruptured capsule, surface tumor, positive cytology
	Stage III	Abdominal or nodal metastasis
	IIIA	Microscopic seeding of adominal-peritoneal surfaces
	IIIB	Abdominal-peritoneal implants < 2 cm, negative nodes
	IIIC	Abdominal-peritoneal implants > 2 cm and/or positive nodes
	Stage IV	Distant metastasis; includes pleural effusion with positive cytology, parenchymal liver metastases
Treatment		Staging laparotomy with tumor debulking (< 1 cm residual disease considered optimal)
		Chemotherapy (six cycles of paclitaxel/platinum-based preferred) for all stages except stage IA and IB with well or moderately well differentiated cancer

15. How does heredity contribute to increased risk for the development of ovarian cancer?

Several familial cancer syndromes contribute to increased risk for the development of ovarian cancer. All are autosomal dominant conditions, but they are relatively rare. The presence of ovarian cancer in two first-degree relatives (mother, sister) may increase the risk for developing ovarian cancer to as much as 50%. In addition, women with family histories of both breast - ovarian cancers and breast-ovarian-endometrial-colon cancers have a higher incidence of ovarian cancer. Despite these positive associations, familial ovarian cancer accounts for less than 5% of all cases of ovarian cancer.

16. Can anything protect women from developing ovarian cancer?

Oral contraceptive pills (OCPs) significantly reduce the risk of ovarian cancer by as much as 50% in women who use them consistently for 5 years. This reduction is attributed to the ovulatory suppression of OCPs. Protection is also obtained from breastfeeding and one or more full-term pregnancies because both situations suppress ovulation. Tubal ligation also gives some protection, although the reasons are unclear.

17. A patient with ovarian cancer is told by her gynecologic oncologist that all visible cancer was removed at the time of her debulking surgery, but she still needs chemotherapy. Why?

Although the removal of all visible tumor markedly improves prognosis, microscopic tumor is still present because of the spread patterns of ovarian cancer. Epithelial ovarian cancer, the most common type of ovarian cancer, arises from the surface of the ovary. The cancer cells can exfoliate and spread throughout the abdominal cavity early in the course of disease. This often results in peritoneal seeding of tumor, which may form microscopic implants of tumor on the peritoneal surfaces. Without the administration of chemotherapy, these implants have the potential to grow and reform bulky tumor. The patient should be informed by her physician that chemotherapy is needed to treat the microscopic tumor.

18. What is a second-look laparotomy? When should a nurse expect a patient to undergo this procedure?

A second-look laparotomy is an exploratory procedure performed after completion of the initial chemotherapy regimen for ovarian cancer. It is initiated when there is no evidence of cancer on physical examination or radiographic evaluation, such as CAT scan. The purpose is to determine whether residual cancer is present. Residual cancer is possible in 50% of women who have undergone debulking surgery and chemotherapy despite the lack of physical evidence of disease. During the procedure, the abdominal and pelvic cavities are thoroughly explored. Visible tumor is removed when possible, and multiple biopsies of the peritoneal surfaces are obtained.

Although it was considered standard practice for many years, second-look laparotomy is no longer routine. Gynecologic oncologists moved to abandon this procedure when it became apparent that as many as 50% of the women with negative second-look surgeries still developed recurrence of disease at a future time. Thus, survival was not positively affected by automatic use of the procedure, and patients were exposed to the increased morbidity and mortality inherent in additional surgery. The procedure occasionally may be used when a patient is enrolled in a study protocol examining the efficacy of existing or new treatment regimens.

19. A patient asks what a borderline ovarian cancer is. How should the nurse explain this type of cancer?

Borderline ovarian cancer is also known as ovarian adenocarcinoma of low malignant potential. These terms can be confusing to both patients and nurses. Pathologically, the cells resemble those of an ovarian carcinoma, but they are not invasive. Patients generally present with symptoms similar to ovarian carcinoma, such as increased abdominal girth, ascites, and enlarged ovaries. These tumors usually occur in the fourth and fifth decades of life, are more commonly confined to the ovary at diagnosis, and are associated with a good prognosis. When they have spread beyond the ovary, which is uncommon, the primary treatment is surgical debulking. In the event that they recur, surgical debulking may be repeated. Chemotherapy is rarely used because few data indicate that it improves survival.

Patients should be informed that borderline ovarian cancer can be extensive and recurrent, but it is treated primarily with surgical excision and has a much more favorable prognosis than epithelial ovarian cancers.

20. How are estrogen and estrogen replacement therapy related to endometrial cancer?

The association of estrogen and endometrial cancer should be known by all nurses caring for women, regardless of practice setting. Endometrial cancer depends on the unopposed supply of estrogen from endogenous (within the body) and exogenous (outside the body) sources. During the reproductive years, neuroendocrine changes occur each month to promote regularity of the menstrual cycle. Cyclical estrogen production in the form of estradiol from the ovary promotes proliferation of the lining of the uterus in anticipation of implantation of a fertilized ovum. After ovulation, secretion of estradiol continues, and progesterone is initiated to maintain the endometrial lining. In the absence of pregnancy and the associated appearance of human chorionic gonadotropin (HCG) from the developing placenta, the level of progesterone falls dramatically. The drop in progesterone causes the organized shedding of the endometrial lining within 1–2 days.

Estrogen production that is not challenged or opposed by progesterone causes ongoing proliferation of the endometrial lining. Continued growth of the endometrial lining favors the development of atypical cells and cancer. When a woman has either increased endogenous sources of estrogen, such as occurs with anovulation and obesity, or increased exogenous sources of estrogen, such as estrogen replacement without progesterone, the associated risk of developing endometrial cancer is greater. Any woman with an intact uterus who is taking estrogen replacement also should receive progesterone either cyclically or daily to counteract the proliferative effects of estrogen on the lining of the uterus. Women who have had the uterus removed do not require progesterone therapy when estrogen replacement is initiated.

Quick Facts—Endometrial Cancer

Incidence	6% of new cancer cases in women annually. In 1997: 34,900 estimated new cases.
Mortality	2% of cancer deaths in women annually. In 1997: 6,000 estimated deaths.
Risk factors	**Unopposed exogenous estrogen**—progesterone "protective"
	Nulliparity, infertility, anovulation
	Late menopause—after age 52
	Obesity—increased levels of endogenous estrogen
	Diabetes mellitus, hypertension
	Family history—breast-ovarian-endometrial-colon cancer
	Complex atypical hyperplasia—thickened endometrium with cytologic atypia of glands

Table continued on following page.

Quick Facts—Endometrial Cancer (Continued)

Histology	Endometrial adenocarcinoma most common; other types include adenosquamous, squamous, mucinous, serous papillary, clear cell, and undifferentiated.
Symptoms	**Abnormal uterine bleeding** in postmenopausal woman occurs in 80% of patients; **Pap smear abnormality,** presence of endometrial cells suspicious; symptoms of uterine enlargement or pelvic pressure may be signs of advanced disease.

Staging	Stage I	Confined to corpus
	IA	Tumor limited to endometrium
	IB	Tumor invades < half of myometrium
	IC	Tumor invades > half of myometrium
	Stage II	Extends to cervix
	IIA	Involves endocervical glands
	IIB	Invades cervical stroma
	Stage III	Involves adjacent structures
	IIIA	Invades uterine serosa, adnexae, or peritoneal cytology positive
	IIIB	Vaginal extension
	IIIC	Positive pelvic or paraaortic lymph nodes
	Stage IV	Distant metastases, including intraabdominal or inguinal lymph nodes, lungs

Treatment	Total abdominal hysterectomy with bilateral salpingo-oophorectomy and lymph node sampling considered gold standard; adjuvant radiation therapy and/or chemotherapy generally recommended for stage IC and above, poorly differentiated tumor, or aggressive histology (i.e., clear cell, serous papillary).

21. How should the nurse respond to the woman who asks if obesity increases the risk for endometrial cancer?

Associations among obesity, excess estrogen levels and endometrial cancer have been documented. As discussed earlier, sources of estrogen may be either endogenous or exogenous. Obese women in general have higher levels of endogenous estrogen because of two mechanisms. First, the adrenal cortex produces androstenedione, which is converted to estrogen by adipose tissue. Consequently, excessive fat tissue leads to excessive production of estrogen. Second, obesity depresses the level of sex hormone–binding globulin (SHBG) and thus leads to higher free, or unbound, levels of estrogen. Unbound estrogen is the hormonally active form. The nurse should explain that obese women face a higher risk for the development of endometrial cancer because increased levels of endogenous estrogen promote proliferation of the uterine lining.

22. A patient who has had a hysterectomy for endometrial cancer is told by her physician that the final surgical pathology report will determine the need for additional radiation or chemotherapy. How may the nurse clarify this statement?

Patients often require clarification when they are informed by their surgeon that the cancer was totally contained in the uterus at the time of the hysterectomy, but they may need additional treatment with radiation or chemotherapy. Several pathologic determinations are required to ascertain the need for adjunctive treatment, including histology, tumor grade, myometrial invasion, cytologic washings, and lymph node status. Adenocarcinomas are the most common histologic types of endometrial cancer. Additional cell types, such as clear cell or papillary serous carcinomas, are considered more aggressive cancers and require adjuvant treatment. Tumor grade is applied to all histologic types and is stated in degree of differentiation—well, moderately, or poorly differentiated cells. A less favorable prognosis is associated with tumors that are moderately to poorly differentiated; thus, adjuvant treatment is desirable.

The extent of myometrial invasion is another important predictor in determining the need for additional treatment after surgery for endometrial cancer. Myometrial invasion refers to the depth of cancer cell penetration into the wall of the uterus. The pathologist provides this information in the form of a measurement on the final pathology report. Myometrial invasion that is less than one-half the thickness of the uterine wall is less likely to have spread beyond the uterus than are tumors that have invaded to the outer half. Such patients require treatment with radiation or chemotherapy. Cytologic washings from the abdominal-peritoneal cavity collected at the beginning of the surgery are checked for the presence of malignant cells that may have disseminated through either the fallopian tubes or the uterine wall before removal of the uterus. Lymph nodes sampled at the time of the surgical procedure are also examined microscopically for evidence of disease. Positive findings in either of these samples require additional treatment, usually chemotherapy or radiation, due to disease spread outside the uterus. Despite the appearance of "normal" tissue at the time of gross visual inspection, any of these pathologic findings may alter the treatment recommendations. The nurse needs to be aware that the treatment plan cannot be determined until the final pathology report has been received so that he or she can offer emotional support to the patient during this time of uncertainty.

23. What resources offer support, counseling, education, and information for women with ovarian cancer?
- National Ovarian Cancer Coalition
  888-OVA-RIAN
- Gilda Radner Familial Ovarian Cancer Registry
  800-OVA-RIAN
  Services include general counseling, data collection registry on the link between heredity and ovarian cancer, support groups, and assistance with genetic screening.

BIBLIOGRAPHY

1. American College of Obstetricians and Gynecologists: Classification and staging of gynecologic malignancies. ACOG Tech Bull No 155:1–6, 1991.
2. Berek JS, Hacker NF (eds): Practical Gynecologic Oncology, 2nd ed. Baltimore, Williams & Wilkins, 1994.
3. DeStefano MS, Bertin-Matson K: Gynecologic cancers. In McCorkle R, Grant M, Frank-Stromberg M, Baird SB (eds): Cancer Nursing: A Comprehensive Textbook, 2nd ed. Philadelphia, W.B. Saunders, 1996, pp 698–728.
4. Dow KH, Hilderley LJ (eds): Nursing Care in Radiation Oncology, Philadelphia, W.B. Saunders, 1992.
5. Markman M, Hoskins W (eds): Cancer of the Ovary. New York, Raven Press, 1993.
6. Parker SL, Tong T, Bolden S, Wingo PA: Cancer statistics, 1997. CA Cancer J Clin 47:5–27, 1997.
7. Shingleton HM, Orr JW: Cancer of the Cervix, 2nd ed. Philadelphia, J.B. Lippincott, 1995.

27. CANCERS OF THE HEAD AND NECK

R. Lee Jennings, MD

Quick Facts—Head and Neck Cancer

Incidence	5–10% of new cases annually; 40,000 new cases in the United States each year
Mortality	2.2% of cancer deaths; one-third of patients die from their disease
Risk factors	Advancing age (more common after age 50)
	Male gender (male-to-female ratio of 3:1)
	Tobacco use (greatest risk factor)
	Alcohol
	Smokeless tobacco (becoming more important)
	Cigars, pipe, marijuana
	Epstein-Barr (EBV) virus (associated with nasopharyngeal cancer)
	Industrial exposure to wood dust, leather, metal (nickel)
	Asbestos
Histology	**Squamous cell carcinomas** (approximately 95% of all head and neck cancer)
	Salivary gland primaries
	Sarcomas (rare)
Symptoms	Pain, tenderness Chronic dysphagia
	Ulceration Unilateral sinusitis
	Neck mass Unilateral nasal obstruction
	Submucosal mass Persistent hoarseness or change in voice
	Unilateral ear pain, not explained by infection
Staging	Tumor, node, metastasis (TNM) system

Primary tumor (T) for lip and oral cavity

T1	Greatest diameter of primary tumor < 2 cm
T2	Greatest diameter of primary tumor 2–4 cm
T3	Greatest diameter of primary tumor > 4 cm
T4	Lip—invades adjacent structures such as bone, tongue
	Oral—invades adjacent structures such as deep muscles of tongue, bone, maxillary sinus

Primary tumor (T) for salivary glands

T1	Greatest dimension of tumor ≤ 2 cm
T2	Greatest dimension of tumor > 2 but ≤ 4 cm
T3	Greatest dimension of tumor > 4 but ≤ 6 cm
T4	Greatest dimension of tumor > 6 cm

All T stages are subdivided into (a) no local extension or (b) local extension.
Local extension is defined as clinical or macroscopic evidence of skin, nerve, or bone.

Cervical node involvement (N), oral cavity and salivary glands

N0	No nodal involvement
N1	Single clinically positive ipsilateral node < 3 cm
N2a	Single clinically positive ipsilateral node 3–6 cm
N2b	Multiple clinically positive ipsilateral nodes, none > 6 cm
N3a	Clinically positive ipsilateral node(s), one > 6 cm
N3b	Bilateral clinically positive nodes
N3c	Contralateral clinically positive node(s) only

Distant metastasis (M)

M0	No known distant metastasis
M1	Distant metastasis present

Table continued on following page.

Quick Facts—Head and Neck Cancer (Continued)

Stage grouping for cancer of lip, oral cavity, and pharynx
Stage I	T1, N0, M0
Stage II	T2–T4, N0, M0
Stage III	Any T, N1–N3, M0
Stage IV	Any T, Any N, M1

Stage grouping for salivary glands
Stage I	T1a or T2a, N0, M0
Stage II	T1b, T2b, or T3a, N0, M0
Stage III	T3b or T4a, N0, M0
Stage IV	T4b, Any N, M0
	Any T, N2 or N3, M0
	Any T, Any N, M1

1. Which sites are usually included in discussions of cancers of the head and neck?

All cancers arising in the upper food and airway passages (upper aerodigestive tract) are included for reporting purposes: lips, oral cavity, pharynx (oropharynx, nasopharynx, hypopharynx), nasal cavity, and paranasal sinuses. Also included are the major and minor salivary glands and the thyroid gland (see chapter on endocrine tumors). Subdivisions of the major sites include buccal mucosa, gingiva, palate, tongue, tonsil, pyriform sinus, and larynx. Each subsite is important because prognosis, treatment, and morbidity of treatment may change dramatically from subsite to subsite. Cancers arising in the skin (melanoma, basal cell and squamous cell carcinoma, skin adnexal tumors) and lymphomas are excluded for reporting purposes but are important in any discussion of malignancies of the head and neck (see chapter on melanoma).

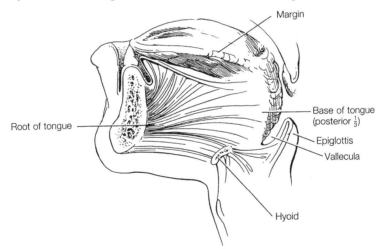

Posterior oral anatomy. (From Jennings RL: Tumors of the head and neck. In Ritchie WP Jr, Steele G Jr, Dean RH (eds): General Surgery. Philadelphia, Lippincott-Raven, 1995, p 35, with permission.)

2. What are the presenting symptoms of head and neck cancer?

Presenting complaints are quite varied because of the complex anatomy of the region and the variety of functions represented in the head and neck. Significant changes in appearance, sight, smell, swallowing, and speech may be early symptoms of cancer. Ulceration and pain at the primary site and referred pain also may be early symptoms. Often the patient consults the dentist first because of one of these symptoms. Pharyngeal primary tumors are the most subtle and varied in presentation and much harder for the patient to detect because these areas are not easily visible.

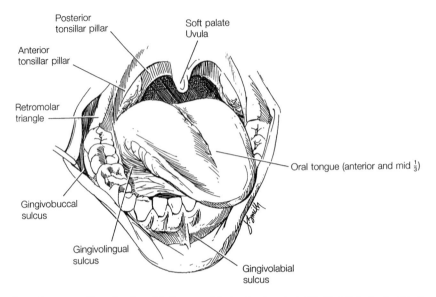

Anterior oral anatomy. (From Jennings RL: Tumors of the head and neck. In Ritchie WP Jr, Steele G Jr, Dean RH (eds): General Surgery. Philadelphia, Lippincott-Raven, 1995, p 35, with permission.)

Symptoms According to Site of Primary Tumor

SITE	PRESENTING SYMPTOMS	LATE SYMPTOMS
Lip	Sore that does not heal	Large ulceration, mass
Oral cavity	See below	Pain, ulceration, foul breath, loss of function; see below
Buccal mucosa	Ulceration or mass, acidic drinks may cause burning	Pain, mass in cheek
Gingiva	Ulceration, dentures do not fit	Pain, loose teeth, trismus (lock jaw)
Oral tongue	Ulceration, mild pain, mass	Decreased range of motion, pain, dysphagia, malnutrition, ear pain
Hard palate	Ulcer or mass	Ulceration, loose teeth
Floor of mouth	Ulceration	Pain, ear pain, mass, invasion of tongue with same symptoms
Pharynx		
Nasopharynx	Nasal stuffiness, nosebleed	Bleeding, nasal obstruction, cranial nerve paralysis, pain, vision changes
Oropharynx	Sore throat, usually unilateral and persistent	Dysphagia pain, difficulty in swallowing, malnutrition, muffled voice
Base of tongue (posterior one-third)	Same	Same
Tonsil, soft palate	Ulceration or mass	Mass or large ulceration, dysphagia
Pharyngoesophageal junction	Possible dysphagia	Same
Hypopharynx (pyriform sinus)	Same	Dysphagia, pain, aspiration, voice change
Larynx	Hoarseness	Severe hoarseness, airway obstruction, aspiration

Table continued on following page.

Symptoms According to Site of Primary Tumor (Continued)

SITE	PRESENTING SYMPTOMS	LATE SYMPTOMS
Salivary gland, major and minor	Preauricular or submandibular mass, mucosa-covered mass in oral cavity (no ulceration)	Enlarged mass, ulceration in oral cavity (minor salivary gland, neck masses, facial nerve paralysis with parotid, mandibular invasion with submandibular gland cancers
Thyroid gland	Thyroid mass	Neck masses, vocal cord paralysis, dysphagia, enlarged mass

3. What are the risk factors for head and neck malignancies?

Malignancies arising on the **skin**, including the lips, are usually caused by prolonged, excessive exposure to sun. **Lip** cancer is more common in outdoor workers, including farmers, construction workers, oil-field workers, and recreation workers (e.g., ski instructors, life guards). Light skin and red or blonde hair are predisposing factors. Tobacco is the most significant factor in cancers of the **oral cavity, pharynx**, and **larynx**. Ninety percent of patients with primaries in these areas have a smoking history. Smokeless tobacco also plays a part but is not as significant as smoking. Alcohol consumption is also linked with these cancers. Heavy alcohol use is common; a high percentage of patients present with cirrhosis of the liver or consumption levels high enough to place them in danger of delirium tremens on sudden withdrawal. Such patients have a lower survival rate and a higher rate of second primaries than nonusers. **Nasopharyngeal** cancers have a more complicated etiology; they are common among Cantonese Chinese and rare among Caucasians. There is a weak link to history of chronic sinusitis and exposure to smoke from cooking fires but a strong link to infection with the Epstein-Barr virus. Cancer of the **turbinates** and **paranasal sinuses** also has a complex etiology. Industrial exposures are significant. However, most patients present without a history of exposure to known environmental carcinogens. No cause has been found for **salivary** cancers. The cause of **thyroid** cancer is mostly unknown. Convincing evidence suggests that radiation exposure, especially in children and adolescents, increases the risk for thyroid cancer. In addition, about one-third of medullary carcinomas of the thyroid (carcinomas arising in the calcitonin-secreting cells) are familial.

4. Describe the initial examination of a patient with a head or neck primary tumor, with an emphasis on clinical staging and treatment planning.

The initial examination should start with a complete history and physical examination. Pay attention to the time that symptoms have been present. Document tobacco and alcohol use. The combination of heavy tobacco and alcohol use may make it impossible for the patient to tolerate radiation therapy to oral mucous membranes. Document weight loss so that nutritional repair can start as the work-up continues. Documenting and understanding the patient's psychosocial history may determine whether the patient accepts treatment and whether rehabilitation is successful. Planning for rehabilitation starts with the initial history.

Physical examination of the oral cavity, pharynx, and larynx requires visualization of all surfaces. The oral cavity, base of tongue, and tonsils are palpated with a gloved finger. The nasopharynx, hypopharynx, and larynx are visualized with a mirror or fiberoptic laryngoscope. All findings are described and documented on a diagram for staging and treatment planning.

5. What instruments are needed for a head and neck examination?

Instruments required for clinical head and neck examination are simple, fairly inexpensive, and easily available in the head and neck surgeon's office but often absent from the hospital unit or outpatient clinic. They include a high-backed chair for the patient and a stool for the examiner. A flashlight is inadequate. Most examiners prefer a headlight to free both hands. Also needed are laryngeal mirrors, a heat source to warm the mirror to prevent fogging, tongue blades, finger cots, local and topical anesthetic, and forceps for biopsy. A fiberoptic laryngoscope may be needed to examine the nasopharynx or for patients with a severe gag reflex. Extensive, complex cancers require several visual examinations and direct palpation to evaluate their extent.

6. How is the suspicious area biopsied?

Diagnosis and staging of any primary site requires a biopsy. Lip, skin, and oral carcinomas are usually biopsied with forceps under local anesthesia at the time of the initial examination. Fine-needle aspiration cytology is helpful in evaluating thyroid and salivary gland masses. Cancers of the pharynx and larynx are examined for staging and biopsy with direct laryngoscopy under general anesthesia. Sinus cancers require general anesthesia for biopsy and staging examination through the nostril or through the anterior wall of the sinus.

7. What diagnostic tests may be ordered?

Selected imaging and laboratory studies are necessary to complete the initial examination, including biochemical survey, complete blood count, urinalysis, and chest roentgenogram for all patients. Selected patients will require computerized tomography or magnetic resonance imaging for oral, pharyngeal, laryngeal, and sinus primaries. Patients with thyroid primaries need radioactive thyroid scans and thyroid ultrasound. Other studies depend on the findings from the history and physical examination (e.g., evaluation for cirrhosis, emphysema, diabetes). More extensive imaging or laboratory evaluation is necessary if any evidence of distant metastasis is found.

8. What types of cancer occur on skin surfaces in the head and neck, including the lip? How are they treated?

Malignant tumors of the skin are the most common cancers requiring surgical care. Over 800,000 skin malignancies are reported each year, along with 2300 deaths. Basal and squamous carcinomas are by far the most numerous, and 85% occur in the head and neck region. Ninety-four percent of recurrent basal cell cancers occur in the head and neck region, with 75% in the central face. The majority of these malignancies are small and are adequately treated by dermatologists and primary care physicians with desiccation and curettage. Biopsy for pathology examination is mandatory. Larger skin cancers, multicentric basal cell cancers, or recurrent skin cancers should be treated with wide excision and pathology confirmation that margins are free of cancer. Wide elliptical excision is usually adequate, but flap reconstruction should be considered if the pathologist reports close or positive margins. Lymph node metastasis is unusual except with large squamous cell skin cancers. Merkel cell cancer and skin appendage cancers are rare but important because nodal metastasis and distant spread are more likely. Wide surgical removal with flap or skin graft reconstruction is necessary, and lymph node dissection may be required, depending on the location of the primary tumor. Melanoma may occur on any skin surface in the head and neck and on mucosal surfaces such as the oral cavity and nasal cavity (see the chapter on malignant melanoma).

9. Name the malignancies that occur in the salivary glands and describe their treatment.

Malignancies may occur in the major (parotid and submandibular) and minor salivary glands. Minor salivary glands are present in all mucosal surfaces in the upper food and airway passages. A mass in one of the major salivary glands has a 20–50% chance of being malignant. A mass covered by intact mucosa in the oral cavity may be a minor salivary tumor; the risk of malignancy is as high as 50%. Complete surgical excision is the treatment of choice, even for biopsy. Most benign tumors of the salivary glands are pleomorphic adenomas (mixed tumors); incomplete excision results in a recurrence rate of 70%.

Treatment of Major Salivary Neoplasms

BENIGN MIXED OR WARTHIN'S TUMOR, NONNEOPLASTIC BENIGN MASSES	T1 OR T2 LOW-GRADE TUMOR MUCOEPIDERMOID OR ACINIC CELL CARCINOMA	T1 OR T2 HIGH-GRADE TUMOR*	T3, N0, OR N+ RECURRENT SALIVARY CANCERS	14
Parotid				
Superficial parotidectomy	Total parotidectomy	Total parotidectomy	Radical parotidectomy	Radical parotidectomy
Preservation of facial nerve	Preservation of facial nerve	Preservation of facial nerve unless involved	Resection of facial nerve	Resection of ear canal, muscle, etc.
	No radiation therapy	No postoperative radiation therapy	Neck dissection if N+	Sacrifice of facial nerve
			Postoperative radiation therapy	Postoperative radiation therapy
Submandibular				
Digastric triangle dissection	Digastric triangle dissection	Digastric triangle dissection	Radical neck dissection	Resection of involved structures
Preserve marginal branch of facial nerve	Preserve marginal branch of facial nerve	Preserve marginal branch of facial nerve unless involved	Removal of marginal branch of facial nerve and lingual nerve as necessary	Radical neck dissection
	No radiation therapy	Neck dissection if N+	Postoperative radiation therapy	Postoperative radiation therapy
		Postoperative radiation therapy		

* Includes malignant mixed, squamous, and poorly differentiated adenocarcinomas and anaplastic and adenoid cysts.

From Jennings RL, Nelson, William R: Tumors of the head and neck. In Ritchie WP Jr, Steele G Jr, Dean RH (eds): General Surgery. Philadelphia, J.B. Lippincott, 1995, with permission.

10. Should surgery be advised for all thyroid masses?

Definitely not. Benign nodular goiter has been calculated to be 500 times more common than thyroid cancer, which makes up only 1% of all malignancies. History and physical examination provide clues that suggest malignancy in a thyroid nodule:

- History of low-dose radiation exposure to thyroid gland
- Risk of malignancy for a new nodule increases with patient age (especially > 40 years)
- Nodule fixation if thyroiditis is excluded
- Rapid growth of a nodule
- Onset of hoarseness
- Palpable cervical lymph nodes
- Solitary thyroid nodule in a male of any age

Surgery is indicated in a patient < 20 years old with a thyroid nodule.

11. What operation is advised when thyroidectomy is necessary for a thyroid nodule?

It is unusual to have a definitive diagnosis of cancer before thyroidectomy. Total thyroid lobectomy on the side of the nodule is the preferred procedure. An attempt at excising the nodule for biopsy is not advised because of the risk of contaminating the surgical field if cancer is found, the greater risk of injury to the recurrent nerve, and the greater difficulty of making a definitive diagnosis from frozen section. A later diagnosis of cancer requires return to surgery to complete the thyroidectomy, again placing the recurrent nerve and parathyroid glands at greater risk. When cancer is identified on frozen section, many surgeons favor total thyroidectomy to allow total thyroid ablation with I^{131} and later radioactive iodine scanning for metastasis. Small (< 2 cm), well-differentiated cancers contained within the thyroid capsule require only total lobectomy. Lymph node dissection for well-differentiated thyroid cancer is necessary only if nodes are clinically involved. Special situations, such as medullary cancer, require total thyroidectomy and node dissection because of a 70% risk of bilateral gland involvement and nodal metastasis. Undifferentiated carcinoma of the thyroid is one of the most malignant of human cancers, but it is rare. Treatment consists of a combination of radical surgery, chemotherapy, and radiation therapy, but it is rarely successful.

12. Describe the types of lip cancer and their treatment.

Most lip malignancies involve the lower lip and are squamous in type. Basal cell carcinoma usually involves the upper lip. The remaining lip malignancies are minor salivary gland cancers treated with wide excision, including the mucosal surface. Postoperative radiation therapy is used for advanced or high-grade malignancies. Basal and squamous cancers are treated with either radiation therapy or surgery; cure rates are the same. Locally advanced cancers or node-positive cancers may require a combination of radiation and surgery. Surgical procedures are usually done in one stage; cancers requiring removal of up to one-third of the lip width are treated with a V excision and primary repair. Cosmetic and functional results are excellent. Upper neck dissection is necessary for the node-positive neck cancers and advanced cancers directly invading skin and bone. Radiation therapy has the disadvantage of requiring 5 weeks of daily treatment, further damaging surrounding skin already damaged by sun exposure, and making surgical care very difficult when the same primary tumor recurs or new skin cancers occur in the same area. Basal cell cancers of the upper lip require special attention; they are more likely to reoccur locally, perhaps because wide excision and cosmetic repair are more difficult.

13. Describe the remaining oral and pharyngeal cancers and their treatment.

Well over 90% of malignancies involving the mucosal surfaces are squamous cell. The remainder are minor salivary gland tumors (see question 9). Small (T1) squamous cancers located in the anterior oral cavity may be treated with radiation therapy or surgery with equal cure rates. Many believe that early cancers with minimal risk of nodal spread are better treated with surgery because it is quickly accomplished, morbidity is usually minimal, and the risk of xerostomia (dryness) is avoided, along with the risk of dental caries and bone loss (osteoradionecrosis).

Many T2 and most more advanced squamous carcinomas are best treated with a combination of surgery and radiation therapy. It is important for both radiation therapist and surgeon to see the patient before treatment begins for treatment planning. When combined treatment is chosen, most surgeons prefer that the surgical procedure be done first if the primary tumor is sufficiently well defined to allow complete excision with free margins. Surgery also may be scheduled between 3 and 7 weeks after completion of radiation therapy. Surgery sooner than 3 weeks usually results in excessive bleeding because of inflammation, and after 7–8 weeks excessive fibrosis increases the risk of poor wound healing.

Advanced cancers of the posterior oral cavity and oropharynx treated with surgery require repair techniques, usually involving flaps, to replace the large amount of functional tissue removed. Repair techniques improve functional and cosmetic results. Microvascular free-flap procedures have allowed bone and soft tissue from distant sites to be used to repair mandible, tonsil, and tongue defects. Nasopharyngeal primary tumors are usually treated with radiation therapy; skull base surgical techniques are reserved for radiation failures and primary tumors with local extension that are not treatable with radiation therapy for cure. Hypopharyngeal and laryngeal cancers are usually treated with primary radiation therapy for malignancies diagnosed early; a combination of surgery and radiation is reserved for advanced-stage primary tumors. Surgical salvage is necessary for radiation failures and usually results in partial or total laryngectomy.

14. Is the postoperative nursing care of patients with head and neck cancer different from the care of other surgical patients?

In 1997 approximately 40,000 cases of cancer of the oral cavity, pharynx, and larynx were reported in the United States. Many patients are treated on an outpatient basis, making it difficult for inpatient nurses to gain adequate experience in caring for patients with head and neck cancer. Major areas of care include the following:

- Patients require assurance of an adequate airway. Many hospitalized patients have a tracheotomy, which should be sutured in place or securely tied at all times. A dislodged tracheotomy may result in hypoxia or death. Attention to secretion clearance is mandatory for airway maintenance, patient comfort, and wound healing. Patients should be taught self-care techniques for airway clearance and wound care as soon as possible after surgery.
- Self-care is particularly desirable for patients with head and neck cancer. The confidence that results from airway assurance, secretion clearance, and wound care allows the patient to gain control of a terrifying situation.
- Speech and swallowing rehabilitation by a speech pathologist is invaluable; it adds to the sense of control and allows recovery to begin.
- Many surgical patients now receive total parenteral nutrition to repair nutritional defects. This method provides excellent short-term support, but it is not the optimal method of feeding for patients with head and neck cancer. Enteral feeding should start as soon as possible. Oral feedings usually start as soon as suture lines allow. Nasogastric or transcutaneous gastric feeding tubes allow patients with long-term swallowing problems to be discharged while outpatient rehabilitation continues.
- The postoperative role of the nurse, speech pathologist, and surgeon changes from caregiver to coach and cheerleader as discharge approaches.

15. What side effects are associated with radiation therapy?

If radiation therapy precedes surgery, take care that the patient's nutritional status is monitored to prevent malnutrition. Prophylactic dental care is necessary because of the risk of radionecrosis and mandibular bone loss. With preoperative radiation therapy, treatment is usually stopped at around 5500 cGy because most patients develop mucositis at this level. Redness and dysphagia usually disappear by 3 weeks. When radiation therapy is the only method of treatment, additional dosage to the primary site is necessary. This boost may be given with external beam or implant techniques. Implants are usually performed under general anesthesia and require hospitalization and often tracheotomy until the implants are removed.

16. How do patients with head and neck cancer differ from patients with cancer in other sites?

The head and neck region is unique among the sites requiring care for cancer. The complex interaction of the face, oral cavity, voice, and air passages in personal presentation, food intake, and comfort makes treatment planning highly demanding. Even the smallest cosmetic or functional defect is viewed with concern by the patient and surgeon. The importance of maintaining acceptable cosmetic and functional results must be balanced with the necessity of adequately treating the primary cancer. Primary tumors of the head and neck create functional and cosmetic problems if not adequately treated and controlled. Good palliation is seldom achieved without cure of the primary cancer.

17. When is chemotherapy used in patients with head and neck cancer?

Chemotherapy is usually reserved for patients with metastatic or recurrent disease. Its role in this setting is palliative with the hope of improving quality of life. The chemotherapy agents showing some responses are methotrexate, carboplatin, cisplatin, and 5-fluorouracil with leucovorin and paclitaxel.

18. Does neoadjuvant chemotherapy minimize a radical resection?

Chemotherapy given before surgery has allowed reduction of the extent of surgery in selected cases of advanced larynx cancer. This has not been true in other primary sites, and neoadjuvant treatment in head and neck cancer remains investigational. Evidence suggests that chemotherapy reduces the rate of distant metastasis, but this advantage affects only a small percentage of patients with head and neck cancer.

19. What is the role of chemoprevention?

Chemoprevention using retinoids, including natural vitamin A and synthetic analogs, beta carotene, and vitamin E, has shown some promise in reversing premalignant lesions and preventing second primary tumors.

20. What is a carotid rupture? How common is it?

Carotid rupture is rare because of improved techniques for both radiation therapy and surgery. The carotid artery may become exposed as a result of flap necrosis, fistula formation and associated infection, or recurrent cancer around the artery. The first hint of this complication may be a trickle of blood hours or even days before rupture. The patient must be moved to a bed near the nurse's station. Blood should be typed and cross-matched, intravenous access assured, tracheotomy established, and hemostat placed in the room. If rupture occurs, the nurse should apply firm pressure over the artery with a towel, initiate oxygen and intravenous fluids, and call for blood—as well as help. When rupture occurs in a palliative setting, surgery is usually not needed, but comfort measures, reassurance, and support are appropriate. The process is not painful but may be terrifying.

21. What additional resources are available to assist patients and family with discharge and coping?

The International Association of Laryngectomies is a program established by the American Cancer Society (1-800-ACS-2345) to assist people who have lost their voice to cancer. Support for People with Oral and Head and Neck Cancer (SPOHNC) is a patient-run support group with a nationwide newsletter (e-mail: Spohnc@lxnetcom.com.). Let's Face It (LFI) (360-676-7325) and the National Foundation for Facial Reconstruction (212-263-6656) are nonprofit organizations that help people to cope with facial disfigurement. Services include referrals for patients unable to afford private reconstructive surgical care.

BIBLIOGRAPHY

1. Jennings RL, Nelson, William R: Tumors of the head and neck. In Ritchie WP Jr, Steele G Jr, Dean RH (eds): General Surgery. Philadelphia, J.B. Lippincott, 1995.
2. Parker SL, Tong T, Bolden S, Wingo PA: Cancer statistics, 1997. CA Cancer J Clin 47:5–27, 1997.
3. Strong EW, Spiro RH: Cancer of the oral cavity. In Suen JY, Myers EN (eds): Cancer of the Head and Neck. New York, Churchill Livingstone, 1981, p 301.

28. LUNG CANCER

*Linda U. Krebs, RN, PhD, AOCN,
and Pamela Williams, RN, BSN, OCN*

Incidence	178,100 newly diagnosed cases estimated in 1997 (98,300 in men, 79,800 in women)
Mortality	160,400 deaths estimated in 1997

Risk factors

Tobacco use	Previous diagnosis of tuberculosis
Environmental tobacco smoke	Asbestos
Air pollution	Nutritional factors
Radon	Genetic predisposition
Occupational respiratory carcinogens	

Histology

Non-small cell lung cancers: 75–80%
　Adenocarcinoma (most common form): 33–50%
　Squamous cell (epidermoid): 30–40%
　Large cell: 5–15%
Small cell (oat cell) lung cancers: 20–25%

Symptoms　Cough, hemoptysis, dyspnea, wheezing, weight loss, fatigue, and chest or shoulder pain

Staging

Stage I	Tumor < 3 cm in greatest dimension or tumor > 3 cm that invades the visceral pleura with or without atelectasis or obstructive pneumonitis; no regional or distant metastasis.
Stage II	Tumor size as for stage I disease plus metastasis to ipsilateral peribronchial and/or ipsilateral hilar nodes, including direct extension; no distant metastasis.
Stage IIIA	Any tumor size with direct extension to adjacent structures (e.g., chest wall) or tumor in the main bronchus within 2 cm, but not involving the carina, with or without local lymph node metastasis.
Stage IIIB	Any tumor size with contralateral mediastinal, contralateral hilar, or ipsilateral or contralateral scalene or supraclavicular nodes or tumor invading mediastinum or other major structure (e.g., heart, esophagus) or malignant pleural effusion; any regional nodal metastasis, no distant metastasis.
Stage IV	Any tumor size or nodal spread with distant metastasis.

Treatment

Non-small cell lung cancer

Stage I	Surgery is treatment of choice; radiation therapy if patient is not surgical candidate.
Stage II	Surgery is treatment of choice; local radiation and systemic chemotherapy have been used both pre- and postoperatively; radiation therapy for nonsurgical candidates.
Stage IIIA	Surgery is treatment of choice; radiation therapy and/or chemotherapy may be added.
Stage IIIB	Radiation therapy is standard treatment; radiation therapy plus chemotherapy also may be used. Radiation therapy plus chemotherapy followed by surgical resection is under investigation for selected cases.
Stage IV	Chemotherapy is treatment of choice for ambulatory patients; radiation therapy may provide palliation.

Small cell lung cancer

Stages I–IV	Combination chemotherapy with or without local radiation therapy, (prophylactic cranial irradiation [PCI] remains controversial).

1. How common is lung cancer?

Lung cancer is the second most common cancer in men and in women, closely following breast cancer in women and prostate cancer in men. The incidence has increased dramatically since the turn of the century. The marked increase in lung cancer in women began in the late 1960s. Lung cancer is the leading cause of death in both men and women; only 13% of patients with lung cancer are alive more than 5 years after diagnosis.

2. What role does cigarette smoking play in the development of lung cancer?

Cigarette smoking is believed to be the chief preventable cause of cancer in the United States. If people would stop smoking (or never start), death rates from cancer would decrease by approximately 25%. It is estimated that 30% of all cancer deaths and approximately 85% of all lung cancer deaths are directly attributable to smoking. The rate for developing lung cancer in nonsmokers ranges between 12/100,000 and 15/100,000 population; for people who smoke less than 1 pack/day the risk is 10-fold greater and for people who smoke more than 1 pack/day the risk is 21-fold greater than for nonsmokers. Tobacco smoke is considered a group A (known human) carcinogen and is both an initiator and promoter of carcinogenesis. A causal link has been established between cigarettes and lung cancer; however, only 10–13% of people who smoke eventually develop lung cancer. The risk for developing lung cancer increases with the number of cigarettes smoked per day and the overall number of years of smoking. The risk of developing lung cancer is higher for people who begin to smoke before age 15 years than for people who begin to smoke after age 25.

Although the overall percentage of Americans who smoke has decreased (approximately 30% of the adult population smoked in 1985, including 10–15% of all physicians and 20–30% of all nurses), it is estimated that 20% of all men and 22% of all women will be smokers in the year 2000. In general, women have a shorter smoking history than men at diagnosis but may be more vulnerable to smoking-related risks than men. Based on current statistics, tobacco-related mortality for women will exceed that for men by 2000. For people who stop smoking, the risk of developing lung cancer drops to about 5-fold after 5 years and approaches the risk level for nonsmokers at 15 years. Because of lung damage during smoking, a slightly increased risk of developing lung cancer is always present in former smokers.

3. Does passive smoke play a role in the development of lung cancer?

Passive smoking or environmental tobacco smoke (ETS) is the involuntary exposure of non-smokers to tobacco smoke. ETS is believed to be qualitatively similar to smoke inhaled by smokers and has been labeled by the Environmental Protection Agency as a group A carcinogen (known to cause cancer in humans). Although significantly fewer cases of lung cancer have been directly attributable to ETS than to smoking, 20% of all lung cancers and 3000 lung cancer deaths are estimated to be related to ETS exposure. This number may well increase when the exact amount of smoke exposure in ETS can be better quantified.

4. Does diet play a role in preventing lung cancer?

Diets high in fruits and vegetables appear to be protective against lung cancer, whereas diets deficient in vitamin A appear to be associated with disease. Current chemoprevention trials have shown no benefit in preventing lung cancer.

5. What are the symptoms of lung cancer?

The most common symptoms of lung cancer include cough, hemoptysis, dyspnea, wheezing, and chest or shoulder pain. Systemic symptoms include anorexia, weight loss, fatigue, and paraneoplastic syndromes such as inappropriate secretion of antidiuretic hormone (SIADH), Cushing's syndrome, and hypercalcemia. Other symptoms include facial swelling (from superior vena cava syndrome), headache or seizures (from brain metastases), pleural effusions, bone pain, clubbing of digits, and hoarseness. Pneumonia that is unresolved after two months of treatment should be investigated as a symptom of lung cancer.

6. How is lung cancer diagnosed?

A combination of history and physical examination, chest radiographs, sputum cytology, and fiberoptic examination is used to diagnose lung cancer. Asymptomatic people often are diagnosed after a chest radiograph for other purposes. Bronchoscopy with washings, brushings, and biopsies of suspicious areas are most common. Transthoracic fine-needle aspiration may be used in unresectable individuals or when a preoperative tissue diagnosis is desired. Additional diagnostic measures include lymph node biopsy, mediastinoscopy, thoracoscopy, and thoracotomy. Chest computed tomography (CT) or magnetic resonance imaging (MRI) also may be used. Fewer than 1% of all lung cancers are diagnosed at an occult stage. One-third to one-half of solitary pulmonary nodules (coin lesions) found on chest radiograph are malignant.

7. What are the differences among the types of lung cancer?

Lung cancer is divided into two histologic classes: non-small cell lung cancer (NSCLC) and small cell lung cancer (SCLC). NSCLC accounts for 75–80% of all lung cancers and has three major subtypes: squamous cell, adenocarcinoma (including bronchoalveolar), and large cell. Squamous cell lung cancer usually arises centrally, grows more slowly, and tends to remain localized. Adenocarcinomas are the most common type of lung cancer and are more frequently found in women and younger people. Large cell lung cancers are associated with an overall poor prognosis. SCLC or oat cell carcinoma accounts for the remaining 20–25%. SCLC is generally a systemic disease at diagnosis; more than 50% of patients present with extensive (widespread) disease. Approximately 25% have regional involvement and less than 10% have only local disease at diagnosis. SCLC metastasizes early and is associated with a poor prognosis.

About 5% of lung cancers can be classified in an "other" category. These types are exceedingly rare and include carcinoid tumors and mucoepidermoid lung cancer.

8. Which lung cancers occur in nonsmokers?

If a nonsmoker develops lung cancer, it more than likely will be adenocarcinoma. Adenocarcinoma also occurs in smokers (particularly women who smoke). Lung cancers most commonly associated with smoking include squamous cell or small cell.

9. Are there any differences in the doubling time for the various types of lung cancer?

The doubling time for SCLC is relatively rapid and averages 45 days, whereas the doubling time for NSCLC averages 90–100 days with a range of 30–150 days. Because of rapid cell division, SCLC tends to be more responsive to both radiation therapy and chemotherapy.

10. How is NSCLC treated?

The mainstay for NSCLC treatment is surgery; however, only 20–25% of patients have localized disease that is amenable for surgery. Surgery is the only modality that offers a chance for cure and is used to treat patients with stage I, stage II, and stage IIIA disease. Occult tumors are rare; 90% are of squamous cell origin. The treatment of choice is lobectomy or pneumonectomy.

Radiation therapy is recommended for stage I and stage II patients who are not surgical candidates and is the standard treatment for stage IIIB disease (however, survival rates are low). Radiation therapy can be used for cure in highly selective, nonsurgical candidates. Chemotherapy has not been shown to improve overall prognosis or survival rates but increases length of survival. Platinum-based regimens are routinely used if chemotherapy is given. Chemotherapy is the treatment of choice for ambulatory stage IV patients, usually with a taxane-based regimen, and has been shown to be of more benefit in improving quality of life than the best supportive care alone. A combination of chemotherapy and radiotherapy is under investigation for stage IIIB disease, and other clinical trials are ongoing for all stages.

11. How is SCLC treated?

SCLC is considered to be a systemic disease at time of diagnosis; thus surgical resection alone is not appropriate. The mainstay of treatment is chemotherapy, with or without the addition of radiation therapy. Regimens including a variety of agents are most commonly used. The standard of care includes treatment with a platinum-based regimen and etoposide. Fewer than 20% of patients survive 2 years. Treatment with a YAG (yttrium, aluminum, garnet) laser may provide palliation, and smoking cessation may improve quality of life but does not necessarily lengthen survival.

12. What is the role of radiation therapy in the treatment of lung cancer?
Radiation therapy (RT) may be used for cure in certain nonsurgical candidates with NSCLC and also may be used to sterilize tumors preoperatively and to treat regional lymph nodes. RT may provide palliation by shrinking tumors and alleviating symptoms.

13. Is adjuvant chemotherapy indicated in the treatment of lung cancer?
Adjuvant chemotherapy is indicated in the treatment of SCLC because microscopic disease is always present. There is no proven benefit of adjuvant chemotherapy for patients with NSCLC; however, clinical trials to ascertain the value of adjuvant chemotherapy currently are being conducted for stage IIIB disease.

14. What are the most common sites of metastasis in lung cancer?
The most common metastatic sites for lung cancer include the liver, adrenal glands, bones, and brain. Both hematogenous and lymphatic spread are common. Local spread of disease includes direct invasion through the walls of lung structures and spread along the inside of the bronchial lumens.

15. Which lung cancers are most likely to have brain metastases?
Approximately 10% of all patients diagnosed with SCLC have brain metastases at diagnosis. Of those who survive for more than 2 years, 50–80% have brain metastases.

16. Should a patient with SCLC receive brain irradiation?
The role of prophylactic brain irradiation remains controversial. The side effects of radiation treatment to the brain must be weighed against long-term survival and quality of life. Currently the rate of brain metastases has been decreased with prophylactic brain irradiation, but no overall survival benefit has been shown.

17. What paraneoplastic syndromes are associated with lung cancer?
Paraneoplastic syndromes are common in lung cancer. SCLC is associated with SIADH, Cushing's syndrome (ectopic production of adrenocorticotropic hormone [ACTH]), Trousseau's syndrome (migratory thrombophlebitis), peripheral neuropathies, Eaton-Lambert syndrome (myasthenia-like transverse myelitis, polymyositis, and weakness), and carcinoid syndrome. Squamous cell lung cancer is associated with hypercalcemia and peripheral neuropathies, whereas adenocarcinoma of the lung is associated with hypercoaguable states and hypertrophic pulmonary osteoarthropathy. Hypercalcemia (rare), hypertrophic pulmonary osteoarthropathy, and peripheral neuropathies are also seen in patients with large cell lung cancers.

18. What oncologic emergencies most commonly occur in lung cancer?
The most common oncologic emergencies seen in patients with lung cancer are superior vena cava syndrome (SVC) and airway obstruction. Seventy-five percent of all instances of SVC are related to obstruction by either squamous cell or small cell lung cancers, whereas partial or complete airway obstruction is seen in 53% of patients with squamous cell, 38% with small cell, and 33% with large cell carcinoma. At thoracotomy, endobronchial lesions are found in approximately 70% of all patients with lung cancer. Pericardial effusions, neoplastic cardiac tamponade (direct extension into the pericardium), and spinal cord compression may occur, and metabolic emergencies, including hypercalcemia and hyponatremia (due to SIADH), are not uncommon.

19. What is Pancoast tumor syndrome?

Named after Henry Pancoast (who described the tumor that bears his name) in 1924, it is a lung tumor usually found after a lengthy investigation associated with severe shoulder and arm pain. Ipsilateral Horner's syndrome, characterized by a small pupil and ptosis of the eyelid, also may be present. The tumor has caused rib destruction and nerve root involvement (C8 or T1). It is located near the brachial plexus, major thoracic vessels, and vertebral bodies. Patients were once considered inoperable; radiotherapy, neoadjuvant chemotherapy, and rib resection may be performed. Neuropathic pain medications are the mainstay of symptomatic treatment.

20. What are the most significant prognostic indicators for patients with lung cancer?

For both SCLC and NSCLC, the single most common prognostic indicator for overall survival and response to treatment is weight loss. Other indicators include tumor bulk, presence and site(s) of metastases, gender (women usually fare better than men), age (patients under 70 years of age tend to do better), and performance status. In addition, an increased level of lactate dehydrogenase (LDH) or alkaline phosphatase and a decreased level of serum sodium are associated with a poorer prognosis in patients with SCLC.

21. Which lung cancers can be cured?

Localized lung cancer has the best chance for cure. Approximately 20–25% of patients with SCLC limited to the hemithorax may be cured by aggressive treatment with chemotherapy and radiation; however, most patients with SCLC present with extensive disease. Up to 90% of all patients with SCLC eventually relapse and die of disease even if complete remission has been achieved with aggressive therapy.

For patients with NSCLC, the potential for cure exists primarily for those with stage I, totally resectable disease. Any patient with distant metastases is not curable, and fewer than 5% of patients with stage III, mediastinal lymph node involvement are cured. Unfortunately, up to 45% of all patients with lung cancer are at risk for developing a second primary lung tumor. Chemoprevention trials to minimize second primaries currently are being conducted.

22. What new treatments are under development for lung cancer?

New chemotherapeutic agents are currently under investigation for the treatment of NSCLC and SCLC, including the taxanes, paclitaxel (Taxol) and docetaxel (Taxotere); vinorelbine (Navelbine); the camptothecins, irinotecan (Camptosar) and topotecan (Hycamtin); and gemcitabine (Gemzar). Combined or multimodal therapy (chemotherapy and radiation therapy), neoadjuvant or preoperative chemotherapy, chemoprevention agents, and internal photodynamic therapies are also under investigation.

23. How does mesothelioma differ from lung cancer?

Mesothelioma, a rare neoplasm commonly involving the pleura or peritoneum, is directly linked to asbestos exposure; people with occupational exposure (e.g., ship builders, pipe fitters, brake repairers, and insulation installers) to asbestos have a 6- to 7-fold greater risk of death from cancer than an unexposed population. Short-term exposure (< 1 month) carries a continued risk for the development of cancer 25 years later. More than 8 million people are believed to be at risk for developing mesothelioma. Cigarette smokers who are concomitantly exposed to asbestos carry a 53-fold increased risk of developing lung cancer. Mesothelioma usually presents with pleural effusion. The three subtypes are epithelial, fibrosarcomatous, and mixed. Disease spreads locally in the mediastinum and chest wall through direct tumor extension. Mesotheliomas rarely metastasize distally.

24. What is the current treatment for mesothelioma?

The primary treatment for mesothelioma is chemotherapy with a platinum-based regimen and the addition of an anthracycline or taxoid. Other regimens may be cyclophosphamide- or platinum-based. Response rates are usually less than 50%. Intrapleural therapy with cisplatin, interferon, or interleukin-2 have been undertaken with mixed results. The role of surgery is controversial, the role of radiation therapy is unclear, and experience with combined modality treatment is limited.

25. What methods are available for early detection of lung cancer?

No cost-effective methods currently exist for early detection of lung cancer. In asymptomatic people, lung cancer is often diagnosed when a chest radiograph is done for another purpose. Routine sputum cytology and intermittent bronchoscopy are under investigation in high-risk individuals. Patient registries and collection of DNA for genetic marker analysis are also components of clinical trials for people at high risk.

26. Does genetics play a role in the development of lung cancer?

It has been postulated that predisposition to lung cancer may be inherited. Amplification of one of the *myc* family of oncogenes is common in lung cancer. Loss, inactivation, or mutations of genes on chromosomes 3p, 13q, and 17p (p53 gene) have been noted.

27. What is the nurse's role in the care of patients with lung cancer?

Because treatment for lung cancer is primarily palliative, the nurse's role is focused on providing support, promoting comfort, and managing cancer- and treatment-related symptoms. Of particular importance are educational and psychosocial interventions to minimize feelings of guilt caused by believing that one has caused one's own disease and to promote quality of life. Role modeling of healthy behaviors and encouraging patients to quit smoking (to minimize further lung compromise) also should be incorporated into nursing care. Comprehensive symptom management, including nutritional interventions, is essential for providing holistic care. The following resources are available to aid the nurse in caring for patients with lung cancer:

- Alliance for Lung Cancer, Advocacy, Support, and Education
  1602 Lincoln Avenue
  Vancouver, WA 98660
  Telephone: 360-696-2436; e-mail: alcase@teleport.com
  National nonprofit organization that provides advocacy, support, education, and rehabilitation programs for people with lung cancer.
- American Lung Association
  1740 Broadway
  New York, NY 10019-4374
  Telephone: 800-LUNG-USA or 212-315-8700
  National nonprofit organization that provides information about cancer for patients and professionals as well as stop-smoking programs.

28. What is the nurse's role in smoking cessation?

Smoking cessation decreases the risk for developing lung cancer or for developing a second primary tumor after an initial diagnosis of lung cancer. In addition, smoking cessation has the potential for improving quality of life in patients undergoing treatment for lung cancer. Of current smokers, 70% want to quit smoking and 34% will actually attempt to quit. However, only 2.5% of people who attempt to quit smoking will be successful. Methods to enhance smoking cessation include (1) behavior modification strategies, such as relaxation techniques, hypnosis, and monitoring and reducing triggers to smoke; (2) group programs that provide skills training, social support, and structure; (3) nicotine replacement therapy (NRT) with gum, transdermal patches, or nasal spray; and (5) self-help programs using videotapes, literature, or brief telephone counseling and advice.

Ninety-five percent of all people who attempt to quit smoking do so without outside help. Of these, 20% will be successful with their first attempt, and up to 60% will be successful with repeated attempts. Multiple modalities (e.g., NRT and counseling) appear to improve smoking cessation efforts. The clinical approach recommended includes the **4 A's**: (1) **ask** about smoking, (2) **advise** to stop smoking, (3) **assist** to quit, and (4) **arrange** follow-up. These recommendations are included in a manual of practical smoking cessation techniques available from the National Cancer Institute, Office of Cancer Communications. Encouragement by health care providers to stop smoking or not to start smoking has been shown to be of benefit and should be incorporated into routine health care practices.

ACKNOWLEDGMENT

The authors thank Adam M. Myers, MD, Chief, Division of Hematology/Oncology, Denver Health Medical Center, Denver, Colorado, for his thoughtful review of this manuscript.

BIBLIOGRAPHY

1. Aisner J, Antman KH, Belani CP: Pleura and mediastinum. In Abeloff MD, Armitage JO, Lichter AS, Niederhuber JE (eds): Clinical Oncology. New York, Churchill Livingstone, 1995, pp 1153–1188.
2. Elpern EH: Lung cancer. In Groenwald SL, Frogge MH, Goodman M, Yarbro CH (eds): Cancer Nursing: Principles and Practice, 3rd ed. Boston, Jones & Bartlett, 1993, pp 1174–1200.
3. Feld R, Ginsberg RJ, Payne DG, Shepherd FA: Lung. In M.D. Abeloff MD, Armitage JO, Lichter AS, Niederhuber JE (eds): Clinical Oncology. New York, Churchill Livingstone, 1995, pp 1083–1152.
4. Glover J, Miaskowski C: Small cell lung cancer: Pathophysiologic mechanisms and nursing implications. Oncol Nurs Forum 21:87–95, 1994.
5. Greco FA, Hainsworth JD: Multidisciplinary approach to potentially curable non-small carcinoma of the lung. Oncology 11:27–36, 1997.
6. Humphrey EW, Ward HB, Perri RT: Lung cancer. In American Cancer Society Textbook of Clinical Oncology, 2nd ed. Atlanta, American Cancer Society, 1995, pp 220–235.
7. Keller SM: Lung cancer: Surgery. In Brain MC, Carbone PP (eds): Current Therapy in Hematology-Oncology, 5th ed. St. Louis, Mosby, 1995, pp 399–404.
8. Lindsey AM, Sarna L: Lung cancer. In McCorkle R, Grant M, Frank- Stromborg M, Baird SB (eds): Cancer Nursing: A Comprehensive Textbook, 2nd ed. Philadelphia, W.B. Saunders, 1996, pp 611–633.
9. Maxwell MB (ed): New developments in lung cancer. Semin Oncol Nurs 12:249–323, 1996 [entire issue].
10. Parker SL, Tong T, Bolden S, Wingo PA: Cancer statistics, 1997. CA Cancer J Clin 47:5–27, 1997.
11. White EJ: Lung cancer. In Varrichio C (ed): A Cancer Source Book for Nurses, 7th ed. Atlanta, American Cancer Society, 1997, pp 284–294.
12. Winn RJ (ed): Oncology practice guidelines. Oncology 10(Suppl 11), 1996 [entire issue].

29. MALIGNANT MELANOMA

Maude Becker, RN, OCN

Quick Facts—Malignant Melanoma

Incidence   40,300 estimated cases in 1997; 3% of all cancers in United States; 9th most common cancer in United States.
Lifetime risk of developing melanoma is increasing: 1991, 1 in 105; 2000, 1 in 75

Mortality   7,300 estimated deaths in 1997

Risk factors   Large number of moles
Family history of melanoma
History of severe sun burning in childhood and adolescence
Light skin type, blue or green eyes, blond hair
Clinically atypical moles, dysplastic nevus syndrome
History of acute and intermittent exposure to sun or ultraviolet radiation

Histology   **Superficial spreading** is the most common followed by nodular melanomas.
Other forms: acral lentiginous melanoma, lentigo maligna melanoma, desmoplastic and uveal melanoma (rare)

Symptoms   Mole that changes in size, elevation, color, surface, surroundings, and sensation

Diagnosis   Biopsy

Microstaging

Clark level	Breslow level (mm)
I and II	0.1–0.75
III (thin)	0.76–1.4
III (thick)	1.2–2.5
IV	2.6–4.0
V	> 4.0

Both level of invasion and maximal thickness determine the T (primary tumor) classification: **Breslow's thickness** = thickness of tumor tissue; **Clark's level** = anatomic level of invasion. Corresponding thickness of Clark and Breslow levels is shown. (From Groenwald S, Frogge M, Goodman M, Yarbro C: Comprehensive Cancer Nursing Review, 2nd ed. Research Triangle Park, NC, Glaxo Wellcome, 1995, with permission.)

Staging   Stage 0   Melanoma in situ
Stage IA   Primary melanoma < 0.75 mm and/or Clark's level II
Stage IB   Primary melanoma 0.76 to 1.50 mm and/or Clark's level III
Stage IIA   Primary melanoma 1.51 to 4.0 mm and/or Clark's level IV
Stage IIB   Primary melanoma > 4 mm and/or Clark's level V
Stage III   Regional lymph nodes and/or in-transit metastases
Stage IV   Systemic metastases

Treatment   Stages I and II: Surgical excision of the primary tumor
Stage III: Surgical excision of the primary tumor with or without radical lymphadenectomy and with or without interferon therapy
Stage IV: No standard treatment; all patients should be encouraged to participate in clinical trials.

1. What is melanoma?

Melanoma is a malignant tumor originating from melanocytes, the pigment (melanin)-producing cells in the skin. Melanocytes are found throughout the skin but are most common in the basal layers of the epidermis. Melanoma may arise from a preexisting nevus or occur spontaneously. It is a tumor that strikes fear because of its unpredictable behavior. For example, a melanoma can be completely excised, recur years later in another site, and cause rapid progression and death in less than 1 year.

2. What is dysplastic nevus syndrome (DNS)?

A dysplastic nevus is a distinct melanocytic lesion that may be a precursor to melanoma. It may occur sporadically or be associated with a personal or family history of melanoma (familial DNS). Regardless of family history, persons with DNS have a higher risk of developing melanoma. Clinically, dysplastic nevi tend to be larger than commonly acquired nevi, often measuring > 5 mm. The lesions may have fuzzy or irregular borders, and the pigmentation pattern is often irregular. Another distinctive feature is a "fried-egg" appearance, which is created when the central nevus component is one color and the peripheral component is another shade. Patients often have dozens or even hundreds of lesions.

3. Where do melanomas commonly occur?

Melanomas can be located anywhere on the body but occur most commonly on the lower extremities in women and on the trunk in men, especially on the back.

4. What type of biopsy should be done if melanoma is suspected?

Because tumor thickness is the most important factor in determining prognosis and treatment, the biopsy should be excisional through the underlying fat, using a punch-type biopsy when possible. After the diagnosis is established, < 1 mm in thickness should be excised with a 1-cm margin, whereas primary lesions of 1–4-mm thickness require a 2-cm margin. Studies have shown that large and disfiguring surgical excisions are unnecessary because they do not improve outcome or decrease local recurrence rates.

5. What are the warning signs of malignant melanoma?

The warning signs of malignant melanoma can be summarized as the **ABCDs:**
- **A**symmetry in shape, color, or appearance of mole; appearance of new pigmented lesion.
- **B**orders that are notched, irregular in shape, or both; bleeding moles.
- **C**olor of mole is variable or contains blue, gray, white, pink, or red.
- **D**iameter exceeds 6 mm in any direction.

6. What preventive measures should be taken to reduce the risk of developing melanoma?

- Avoid peak times of intense ultraviolet (UV) radiation exposure (10 a.m.–3 p.m.).
- Use sunscreen with a sun protection factor (SPF) of at least 15; reapply if swimming, perspiring, or outdoors > 2 hours.
- Apply 1 ounce of sunscreen evenly over the body at least 30 minutes before sun exposure.
- Wear protective clothing while outdoors.
- Do not use artificial suntanning lamps.
- Do regular self-examinations of skin and evaluate suspicious lesions using the ABCDs.

7. What is the relationship between melanoma and sunlight?

Sunlight is composed of UV radiation that damages the DNA of the skin cells. This damage may result in mutations that lead to the development of all forms of skin cancer, including melanoma. The same process occurs with the use of tanning booths. There is no such thing as a safe tan. The damaging effects of sunlight may occur many years before tumors appear; therefore, sun protection during childhood and youth is particularly important.

8. What does sun protection factor (SPF) mean?

Minimal erythematous dose (MED) is the minimal dose of UV that causes erythema. SPF is the relative protection offered by a sunscreen vs. no sunscreen protection. For example, a person who can be exposed to the sun for only 20 minutes without developing erythema can apply sunscreen with an SPF of 8 and stay outside for 160 (20 × 8) minutes without burning. More sun protection is offered by sunscreens with higher SPF numbers. A sunscreen with a SPF of 15 offers complete protection in most cases; it is recommended that patients use > 15 SPF for protecting skin after chemotherapy and radiation therapy.

9. What role do sentinel lymph node mapping and biopsy play in melanoma?

Because the role of elective lymph node dissection remains controversial, sentinel lymph node mapping and biopsy are available to help with the management of regional lymph nodes. The draining lymphatic vessels from a high-risk primary melanoma are identified by injecting dyes such as isosulfar blue and patent blue-v. The first ("sentinel") lymph node that takes up the dye is surgically removed and subjected to histologic analysis. If this node is not involved with melanoma, there is a less than 5% chance that any lymph node in that drainage site is pathologically involved. After further study, this technique may prove to be the best way to determine optimal surgical and medical management of intermediate- and high-risk primary melanomas.

10. Is there a benefit to prophylactic lymph node dissection?

An elective or (prophylactic) lymph node dissection is generally performed in patients with deep primary tumors under the assumption that they have a higher risk of regional nodal involvement and that early surgical treatment of the regional nodal basin will improve prognosis. Although this approach seems intuitively reasonable, two large randomized studies failed to demonstrate benefit; thus, its use remains controversial. Most melanoma experts do not recommend prophylactic lymph node dissection. In contrast, a therapeutic lymph node dissection is one in which the involved lymph nodes are removed; this technique remains a cornerstone of treatment for patients with stage III melanoma.

11. What are the histologic subtypes of melanoma?

Malignant melanoma has four major subtypes, each with unique clinical features.

Common Melanoma Types

TYPE (%)	INCIDENCE	COLORS AND CHARACTERISTICS	GROWTH	LOCATION
Superficial spread (70–75%)	Male:female ratio of 1:1 5th decade	Tan, brown Flat, crusty, irregular borders	Radial growth 1–5 years; vertical growth rapid	Women: legs Men: upper back
Nodular (10–15%)	Male:female ratio of 2:1 5th decade	Blue-black, blue-gray, red-blue Raised, bleeding may occur	No radial growth All vertical growth (< 1 year; aggressive)	Head, neck, trunk
Acral lentiginous (5–10%)	African-American Oriental Hispanic	Tan, brown, black	Radial growth: months to years	Palms, soles, subungual
Lentigo maligna (5%)	Male:female ratio of 1:3 7th decade	Tan, brown Mottling, irregular borders	Radial growth: decades; slow-growing; best prognosis of all melanomas	Head, neck, cheek, temple, hands

12. What are the most common sites of metastases?

Malignant melanoma can metastasize to almost any organ in the body. The most frequent sites for metastases are the regional lymph nodes, followed by the lungs. Other sites include skin, subcutaneous tissue, liver, brain, and bone.

13. What is the prognosis of a patient who presents with brain metastases?

Melanoma ranks with small cell lung cancer as the most common tumor that metastasizes to the brain. Headache, seizures, and neurologic deficits are the most common symptoms. The median survival once a patient develops brain metastases is < 6 months; without treatment it can be less than 6 weeks.

14. Does melanoma always occur on the skin?

No. Melanoma may originate in any area of the body that contains pigment cells. Unusual variants of melanoma include ocular melanoma (originating in the pigment cells of the retina or iris); conjunctival melanoma; and mucosal melanomas, such as nasopharyngeal, oral, vulvar, and anorectal melanomas. Between 1 and 12% of patients present with metastatic disease originating from an unknown primary site.

15. Where do ocular melanomas commonly spread?

The liver.

16. What tests are used for diagnosis and staging?

For stage I and II melanoma, a chemistry panel and chest radiograph are recommended. Patients with stage III and IV melanoma may also need a magnetic resonance (MR) brain scan, chest radiograph, computed tomography (CT) scan of the abdomen and pelvis, and chemistry profile because of the higher risk for metastases.

17. What is the role of interferon in the treatment of melanoma?

Alpha-interferon is currently indicated for postsurgical adjuvant therapy in patients with tumors > 4 mm in thickness and after therapeutic lymph node dissection. Interferon $\alpha 2A$ and $\alpha 2B$ are clinically indistinguishable and are interchangeable in the treatment of melanoma. Interferon is also commonly used alone or in combination for treatment of metastatic disease. As a single agent, it produces a 15–20% response rate. The use of interferon is currently under evaluation for the treatment of earlier-stage melanoma.

18. What is the optimal dose of interferon?

The best dose and optimal length of treatment remain controversial. The Food and Drug Administration (FDA) has approved a regimen of high-dose interferon for 1 year based on a large randomized study that showed improved disease-free and overall survival in treated patients. However, side effects such as fatigue were substantial, and approximately 40% of patients were unable to complete the prescribed regimen. Some evidence suggests that lower-dose regimens for longer periods of time also may be efficacious. The results of a large study to address this issue have not yet been analyzed.

19. What is the role of chemotherapy in melanoma?

Chemotherapy has generally been considered ineffective in the treatment of melanoma. Studies have shown no benefit in the adjuvant setting in patients at high risk for relapse. In advanced melanoma the only FDA-approved chemotherapy agent is dacarbazine (DTIC), which in many parts of the country remains the standard treatment. The response rate to DTIC is a dismal 15–20%, with a median duration of response of 5–6 months. Complete responses were observed in only 5% of 580 patients entered into phase III trials. Only 3% of patients who achieved a complete response remained disease-free at 6 years. Several multidrug regimens containing

DTIC and cisplatin, in combination with vinblastine or 1,3-bis-(2-chloroethyl)-1-nitrosourea (BCNU) and tamoxifen, have resulted in somewhat higher response rates. Nevertheless, the role of combination chemotherapy remains controversial, and its impact in long-term survival remains disappointing.

20. What are the latest treatment options for melanoma?

Newer modalities of diagnosis and treatment are currently under investigation, including lymphoscintigraphy and sentinel node biopsy, stereotactic radiation either with a gamma knife or linear accelerator for brain metastases, hyperthermic limb perfusion, and chemoembolization for liver metastases. Several new systemic agents and regimens are in various stages of development, including interleukin-2 (IL-2), temazolamide (an oral analog of DTIC), bryostatin (biologic agent), combinations of biologic agents and chemotherapy, gene therapy, and various melanoma vaccines.

21. Why should patients with melanoma enroll in clinical trials?

Although substantial progress has been made over the years, all too often patients are confronted with an advanced malignancy, a median survival time of 6–12 months, and no currently available effective treatment. In this circumstance the best option is to enroll in a clinical trial, which provides the hope of more effective treatment and often is the only way to obtain access to experimental drugs. By participating in clinical trials patients also contribute to the rapid progress of science, provide earlier access to new treatment modalities for future patients, and may facilitate the eventual discovery of a cure.

22. Who is at the risk for recurrent melanoma?

Patients who have had one melanoma are at greater risk for developing a second melanoma. The lifetime risk of developing a second primary tumor ranges from 3–6%. Patients who have multiple dysplastic nevi or a familial form have an even greater risk of developing multiple primary melanomas. Persons with familial melanoma account for approximately 10% of all patients with melanoma.

23. What is the relationship between pregnancy and melanoma?

The precise influence of pregnancy on melanoma is unknown. During pregnancy, the level of melanocyte-stimulating hormone is higher than normal, and nevi may show an increase in pigmentation. This suggests that hormonal changes secondary to pregnancy may have an abnormal effect on or accelerate melanocyte growth. Other issues to be considered are:

1. The effect of the pregnancy on the outcome of the melanoma.
2. The effects of the melanoma on the fetus and outcome of the pregnancy.
3. The effects of treatments on the fetus and outcome of the melanoma.

In the absence of specific answers to these questions, the decision to become pregnant or to terminate a pregnancy should be left to the patient and her doctor.

24. Does melanoma respond to radiation therapy?

Radiotherapy has a limited role in the management of metastatic disease. It is used mainly for palliation of central nervous system (CNS) or bone metastases. Stereotactic radiation may be beneficial in selected cases with CNS involvement.

25. What follow-up care should a patient have after a diagnosis of melanoma?

All experts agree that lifetime follow-up is indicated because local recurrences and metastases are always possible. Follow-up should include a thorough skin and lymph node examination. The following schedule is recommended: for years 1, 2, and 3, every 3–4 months; for years 4 and 5, every 6 months; and annually thereafter.

26. What are the 10-year survival rates for the various stages of melanoma?

AJCC Stage	10-year Survival Rate
I	85%
II	60%
III	20%
IV	< 5%

ACKNOWLEDGMENT

The author thanks Rene Gonzalez, MD, Assistant Professor, Division of Medical Oncology, UCHSC, for his thoughtful review of this manuscript.

BIBLIOGRAPHY

1. Anderson C, Tabacof J, Legha S: Malignant melanoma: Biology, diagnosis, and management. Med Oncol Compr Rev 32:493–509, 1995.
2. Balch C, Houghton A, Milton G, et al: Cutaneous Melanoma, 2nd ed. Philadelphia, J. B. Lippincott, 1992.
3. Dhawan M, Kirkwood J: Contemp Oncol 4(9):40–50, 1994.
4. Groenwald S, Frogge M, Goodman M, Yarbro C: Comprehensive Cancer Nursing Review, 2nd ed. Research Triangle Park, NC, Glaxo Wellcome, 1995.
5. Hoffman S, Yohn J, Norris D, et al: Cutaneous malignant melanoma. Curr Probl Dermatol 5:7–41, 1993.
6. Parker SL, Tong T, Bolden S, Wingo PA: Cancer statistics, 1997. CA Cancer J Clin 47:5–27, 1997.
7. Reintgen D, Albertini J, Berman C: Accurate nodal staging of malignant melanoma. Cancer Control 2:405–413, 1995.
8. Urist M: Surgical management of primary cutaneous melanoma. Cancer J Clin 46: 217–224, 1996.

30. PROSTATE CANCER

Susanne K. Cook, RN, BSN, OCN

Incidence	No. 1 cancer in men; 334,500 estimated new cases in 1997
Mortality	Second leading cause of cancer deaths in men; 41,800 deaths estimated in 1997
Etiology	Unknown
Risk factors	Increased risk with increasing age African-American Family history
Histology	95% adenocarcinoma

Symptoms

Early	**Late**
May be asymptomatic	Bone pain
Urinary frequency	Painful defecation
Nocturia	Obstructive urinary symptoms
Dysuria	Weight loss
Slow urine stream	
Hematuria	
Urinary retention or hydronephrosis	

Screening	Digital rectal examination Prostate-specific antigen (PSA)
Diagnosis and staging studies	Core biopsy Transrectal ultrasound (TRUS) is controversial Abdominal CT Complete blood count, acid phosphatase, chemistry screen Bone scan
Staging	Tumor, node, metastasis (TNM) and American Urological Association (AUA) systems

STAGE	TNM	AUA	EXTENT OF DISEASE	TREATMENT
I	T1–T1b	A–A2	Incidental histologic findings of cancer; prostate normal to palpation	Radical prostatectomy, radiation therapy (external beam + brachytherapy), cryosurgery, hormonal therapy, watchful waiting
	T1c		PSA elevation only	
II	T2–T2c	B–B2	Tumor palpable but confined to prostate	Same as above
III	T3–T3c	C–C2	Tumor localized to periprostatic area, may be fixed, and invades structures	Radical prostatectomy, radiation therapy, hormonal therapy, watchful waiting
IV	T4–M+	D–D2	Advanced disease (pelvic lymph node and distant metastasis)	Hormonal therapy, chemotherapy, strontium, radiation therapy

Adapted from American Joint Committee on Cancer: Manual for Staging of Cancer, 4th ed. Philadelphia, J.B. Lippincott, 1992.

1. How common is prostate cancer?

Prostate cancer has doubled in the last two decades, partly as a result of early detection as well as aging of the U.S. population. In men, it is currently the number one cancer and the second leading cancer cause of death. The American Cancer Society estimates that approximately 334,500 new cases of prostate cancer and approximately 41,800 deaths will be associated with this disease in 1997. African-American men have the highest incidence in the world (60% increase in incidence), whereas Asian men have the lowest, excluding Asian men who have migrated to Western countries. Although this distinction points to an environment risk, studies show that Japanese men may have differences in androgen levels that account for the decreased incidence.

2. How much research funding is provided for prostate cancer?

Until recently prostate cancer has received dramatically less publicity and funding than breast cancer and AIDS. Only $59 million was allotted for prostate cancer research in 1994, whereas $500 million was made available for breast cancer and $1.3 billion for AIDS. To increase public awareness, politicians, actors, musicians, and athletes have been speaking about their experiences with prostate cancer. Michael Milken, a prominent financier who was diagnosed with prostate cancer while incarcerated, founded CaPCURE (Cure for Prostate Cancer) and pledged $25 million over the next 5 years for research. The government has granted funding of $7.5 million annually for the next 3–5 years for Specialized Programs of Research Excellence (SPORE) in prostate cancer. Additional government funding of $100–$130 million between 1996 and 1999 has been awarded.

3. Can we predict who is at risk for developing prostate cancer?

The strongest predictors for prostate cancer are age, race, and family history. Eighty percent of men are 65 years or older when initially diagnosed. In comparison with Caucasian men, African-American men have a 37% higher chance of being diagnosed with prostate cancer, develop it at an earlier age, have a greater extent of disease at time of diagnosis, and have a mortality rate two times higher. Availability of health care services and beliefs about the health care system may be contributing factors to the disparities.

Family history may genetically predispose men to prostate cancer. A man whose father or brother has been diagnosed with prostate cancer has two times the risk of developing it. Men with two or three first-degree relatives who are affected have a 5- or 11-fold increased risk, respectively.

There seems to be no correlation between prostate cancer and venereal disease, infections, or sexual habits. Exposure to cadmium (a trace mineral found in cigarette smoke and alkaline batteries) has been correlated with prostate cancer. The relationship between prostate cancer and tobacco smoking or vasectomy is inconclusive.

4. Are there any ways to prevent prostate cancer?

Numerous variables have been evaluated, but there is no consensus. Some research suggests that decreasing dietary fat is probably beneficial. It is currently undetermined whether dietary intake of retinoids and carotenoids offers any benefit. Synthetic retinoids are under investigation because the therapeutic doses of natural vitamin A necessary to inhibit carcinogenesis are toxic. Selenium supplementation in low doses (200 mg/day) decreases the prostate cancer rate fourfold.

5. Does Proscar or Hytrin prevent prostate cancer?

The goal of the NCI-funded Prostate Cancer Prevention Trial (PCPT) is to determine whether finasteride (Proscar) will decrease a man's chance of developing prostate cancer. Proscar prevents the conversion of testosterone into dihydrotestosterone (DHT), a hormone believed to contribute to the development of prostate cancer. A recent study compared the safety and efficacy of placebo, terazosin (Hytrin), finasteride (Proscar), and the combination of both drugs in 1229 patients with benign prostatic hyperplasia (BPH). Only Hytrin was effective in reducing symptoms. However, men currently taking Proscar on protocol should not discontinue the drug.

Hytrin and Proscar have different mechanisms of action. Hytrin improves urinary flow by relaxing smooth muscle in the glands and does not affect DHT levels. Hytrin helps men whose problem with urinary flow is related to smooth muscle contraction, whereas Proscar helps men with larger prostate glands whose urinary problems are associated with a large amount of epithelial tissue. Hytrin and Proscar offer different options for treatment and have potential for prevention of prostate cancer.

6. What are the current recommendations or guidelines for prostate cancer screening?

American Cancer Society guidelines: Normal-risk men older than 50 years and high-risk men older than 40 years should have both a digital rectal exam (DRE) and prostate-specific antigen (PSA) test annually.

American Urological Association guidelines: All men older than 40 years should have an annual DRE and PSA test.

The National Cancer Institute is currently conducting a large prospective, randomized trial to study whether early detection increases survival and decreases disease-related mortality. Results will not be available for 15 years.

7. What is the debate over using PSA for screening?

Whether survival is increased by early detection and whether morbidity is increased by taking an aggressive approach based on PSA levels are controversial issues. PSA is a glycoprotein that acts as an enzyme in liquidating semen. Manufactured in the prostate, it is considered to be elevated when it is > 4.0 (normal: 0–4.0 mg/ml). PSA blood screening first became available in 1987 and meets the requirement for sensitivity. Specificity, however, is not as high; 36% of patients with a moderately increased PSA have nonmalignant disease. In addition to detecting prostate cancer cells, the PSA also may give a false-positive result secondary to benign prostatic hypertrophy, prostatitis, cystoscopy, TURP, and needle biopsy. Manipulating the prostate gland for DRE before drawing the blood sample does not cause significant changes in the PSA level. Because the PSA results do not help to decipher between fast-growing and slow-growing tumors, PSA levels alone may be misleading for determining treatment. Approximately 20% of patients with prostate cancer (confined or metastatic) have a normal PSA level (nonsecreting tumor). Many health maintenance organizations, including Medicare, will not pay for a PSA screen.

8. What is meant by age-specific PSA reference ranges?

Because normal PSA levels increase as men become older, many researchers suggest that age-specific reference ranges should be used to increase the sensitivity of the PSA test among younger men and increase the specificity for older men. These ranges have not been approved or accepted by all urologists and clinicians.

Age (yr)	PSA Reference Range (ng/ml)
40–49	0–2.5
50–59	0–3.5
60–69	0–4.5
70–79	0–6.5

9. Should all patients with elevated PSA be treated aggressively?

Watchful waiting has gained the interest of health care providers and patients. This approach defers treatment until the tumor becomes more aggressive, i.e., increasing PSA levels, marked change in DRE, or patient-identified symptoms. Currently the NCI has initiated a research trial called PIVOT (Prostate Cancer Intervention vs. Observation Trial) to determine whether radical prostatectomy leads to a sufficiently significant decrease in mortality to choose surgery over watchful waiting. Because radical prostatectomy is associated with a 1% mortality rate, total urinary incontinence (1–5%), and impotence in at least 50% of older patients, some men prefer the watchful waiting approach because of the decreased morbidity and improved quality of life.

10. What are the signs and symptoms of prostate cancer?

Generally, early-stage prostate cancer is asymptomatic. However, as the tumor progresses, the patient may complain of symptoms consistent with urinary obstruction: nocturia, hesitancy, straining to void, or irritative symptoms such as urgency, dysuria, feeling of incomplete voiding, or hematuria.

Symptoms of late-stage prostate cancer are often associated with bone metastasis; consequently, pain is the most common complaint of patients with metastatic disease. Pain is frequently located in the pelvis and femur areas. The quality of the pain is commonly described as migratory; e.g., pain that radiates from one site to another. Complaints of back pain require thorough assessment for possible spinal cord compression. Liver involvement is manifested by elevated liver function tests, tenderness on palpation, anorexia, and nausea. Rarely, coagulopathies, such as thrombophlebitis and disseminated intravascular coagulation, may occur in the late stages. Lung metastasis is rare but may be manifested by shortness of breath.

11. What are the survival rates for prostate cancer?

AUA Stage	5-Year Survival Rate
A	90–94%
B	74–90%
C	55–72%
D	1–4 years survival

12. What questions should the patient ask about proposed treatments?
- What is my chance of being cured?
- What is the survival rate with each proposed treatment?
- Is the cancer confined to the prostate? How can you tell?
- Are there fewer complications with surgery or radiation?
- What is the risk of impotence?
- What is the chance of incontinence?
- What can I expect from taking hormones?

13. What is a radical prostatectomy?

Radical prostatectomy is an option when the tumor is confined to the prostatic capsule. It involves removal of the entire prostate, including the true prostatic capsule, seminal vesicles, and a portion of the bladder neck. It can be performed by the perineal or retropubic approach. Stress incontinence occurs after 10–15% of procedures. Loss of potency after radical prostatectomy, regardless of approach, may be as high as 90% but is age-dependent and associated with erection capabilities before treatment. Sparing one or both of the neurovascular bundles that control sexual function helps to preserve potency.

14. What are the usual complications associated with surgery for prostate cancer?

Atelectasis, wound infection, and bleeding may occur. After lymph node dissection, edema of the penis or lower extremities and deep vein thrombosis may result. Patients remain in the hospital for 2–6 days and usually go home with a Foley catheter in place for 2 weeks.

15. When is treatment with radiation therapy a consideration?

Radiation therapy may be used in any stage from A to C. It is an option for organ-confined disease and for patients who are considered a poor surgical risk. When positive margins have been identified, radiation therapy may be used alone or postsurgically in combination with interstitial or hormonal therapy. Recent evidence also suggests that use of neoadjuvant hormonal suppression in combination with radiation therapy improves disease-free survival.

The most recent advance in radiation therapy is three-dimensional conformal radiation, which gives a prescribed radiation dose to the entire target volume while conforming to the anatomic boundaries of the tumor in its three-dimensional shape. This computerized therapy has the advantage of delivering a higher dose of radiation to a precise area, thereby increasing tumor kill while decreasing damage to surrounding tissue.

16. What are the side effects of radiation therapy for prostate cancer?

Radiation therapy may cause cystitis and diarrhea during treatment. Incontinence is possible as a more immediate side effect but may not resolve completely in 4–6% of patients. Rather than stress incontinence, it is bladder irritation that precipitates feelings of urgency. Recently, the severity of urinary incontinence has decreased secondary to linear accelerators, careful simulation, and treatment planning. Lymphedema and impotence may occur as delayed effects secondary to fibrosis. The incidence of impotence is less than with surgery. New techniques for brachytherapy and selection of favorable patients have been instrumental in maintaining potency in approximately 70% of patients, similar to the rate with radical prostatectomy.

17. What is the significance of the PSA level after primary treatment?

If the PSA returns to low levels of normal (≤ 1.0 ng/ml) after radical prostatectomy or radiation therapy, patients are less likely to have a subsequent relapse than patients with levels > 1.0 to ≤ 4.0 ng/ml.

18. What is cryosurgery? When is it used?

Cryosurgery is used for localized prostate cancer. This procedure consists of implanting rods into the prostate gland and injecting liquid nitrogen to freeze and kill the cancerous cells. Urethral freezing may be a consequence. To prevent this undesired side effect, a warming fluid is injected simultaneously into the urethra. Because cryosurgery is a new treatment option, few long-term data are available. Some responses to treatment have lasted approximately 2 years. At that time 15% of biopsy results are positive for prostate cancer. One advantage of cryosurgery over radiation therapy is the option to repeat treatment.

19. What are the side effects of cryosurgery?

More than 50% of patients who have undergone cryosurgery experience at least one side effect. The damage may be to the urethra; in rare cases, urethral strictures (i.e., urethral fistula) and prostatitis may develop. Incontinence occurs in only 3% of patients, unless cryosurgery is used after failure of radiation therapy; then the incontinence rate increases dramatically to 20–30%. Potency is regained at 6–12 months after treatment in 20% of patients who were potent before treatment.

20. What is hormonal therapy for prostate cancer? How does it work?

Hormonal therapy is usually reserved for patients with symptomatic, metastatic disease and is generally used in the palliative setting. Men who are potent at the time of initiating therapy need to know that the risk of losing potency is almost 100%. In addition, hot flashes, weight gain, loss of bone density, and gynecomastia may occur.

Approximately 95% of testosterone comes from the testicles; the other 5% is produced by the adrenal glands. The goal of endocrine manipulation is to inhibit the formation of testosterone. This goal can be achieved surgically by orchiectomy or pharmacologically with oral hormones or injections that inhibit testosterone formation. Response rates are equal. Therapy can be aimed at one or both testosterone-producing systems. Single-agent androgen blockade can be achieved by surgical orchiectomy or by injections of analogs of luteinizing hormone-releasing hormone (LHRH), such as a leuprolide (Lupron) or goserelin acetate (Zoladex) implant that interferes with the pituitary feedback system. Analogs can be given as a depot injection monthly or every 3 months. The hormone injections "trick" the pituitary into thinking that testosterone production does not need to be initiated.

Combined therapy, or total hormone blockade, consists of treatment aimed at both the pituitary and adrenal glands. Flutamide and Casadex are oral antiandrogens that inhibit testosterone effects at the target tissue level. In combination with surgical or pharmacologic orchiectomy, both drugs achieve total hormone blockade. Combination hormonal therapy may delay time to relapse in comparison to single-agent therapy; however, it has no advantage over orchiectomy alone. Relapse may occur from 18–36 months after treatment.

21. What are the newer uses of hormone therapy?

Hormonal therapy is used in the neoadjuvant setting to downstage and downsize the tumor. Hormonal therapy also has been used intermittently in patients with prostate cancer whose PSA levels are < 0.2 ng/ml so that sexual function can be resumed and other side effects decreased. The LHRH analog is withdrawn until the first sign of PSA elevation occurs and then restarted. If a patient has been on complete androgen blockade and is noted to have a rising PSA, sometimes the antiandrogen therapy may be withdrawn. This approach has caused a decrease in PSA and occasional improvement of a positive bone scan. Remission, however, is brief.

22. When is chemotherapy indicated?

Chemotherapy for prostate cancer is not curative, but it may be used to palliate metastatic disease. Side effects are minimal with most therapies. Estramustine, vinblastine, and novantrone have been the most effective drugs. Floxuridine has been used alone or in combination with oral leucovorin; mucositis and diarrhea are the dose-limiting toxicities. Recent studies have looked at paclitaxel and ketoconazole in combination with vinblastine and estramustine. A consideration in prescribing oral chemotherapeutics is that patients with prostate cancer are frequently funded through Medicare, which does not cover outpatient treatment. Consequently, unless they have supplemental insurance, the expense of chemotherapy may be prohibitive. Novantrone is the only agent approved by the Food and Drug Administration (FDA) for painful hormone-refractory disease.

23. What treatments are available to treat erectile dysfunction?

The most common treatments, in order of patient ease, are vacuum devices, injectable drugs, and implants. Recently the FDA approved a urethral suppository (MUSE) for erections. Vacuum devices work by assisting the penis to become erect by suction. A combination of drugs can be injected subcutaneously by the patient or significant other into the corpus cavernosum to attain penile erection. Patients must be counseled about potential priapism. Penile implants require surgical intervention. Thus, infection is a potential complication. Hollow tubes are placed in the corpus cavernosum, and erection results from pumping a reservoir that inflates the tubes with normal saline. In addition, rods may be surgically placed in the corpus cavernosum to maintain a permanent erection.

24. How are hot flashes controlled?

Controlling hot flashes is a challenge. Severity may be diminished, but total eradication is rare. Commonly prescribed medications are vitamin E, clonidine, and Megace. Vitamin E may be obtained over the counter and is recommended in doses of 400 I.U. twice daily. Clonidine patches may be prescribed if the patient has no history of hypotension or syncope. Blood pressure is monitored and, if tolerated, an increase in dosage is prescribed. The most effective drug is Megace at doses of 20 mg/day orally. Studies have not shown this dose to cause thrombophlebitis.

25. Is strontium a useful treatment for bone metastases?

Strontium-89 is a radioisotope that is administered intravenously to patients with far advanced prostate cancer who have failed all other therapy and have a life expectancy > 2 months. It travels to areas of bone that have become infiltrated by the metastatic process, follows the biochemical pathways of calcium in the body, and is taken into the mineral structure of the bone. Initially it may cause flare pain and myelosuppression. It also has been noted to cause prolonged anemia and thrombocytopenia. Patients should be instructed to continue taking their prescribed pain medication for approximately 2–3 weeks after receiving strontium-89 because of the delayed response before pain relief occurs. Pain relief can be maintained for 4–15 months. Response rates have been shown to be 70–80%. Patients also may benefit from a second injection; however, caution must be used because of the prolonged side effects. Use of strontium 89 may compromise further chemotherapy.

26. What resources are available to support men and their families in dealing with prostate cancer?

The American Cancer Society (800-ACS-2345) offers a group program (Man-to-Man) to men and their partners in a supportive atmosphere with the assistance of qualified health care professionals. The support group provides information about prostate cancer and related issues. US TOO is an international network of chapters providing support and service to survivors of prostate cancer and professional education for health care workers (1-800-808-7866). The American Foundation for Urological Diseases (AFUD) provides public education materials (410-727-2908).

ACKNOWLEDGMENTS

The author thanks E. David Crawford, MD, Professor of Surgery, Division of Urology, and L. Michael Glode, MD, Professor of Medicine, Division of Hematology/Oncology, University of Colorado Health Sciences Center, for their thoughtful review of this manuscript.

BIBLIOGRAPHY

1. Abeloff MD, Armitage JO, Lichter AS, Niederhuber JE (eds): Clinical Oncology. New York, Churchill Livingstone, 1995.
2. American Joint Committee on Cancer: Manual for Staging of Cancer, 4th ed. Philadelphia, J.B. Lippincott, 1992.
3. Brenner ZR, Krenzer ME. Update on cryosurgical ablation for prostate cancer. Am Nurs 4:44–48, 1995.
4. Cher ML, Carroll PR: Screening for prostate cancer. West J Med 162:235–242, 1995.
5. Colditz GA: Selenium and cancer prevention: Promising results indicate further trials required. JAMA 276:1984–1985, 1996.
6. Held JL, Osborne DM, Volpe H, Waldman AR: Cancer of the Prostate: Treatment and Nursing Implications. Oncol Nurs Forum 21:1517–1529, 1994.
7. Garnick MB, Fair WR: Prostate cancer: Emerging concepts. Parts I and II. Ann Intern Med 125:118–125, 205–211, 1996.
8. Greco KE, Held JL, Waldman AR, et al: Prostate cancer: Controversies Surrounding Risk, Screening, and Management. Oncol Nurs Forum 21:1503–1511, 1994.
9. Jaroff L: The man's cancer. Time April 1, 1996, pp 58–65.
10. Lepor H, Williford WO, Barry MJ, et al: The efficacy of terazosin, finasteride or both in benign prostatic hyperplasia. N Engl J Med 335:533–539, 1996.
11. Maxwell MB: Cancer of the prostate. Semin Oncol Nurs 9:237–251, 1993.
12. Parker SL, Tong T, Bolden S, Wingo PA: Cancer statistics, 1997. CA Cancer J Clin 47:5–27, 1997.
13. Steinberg GD, Carter BS, Beauty TH, et al: Family history and the risk of prostate cancer. Prostate 17:337–347, 1990.
14. Waldman AR, Osborne DM: Screening for prostate cancer. Oncol Nurs Forum 21:1512–1516, 1994.
15. Zelefsky MJ, Leibel SA, Wallner KE, et al: Significance of normal serum prostate-specific antigen in the follow-up period after definitive radiation therapy for prostatic cancer. J Clin Oncol 13:459–463, 1995.

31. RENAL CELL CARCINOMA

Patrick Judson, MD

1. Discuss the incidence and mortality rate of kidney or renal cell carcinoma.

In 1997, there will be an estimated 28,800 new cases of renal cell carcinoma (also called hypernephroma or renal adenocarcinoma) and 11,300 deaths. Males are affected twice as often as females. The median age at diagnosis is 57 years.

2. What risk factors have been associated with renal cell carcinoma?

- Smoking
- Exposure to asbestos
- Von Hippel-Lindau syndrome (VHL)
- Patients who develop renal cystic disease while on renal dialysis

3. Is renal cell carcinoma associated with genetic predispositions?

Families with an inherited autosomal-dominant predisposition to renal cell carcinoma have a translocation involving chromosome 3. Members of the family without the disease do not have this translocation. Another form of hereditary renal cell carcinoma is seen with von Hippel-Lindau disease, which is characterized by multiple, bilateral renal cysts and carcinomas, pheochromocytomas, retinal angiomas, hemangioblastomas of the central nervous system, pancreatic cysts and tumors, and epididymal cysts.

4. What are the pathologic findings in renal cell carcinoma?

- 2–4% are bilateral.
- 4–10% have extension into the renal vein or the inferior vena cava.
- Approximately 85% of cases are adenocarcinomas, which are separated into clear cell (most common) and granular cell carcinomas. The two types also may occur together. The remainder of cases are papillary (sarcomatoid) or transitional cell carcinomas.
- Expression of multidrug-resistant (MDR) phenotype

5. What are the signs and symptoms of renal cell carcinoma?

The classic triad of flank pain, flank mass, and hematuria is unusual (10–15% of cases) and indicates advanced disease. An increasing number of cases (25–30%) are found serendipitously in imaging studies obtained for unrelated reasons. Renal cell carcinoma (RCC) also may present as distant metastases (primary adenocarcinoma undetermined).

6. What is unique about renal cell carcinoma?

A unique aspect of RCC is that paraneoplastic syndromes are relatively common. These syndromes include an increased erythrocyte sedimentation rate, polycythemia, hypertension, anemia, cachexia and weight loss, fever, hepatic dysfunction (Stauffer's syndrome), hypercalcemia, erythrocytosis, neuromyopathies, and amyloidosis.

Another unique aspect is that RCC tumors may regress spontaneously without therapy. Documented cases of spontaneous regressions are rare and do not necessarily lead to long-term survival.

7. Where are the usual sites of metastases?

About one-third of patients present with metastatic disease. Frequent sites include the lung, liver, bones, lymph nodes, and central nervous system.

8. What should the evaluation of a patient with renal cell carcinoma include?

History and physical examination	Ultrasound
Complete blood count and chemistry profile	CT of chest and abdomen

Consider venogram of inferior vena cava (IVC) or MRI to evaluate IVC involvement

9. What is the staging system for renal cell carcinoma?

The TNM system for RCC is unwieldy. The American Joint Committee on Cancer (AJCC) described four stages that incorporate the TNM system. The staging system modified by Robson is generally used:

I　　Tumor is confined within the renal capsule

II　　Tumor invades through the renal capsule but is confined by Gerota's fascia

III　Tumor has invaded the renal vein or inferior vena cava (A), regional lymph nodes (B), or both (C)

IV　Distant metastases or involvement of local organs other than ipsilateral adrenal gland

10. Which type of renal cancer has the worst prognosis?

Prognosis depends on the tumor's size, stage, and grade. Sarcomatoid variants are more aggressive and have a poorer prognosis.

11. What is the primary treatment for renal cell carcinoma?

Resectable, early-stage disease is curable only with surgery. With surgery, patients with stage I tumors have a 5-year survival rate of approximately 80%. Selected patients with stage I disease may have a radical, simple, or partial nephrectomy. Radical resection involves removal of the kidney, adrenal gland, perirenal fat, and Gerota's fascia with or without dissection of regional lymph nodes. Surgical excision of solitary or multiple metastatic lesions also may have a beneficial role.

12. Is there a role for adjuvant therapy outside clinical trials?

There is no proven benefit for adjuvant systemic or radiation therapy.

13. What is the treatment for metastatic disease?

Patients with advanced local or metastatic disease have a 5-year survival rate of approximately 15%. In the past, no chemotherapy regimen has had significant benefit (< 10% response) for metastatic renal cell carcinoma.

Immunotherapy with agents such as interleukin-2 (IL-2) holds promise, as does therapy with interferon (IFN). IL-2 has a response rate of approximately 15-20%. The good news is that one-half of responders have long unmaintained remission or potential cure. Recent combinations of IL-2, IFN, and 5-fluorouracil (5-FU) have yielded response rates of approximately 40%. External beam radiation can be used to palliate metastatic renal disease (bone and brain lesions).

14. What resources are available for patients with renal cell cancer?

The American Kidney Fund (800-638-8299) provides assistance with finances and medical referrals for people with renal cancer and other kidney diseases.

The National Kidney Cancer Association (800-850-9132; E-mail: nkca@merle.acns.nwu.edu) advocates for patients with kidney cancer and provides research funds and professional or patient information.

BIBLIOGRAPHY

1. Bossinger SO, Messing EM: Genitourinary cancer: Early stage cancers of the prostate, bladder, and kidney. In Brain MC, Carbone PP (eds): Current Therapy in Hematology-Oncology, 5th ed. St. Louis, Mosby, 1995, pp 423–436.
2. Fonseca GA, Ellerhorst J: Renal-cell carcinoma. In Padzur R (ed.): Medical Oncology: A Comprehensive Review, 2nd ed. Huntington, NY, PRR, 1995. pp 459–466.
3. Parker SL, Tong T, Bolden S, Wingo PA: Cancer statistics, 1997. CA Cancer J Clin 47:5–27, 1997.

32. TESTICULAR CANCER

Jeffrey L. Berenberg, MD, COL, MC

Incidence	7200 new cases are estimated in 1997 (accounts for 1% of all cancers in men). Most common tumor in men between the ages of 20–34 years. Patients with seminoma present one decade later. Incidence is rising in the United States and Europe. Less common in both African-Americans and Africans. 1–2% of all germ cells are bilateral; both tumors may occur synchronously or second tumor may occur years later.
Mortality	350 deaths estimated in 1997 Mortality in white U.S. men has decreased from 37% in 1960–1963 to 5% in 1986–1991.
Etiology	Unknown; testicular germinal cell tumors probably start in utero.
Risk factors	History of cryptorchid testis (20–40-fold increased risk); successful orchiopexy performed before 6 years of age reduces the risk. Klinefelter's syndrome History of previous testis tumor Isochrome of short arm of chromosome 12, i(12p) (80% of germ cell cases).

Histology	**Germ cell neoplasms** make up more than 95% of tumors; the remaining 5% are non-germ cell types (e.g., Sertoli and Leydig cells).
	 Two categories
	   Seminoma (40%)
	   Nonseminoma (60%)
	     • Embryonal
	     • Teratoma
	     • Yolk sac (endodermal sinus—most common in children)
	     • Choriocarcinoma (rare—1%)
	 40% of tumors are mixed (seminoma ± nonseminoma)

Symptoms	Patients usually present with mass, with or without pain. Often swelling has been present for > 3 months. Differential diagnosis includes varicocele, hydrocele, spermatocele, torsion, and epididymitis. Gynecomastia and low back pain (secondary to retroperitoneal lymph node involvement) are less common at presentation. Advanced disease: cough, dyspnea, headache, seizures.
Diagnosis and evaluation	Testicular examination: tumor is unlikely if the mass clearly separates from the body of the testis. Ultrasound examination Radical inguinal orchiectomy (removal of testis, epididymis, part of vas deferens, and parts of gonadal lymphatics and blood vessels) Tumor markers: beta human chorionic gonadotropin (BHCG), alpha-fetoprotein (AFP), and lactate dehydrogenase (LDH) Chest radiograph, CT scan of chest, abdomen, and pelvis Lymphangiogram (still done at times in some centers) for seminoma radiation planning
Staging	Tumor, node, metastasis (TNM) classification of the American Joint Committee on Cancer (AJCC)

Table continued on following page.

Quick Facts—Testicular Cancer (Continued)

Primary tumor (T)

The extent of primary tumor is classified after radical orchiectomy.

TX	Primary tumor cannot be assessed (if no radical orchiectomy has been performed, TX is used)
T0	No evidence of primary tumor (e.g., histologic scar in testis)
Ti	Intratubular tumor; preinvasive cancer
T1	Tumor limited to testis, including rete testis
T2	Tumor invades beyond tunica albuginea or into epididymis
T3	Tumor invades spermatic cord
T4	Tumor invades scrotum

Regional lymph nodes (N)

NX	Regional lymph nodes cannot be assessed
N0	No regional lymph node metastasis
N1	Metastasis in a single lymph node, 2 cm or less in greatest dimension
N2	Metastasis in a single lymph node, > 2 cm but not > 5 cm in greatest dimension, or multiple lymph nodes, none > 5 cm in greatest dimension
N3	Metastasis in lymph node > 5 cm in greatest dimension

Distant metastasis (M)

MX	Presence of distant metastasis cannot be assessed
M0	No distant metastasis
M1	Distant metastasis

AJCC stage groupings

Stage 0	Tis, N0, M0	
Stage I (40%)	Any T, N0, M0	Tumor limited to testis and adjacent structures
Stage II (40%)	Any T, N1, M0	Tumor beyond testis but not beyond regional retroperitoneal lymph nodes
	Any T, N2, M0	
	Any T, N3, M0	
Stage III (20%)	Any T, any N, M1	Disseminated metastasis beyond lymphatic drainage or above diaphragm

In addition to the clinical stage definitions, surgical stage may be designated based on the results of surgical removal and microscopic examination of tissue.

---

1. What is unique about testicular cancer?

Testicular carcinoma is the most curable solid tumor in adults (> 90% cure rate in patients with stage I or II disease). It is unique because even in late stages, testicular carcinoma can still be cured.

2. How often are patients with testes cancer diagnosed correctly on presentation?

Only 33% in one series. Delay in diagnosis from 1–3 months is not unusual because signs or symptoms are mistaken for benign abnormalities and patients delay seeking medical attention.

3. Is screening for testicular cancer of proven value?

The American Cancer Society recommends monthly testicular self-examination (TSE) starting at puberty; this approach has not been validated and continues to be controversial. Some researchers believe that the potential yield from TSE is outweighed by increased anxiety in an already body-conscious age group. Others believe that testicular examination provides an opportunity to initiate education and discussion about male sexuality and sexually transmitted diseases.

4. What raises the suspicion of cancer when a patient presents with a testicular mass?

The combination of gynecomastia, a swollen left supraclavicular lymph node, and testicular mass almost always means testicular cancer.

5. **How is an intrascrotal mass evaluated?**

Trauma and infection should be ruled out as a cause of intrascrotal pain or swelling.

1. Examine the patient for
   - Varicocele—vein engorgement within scrotum
   - Spermatocele—irregular grapelike sac
   - Hydrocele—accumulation of scrotal fluid
   - Torsion—swelling

2. Transilluminate the scrotum with a flashlight. Cysts such as hydroceles often appear transparent, whereas tumors appear dense.

6. **Why are needle biopsy and transscrotal orchiectomy contraindicated?**

Because of the dual risk of scrotal recurrence from implantation and inguinal spread from change in lymphatic drainage.

7. **Where does testis cancer spread?**

Retroperitoneal nodes are usually the first area of spread. With the exception of choriocarcinoma, hematogenous spread occurs later to lung, liver, and brain.

8. **What is the value of tumor markers?**

Tumor markers, such as AFP and BHCG help to identify nonseminomatous elements, predict prognosis (very high levels), determine residual disease after orchiectomy or retroperitoneal lymph node dissection (RPLND), confirm response to treatment, and detect recurrence. Almost 90% of nonseminomatous tumors have at least one abnormal marker. Patients with pure seminoma do not usually have elevated tumor markers. Occasionally BHCG is mildly elevated in seminoma (< 10% of patients). AFP elevations in seminoma indicate other nonseminomatous elements, whether or not the pathologist can confirm their presence. False-positive results are extremely rare except in marijuana users (BHCG may be elevated). AFP may be elevated in hepatoma or liver inflammation due to cirrhosis or hepatitis. Increased LDH levels may correlate with widespread disease.

9. **How reliable is the CT scan in staging retroperitoneal disease in patients with nonseminomatous tumors?**

About 20–25% of patients with clinical stage I disease are downstaged after RPLND. A similar percentage of patients with clinical stage II disease is upstaged.

10. **What prognostic factors are useful in patients with stage I nonseminoma?**

Vascular or lymphatic invasion, embryonal histology, and absence of yolk sac tumor/AFP negativity predict a higher relapse rate when patients are observed without RPLND after orchiectomy.

11. **When is observation after orchiectomy a reasonable treatment choice?**

Orchiectomy followed by RPLND yields an anticipated cure rate of 80–90% in patients with nonseminomatous disease and is under study in patients with seminoma. However, the morbidity associated with RPLND includes injury to nerves supplying the prostate, seminal vesicles, vasas, and bladder neck. Even if erectile potency is preserved, there may be reduction or loss of ejaculate. A nerve-sparing lymphadenectomy may be done to preserve ejaculation.

Observation with assessment of tumor markers every month and chest radiographs and CT scans every 2 months for 2 years yields a relapse rate of 27% and a salvage rate of > 90% with 3 or 4 cycles of platinum-based chemotherapy. However, this approach requires patient commitment and personal involvement of both nurses and physicians in follow-up.

12. **What prognostic classifications are commonly used for advanced testis cancer?**

Both Indiana University and Memorial Sloan-Kettering Cancer Center have classification systems based on a combination of tumor marker elevation, histology, and metastatic sites (number, size, and location). These systems are useful because patients with low risk or minimal disease (serum marker elevations only, small volume of infradiaphragmatic or supradiaphragmatic involvement) may need only three courses of chemotherapy. High-risk patients have disseminated testicular cancer and present with advanced pulmonary metastases; liver, bone, or central nervous system metastases; and palpable abdominal masses.

13. What is the standard treatment for seminoma?

A diagnosis of seminoma carries a good prognosis; the tumor is usually localized and is especially radiosensitive. All stages of seminoma require removal of the testicle by radical inguinal orchiectomy. After surgery, stage I and II patients have radiation therapy, and stage III patients receive combination cisplatin-based chemotherapy or radiation to the abdominal and pelvic lymph nodes.

14. Does radiation therapy still have a role in primary treatment of testis cancer?

Yes—in seminoma. Stage I patients typically receive radiation to the ipsilateral iliac and retroperitoneal lymph nodes. This treatment is curative in more than 95% of patients. Stage II nonbulky tumors (< 5 cm) are cured in more than 90% of patients by irradiation.

15. What is the impact of testis cancer and its treatment on fertility?

Sterility from chemotherapy, radiation therapy, and surgery are of major concern to young men diagnosed with testicular cancer. For unknown reasons, oligospermia, azoospermia, and Leydig cell dysfunction are often seen before treatment is initiated. Sperm banking may not be an option because of the urgency of chemotherapy and rapid tumor growth. Chemotherapy may affect spermatogenesis. Patients remain azoospermic for almost 1 year after therapy. Approximately 50% of patients regain both spermatogenesis and Leydig cell function within 2 years. About 33% of patients are able to father children. Oligospermia after radiation is usually reversible. Congenital malformations are not increased.

The size and location of the tumor may preclude the use of nerve-sparing retroperitoneal lymph node dissections. Fertility may be affected by retrograde "dry" ejaculation (ejaculate enters the bladder upon orgasm) due to the severing of the sympathetic plexus, which occurs in many patients undergoing retroperitoneal lymph node dissection.

16. When should chemotherapy be the initial treatment?

Patients with bulky seminoma and patients with stage III or bulky stage II (> 5 cm or palpable mass) nonseminomatous disease should receive treatment with 3–4 cycles of bleomycin, etoposide, and cisplatin (BEP). Three cycles should result in a long-term disease-free survival rate of > 85% if minimal metastatic disease is present. A recent trial comparing etoposide and cisplatin with either bleomycin or ifosfamide showed that high-risk patients need to receive four cycles and have a disease-free survival rate of > 50%.

17. What is the role of retroperitoneal lymph node dissection in nonseminomatous patients after orchiectomy?

Retroperitoneal lymph node dissection (RPLND) as part of the initial therapy is controversial because of its morbidity and lack of survival benefit in comparison with chemotherapy. Many oncologists believe that it is adequate simply to follow the tumor markers after orchiectomy. If weekly tumor marker values return to normal after orchiectomy, monthly follow-up (e.g., tumor markers, frequent radiologic exams) for 2–3 years should be sufficient. However, if the marker does not return to normal after orchiectomy or rises after an initial decrease, chemotherapy may be instituted immediately even if no discernible disease can be found. RPLND is indicated after chemotherapy when discernible residual disease is found and markers are normal. Fibrosis/necrosis, cancer and/or teratoma may be found during this surgical procedure. Unresected teratoma may transform into malignancy and needs to be removed.

18. What acute and long-term toxicities are associated with chemotherapy for testicular cancer?

Gastrointestinal effects (nausea and vomiting), renal effects (decreased creatinine clearance and tubular loss of sodium, potassium, and magesium), and bone marrow depression are the major acute toxicities associated with chemotherapy. Long-term toxicities include:

- Bleomycin pneumonitis
  (rarely fatal if < 400 units are given)
- Peripheral neuropathies
- Cisplatin-induced hearing loss
- Sterility
- Secondary acute myelogenous leukemia
  (related to etoposide; typically shows 11q23 translocation; incidence < 5% at 5 years).

19. If a patient has persistent disease after therapy with BEP, what are the options for salvage treatment?

Patients who fail primary chemotherapy may be salvaged with vinblastine, cisplatin, and ifosfamide (20–45%). Surgery also may have a role. High-dose chemotherapy with peripheral stem cell transplant using etoposide/carboplatin with or without cyclophosphamide or ifosfamide offers a limited potential for cure.

20. What are the significant nursing implications in caring for patients with testicular cancer?

Because all types of testicular cancer require that patients undergo radical inguinal orchiectomy for diagnostic and therapeutic purposes and possibly RPLND for nonseminoma, nurses need to address concerns about body image and fear of sexual dysfunction. Patients are scared of the surgical consequences and toxicities of radiation or chemotherapy. They need careful exploration of fears, explanation and correction of unfounded concerns, and reassurance of positive outcomes. Patients may be so afraid of sexual dysfunction that they refuse potentially curative therapies. Patients need to be prepared about the effect of the orchiectomy on genital appearance and about the possibility of retrograde ejaculation after RPLND. Inform patients about testicular prostheses and, if indicated, make appropriate referrals. (See chapter 43 for information about sexual counseling, retrograde ejaculation, and sperm banking.)

The views contained in this manuscript are solely those of the author and do not reflect the views or policies of Tripler Army Medical Command, the Department of Defense, or the U.S. Government.

BIBLIOGRAPHY

1. American Cancer Society: Cancer Facts and Figures 1997. Atlanta, American Cancer Society, 1997.
2. Bajorin DF, Bosl GJ: The use of serum tumor markers in the prognosis and treatment of germ cell tumors. Cancer: Principles and Practice of Oncology Updates 6:1–11, 1992.
3. Beahrs OH, Henson DE, Hutter RVP, Kennedy BJ: Manual for Staging of Cancer. Philadelphia, J.B. Lippincott, 1992.
4. Bokemeyer C, Schmoll H: Treatment of testicular cancer and the development of secondary malignancies. J Clin Oncol 13:283–292, 1995.
5. Brock D, Fox S, Gosling G, et al: Testicular cancer. Semin Oncol Nurs 9:224–236, 1993.
6. Droz JP, Kramer A, Rey A: Prognostic factors in metastatic disease. Semin Oncol 19:181, 1992.
7. Fox EP, Weathers TD, Williams SD, et al: Outcome analysis for patients with persistent nonteratomatous germ cell tumor in postchemotherapy retroperitoneal lymph node dissections. J Clin Oncol 11:1294–1299, 1993.
8. Hawkins C, Miaskowski J: Testicular cancer: A review. Oncol Nurs Forum 23:1203–1213, 1996.
9. Loerher PJ, Einhorn LH, Elson P, et al: Phase II study of cisplatin plus etoposide with either bleomycin or ifosfamide in advanced stage germ cell tumors: An intergroup trial. Proc Am Soc Clin Oncol 12:262, 1993.
10. Munshi NC, Loehrer PJ, Roth BJ, et al: Vinblastine, ifosfamide and cisplatin (VeIP) as second line chemotherapy in metastatic germ cell tumors (GCT). Proc Am Soc Clin Oncol 9:A-520, 134, 1990.
11. Parker SL, Tong T, Bolden S, Wingo PA: Cancer Statistics, 1997. CA Cancer J Clin 47:5–27, 1997.
12. Sesterhenn IA, Weiss RB, Mostofi FK, et al: Prognosis and other clinical correlates of pathologic review in stage I and II testicular carcinoma: A report from the Testicular Cancer Intergroup Study. J Clin Oncol 10:69–78, 1992.
13. Stephenson WT, Poirier SM, Rubin L, et al: Evaluation of reproductive capacity in germ cell tumor patients following treatment with cisplatin, etoposide, and bleomycin. J Clin Oncol 13:2278–2280, 1995.
14. Williams SD, Birch R, Einhorn LH, et al: Treatment of disseminated germ-cell tumors with cisplatin, bleomycin, and either vinblastine or etoposide. N Engl J Med 316:1435–1440, 1987.

V. Symptom Management

33. CONSTIPATION

Leslie Tuchmann, RN, MSN

1. Define constipation. How common is it in patients with cancer?
Constipation is defined as a decrease in frequency of defecation accompanied by difficulty and discomfort. Some define constipation as the passage of fewer than three stools per week. As a subjective symptom, assessment *must* take into account the individual's previous elimination pattern. In comparison, obstipation is a more severe degree of constipation with no bowel movement and large volumes of stool are present throughout the bowel. Constipation occurs in approximately one-half of patients with cancer and in over three-fourths of terminally ill patients. It is more common in women and elderly patients.

2. How are the causes of constipation classified?
Primary: related to extrinsic factors, such as lifestyle factors. Examples: age, inadequate privacy or time to defecate, low-fiber diet, depression, dehydration, decreased activity and exercise, weakness and poor muscle tone, lack of energy to defecate.

Secondary: related to another primary problem or disease process, such as cancer. Examples: tumors that compress spinal nerve roots innervating the bowel; spinal cord compression at T8–L3; cauda equina compression from epidural metastases; metabolic effects (hypercalcemia, hypokalemia, uremia, hypothyroidism); and diseases other than cancer (e.g., diabetes).

Iatrogenic: resulting from the use of pharmacologic agents or medical interventions (probably the most common type in patients with cancer). Examples: opioids, radiation therapy complications, surgical anastomosis (may lead to narrowing of the colon lumen from scarring).

3. What are the major consequences of constipation?

Abdominal discomfort	Inflammation of hemorrhoids
Nausea and/or vomiting	Rupture of the bowel
Rectal fissures and tears	Obstruction

Reluctance or refusal to take opioids because of constipating effects, which results in poor pain control and decreased quality of life.

4. What factors should be included in assessing the potential for and evaluating the severity of constipation?
- Comprehensive history and physical examination, including extent of the patient's cancer and understanding of past and current therapy
- Previous pattern of bowel elimination: frequency, amount, timing
- Last bowel movement: when, amount, consistency, color, presence of blood
- Abdominal discomfort: pain, cramping, nausea, vomiting, excessive gas, rectal fullness
- Type of diet
- Amount of fluids and what type
- Previous regular laxative or enema use and its effect
- Present medications: dosages and frequency

- Whether symptom is a recent change
- Patient's understanding and compliance with fluid, fruit, and fiber intake
- Exercise, functional status, and level of mobility

5. What should be incorporated into the physical examination of constipated patients?
- Abdomen should be assessed for bowel sounds, tenderness, masses, or palpable stool-filled colon.
- The perineal region should be evaluated. Rectal (or stoma) exam is indicated to rule out hemorrhoids, fecal impaction, or rectal malignancy.
- Hemoccult test may be helpful. A positive result may be an early warning of an intraluminal lesion.
- Laboratory tests (electrolytes, complete blood count, renal and liver tests, levels of thyroid-stimulating hormone) assist in metabolic evaluation.
- Radiographs in both supine and upright positions may help to differentiate between mechanical obstruction and decreased motility from an ileus.
- Ultrasound and/or CT scan of abdomen and pelvis is usually ordered if an extraluminal site is suspected.
- Barium enema and endoscopy are tests of choice if intraluminal site is suspected.

6. How is constipation best managed?
Prevention is the key to effective management of constipation. It is important to identify the cause and its relationship to cancer and to reverse the cause if possible. Treatment may involve nonpharmacologic and pharmacologic interventions.

7. What nonpharmacologic interventions help to prevent constipation?
Teaching patients and families the following interventions can be helpful; most people are unaware of how these factors relate to constipation.

1. **Increase fiber in the diet.** Warn patients that they may experience abdominal discomfort, flatulence, or erratic bowel habits in first few weeks. Tolerance will develop, and such effects can be minimized by slowly titrating fiber upward, starting with the addition of 3–4 gm of fiber/day and increasing to 6–10 gm/day. This approach may be contraindicated in patients whose constipation results from structural blockage of the bowel because increasing bulky intraluminal contents may increase the obstruction.

2. **Increase fluid intake.** Increasing fluids may be difficult for patients experiencing nausea, vomiting, anorexia, and/or fatigue. However, an increase of approximately 6–8 glasses of water/day (1–2 L) helps to keep stool soft. Suggest carrying a water bottle at all times to sip on fluids (especially between meals). Coffee, tea, and grapefruit juice are usually discouraged because they act as diuretics. However, some form of warm liquid before a defecation attempt may be helpful.

3. **Establish a routine.** Regular toilet activities after breakfast are most productive because propulsive contractions in the intestine are strongest. The use of raised toilet seats, footstools, and bedside commodes may be helpful. Ensure privacy.

4. **Increase exercise.** Gastrointestinal motility is diminished by immobility and stimulated by regular exercise (e.g., 30-minute walk/day). Teaching patients simple diaphragmatic breathing and abdominal muscle exercises, which may assist in strengthening and increasing muscle tone, is necessary for defecation.

8. Which home remedies are useful for treating constipation?
Anti-Constipation Fruit Paste
  3 cups prune juice
  3 cups applesauce
  ½ cup bran
Mix ingredients together and keep in refrigerator. Take 30–60 cc daily.

Anti-Constipation Fruit Paste
   Dose: 1–2 tablespoons per day
      1 lb prunes   4 oz senna tea
      1 lb raisins—pitted   1 cup brown sugar
      1 lb figs   1 cup lemon juice
   1. Prepare tea. Use about 2½ cups boiled water added to tea and steep 5 minutes.
   2. Strain tea to remove tea leaves, and add only 1 pint tea to a large pot; then add fruit.
   3. Boil fruit and tea for 5 minutes.
   4. Remove from heat, and add sugar and lemon juice. Allow to cool.
   5. Use hand mixer or food processor to turn fruit mixture into smooth paste.
   6. Place in glass jars or plasticware, and place in freezer. (Paste will not freeze but will keep indefinitely in freezer.)

9. Are prunes or prune juice the best items to increase dietary fiber and aid in constipation?
   A common misconception in treating constipation is the belief that patients should consume prunes or prune juice as their primary source of increased dietary fiber. In fact, prunes contain only 2 gm of fiber, and prune juice contains very little. Prunes also contain phenolphthalein and may cause cathartic colon (narrowing of the ileum and proximal colon in addition to loss of colonic muscle tone) with prolonged use. Better high-fiber recommendations include wheat bran (in breads and cereals), beans, broccoli, sweet potatoes, carrots, and dried apricots.

Food	Dietary fiber
Wheat bran (3 tbsp)	10 gm
Bran flakes (100 gm)	2.7–6.5 gm
Whole wheat bread (1 slice)	1–2 gm

10. List the common laxatives and cathartics, their mechanism of action, contraindications, adverse effects, and drug interactions.
   See table on pages 220–223.

11. What helpful hints may optimize the administration of specific constipation medicines?
   Psyllium, methylcellulose, and polycarbophil. Give with adequate (8 oz) fluid to minimize risk of intestinal or esophageal obstruction. Allow at least 3 hours before and after administration of other drugs to minimize potential interactions. Citrucel is the least gritty of these agents; it is also sodium-free and should be used for patients on a sodium-restricted diet.
   Diphenylmethanes. Phenolphthalein is more potent than bisacodyl. Because bisacodyl is packaged as enteric-coated tablets, it should not be given within 1 hour of ingesting milk or antacids; it should be swallowed whole and not chewed. Bisacodyl also has a strong stimulatory effect, which may be helpful for refractory opioid-induced constipation.
   Anthraquinones. One Senekot tablet reverses the constipating effect of 120 mg of codeine. Warn patients of urine discoloration (yellowish brown or reddish, depending on urinary pH). Cascara sagrada fluid extract is 5 times more potent than cascara sagrada aromatic fluid extract. Cascara is the mildest form of anthraquinone and rarely causes colic.
   Lactulose, sorbitol, and polyethylene glycol electrolyte solutions. Lactulose's sweet taste may be more palatable mixed with fruit juice, water, or milk; it also may be given as an enema. If lactulose is administered through gastric or feeding tubes, it should be diluted in 60–120 ml of water. Chronulac is the preferred form for chronic constipation. Sorbitol is equally effective but less expensive—and may be less nauseating than lactulose. Golytely (8–16 oz/day) is reserved for resistant chronic constipation; it should be used within 48 hours of preparation. Chill before use.
   Glycerin. Glycerin is usually given high in the rectum and held for 15 minutes.
   Mineral oil. Mineral oil should be taken on an empty stomach.

Docusate. Surfak (docusate calcium) is preferred over Colace (docusate sodium) for patients with salt and fluid retention. It should be taken with a full glass of water, and total daily fluid intake should be increased.

Magnesium salts. Magnesium salts should be chilled and the taste disguised in fruit juice or a citrus-flavored carbonated beverage. Magnesium citrate is best taken on an empty stomach (e.g., on rising in the morning, 30 minutes before meals, or at bedtime for overnight action.)

12. How do you know which laxative to start with?

A stepwise approach to using laxatives for constipation begins with bulk-forming agents (not recommended in counteracting bowel effects of opioids); then add or change to docusate. Although some providers believe doses of docusate > 200 mg may yield little benefit, the palliative care literature notes use of up to 300 mg 3 times/day with positive effect. If docusate produces no result, add senna or cascara (docusate and senna are frequently used in combination for opioid-induced constipation). If these combinations are ineffective, switch to lactulose or sorbitol. The last step is use of magnesium citrate or Golytely; however, referral to a gastroenterologist may be indicated before using either agent. Drug and dosage selection should be based on patient condition, drug response, and tolerance of side effects. Once medications have been used at maximal doses with little effect, switch to medications in the next step of the ladder rather than adding several medications from different steps. It is usually best to allow 2 days for the intervention to work. Titrate the regimen to produce a bowel movement every 1–2 days. For patients who have not had a bowel movement in 3 days, a rectal exam is indicated. Digital disimpaction, followed by suppositories or enemas, may be necessary. After success with this type of treatment, escalate the maintenance regimen.

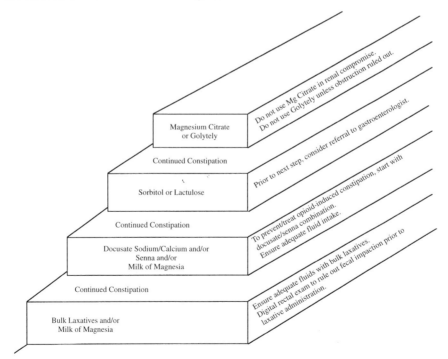

Ladder indicating appropriate steps in the use of constipation medications. Advance to the next step after exceeding the upper-limit dose. Allow two days for intervention to work. (Chart created by Thomas Loughney, MD, and Leslie Tuchmann, RN.)

Constipation Medications: Laxatives and Cathartics

	DRUG	MECHANISM OF ACTION
Bulk Formers	Psyllium (Metamucil) Methylcellulose (Cologel, Citrucel) Polycarbophil Onset of effect: 12 hr–3 days	Nondigested plant cell walls absorb water in feces; softens, increases stool size, thus increasing peristalsis; acts in small and large intestines.

Bowel Stimulants	**Diphenylmethanes**
	  Phenolphthalein (in Ex-lax, Feen-a-mint, Correctol, Doxidan)
	  Bisacodyl (Dulcolax): 5 mg enteric-coated tablet orally 1–3 times/day; 10-mg suppository (single dose as needed)
	Onset of effect: 6–10 hr; Rectally: 15–60 min
	
	Arthraquinones
	  Senna (Senekot, X-Prep): 187 mg tablet; daily maximum of 8 tablets or 4 tsp granules (326 mg)/day
	  Cascara Sagrada (aromatic): 5 ml or 1 tablet (325 mg) at bedtime as needed
	  Casanthranol (cascara derivative): 30 mg, usually in combination with docusate
	Onset of effect: 6–12 hours
		Directly stimulates nerve plexus of colon.
		Irritates smooth muscle of intestine, stimulating peristalsis.
		Phenolphthalein and Bisacodyl first metabolized in liver, then colon; effect may be prolonged.
		
		Exact mechanism unknown; may stimulate colon and myenteric plexus.
		Senna stimulates submucosal nerve plexus and peristalsis in transverse and descending colon, decreases sodium and water absorption; produces semiliquid or formed stool
		Cascara directly irritates intestinal mucosa, results in motility and changes in fluid and electrolyte secretion

Osmotic Laxatives	Lactulose
	  Cephulac: 30–45 ml 3 or 4 times/day or hourly to induce rapid effect in initial phase
	  Chronulac: 15–30 ml/day; may increase to 60 ml/day
	  Sorbitol: 3–150 ml/day (70% solution)
	
	Polyethylene glycol electrolyte solution (Colyte, Golytely): 8 oz orally every 15 min as tolerated over 3–4 hr until 1 L taken or diarrhea results
	Onset of effect:
	  Lactulose: 24–48 hr
	  Polyethylene glycol: first bowel movement within 1 hr
	Glycerin: rectal suppositories, 1–2/day as needed, or 5–15 ml as enema
	Onset of effect: within 30 min of use
		Lactulose/Sorbitol: nonabsorbable sugars; exert osmotic effect mostly in large bowel
		Lactulose also used in hepatic encephalopathy to lower serum ammonia
		
		Polyethylene glycol: catharsis by strong electrolyte and osmotic effects
		
		Lubricates and softens
		Stimulates defecation osmotically; sodium stearate in suppository may irritate rectal membranes

Lubricants	Mineral oil: 15–40 ml/day orally (once or in divided doses); as retention enema: 60–150 ml/day as single dose Onset of effect: within 8 hr	Lubricates intestinal mucosa and feces; softens stool by preventing loss of water from feces

Columns continued on following page.

Constipation Medications: Laxatives and Cathartics (Columns Continued)

CONTRAINDICATIONS	ADVERSE EFFECTS	DRUG INTERACTIONS
Intestinal strictures, partial or total bowel obstruction or fecal impaction, phenylketonuria Advanced cancer with early satiety, nausea, anorexia Caution in diabetics due to sugar content	Flatulence, erratic habits, abdominal discomfort or initiation	May decrease effects of tetracycline, anticoagulants, digitalis glycosides or salicylates, nitrofurantoin
Bowel obstruction Phenolphthalein less suitable in cancer patient because major GI peristaltic effect difficult to predict and control Bisacodyl: abdominal pain	Phenolphthalein: diarrhea, cramps, skin reactions, photosensitivity, hypersensitivity-type encephalitis Bisacodyl: cramps, urgency, incontinence	Bisacodyl decreases effect of warfarin
Bowel obstruction	Cathartic colon, may result in intestinal atony Fluid and electrolyte disturbances	Cascara decreases effect of oral anticoagulants
Lactulose/Sorbitol: avoid with fecal impaction or intestinal obstruction Caution with severe cardiopulmonary and renal impairment (contraindicated in anuria) May cause elevations in blood glucose levels in diabetics	Lactulose: cramps, flatulence, nausea, vomiting; excessive use may cause electrolyte losses, diarrhea Chronulac: gas from bacterial degradation Sorbitol: edema, nausea, vomiting, diarrhea, abdominal discomfort, potential fluid and electrolyte loss	Decreased effect of neomycin, other anti-infectives, and antacids
Golytely: do not give with bowel obstruction (high risk for perforation), toxic colitis, megacolon, gastric retention, bowel perforation	Polyethylene glycol: nausea, abdominal fullness, bloating, cramps	Do not give oral medications within 1 hr of Golytely
Abdominal pain, nausea, vomiting	May cause rectal irritation if used too frequently; headache	
Known reflux, dysphagia (risk of lipid pneumonia or aspiration pneumonitis, especially in elderly)	Excessive use may lead to anal leakage and irritation Chronic use reduces absorption of fat-soluble vitamins Lipid pneumonitis with aspiration	Docusate sodium increases absorption and risk of lipid granuloma of gut wall Alters absorption of antibiotics, anticoagulants, oral contraceptives, digitalis glycosides

Table continued on following page.

Constipation Medications: Laxatives and Cathartics (Continued)

DRUG	MECHANISM OF ACTION
Detergent Laxatives Docusate: 50–500 mg/day in 1 to 4 doses Docusate sodium = Colace Docusate calcium = Surfak Onset of effect: 24–72 hr	Decreases surface tension and allows water and fat penetration of hard stool Mucosal contact effect decreases electrolyte and water reabsorption in small and large intestines

Saline Laxatives Magnesium (Mg) salts
   Mg citrate: 1/2–1 full bottle (120–300 ml) orally as needed
   Mg hydroxide (e.g., Milk of Magnesia Regular Strength): 30–60 ml/day orally or in divided doses
Sodium (Na) salts
   Sodium phosphate
      Fleet Phospho-soda: 20–30 ml as single dose
      Fleet enema: 4.5 oz enema; may repeat
Onset of effect:
   Mg citrate: 30 min–6 hr, depending on dose
   Mg hydroxide: 4–8 hr
   Sodium phosphate: Oral: 3–6 hr
      Rectal: 2–5 min
	Mg increases gastric, pancreatic, small intestine secretion and motor activity of small and large intestines
	Mg and Na salts are poorly absorbed and draw water into lumen, thus increasing stool water content and frequency

Columns continued on following page.

13. How do opioids affect the bowel?

Opioids are a *major* cause of cancer-related constipation. Opioid-induced constipation is thought to be dose-related, but variability among individual patients is considerable. Opioids affect the bowel by activation of specific opioid receptors in both the gastrointestinal tract and central nervous system. Activation of these receptors results in increased tone and nonpropulsive motility in the ileum and colon, resulting in increased transit time and water absorption. Difficult passage of hard dry stool is the end result. Morphine-induced insensitivity to rectal distention further contributes to slowed defecation.

14. Do patients develop a tolerance to the constipating effects of opioids?

Tolerance to this side effect of opioids develops extremely slowly, if at all. It is not uncommon for patients to require laxative therapy for as long as they are taking opioids.

15. Other than opioids, what medications cause constipation?

Numerous medications contribute to constipation. Unfortunately, patients frequently take more than one at a time, further compounding the problem:

Chemotherapy (vinca alkaloids, cisplatin, etoposide)   Diuretics
Antiemetics (serotonin antagonists, phenothiazines)   Calcium channel blockers
Anticonvulsants   Antiparkinsonian agents
Anticholinergics   Iron supplements
Tricyclic antidepressants

16. How do the vinca alkaloids cause constipation?

Vincristine may damage the myenteric plexus of the colon. Severe constipation may occur in up to 35% of patients. It is more common in elderly patients and may lead to bowel obstruction. Constipation has been reported in 20% of patients receiving vinblastine, especially in high doses or with prolonged treatment. Both vincristine and vinblastine may cause neurotoxicity of smooth muscles of the gastrointestinal tract, which may lead to decreased peristalsis or paralytic ileus. The bowel effects of vinca alkaloids may be unaccompanied by peripheral nerve dysfunction.

Constipation Medications: Laxatives and Cathartics (Columns Continued)

CONTRAINDICATIONS	ADVERSE EFFECTS	DRUG INTERACTIONS
Intestinal obstruction, acute abdominal pain, nausea, or vomiting	Diarrhea, abdominal cramps Prolonged use may lead to dependence or electrolyte imbalance	Increases mineral oil absorption Decreases effect of Coumadin and aspirin
Fecal impaction, intestinal obstruction, nausea, vomiting, abdominal pain Avoid Mg salts in renal failure, myocardial damage, heart block, hepatitis, ileostomy, colostomy Avoid Na salts in cardiac or renal disease, hyperphosphatemia, hypernatremia, hypocalcemia; use with caution if diet is sodium-restricted	Mg salts: excessive use may cause electrolyte losses, hypermagnesemia, diarrhea, cramps, gas Na salts: nausea, vomiting, diarrhea, edema, hypotension; excessive use may cause dependence	Effects of Mg counteracted by aluminum salt in many antacids Milk of Magnesia decreases absorption of tetracyclines, digoxin, indomethacin, or iron salts Na phosphate: do not give with Mg or aluminum-containing antacids or sucralfate; they may bind with phosphate

Vinorelbine causes mild-to-moderate constipation with an overall incidence of 34%. Vindesine, which is currently under investigation, is a semisynthetic vinca alkaloid known to have constipating effects but to a lesser extent than vincristine. Combinations of a laxative and stool softener may be used prophylactically with the vinca alkaloids to avoid constipation.

17. How should constipation be managed in neutropenic or thrombocytopenic patients?

Constipation in neutropenic or thrombocytopenic patients requires an increase in fluids and fiber and management with oral medications. Avoid manipulation (rectal exams, suppositories, enemas) of the anus or stoma in neutropenic patients, because it may lead to anal fissures or abscesses, which serve as a portal of entry for infection. Manipulation also may put the thrombocytopenic patient at risk for bleeding. If the anal area must be manipulated, it should be done gently, using a generous amount of lubricant. The use of suppositories or enemas is contraindicated.

18. What is the origin of laxative misuse?

The belief that one needs to have a "normal" number of bowel movements per day, as well as the myth that laxatives "cleanse the blood" or eliminate "corrupt humors" from absorbed colonic contents, has led to the steady sales of laxative agents. However, as long as the liver is functioning properly, intoxication does not result from intestinal contents. The use of bulk substances as a supplement to low-residue diets is not a problem. However, chronic use of irritant purgatives or cathartics may be dangerous because of potentially serious electrolyte imbalances (e.g., hypokalemia resulting in cardiac arrhythmias).

19. Discuss the physiological and psychological bases of laxative dependence.

The natural defecation reflex, which empties the large bowel from the descending colon downward, is triggered when the sigmoid colon and rectum are full. The reflex is not triggered again until the colon segments are refilled. Unlike the natural reflex, large-bowel irritant purgatives (anthraquinone derivatives such as senna and diphenylmethane derivatives such as bisacodyl and phenolphthalein) clear the entire colon. As a result, the interval to refill the sigmoid colon and rectum lengthens; in this interval, patients become concerned that they are constipated and believe they need the assistance of a laxative to move their bowels. Thus, they use the laxative repeatedly; repeated use continues to empty the entire colon; and a vicious cycle begins. It is important to instruct patients to expect a "compensatory pause" after discontinuing laxative therapy. In addition, an actual physiologic bowel inertia may result from laxative-induced hypokalemia, leading the person to mistake decreased peristalsis for constipation and to reinitiate laxative therapy.

20. Why are combination laxatives, such as Senekot-S or Peri-Colace, better than Colace alone for opioid-induced constipation?

Colace softens the stool but usually does not provide the peristaltic stimulation needed to counteract opioid-induced constipation. By combining the softening action of docusate with the peristaltic stimulant effect of the anthraquinone derivatives (i.e., senna concentrate, casanthranol), success in managing opioid-induced constipation may be achieved. Patients need to be instructed to consume adequate amounts of fluids while using these medications. Examples of combination medications include the following:

Senekot-S = senna concentrate and docusate sodium

Peri-Colace = casanthranol and docusate sodium

A useful formula for the prevention of opioid-induced constipation is:

1 Senekot tablet + 100-mg tablet of Colace per 30-mg tablet of MS Contin

Titrate to effect.

21. What types of enemas can be used safely in patients with cancer?

Enemas tend to be used for the management of acute constipation or fecal impaction. Use caution in administering enemas, because they may place the patient at risk for bowel perforation due to previous bowel wall irritation from impaction and electrolyte imbalance, particularly in the setting of renal failure.

Commonly recommended enemas
- Tap water or saline enemas
- Water-soluble lubricant enema. Fill a 60-ml syringe with water-soluble lubricant (Surgilube), replace plunger, and attach rectal tube to syringe. Lubricate tip of tube and place tip inside rectum. Slowly inject, as for retention enema. Retain for one-half hour.
- Milk and molasses enema. To 1 liter of warm water, add 1 cup of powdered milk and 1 cup of molasses or corn syrup.

Enemas that should be avoided or used with caution
- Fleet enemas are reported to cause tissue necrosis and are not safe in patients with renal or cardiac disease.
- Soap suds enemas are no longer used because of the risk of acute colitis (usually self-limiting). More serious potential complications include anaphylaxis, hemorrhage and rectal gangrene.

22. What is the safest way to treat impaction?

The first step in treatment for impaction is softening the stool so that it can be gently removed or passed. Enemas (oil retention, tap water, or hypertonic phosphate) or glycerin suppositories assist in lubrication of bowel and softening of stool. Laxatives that stimulate the bowel or cause cramping should be avoided to prevent further damage to the bowel wall. Digital disimpaction, if needed, is best done after lubrication with an enema or glycerin suppository. Because of the discomfort associated with disimpaction, some form of analgesia is recommended before the procedure; a light sedative may be indicated as well.

The views contained in this manuscript are solely those of the author and do not reflect the views or the policies of Tripler Army Medical Command, the Department of Defense, or the U.S. Government.

ACKNOWLEDGMENT

The author thanks Thomas Loughney, MD, Department of Medicine, Gastroenterology Service, Tripler Army Medical Center, for his critical review and assistance.

BIBLIOGRAPHY

1. Billings JA: Outpatient Management of Advanced Cancer: Symptom Control, Support and Hospice-in-the-Home. Philadelphia, J. B. Lippincott, 1985.
2. Brogden JM, Nevidjon B: Vinorelbine tartrate (Navelbine): Drug profile and nursing implications of a new vinca alkaloid. Oncol Nurs Forum 22:635–646, 1995.
3. Lacy C, Armstrong LL, Ingrim N, Lance LL: Drug Information Handbook, 3rd ed. Hudson, OH, Lexi-Comp Inc., 1995
4. Levy M: Constipation and diarrhea in cancer patients. Cancer Bull 43:412–422, 1991.
5. Lullmann H, Mohr K, Ziegler A, Bieger D: Pocket Atlas of Pharmacology. New York, Thieme Medical Publishers, 1993.
6. Maguire LC, Yon JL, Miller E: Prevention of narcotic-induced constipation. N Engl J Med 305:1651, 1981.
7. Perry MC: The Chemotherapy Source Book, 2nd ed. Baltimore, Williams & Wilkins, 1996.
8. Portenoy R: Constipation in the cancer patient: Causes and management. Med Clin North Am 71:303–311, 1987.
9. Rousseau P: Treatment of constipation in the elderly. Postgrad Med 83:339–349, 1988.
10. Storey P: Primer of Palliative Care. Gainesville, FL, Academy of Hospice Physicians, 1994.
11. Yakabowich M: Prescribe with care: The role of laxatives in the treatment of constipation. J Gerontol Nurs 6(7):4–11, 1990.
12. Yasko JM (ed): Nursing Management of Symptoms Associated with Chemotherapy, 3rd ed. Philadelphia, Meniscus Health Care Communications, 1993, pp 118–120.

34. DIARRHEA

Leslie Tuchmann, RN, MSN

1. How is diarrhea defined? What are the clinical signs?

Diarrhea is an increase in the liquidity and frequency (> 3 stools/day) of stool and passage of > 200 gm of stool/day. High volumes of stool output, up to 8–10 L/day, may occur in bone marrow transplant patients and patients with graft vs. host disease. Diarrhea may result in signs of volume depletion, such as orthostatic hypotension, decreased skin turgor, and dry mouth. Uncontrolled diarrhea may result in massive potassium and bicarbonate loss and severe perianal irritation.

2. How prevalent is diarrhea in patients with cancer? What are the major causes?

Diarrhea is found in 6% of hospitalized cancer patients, 10% of advanced cancer patients, and 43% of patients undergoing bone marrow transplant. Causes of acute diarrhea (sudden onset lasting a few days) include infection, drug-induced reactions, diet alterations (antacid use), heavy metal poisoning, and fecal impaction. Causes of chronic diarrhea (persisting over 3 weeks) include colon cancer; neuroendocrine tumors such as tumors of the parathyroid, pituitary, pancreatic islet cells (vipoma, gastrinoma), pheochromocytoma, medullary thyroid carcinoma; carcinoid syndrome; radiation enterocolitis; malabsorption diseases; laxative abuse; and chemotherapeutic agents. The most common type of large-volume diarrhea in patients with cancer is iatrogenic (e.g. chemotherapy, radiation therapy, surgery, antibiotics). The most common type of diarrhea in the palliative care setting is related to imbalance of laxative therapy.

3. What are the common mechanisms of diarrhea?

Up to 90% of patients receiving radiation therapy and/or chemotherapy experience diarrhea, which commonly presents as a mixture of osmotic and secretory types.

- **Osmotic.** Unabsorbable substances draw water into the intestinal lumen by osmosis and result in increased stool volume and weight. Osmotic diarrhea typically lessens after stopping the causative drug or fasting for 2–3 days. Osmotic diarrhea may be caused by insufficient lactase related to genetic deficiency (lactose intolerance) or prolonged absence of lactase due to infection, obstruction, or mucosal damage from either chemotherapy or radiation. Pancreatectomy may result in fat malabsorption and thus osmotic steatorrhea.
- **Secretory.** Excessive intestinal mucosal secretion of electrolytes and fluids is usually caused by toxins from bacteria (*Escherichia coli* or *Clostridium difficile*) or hormone-producing neoplasms. Because secretory diarrhea usually has nothing to do with food intake, it persists despite fasting.
- **Hypermotility.** Suspected after osmotic or secretory diarrhea is ruled out, hypermotility diarrhea usually results from disorders that affect motility of the intestine such as irritable bowel syndrome, neurologic diseases, and medications (e.g., metoclopramide, cisapride). Excessive fatty acids can also stimulate motility diarrhea, whereas incomplete fat digestion in the small intestine acts as an osmotic agent.
- **Exudative/inflammatory.** The mechanism may be malabsorption or intestinal secretion. Positive test for cell count or occult blood suggests an exudative mechanism as in infective diarrhea, radiation colitis, or colonic neoplasm.

4. Which chemotherapy or biotherapy drugs cause diarrhea?

Chemotherapy-induced diarrhea is related to destruction of actively dividing epithelial cells of the gastrointestinal tract. Degree and duration depend on agents used, dosage, and frequency of administration. Chemotherapy agents with the highest risk for diarrhea are 5-fluorouracil (in high doses or in combination with leucovorin, methotrexate, or interferon), actinomycin D, and topoisomerase inhibitors (irinotecan, topotecan), and paclitaxel (Taxol). Other agents that cause diarrhea (> 10%) are fludarabine, cytarabine, idarubicin, mithramycin, mitoxantrone, pentostatin, and floxuridine. Diarrhea occurring with administration of 5-FU and floxuridine is a sign of toxicity. Temporary discontinuation of these drugs is required. With other agents, dose reduction on subsequent cycles or discontinuation may be indicated, depending on chemotherapy schedule and diarrhea severity. Biotherapy drugs that cause diarrhea include interleukin-2, interleukin-4, and interferons.

5. What is *Clostridium difficile* diarrhea?

C. difficile diarrhea is an example of infection-induced diarrhea and should be suspected after any antibiotic therapy, particularly ampicillin, cephalosporins, and clindamycin. *C. difficile* makes enterotoxins that produce watery diarrhea associated with pseudomembranous colitis; symptoms range from mild diarrhea to life-threatening illness. *C. difficile* is the cause of > 50% of nosocomial infectious diarrhea. After a patient has tested positive for *C. difficile* and production of toxin A, precautions should be taken to prevent nosocomial transmission. An important point in treating infectious diarrhea is to *avoid* anticholinergic agents or opiates because they slow peristalsis and inhibit elimination of pathogens from the gastrointestinal system, causing prolonged and severe symptoms. *C. difficile* diarrhea is usually treated with metronidazole or oral vancomycin.

6. How is the severity of diarrhea determined?

Assessment parameters for diarrheal stools include duration, frequency, consistency, and amount (total stool volume); presence of blood, mucus, or pus; and incontinence. The table below outlines the National Cancer Institute (NCI) criteria for grading the severity of diarrhea.

National Cancer Institute Criteria for Grading the Severity of Diarrhea

	GRADE 0	GRADE 1	GRADE 2	GRADE 3	GRADE 4
Increased number of loose stools per day	Normal	2–3	4–6	7–9	10
			and/or	*and/or*	*and/or*
Symptoms			Nocturnal stools	Incontinence	Grossly bloody diarrhea
			and/or	*and/or*	*and/or*
			Moderate cramping	Severe cramping	Need for parenteral support

7. What factors are important to consider in the assessment of diarrhea?

For all patients, obtain a thorough history and physical examination with particular attention to the primary neoplasm, sites of metastases, associated diseases, body weight, and skin condition. Laboratory analysis is also recommended to determine electrolyte levels, nutrition, and hydration status. Patients should be assessed for the following:

Infection. Obtain stool cultures from all outpatients for enteric pathogens, including *Shigella, Campylobacter,* and *Salmonella.* A stool sample for *C. difficile* is recommended along with samples for ova and parasites. For hospitalized bone marrow transplant patients, viral agents (adenoviral, rotaviral coxsackie viruses) may be implicated, and the cause of significant morbidity and mortality.

Medication history. Antibiotics (especially ampicillin, clindamycin, and broad-spectrum antibiotics) may cause diarrhea due to alteration of normal gastrointestinal flora or inflammation of intestinal mucosa. Chemotherapeutic agents, antacids (especially magnesium-containing compounds), antihypertensives, potassium supplements, diuretics, caffeine, theophylline, nonsteroidal antiinflammatory drugs (NSAIDs), and antiarrhythmic drugs also may cause diarrhea. Other causes related to medications include overuse of laxatives and opioid withdrawal.

Diet history. Assess for change in diet habits, food or lactose intolerances or allergies, alcohol consumption, and sorbitol-based gum. Cramping, flatulence, and diarrhea may indicate lactose intolerance.

Malnutrition. Malabsorption of nutrients may lead to diarrhea, creating a negative cycle in which diarrhea worsens malnutrition.

Fecal impaction. Diarrhea results when liquid stool from the proximal colon is forced around the impaction. Impaction should be suspected after a period of absent bowel movement. Other clues include anorexia, hypoactive bowel sounds, and an abdomen dull to percussion. A rectal examination is required.

Neurologic lesions. Incontinence may be mistaken for diarrhea.

8. How is diarrhea best managed?

Diarrhea in patients with advanced cancer is usually managed with symptomatic, nonspecific antidiarrheal treatments (see table, pages 230–231) as long as infection or an inflammatory disorder is not suspected. In other patients, a reasonable attempt should be made to determine the cause and to tailor the treatment accordingly. While the patient is evaluated for specific causes of diarrhea, nonspecific therapy, such as administration of stool binders (e.g., fiber psyllium, 1 tbsp twice daily; aluminum-containing antacids, 30 cc 3 times/day), intravenous hydration, and antimotility agents (e.g., Imodium, 2 mg 4 times/day) may be instituted. Other suggestions include oral therapy with glucose, electrolyte, and water solutions; however, patients experiencing nausea and vomiting may require parenteral replacement. Bowel rest is recommended, especially after chemotherapy-induced diarrhea, to allow the gastrointestinal tract to heal. Patients are then started on a liquid diet and gradually increased to low-residue foods as tolerated (usually proteins first, then fats).

9. How does radiation cause diarrhea?

Abdominal or pelvic radiation therapy can damage the epithelial lining of the gastrointestinal tract and result in mild-to-severe diarrhea. Radiation-induced bowel injury occurs despite efforts to minimize incidental damage. Radiation causes sloughing of epithelium and shortening of villi in intestinal walls; thus lactase (an enzyme necessary for disaccharide digestion) is decreased or absent, and patients become lactose intolerant. Unabsorbable lactose in the small intestine causes an osmotic fluid shift that results in accelerated movement of contents and cramping abdominal pain. A lactose-free diet may be recommended, but once healing has occurred, the patient may return to a normal diet. Ischemic enteritis (potentially resulting in malabsorptive/osmotic or hypersecretory diarrhea) may result from chronic radiotherapy, but this is rare with modern radiation techniques.

10. At what point after radiation therapy does diarrhea occur?

Diarrhea may begin at any time after administration of high-dose (750 cGy) radiation. The incidence is increased in patients with a history of abdominal surgery, adhesions, vascular insufficiency, and prior chemotherapy. The likelihood of diarrhea increases with the volume of bowel treated and daily dose delivered. For example, in patients with seminoma an average of 2500 cGy is delivered to the majority of small bowel and virtually always leads to diarrhea. In comparison, in a patient with prostate cancer 7000 cGy may be delivered with conformal technique to the prostate only and cause no diarrhea at all. The incidence of diarrhea after radiotherapy to the abdomen or pelvis peaks at 1–3 weeks after initiation of treatment; symptoms may persist for quite a while. Patients receiving radiation to the abdomen, pelvis, or lower thoracic or lumbar spine are at greater risk for acute diarrhea. Chronic enterocolitis may develop 6–12 months after treatment is administered. Chronic diarrhea may occur as late as 5–15 years after radiation treatment.

11. How is radiation-induced diarrhea managed?

Patients are instructed to maintain a bland, low-residue diet for the duration of treatment and until bowel habits return to normal (approximately 2–6 weeks after completion of radiation).

Diarrhea-related cramping, tenesmus, and peristaltic activity are most commonly treated with the belladonna derivatives (atropine) in combination with an opioid. The combination agent Lomotil is usually prescribed at a dose of 2.5 mg for moderate diarrhea (> 3 stools/day) and administered orally as 1–2 tablets after each loose stool to a maximum of 8 tablets/day. Lomotil may be clustered around a certain time of day if the patient notices a pattern to the diarrhea. Imodium is also frequently used for radiation-induced diarrhea. Given that Lomotil decreases intestinal peristalsis and Imodium increases absorption of fluid and electrolytes in the small intestine, the two medications may be used simultaneously for a synergistic effect by alternating doses of each, not in excess of 8 total tablets/day. Tincture of opium, which directly acts on intestinal musculature to decrease peristalsis and secretions, also may be used for radiation-induced diarrhea. Patients who have received doses (3000–5000 cGy) may no longer respond to dietary interventions, Lomotil, and Imodium.

12. How is good skin care maintained in patients with diarrhea?

Good skin care is essential. Watery stool contains bile and enzymes and frequently is heme-positive; it contributes to skin breakdown. The following tips should be taught to patients and caregivers to ensure proper care of the skin and mucous membranes of the rectal area:

- Wash perineal and rectal area after each bowel movement with mild soap and water; rinse well and pat dry with soft towel.
- Apply a topical moisture-barrier cream (e.g., A&D ointment, zinc oxide) to promote skin healing. For patients with moderate-to-severe diarrhea, cream should be applied at least ¼ inch thick to provide adequate protection from enzymatic activity.
- To relieve pain related to inflammation, use a corticosteroid spray or cream. Suggest frequent sitz baths or bathing in a tub of warm water. A mixture of 1000 ml physiologic bicarbonate, 100 ml of diphenhydramine HCL elixir, and 1 bottle of viscous lidocaine HCL may be used in the sitz bath to relieve pain and itching every 4 hours as needed.
- To promote healing and treat desquamation, add aluminum acetate solution (Domeboro), 1 package to 1 quart of water, to sitz bath.
- Wear loose-fitting clothing and expose rectal area to air frequently.

13. What is octreotide? When is it used?

Octreotide is a somatostatin analog (synthetic derivative of somatostatin, a naturally occurring peptide hormone) with antisecretory and motility-inhibiting properties. Its mechanism of action is related to inhibition of gastrointestinal hormone secretion (e.g., vasoactive intestinal peptide [VIP], gastrin, motilin, secretin); thus, octreotide prolongs intestinal transit time and increases net sodium and water absorption. It is useful for chemotherapy-induced diarrhea, secretory diarrhea (as with carcinoid and VIPomas), short-bowel syndrome, and high-output ostomies. Whether octreotide is better than conventional therapy with loperamide for treatment of chemotherapy-related diarrhea is under investigation in patients with advanced colorectal cancer treated with 5-fluorouracil-based regimens. Patients who experience refractory diarrhea may be started on octreotide at a dose of 50 µg subcutaneously 3 times/day.

14. What dietary tips should be given to patients with diarrhea?

- Lactose-intolerant patients should maintain a lactose-free diet or use lactobacillus preparations to aid digestion. Patients taking oral nutritional supplements to maintain calorie and protein levels also may benefit from lactose-free preparations (e.g., Vivonex T.E.N., Osmolite).
- Use isosmotic (300 mOsm/kg water) and lactose-free enteral feedings and administer at room temperature.
- Eat foods containing pectin, such as bananas, avocados, asparagus tips (all three of which are also high in potassium), beets, unspiced applesauce, or peeled apples.
- Add nutmeg to foods, because it decreases gastrointestinal motility.
- Avoid foods that are stimulating or irritating to the gastrointestinal tract (e.g., whole grain products, nuts, seeds, popcorn, pickles, relishes, rich pastries).

Antidiarrheal Agents

DRUG AND DOSAGE	MECHANISM OF ACTION	CONTRAINDICATIONS
Opioids *Lomotil* (2.5 mg diphenoxylate with 0.025 mg atropine sulfate tablet): May load: 10 mg, then 1–2 tablets 3 or 4 times/day. Maximal dose: 20 mg/day *Imodium (loperamide)*: 2-mg capsules. May load: 4–8 mg orally, then 2 mg after each loose stool. Maximal dose: 16 mg/day *Codeine:* 15– 60 mg orally every 4–6 hr as needed *Opium tincture* (10% opium liquid: 10 mg morphine/ml with 19% alcohol): 0.3–1 ml every 2–6 hr until controlled. Maximal dose: 6 ml/24 hr *Paregoric* (0.4 mg morphine/ml with 45% alcohol): 5–10 ml orally 1–4 times/day or 4 ml every 4 hr	*All opioids* act as agonists at opiate receptors in smooth muscle of GI tract, reducing secretion and peristalsis. Also increase ileocecal valve and anal sphincter pressure; improving continence. *Atropine* (in Lomotil) blocks muscarinic receptors, inhibiting peristalsis and reducing gastric secretions. It is added for prevention of abuse more than treatment of diarrhea.	*All opioids:* parasitic or bacterial infections accompanied by fever, obstructive jaundice *Diphenoxylate* (in Lomotil): advanced liver disease (e.g., cirrhosis); may precipitate hepatic coma *Lomotil and Imodium:* not recommended in children younger than 2 yr *Paregoric:* convulsive states
Adsorbents *Bismuth subsalicylate* (Pepto-Bismol): chewable tablets: 262 mg, and suspensions: 262 mg/15 ml or 524 mg/ 15 ml (maximal strength). Usual dose: 524 mg every 30 min up to 5 gm/day	Adsorbs (binds) toxins produced by bacteria and other GI irritants, allowing them to be inactivated or eliminated; direct antimicrobial effect on *E. coli.*	Aspirin sensitivity
Kaopectate (5.85 gm kaolin and 130 mg pectin per 30 ml suspension). Usual dose: 2–6 gm every 6 hr as needed	Pectin produces a viscous colloidal solution with both adsorbent and absorbent properties.	Obstructive bowel lesions Children younger than 3 yr
Cholestyramine (Questran)	Nonabsorbable resin; adsorbs bile salts/acids, which cause diarrhea by effect on large intestine; adsorbs *C. difficile* toxin.	
Anticholinergics *Atropine* *Dicyclomine* (Bentyl) *Pro-Banthine* (15 mg orally 3 or 4 times/day)	Muscarinic agonists; inhibit GI secretions and peristalsis; decrease spasm of small intestine lining	Closed angle glaucoma Prostate hypertrophy Heart disease Obstructive bowel disease
Somatostatin analog *Octreotide acetate* (Sandostatin): 50–200 µg 2 or 3 times/day subcutaneously	Inhibits GI hormone secretion, thus prolonging intestinal transit time and increasing net sodium and water absorption	

Table continued on following page.

Antidiarrheal Agents *(Columns continued)*

ADVERSE EFFECTS	DRUG INTERACTIONS	ADMINISTRATION TIPS
Atropine (in Lomotil): limited use due to dry mouth, urinary retention, blurred vision *Imodium:* uncommon effects include cramping, gastric upset, dry mouth, skin rash, dizziness, drowsiness *All opioids:* potential constipation, abdominal and bowel distention, nausea	*Diphenoxylate* (in Lomotil), *codeine, paregoric:* potentiate CNS depressants *Diphenoxylate* (in Lomotil): increases risk of hypertension with monoamine oxidase inhibitors; increases risk of paralytic ileus with antimuscarinics	*Lomotil* favored in partial bowel obstruction due to shorter action *Atropine* useful in diarrhea associated with painful cramping *Imodium* is DRUG OF CHOICE for nonspecific antidiarrheal therapy; unlike codeine and diphenoxylate, it has no central opioid effect at therapeutic doses. Titrated to effect; treat overdose with naloxone. *Opium tincture* for severe diarrhea; prolonged use may result in dependence. Measured by drops; must be diluted in juice or water. *Oral equianalgesic doses:* Imodium: 4 mg/day Lomotil: 10 mg/day Codeine: 200 mg/day
Impaction	Potentiates oral anticoagulants and hypoglycemics Reduces uricosuric effects of probenecid and sulfinpyrazone Decreases absorption and bioavailability of tetracyclines Can interfere with radiologic exams because it is radiopaque	Prophylaxis for traveler's diarrhea, but large doses limit utility Useful in secretory diarrhea for enterotoxic bacteria, radiotherapy, prostaglandin-secreting tumors (acts as mucosal antiprostaglandin) Indicated for mild diarrhea
May increase K^+ loss or interfere with absorption of of nutrients and drugs	Decreases absorption of many drugs	Indicated for mild diarrhea
Constipation	Binds with and decreases absorption of many drugs (e.g., warfarin sodium, aspirin, thyroxin, digoxin, phenobarbital)	Helpful in radiation-induced diarrhea and ileal surgery. Give with meals; use limited by taste; onset of action: 12–24 hr
Decreased memory and concentration. Drowsiness, dry mouth, urinary retention, tachycardia	Antacids interfere with absorption of these drugs.	Useful in diarrhea due to peptic ulcer disease or irritable bowel syndrome and refractory diarrhea
Nausea, abdominal cramps, flatulence, steatorrhea. Biliary sludge and gallstones after 6 months. Transient deterioration in glucose tolerance at start		Useful in secretory diarrhea associated with endocrine tumors, AIDS, graft vs. host disease, GI resection, diabetes.

• Avoid alcohol, caffeine-containing products, and tobacco.
• Avoid greasy, spicy (curry, chili powder, garlic), and fried foods.
• Avoid raw vegetables.
• Eat food at room temperature.

15. Why should water or carbonated drinks not be the primary fluid replacement for patients with diarrhea?

Water lacks the necessary electrolytes (e.g., potassium) and vitamins. Carbonated caffeine drinks have low electrolyte content and extremely high osmolality, which in fact may worsen acute diarrhea. Better choices for fluid and electrolyte replacement include bouillon, fruitades, cranberry juice, grape juice, Gatorade or other sport drinks, weak tepid tea, and gelatin. Fluids with glucose are useful because glucose absorption drives sodium and water back into the body, supporting oral rehydration therapy.

16. Why is perineal pouching preferred over rectal tubes and Foley catheters for excessive partial fecal incontinence?

Perineal pouching protects the skin by containing liquid stool (as well as odor) and minimizes cross-contamination. The use of rectal tubes and large balloon-tipped Foley catheters for internal drainage systems are contraindicated. Rectal tubes in place for > 20 minutes decrease rectal sphincter responsiveness, and balloon Foley catheters produce pressures (250–300 mmHg) associated with rectal perforation.

17. How is a perineal pouch applied?

1. Trace a circle of 1¾ inches onto both a pouch adhesive faceplace and a skin barrier wafer; then cut out the circles.

2. After removal of adhesive pouch backing, lay skin barrier onto pouch adhesive and center openings. Press together firmly, and avoid wrinkles. Set aside.

3. Cleanse perineal area and clip perineal hair. Rinse and dry area.

4. After removing paper backing from skin barrier, have assistant hold buttocks apart and apply pouch to perineum with opening centered over anus (must be sealed to skin, especially in crease of buttocks). Hold a hand over the pouch; the warmth of the hand promotes adhesiveness.

5. Apply liquid skin sealant around edges of pouch, and allow to dry. Frame the edges of the pouch with 1-inch paper tape.

The views contained in this manuscript are solely those of the author and do not reflect the views or the policies of Tripler Army Medical Command, the Department of Defense, or the U.S. Government.

ACKNOWLEDGMENT

The author thanks Thomas Loughney, MD, Department of Medicine, Gastroenterology Service, Tripler Army Medical Center, for his critical review of this chapter.

BIBLIOGRAPHY

1. Bond JH: Office-based management of diarrhea. Geriatrics 37:52–64, 1982.
2. Culhane MB, Rust DM, Horbal-Shuster M: Bowel function alterations. In Yasko J, Dudjak L (eds): Biological Response Modifier Therapy: Symptom Management. Emeryville, CA, Park Row Publishers, 1990, pp 97–105.
3. Krejs C, Fordtran JS: Diarrhea. In Sleisenger MH,Fordtran JS (eds): Gastrointestinal Disease: Pathophysiology, Diagnosis, Management, 3rd ed. Philadelphia, W.B. Saunders, 1983, pp 257–277.
4. Halpin JE: Understanding and controlling fecal incontinence. Ostomy/Wound Manage 13:28–36, 1986.
5. Hassey-Dow, K, Hilderley LJ: Nursing Care in Radiation Oncology. Philadelphia, W.B. Saunders, 1992.
6. Kochman ML, Traber, PG: Bowel dysfunction in the cancer patient. In MacDonald JS, Haller DG, Mayer RJ (eds): Manual of Oncologic Therapeutics, 3rd ed. Philadelphia, J.B. Lippincott, 1995, pp 444–449.

7. Lankford TR, Jacobs-Steward PM: Foundations of Normal and Therapeutic Nutrition. New York, John Wiley & Sons, 1986.

8. Levy M: Constipation and diarrhea in cancer patients. Cancer Bull 43: 412–422, 1991.

9. Mercadante S: Diarrhea in terminally ill patients: Pathophysiology and treatment. J Pain Symptom Manage 10(4):298–309, 1995.

10. Preston F: Comfort measures for perineal excoriation. Oncol Nurs Forum 13:71, 1986.

11. Portenoy R: Constipation in the cancer patient: Causes and management. Med Clin North Am 71:303–311, 1987.

12. Skeel RT, Tipton J: Symptom management. In Brain MC, Carbone PP (eds): Current Therapy in Hematology-Oncology, 5th ed. St. Louis, Mosby, 1995, pp 582–584.

13. Sykes NP: Constipation and diarrhoea. In Doyle D, Hanks GWC, Macdonald N: Oxford Textbook of Palliative Medicine. Oxford, Oxford University Press, 1993, pp 299–310.

14. Twycross RG, Lack SA: Diarrhoea. In Control of Alimentary Symptoms in Far Advanced Cancer. Edinburgh, Churchill Livingstone, 1986, pp 208–229.

15. Wadler S: Secretory Diarrhea: Induction by Chemotherapy. East Hanover, NJ, Sandoz, 1994.

16. Wright PS, Thomas SL: Constipation and diarrhea: The neglected symptoms. Semin Oncol Nurs 11(4): 289–297, 1995.

17. Yasko JM (ed): Nursing Management of Symptoms Associated with Chemotherapy, 3rd ed. Meniscus Health Care Communications, Philadelphia, 1993, pp 118–120.

18. Yolken RH, Bishop CA, Townsend RT, et al: Infectious gastroenteritis in bone marrow transplant recipients. N Engl J Med 306: 1010–1012, 1982.

35. FATIGUE

Lillian M. Nail, PhD, RN, FAAN

1. Is fatigue a major problem for patients with cancer?

Cancer treatment–related fatigue (CRF) is the most frequently reported side effect of treatment. All types of treatment produce CRF, and the most severe, dose-limiting form occurs with biologic response modifiers (e.g., interferon, interleukins). The percentage of patients experiencing CRF as a side effect of cancer treatment ranges from < 10–100%, depending on the type of treatment, dose of therapy and method used to measure fatigue. CRF is poorly understood and often ignored in clinical practice.

2. Define cancer treatment-related fatigue.

CRF includes sensations of physical tiredness, mental slowness, and lack of emotional resilience. It fluctuates in intensity over the course of the day, often exhibits a pattern that it is tied to administration of treatment, and can be overcome in an emergency. Although patients with CRF may experience muscle weakness, CRF is not synonymous with weakness. In contrast to patients with neurologic problems, patients with CRF may have normal muscle strength and endurance and still experience an overwhelming feeling of tiredness.

3. How is CRF different from the fatigue experienced by healthy people?

In comparison with the fatigue experienced by healthy people, CRF is overwhelming, persistent, and relentless. Fatigue in healthy people is eventually fully relieved by sleep and rest, even if it takes more than one or two nights to achieve relief. In contrast, people with CRF wake up tired no matter how much rest they get. CRF also may cause patients to redefine the level of fatigue that they label as "not tired." Thus, what they formerly thought of as feeling tired is now defined as "not tired," and a new sensation of overwhelming fatigue replaces "severe fatigue."

4. What is the impact of CRF?

Patients describe themselves as being too tired to do anything, unable to concentrate, frustrated by feeling that they are not themselves, concerned that fatigue means that they are not doing well or that the cancer is progressing, and depressed because of the feeling of tiredness. The limitations imposed by fatigue are dramatic. The person experiencing CRF may not be aware of the magnitude of the negative impact on usual activities until the fatigue resolves.

5. What are the probable causes of CRF?

People with cancer are likely to experience many potential causes of fatigue, such as electrolyte imbalance, poor nutritional status, anemia, hormone shifts, volume depletion, sedation as a side effect of analgesics, hypoxia, and infection. Other contributors include sleep disruption, increased demands for physical activity, emotional strain, interpersonal demands, and increased need for vigilance and concentration. Symptoms, side effects, anxiety, hospital noise, and interpersonal demands at home have the potential to disrupt sleep and rest. Multiple visits to health care providers, travel to appointments, physical demands of surgery and other forms of treatment, processing information about treatment options to make an informed decision, establishing relationships with new health care providers, explaining the diagnosis and treatment to friends and family members, and monitoring the care provided by others are potential contributors to fatigue that are not fully understood by health care providers or friends and family.

6. What physiologic mechanisms are responsible for CRF?

The physiologic causes of CRF are unknown. Multiple causes are likely, given the variation in the intensity and characteristics of CRF experienced with different types of treatment. Various hypotheses have been proposed, including toxic effects of accumulated products of cell death, neurohormonal changes, depletion of essential neurotransmitters, bone marrow suppression, and accumulation of cytokines. However, no definitive tests of these hypotheses have been reported.

7. How should the nurse assess CRF?

The clinical assessment of fatigue should be modeled on the approach to pain in the practice setting. For example, "On a scale of 0 to 10 where 0 is no fatigue and 10 is the most fatigue possible, how much fatigue have you had today?"

Both the time frame (now, today, during the past week, during the past month) and the reference point (highest level of fatigue, lowest level of fatigue, usual level of fatigue) can be altered to accommodate the type of treatment. Patients receiving cyclic chemotherapy often arrive for treatment on a day when they have the lowest level of fatigue during the treatment cycle. Assessment based on the "today" approach does not fully describe their experience after treatment because the peak time of CRF is not captured. Patients assessed on the day of the next treatment should be asked about level of fatigue over the week following the previous treatment as well as "today." The average level of fatigue over each week since the previous treatment may also be assessed to evaluate rate of recovery. Weekly assessment focused on the past week and beginning of the second week of treatment is appropriate for most patients receiving radiation therapy.

Potential treatable causes should be evaluated, especially when (1) the pattern of CRF is unusual for the type of treatment delivered, (2) the intensity of fatigue increases suddenly and dramatically, or (3) the impact of fatigue on quality of life is beyond the patient's level of tolerance. In addition to standard laboratory tests and physical examination, daily activity level, sleep patterns, and new demands imposed as a result of cancer should be assessed.

8. What are major barriers to effective management of CRF?

- Assumption by health care providers that CRF is the same as the fatigue that all healthy people encounter in day-to-day life
- Lack of knowledge of the underlying mechanisms of CRF
- Erroneous belief that nothing can be done about CRF
- Confusing CRF with depression
- Failure to appreciate the negative impact of CRF on quality of life

9. What interventions are used to manage CRF?

The approach to managing CRF is multifaceted:
- Assessing level of fatigue
- Delivering preparatory information
- Managing treatable causes
- Controlling symptoms and side effects
- Providing instructions about energy conservation and appropriate exercise
- Promoting sleep and rest
- Evaluating effectiveness of interventions

10. Why should patients get preparatory information?

Preparatory information helps patients (1) to understand that CRF is a side effect of treatment, not an indication that the cancer is progressing; (2) to plan for CRF by using information about onset, pattern, and resolution in planning activities; and (3) to increase confidence in dealing with CRF. Research about informational interventions in patients undergoing stressful medical procedures demonstrates that preparatory information does not "cause" patients to experience side effects by power of suggestion. Patients who are aware of potential side effects but do not experience them describe themselves as "lucky" and appreciate being prepared.

McHugh, Christman, and Johnson developed specific guidelines for preparatory informational interventions. Their guidelines include objective or factual information about CRF from the patient's perspective rather than value judgments, based on experiences reported by others who have had the same treatment. For example, a message to prepare men for receiving radiation treatment for prostate cancer included information about the time of day when CRF was likely to occur, the week of treatment when it began, and how long the fatigue persisted after treatment.

11. What are the common treatable causes of fatigue and sleep disruption?

- Pain is an important contributor to fatigue in patients with cancer. Pain disrupts sleep and rest, increases the energy needed to perform day-to-day activities, restricts mobility, and constitutes an emotional burden. Pain relief should improve fatigue unless the management technique disrupts sleep (e.g., drugs administered every 4 hours around the clock), requires extensive energy investment (e.g., frequent changes of hot or cold packs), or has a sedative effect.
- Symptoms related to tumor involvement (e.g., obstruction, fever, pruritus, coughing, dyspnea)
- Side effects related to therapy (e.g., nausea, vomiting, hot flashes, dry mouth, stomatitis, constipation, diarrhea)
- Urinary frequency, incontinence, retention, spasms, or genitourinary irritation can disrupt sleep as often as every hour.
- Anxiety and depression
- Drugs or other substances that interfere with sleep, such as steroids, sedatives or hypnotics, caffeine or nicotine, and some antidepressants
- Primary sleep disorders (e.g., sleep apnea, narcolepsy, restless leg syndrome)

12. How can patients conserve energy and manage activity?

Patients with cancer are often advised to conserve energy by decreasing activity. This approach to managing CRF has not been tested, although energy conservation techniques are commonly used by patients with physical illness. The appeal of this approach is derived from patients' perceptions that they have a limited amount of available energy and the assumption that conserving energy allows it to be redirected to other activities. There are no standard guidelines for energy conservation in patients with cancer.

Current recommendations include assisting patients to prioritize activities by identifying those that are essential and those that are optional. Some essential activities can be delegated to others while the patient maintains involvement in activities that are highly valued. Nonessential activities that are not valued by the patient can be eliminated. Finding different ways to perform activities is also helpful in energy conservation. Simple suggestions such as sitting in a firm chair with arms to aid getting out of the chair, adding a raised toilet seat in the bathroom, using a wheelchair if walking is difficult, arranging commonly used supplies and equipment within easy reach of a workspace, and sitting rather than standing to perform repetitive tasks are examples of energy conservation techniques. Physical and/or occupational therapy referrals are important both in evaluating a patient's physical capacity and in identifying appropriate energy conservation techniques.

13. How is exercise used in managing CRF?

The conceptual basis for using exercise as a strategy for managing CRF is derived from principles of energetics and muscle physiology. Decreased activity leads to deconditioning, which results in less efficient muscular work. Furthermore, energy use is an important component of energy regulation. No research has explicitly tested the the principles behind this concept of the relationship between exercise and CRF. However, research with women receiving adjuvant chemotherapy for breast cancer demonstrates that both supervised and self-administered exercise programs are feasible and safe in this clinical population and suggests that exercise holds promise as a means of preventing or treating CRF.

14. How does sleep disruption contribute to CRF?

In healthy adults, sleep disruption produces varying levels of fatigue, mood disturbance, attention deficit, and daytime performance problems. Inadequate sleep and rest in patients with cancer probably has the same effects. Patients may have difficulty in processing information, adhering to treatment regimens, or implementing self-care instructions. Irritability, depression, and despair are potential consequences of prolonged sleep disruption. Increasing sleep and rest are the most common self-care strategies used by patients with cancer, but they do not fully relieve the symptoms of CRF. The suggestion that sleep and rest may be used to treat CRF is based on a few descriptive studies with cancer patients, findings of the more extensive research on healthy adults, and best clinical judgment.

15. How are sleep disturbances assessed?
- Determine whether the sleep pattern has changed from the patient's precancer pattern.
- Document current sleep patterns by having the patient keep a sleep log to record time to sleep onset, duration of sleep, sleep habits, frequency and reason for awakenings, naps, and use of sleep aids.
- Ask patients about amount and quality of sleep, current medications, and history of sleep disorders.

16. How are sleep disturbances managed?
- Controlling pain and other symptoms or side effects of therapy.
- Reducing anxiety (manifested by frightening thoughts, worries, or nightmares) with use of pharmacologic or cognitive/behavioral treatments. Specific cognitive/behavioral treatments, such as biofeedback and relaxation, are established interventions for problems with delayed sleep onset, frequent awakening, and shortened sleep periods.
- Recommending appropriate pharmacologic management (e.g., mild barbiturates, benzodiazepines, antihistamines, chloral hydrate, or antidepressants).
- Making appropriate referrals if a primary sleep disorder is suspected.
- Instructing patients about sleep hygiene.

17. What practical tips may promote sleep hygiene or help patients to get a better night's sleep?
- Develop a standard, predictable bedtime ritual.
- Go to bed when drowsy, but do not stay in bed if you are not sleeping.
- Sleep in a dark, well-ventilated, quiet room maintained at a comfortable temperature.
- Avoid stimulants (caffeine, chocolate, nicotine), alcohol, heavy meals, and exercise in the period prior to sleep.
- Avoid disrupting sleep by delegating the care of others to someone else, trying not to ruminate on worries, and turning down telephones.
- Take a warm bath or hot drink before bedtime or get a backrub or massage.
- Ensure comfort by using a mattress and pillow of appropriate firmness and extra pillows for support, by sleeping in comfortable, loose clothing, and by straightening the bed linen.
- Sleep in a familiar environment whenever possible.

18. What drugs interfere with sleep?
Opioids, some hypnotics, and other medications such as hormones, steroids, and nonsteroidal antiinflammatory drugs may affect the quality of sleep. Any medication that produces respiratory depression may induce the type of breathing problem identified as a cause of chronic insomnia.

19. What medications are commonly used to help sleep?
Expert recommendations for the use of hypnotics include limiting use to relatively brief periods (a few weeks), beginning at a low dose, choosing a drug that does not impair alertness or performance the next day, and considering the duration of action in relation to the specific sleep problem (delayed onset of sleep, frequent awakening, or early wakening). When pain is a problem, adequate analgesia is essential for sleep.

In patients with cancer, adequate symptom management and an environment conducive to sleep form the foundation of sleep promotion. When these interventions do not solve the problem, short-term or intermittent use of pharmacologic agents should be considered. Factors that influence the choice of agent include age of patient, desired duration of effect, nature of the problem, potential side effects, comorbidity, and drug interactions. Benzodiazepines are usually the first class of drugs considered, because they disrupt rapid eye movement sleep less than other hypnotics. Temazepam (15-30 mg for adults; limit dose for elderly to 50% adult dose) is the benzodiazepine most often recommended because of its rapid onset, 6–8 hour duration of action, and relatively low incidence of side effects when used in low doses for short periods. Because antihistamines contribute to relief of nausea or itching, diphenhydramine (25 mg) or hydroxyzine (10–100 mg) may be especially useful for some patients.

20. What about depression?

Patients, family members, and care providers often wonder whether CRF is a manifestation of depression. Historically, the diagnosis of depression depends on the presence of vegetative symptoms such as anorexia, sleep disturbance, decreased activity, constipation, and weight loss. All of these symptoms are likely to occur as side effects in patients undergoing treatment for cancer, potentially confounding the diagnosis of depression. Recent revisions to the diagnosis of depression state that symptoms of physical illness and side effects of treatment are not appropriate considerations in making a diagnosis of depression. The incidence of depression in patients with cancer is comparable to that of the general population of the same age when symptom-free measures of depression are used.

In patients with cancer, feelings of sadness and inability to feel pleasure, which are present all or most of the time for several weeks, are the hallmarks of depression. The most important risk factor is a previous episode of depression. Depression in patients with cancer can be treated effectively, but CRF may interfere with attendance at support groups or participation in therapy sessions. However, pharmacologic management is appropriate for many patients if the therapy does not interact with other medications or adversely influence responses to cancer treatment.

21. Do patients with cancer use alternative therapies to treat CRF?

Vitamins, mineral supplements, herbal remedies, and hormones are used by patients with cancer. No published reports confirm the efficacy of any of these agents in preventing or ameliorating CRF. Patients who experience sleep problems may use melatonin as a sleep promoter. Research into the effects of melatonin on sleep and CRF is ongoing, but the results reported at this time are contradictory.

22. What should care providers do about CRF?

The practices that need to be implemented immediately include:
- Recognizing that fatigue is a side effect of treatment
- Assessing patients for CRF
- Preparing patients for the experience of CRF
- Understanding that the fatigue experienced by "healthy" people is not the same as CRF
- Recognizing that CRF has a major negative impact on quality of life
- Pursuing treatment to maximize quality of life

BIBLIOGRAPHY

1. Breetvelt IS, Van Dam FS: Underreporting by cancer patients: The case of the response-shift. Soc Sci Med 32:981–987, 1991.
2. Cimprich B: Symptom management: Loss of concentration. Semin Oncol Nurs 11:279–288, 1995.
3. Ferrell BR, Grant M, Dean GE, et al: "Bone tired": The experience of fatigue and its impact on quality of life. Oncol Nurs Forum 23:1539–1547, 1996.
4. Foltz AT, Gaines G, Gullatte M: Recalled side effects and self-care actions of patients receiving inpatient chemotherapy. Oncol Nurs Forum 23:679–683, 1996.

5. Graydon JE, Bublia N, Irvine D, et al: Fatigue-reducing strategies used by patients receiving treatment for cancer. Cancer Nurs 18:23–28, 1995.

6. Johnson JE: Coping with elective surgery. Annu Rev Nurs Res 2:107–132, 1984.

7. Johnson JE: Coping with radiation therapy: Optimism and the effect of preparatory inventions. Res Nurs Health 19:3–12, 1996.

8. Johnson JE, Nail LM, Lauver D, et al: Reducing the negative impact of radiation therapy on functional status. Cancer 61:46–51, 1988.

9. Kurtz ME, Kurtz JC, Given CW, Given B: Loss of physical functioning among patients with cancer: A longitudinal view. Cancer Pract 1:275–281, 1993.

10. MacVicar MG, Winningham ML, Nichel JL: Effects of aerobic interval training on cancer patients: Functional capacity. Nurs Res 38:348–351, 1989.

11. Massie MJ, Holland JC: Overview of normal reactions and prevalence of psychiatric disorders. In Holland JC, Rowland JH (eds): Handbook of Psychooncology: Psychological Care of the Patient with Cancer. New York, Oxford University Press, 1990, pp 273–383.

12. McHugh NG, Christman NJ, Johnson JE: Preparatory information: What helps and why. Am J Nurs 82:780–782, 1982.

13. Mock V, Barton Burke M, Sheehan P, et al: A nursing rehabilitation program for women with breast cancer receiving adjuvant chemotherapy. Oncol Nurs Forum 21:899–907, 1994.

14. Nail LM, Jones LS: Fatigue as a side effect of cancer treatment: Impact on quality of life. Qual Life Nurs Chall 4:8–13, 1995.

15. Nail LM, Jones LS, Greene D, et al: Use and perceived efficacy of self-care activities in patients receiving chemotherapy. Oncol Nurs Forum 18:883–887, 1991.

16. Nail LM, Winningham ML: Fatigue and weakness in cancer patients: The symptom experience. Semin Oncol Nurs 11:272–278, 1995.

17. Nicholson AN: Hypnotics: Clinical pharamacology and therapeutics. In Kryger MH, Roth T, Dement WC (eds): Principles and Practices of Sleep Medicine, 2nd ed. Philadelphia, W.B. Saunders, 1994, pp 355–363.

18. NIH Technology Assessment Panel: Integration of behavioral and relaxation approaches to the treatment of chronic pain and insomnia. JAMA 276:313–318, 1996.

19. Pearce S, Richardson A: Fatigue in cancer: A phenomenological perspective. Eur J Cancer Care 5:111–115, 1996.

20. Richardson A: Fatigue in cancer patients: A review of the literature. Eur J Cancer Care 4:20–32, 1995.

21. Winningham M, Nail LM, Burke MB, et al: Fatigue and the cancer experience: The state of the knowledge. Oncol Nurs Forum 21:23–26, 1994.

36. LYMPHEDEMA SECONDARY TO CANCER TREATMENT

Jean K. Smith, RN, MS, OCN

1. Why do we usually think of breast cancer when we hear the word lymphedema?

Lymphedema is the accumulation of lymph fluid in interstitial spaces, primarily in subcutaneous fat. It is an abnormal collection of excessive tissue proteins, edema, fibrosis, and inflammation. In the United States, breast cancer treatment causes significantly more lymphedema than any other single factor. Twenty to thirty-three percent of patients diagnosed with breast cancer and treated surgically will develop lymphedema. A more open public and media discussion has increased the association of lymphedema with breast cancer despite the fact that other cancers and health problems also cause lymphedema.

2. How relevant is lymphedema prevention in view of more conservative breast cancer surgeries?

The trend in the past 10 years has been to forego lymphedema prevention because more conservative breast cancer surgeries appear to have decreased the incidence and severity of lymphedema. In 1981, Markowski reported the incidence of lymphedema as ranging between 6.7–62.5%. In 1996, Kiel and Rademacker described an incidence of 35% in 183 patients with early-stage breast cancer who underwent breast conservation surgery accompanied by radiation therapy with a median follow-up of 20 months. Clearly, lymphedema continues to develop as a sequelae to lymph node dissection. Therefore, as long as node dissection remains a gold standard for staging and treatment decision-making, approximately one-third of patients will develop lymphedema. Organized, effective prevention of lymphedema is inexpensive, saves costs, provides lower posttreatment morbidity, and increases patient functional outcomes.

3. What other cancers and factors are associated with lymphedema? Why?

Any surgery with or without radiation therapy that involves large node dissections or dissections seriously interrupting lymph flow is associated with a high risk for lymphedema. In addition to breast cancer, treatment for prostate cancer, lymphoma, sarcoma, melanoma, head and neck cancers, and pelvic cancers commonly lead to an increased risk of lymphedema. Any cancer that metastasizes to lymph nodes is likely to cause lymphedema if treatment is either not given or ineffective. Radiation therapy to dissected nodal areas also has been associated with lymphedema.

4. How is lymphedema diagnosed?

Lymphedema in patients with cancer is often diagnosed by the process of elimination combined with a careful history and physical examination. Imaging can be extremely useful, but certain precautions must be kept in mind. Lymphedema experts universally discourage the use of lymphangiography or venography for people with or at a high risk for lymphedema. Lymphscintigraphy is considered safe and helpful in the diagnosis of lymphedema; however, it is relatively expensive and requires a radiologist experienced in the procedure.

5. What are the essentials of lymphedema prevention for high-risk cancer patients?

People at high risk for lymphedema seem to be most compliant and participatory when they have been taught (1) the transport and immune function of lymph vessels and nodes, (2) the inability of the body to replace lymph vessels that have been damaged or removed, (3) the lifelong need for risk prevention, and (4) specific prevention practices (taught verbally and reinforced in writing).

6. What helpful hints can patients be taught to reduce, prevent, or control lymphedema?

1. Elevate affected limb above the level of the heart whenever possible.
2. Clean skin and use oil or skin cream daily.
3. Keep pressure off affected arm or leg.
   - Don't cross affected legs; change position often.
   - Wear loose jewelry, watches, and clothes
   - Carry bags with unaffected arm.
   - Do not have blood pressure taken on affected arm.
4. Avoid injuries and infection.
   - Use electric razor to shave legs.
   - Wear gloves when gardening and cleaning.
   - Wear thimbles when sewing.
   - Take good care of nails; see a podiatrist for problems; do not cut cuticles.
   - Use insect repellent, and avoid insect bites by wearing protective clothing.
   - Clean any cuts with soap and water followed by antiseptics or antibacterial ointment.
   - Avoid extreme heat or cold on the affected limb.
   - Try to avoid blood draws or intravenous starts on affected arm.
5. Check for changes daily and notify doctor if *any* of the following symptoms develops:
   - Redness   • Heat   • Fever
   - Pain   • Swelling
6. Practice drainage promotion exercises.

7. What is the single most likely situation to precipitate lymphedema?

Infection is the most prevalent precipitator of lymphedema in patients with cancer. Infections may be acute with dramatic symptoms that require intravenous antibiotic therapy and progress to life-threatening severity within a few hours. Subclinical infections are not apparent but respond to a short course of antibiotic therapy with a resultant decrease in edema.

8. Is there a relationship between exercise or heavy lifting and lymphedema?

People at high risk for lymphedema have long been encouraged to avoid strenuous, repetitive exercise and heavy lifting with the affected limb. This recommendation is based on case studies in which no other precipitating cause was found and/or such activities clearly increased edema and discomfort. Medical staff have found that each patient with or at high risk for lymphedema seems to have an individual tolerance to strenuous exercise and weightlifting. Gradually increasing exercise and weightlifting while carefully monitoring limb size and status is a safe way to establish individual tolerance.

9. How do staff and patients decide when a limb at high risk for lymphedema must be used for intravenous therapy?

This is a difficult and controversial issue. Experts recommend that affected limbs should not be used for any IV infusions, especially chemotherapy. The reality of patient needs may complicate this recommendation. Development of a set protocol or Lymphedema Prevention Standard of Care is recommended. Suggested decision-making criteria for these patients include the following: (1) venipuncture by experienced phlebotomists only; (2) approval process required for use of suggested limb (e.g., by a physician, clinical nurse specialist); (3) central venous catheter (VAD) considered for any patient requiring more than a few days of IV infusion; (4) established procedure for venipuncture skin preparation and monitoring of infusions when affected limb must be used.

10. List the three conditions that must be ruled out when a patient presents with unexplained limb edema before beginning any lymphedema treatment.

Infection, thrombus, and new or metastatic cancer must be detected and treated before beginning lymphedema therapy. Often one of these three conditions is the cause of new lymphedema or of progression of established lymphedema. Proper treatment of these three conditions may lead to resolution or at least significant improvement of edema.

11. How helpful are diuretics in the treatment of lymphedema?

Diuretics remove excessive fluid from the body; they generally regulate sodium and potassium excretion and reabsorption. Fluid collection from lymphedema is related to inadequate lymphatic function and increased extravascular protein. Diuretics sometimes seem helpful for immediate relief of newly found lymphedema that is pitting and does not contain protein-hardened areas. Many experts, especially in Europe and Australia, do not believe in the use of long-term diuretics for people with lymphedema. Theory suggests that removal of fluid without removal of protein is likely to cause greater tissue inflammation and injury than when protein is diluted by fluid and that long-term deleterious effects, such as progression of lymphedema, are likely.

12. Is the use of antibiotics for every infection truly warranted in all patients at high risk for lymphedema?

Antibiotics have been recommended prophylactically at the first sign of infection or when a specific injury presents a substantial risk of infection in high-risk patients. Because antibiotics are used for prevention, outcomes without their use are unknown. Caregivers who have observed the development of severe, life-threatening infection from something as minor as a hangnail recommend antibiotic prevention for everyone because there currently is no way to determine which patients will develop such infections. Patients must be educated about the purpose and possible excesses of prevention as well as the *lifelong* nature of lymphedema.

13. What is manual lymph drainage? Why has it become popular only recently in the United States, although it has been used for decades in Europe?

Manual lymph drainage (MLD) is a gentle massage technique, based on lymphatic anatomy and physiology, that increases lymph flow out of edematous areas to body areas with healthy lymphatic activity. Edema is reduced by helping lymph fluid return to the bloodstream. Probably because of emphasis on high technology, combined with a desire for efficiency and greater patient autonomy, the time-consuming, expensive, and tedious nature of MLD was not appealing to the American medical community. Years of disappointing treatment outcomes led experts to seek new treatment solutions, such as MLD. Significant results from combining MLD with other modalities have been reported in Europe, Australia, and the U.S.

14. What are the standard components of state-of-the-art lymphedema care in the U.S.?

There are four elements to sound lymphedema care: skin care, exercise, external compression, and manual lymph drainage. Different treatment centers have different names for the combination of these basic components. One other component essential for high-quality treatment is a program that produces educated, empowered patients who know how to manage lymphedema and when and where to seek assistance.

15. Is the skin care component of lymphedema similar to diabetic skin care?

Skin care for both conditions focuses on preventing decreased oxygenation of tissues and promoting skin integrity. Skin problems in lymphedema are caused by excessive extravascular fluid and protein. The care for both conditions is similar: daily cleansing; gentle, thorough drying; lubrication; and monitoring for problems.

16. How is the exercise component of treatment unique to lymphedema?

Exercise is one of several ways of stimulating lymphatic flow. Muscle contractions encourage lymphatic contractions that increase lymph transport. Even deep breathing, which is recommended in supervised exercise, is useful in improving lymphatic function. The unique component is that excessive exercise results in increased accumulation of fluid and worsening of edema. The sign of excessive exercise is increased edema after completion of exercises. No known exercise rules can be applied to all patients; each patient must establish an individual exercise program with the help of an expert familiar with lymphedema, such as an occupational, physical, or exercise therapist.

17. What are the advantages and disadvantages of the use of gradient sequential compression pumps vs. manual lymph drainage?

Gradient sequential compression pumps became popular in our high-technology society because better treatment solutions were not known and pumps provided a way for patients to be treated at home either by themselves or with the assistance of a significant other. Although a number of pumps were costly, treatment expenses were fixed and patients were in charge of their own problem. Pump usage has a number of disadvantages. Patients often receive minimal instruction from nonmedical retailers who are interested mainly in making a profit; they may prescribe protocols that have not been established by research or recommend pressures high enough to occlude lymph vessels. The patient lacks the knowledge needed to evaluate lymphatic activity and problems or to know when to seek appropriate assistance. Most importantly, pump compression is limited to the arm or leg and does not ensure lymphatic flow into the center of the body, where it can be returned to the bloodstream to provide long-term benefit. Manual lymph drainage is expensive, time-consuming, and tedious, but when combined with the three other components of treatment, it provides lasting benefit for most patients. Future research could determine ways to effectively combine pump use with other standard treatment modalities.

18. What is the difference between bandaging and compression garments?

Both techniques provide essential external compression to an area with lymphedema, encouraging the return of lymph to the center of the body. Bandaging (also called wrapping) is designed to provide nonstretch compression that is easily adapted to varying limb size at each application. Ace bandages are not appropriate for lymphedema bandaging. Nonstretch compression has been more effective at preventing fluid build-up, especially in cases of severe lymphedema. Bandaging is particularly effective during an intensive treatment program and at night. Compression garments, including stockings and sleeves, are less bulky and time-consuming than bandaging; thus, they are more expedient and cosmetically attractive. Such garments are ideal for maintaining limb size once intensive treatment has been completed. A new product that has been helpful to some patients is CircAid, a semirigid support device that combines nonelastic support with Velcro to make application quick and easy while reducing bulk.

19. Must a patient with lymphedema wear a compression garment day and night?

Patients with severe lymphedema need external compression for as many hours of the day as possible. For other levels of lymphedema, opinions vary; there is no standardized way to compare outcomes of various treatment centers. Until research is completed, one logical approach to determining extent of use is for patients and caregivers to base decisions on limb measurements, limb functionality, and overall edema control in view of the patient's daily lifestyle and quality-of-life needs.

20. Is lymphedema painful?

Pain occurs in a small percentage of patients. Because cancer, thrombosis, and infection can also cause pain, careful evaluation is imperative. Lymphedema pain may be due to pressure on nerve endings, atrophy of muscles, or muscle contractures during movement. Pain can be managed with nonopioid analgesics; adjuvant drugs such as antidepressants, muscle relaxants, and opioid analgesics; transcutaneous electrical nerve stimulation (TENS); or relaxation techniques.

21. Are there any serious long-term complications for people with lymphedema?

The most common serious complications of lymphedema are severe infections and loss of limb function accompanied by immensely decreased quality of life and emotional distress. A rare and generally fatal complication associated with long-term lymphedema is lymphangiosarcoma.

Less than 1% of patients with lymphedema develop lymphangiosarcoma. The median survival time is 1.3 years.

22. What kind of support is available for people with lymphedema?

The National Lymphedema Network (NLN) has contributed immensely to education and treatment for patients and medical staff. This nonprofit organization, located in San Francisco, provides a toll-free hotline, a quarterly newsletter for patients and medical staff, international conferences for patients and caregivers, various low-cost educational materials, and several patient networking programs. Call 1-800-541-3259 for access to NLN.

BIBLIOGRAPHY

1. Boris M, Weindorf S, Lasinski B, et al: Lymphedema reduction by noninvasive complex lymphedema therapy. Oncology 8(9):95–106, 1994.
2. Brennan M, DePompolo R, Garden F: Focused review: Postmastectomy lymphedema. Arch Phys Med Rehabil 77(Suppl 3):95–106, 1996.
3. Foldi E, Foldi M, Clodius L: The lymphedema chaos: A lancet. Ann Plast Surg 22:505–515, 1989.
4. Jeffs E: Management of lymphoedema: Putting treatment into context. J Tiss Viabil 2(4):127–131, 1992.
5. Kiel KD, Rademacker AW: Early stage breast cancer: Arm edema after wide excision and breast irradiation. Radiology 198:279–283, 1996.
6. Markowski J, Wilcox JP, Helm PA: Lymphedema incidence after specific postmastectomy therapy. Arch Phys Med 62:449–452, 1982.
7. Miller L: Lymphedema: Unlocking the doors to successful treatment. Innovat Oncol Nurs 10(3):58–62, 1994.
8. Simon MS, Cody RL: Cellulitis after axillary lymph node dissection for carcinoma of the breast. Am J Med 93:543–548, 1992.
9. Thiadens S: Eighteen Prevention Steps for Lower Extremities. San Francisco, National Lymphedema Network, 1995.

37. MUCOSITIS

Janet Kemp, RN, MS, and Harri Brackett, RN, BSN, OCN

1. What is the difference between stomatitis and mucositis?

Stomatitis and mucositis mean inflammation and ulceration of the oral cavity. Stomatitis is usually associated with chemotherapy drugs, mucositis with radiation therapy. Currently mucositis refers to any oral mucosal inflammation, regardless of cause. Mucositis may progress from dry, red, inflamed, cracked areas to open sores and bleeding ulcers not only in the mouth but also in the esophagus, vagina, and rectum.

2. What causes mucositis in patients with cancer?

Mucositis is a side effect of chemotherapy, radiation therapy to the head and neck area, surgery of the oral cavity, and some of the biologic response modifiers (interleukin 2 and lymphokine-activated killer [LAK] cells). Mucous membranes are susceptible to toxicity from anticancer therapy because of their high mitotic index and rapidly proliferating epithelial cells. Chemotherapeutic agents associated with a high incidence of oral complications are 5-fluorouracil (5-FU) with or without leucovorin, methotrexate, and bleomycin. Other drugs include cytarabine, daunorubicin, doxorubicin, hydroxyurea, mitomycin, mitoxantrone, vinblastine, vincristine, and high doses of alkylating agents.

3. What subgroups of patients are at highest risk of developing oral complications?

Patients who are exposed to multiple therapies and have other predisposing risk factors, such as poor oral hygiene, dental caries, or tobacco and alcohol use, are more likely to develop mucositis. For example, many patients with head and neck cancer are at high risk for mucositis related to multiple causes, such as surgery followed by radiation therapy, history of alcohol and tobacco use, poor nutritional habits, and therapy with 5-FU (stomatoxic agent). Patients with leukemia and lymphoma and candidates for bone marrow transplant are also at high risk because they not only receive drugs with great potential to produce mouth sores but also remain neutropenic for lengthy amounts of time, which predisposes them to secondary opportunistic infections.

4. When does mucositis occur?

Stomatitis usually occurs 2–5 days after chemotherapy administration, persisting up to 14 days. Mucositis associated with radiation therapy begins 1–2 weeks after therapy is started and may persist for many weeks. The intensity and duration of mucositis are influenced by type and dosage of chemotherapy drug or depth of penetration, number, and frequency of radiation treatments.

5. What are the consequences of mucositis?

- Pain
- Malnutrition
- Volume depletion
- Electrolyte imbalances
- Taste changes
- Infection
- Bleeding (platelet count < 20,000)

6. How is mucositis assessed?

The mouth should be assessed daily and after treatment with a tongue blade and light because beginning lesions are difficult to visualize. Carefully inspect all areas of the mouth, including the tongue and underneath the tongue and the sides and roof of the mouth. Look as far back into the throat as can be visualized and in the front and back around the lips. Pay particular attention to the appearance of any lesions and the color of the mucous membranes. Early signs and symptoms of oral mucositis include mild redness and swelling along the gumline and sensations of mild burning and dryness. The presence of redness or white patches indicates a problem. Note the color, amount, and consistency of saliva; adequate moisture is important to prevent irritation. Check for swelling, ulcerations, cracks, fissures, and bumps both in the mouth and on the lips. Ask patients if they are having pain, taste changes, swallowing problems, or sore throat.

7. What common tools are available to assess and document the incidence of mucositis?

In an effort to standardize measurements and descriptions of mucous membrane integrity, several oral assessment tools have been developed to grade the level of mucositis. A commonly used tool is the University of Nebraska Medical Center's *Oral Assessment Guide* (OAG). The OAG contains eight categories, each with three levels of descriptive ratings. The eight categories describe quality of the voice, swallow, and saliva, and integrity of the lips, tongue, mucous membranes, gingiva, and teeth. The three descriptive levels rate each category from most normal (1) to most abnormal (3). In addition, the OAG includes a narrative description of each category of assessment.

The U.S. Cancer Cooperative Groups grade stomatitis according to common toxicity criteria (CTC) developed by the National Cancer Institute:

0   None
1   Painless ulcers, erythema, or mild soreness
2   Painful erythema, edema, or ulcers, but patient can eat solids
3   Painful erythema, edema, or ulcers, and patient cannot eat solids
4   Requires parenteral or enteral support

8. What do infected lesions look like? How are they treated?

Signs and symptoms of oral infection in immunosuppressed patients may be minimal. Pain and tenderness may be the only symptoms of oral infection. If **odynophagia** (painful swallowing localized to the esophagus) is present, simultaneous involvement of the esophagus must be assumed and systemic therapy is necessary. For example, thrush and odynophagia usually mean candidal esophagitis; oral herpes and odynophagia usually mean herpetic esophagitis. Likewise, bacterial ulcerations and odynophagia, although fortunately rare, may indicate devastating bacterial involvement of the esophagus.

Infection	Appearance/Symptoms	Treatment
Candida albicans	Cottage cheese-like to pearly white patches may coat tongue, roof, and side of mouth; may be discolored by food or tobacco; scrapes off easily, revealing ulcerated, sometimes bleeding surfaces. Early symptoms: burning sensation or metallic taste	**Topical:** nystatin (Mycostatin) oral suspension, 400,000–600,000 units, swish and swallow 4 times/day; or clotrimazole (Mycelex) troches, 10 mg 5 times/day **Systemic:** ketoconazole (Nizoral), 200 mg/day, or fluconazole (Diflucan), 100 mg/day; amphotericin B may be necessary.
Herpes simplex	Usually appears first on lips as painful, annoying, itchy vesicle. After 6–8 hr vesicles rupture and become encrusted, painful ulcerations. Lesions may progress to involve other oral mucosa May present as ulcerations only	Acyclovir (Zovirax), 400 mg orally every 8 hr or 5 mg/kg intravenously every 8 hr.
Bacterial infection (e.g., *Pseudomonas* and *Klebsiella* spp., *Escherichia coli*)	Raised yellow or yellow-white lesions encircled by reddened halo; ulcerated and painful. Fever often present. May present as ulcerations only. Blood cultures may be positive. Tooth pain with manipulation may be clue to dental involvement.	Topical or systemic antibiotic therapy based on culture results. Empiric therapy should cover *Pseudomonas* sp.

9. How should oral or topical medication be administered?

Fungal infections (50% of oral infections) may be treated with topical agents such as nystatin (Mycostatin) oral suspension or clotrimazole (Mycelex) troches. To facilitate drug contact of topical agents with mucosal surfaces, instruct the patient to do a mouth rinse (normal saline or water) before the medication is given and to avoid eating or drinking for at least 30 minutes after taking the topical agent. The suspension must be swished around the mouth for 5 minutes, 4 times/day. It may be spit or swallowed; swallowing is recommended because of coating of the back of the throat, where fungal lesions can hide. Troches need to be sucked and held in the mouth until they dissolves (about 5 minutes). Ketoconazole absorption is greatly enhanced by an acidic gastric fluid and should be taken on an empty stomach. The patient should not be taking antacids, H-2 blockers, or proton pump inhibitors (e.g., omeprazole). If hypochlorhydia (inadequate stomach acid) is suspected, absorption can be improved by taking ketoconazole with a cola beverage. Beware that ketoconazole may increase cyclosporine levels. Fluconazole is more expensive, but oral bioavailability is 90% and absorption is not influenced by food or antacid preparations.

For patients with limited **oral herpes involvement** around lip area, acyclovir (Zovirax) ointment can be applied topically as needed every 4 hours. Patients should be taught to apply the ointment wearing gloves or using cotton swabs to avoid spread to other areas. Often, topical therapy is inadequate and systemic therapy is needed. Oral acyclovir at 400 mg every 8 hr works as well as 200 mg 5 times/day and is more convenient.

10. How can oral mucositis be prevented?

There is no standard oral care protocol to prevent mucositis; however, studies show that, regardless of agents used, a protocol emphasizing adequate teaching, consistent documentation, and reinforcement of mouth care alone decreased the incidence of mucositis. Individualized and regular oral care protocols consisting of cleaning, lubricating, and adequate pain control are essential. Mouth care should be done at least every 4 hours while awake. Other helpful interventions include:

- Dental evaluation and crucial dental work should be done before chemotherapy is started. Prophylactic cleanings may be helpful, but dental work should be avoided during therapy, unless scheduled when blood counts are normal.
- Dietary intake should emphasize high-protein foods and lots of fluids (> 1500 ml/day) to encourage oral mucous membrane regeneration.
- The use of cryotherapy (chewing ice during chemotherapy infusion) has been shown to prevent mucositis.

11. Which is the better rinsing agent—normal saline or sodium bicarbonate?

Frequent oral rinsing of the mouth is encouraged throughout the day, particularly after eating. Because the optimal mouthwash is not yet determined, the choice often depends on patient preferences. There is no statistically significant difference in the efficacy of normal saline vs. sodium bicarbonate.

Normal saline controls mechanical plaque. It removes and washes away loose debris while moistening and soothing the oral mucosa. It is generally nonirritating, inexpensive, and readily available. Normal saline is prepared by dissolving 1 tsp of salt in a quart of warm water.

Sodium bicarbonate solution also controls mechanical plaque while neutralizing acidity and decreasing redness. It is prepared by mixing 1 tsp of baking soda in 8 ounces of warm water. Some patients prefer mixing baking soda (1 tsp) and salt (½ tsp) together in 1 cup of warm water.

12. Is hydrogen peroxide useful in the treatment of mucositis?

The use of hydrogen peroxide is controversial. Although it loosens debris and mucus and has a good antimicrobial effect, it may cause overgrowth of filiform papillae on the tongue, which enhances growth of candida. Patients also complain that hydrogen peroxide (1.5% concentration) causes increased thirst, dry mouth, and a bad taste. Peroxamint, a mint-flavored solution, may improve the taste problem.

13. Is chlorhexidine helpful in preventing infection?

Chlorhexidine gluconate, a broad–spectrum antibiotic, binds to glycoproteins coating the oral mucosa and teeth. It has been found to reduce microbial burden in patients with gram-positive or gram-negative organisms, yeast, and fungi. Chlorhexidine gluconate (0.12%) mouthwash is commercially available as Peridex. The usual dose is 15 ml, swished 2 or 3 times daily for 30 seconds after brushing teeth. Peridex can be used prophylactically as well as with moderate-to-severe stomatitis. A drawback to chlorhexidine is that it contains 11.6% alcohol glycerin leading to drying and burning. Other disadvantages include teeth staining, dysgeusia, need for a prescription, and expense.

Chlorhexidine gluconate (0.12%) mouthwash has been reported to reduce oral infection, specifically gram-positive organisms (streptococci) and yeast, in patients treated with chemotherapy. However, a recent study by Dodd et al. showed no significant differences in the incidence and severity of mucositis in a large group of patients randomized to the use of sterile water vs. 0.12% chlorhexidine to prevent chemotherapy-induced oral mucositis. Of significance, all study patients were educated in oral assessment; routine, systematic mouth care; and when to report findings to health care workers. Patients receiving high-dose head and neck irradiation show little or no reduction in stomatitis because chlorhexidine does not bind directly to epithelial tissues; instead, it binds to negatively charged salivary mucins or glycoproteins, which are decreased by radiation-induced xerostomia.

14. What can be done for vaginal or perianal mucositis?

Patients should be educated to report pain, itching, ulceration, or bleeding and be alerted to signs and symptoms of fungal or herpes infections. Management and prevention include frequent and meticulous perianal and vaginal cleansing, especially after voiding. Witch hazel (Tucks) pads may be used for the perianal area if the patient does not have skin breakdowns and can tolerate the potential stinging sensation. Water-soluble lubricants can be applied to prevent dryness and to protect the mucous linings. Sitz baths of warm water may provide comfort in patients without extensive skin breakdown.

15. What helpful hints may be shared with patients?

1. **Keep mouth moist.**
   - Rinse mouth frequently with water.
   - Use spray bottle and mist often; humidifying the room is also helpful.
   - Use commercially available salivary substitutes or supplements (e.g., Salivart, Oral balance, Salagen, MoiStir).
   - Apply lip lubricant generously.
2. **Keep mouth and teeth clean.**
   - Use soft-bristled toothbrushes or sponge-covered oral swabs with nonabrasive toothpaste to brush teeth 30 minutes after each meal and at bedtime. A tongue blade wrapped in gauze and moistened may be used as an alternative to a toothbrush.
   - Gently floss teeth with unwaxed floss (if platelet count > 20,000).
   - Remove dentures and bridges and clean after meals; do not replace if stomatitis is severe.
   - Avoid alcohol-based mouthwashes and lemon glycerin swabs because of drying and unpleasant taste.
   - Frequently rinse mouth (every 2 hr during day and at least once during night). Try alternating mouth rinses (e.g., baking soda or saline rinses at 8 AM and Peridex at 10 AM), followed by topical analgesics.
3. **Maintain integrity of oral mucosa.**
   - Apply liquid from punctured vitamin E capsule to provide natural protective action to mucous membranes and lesions, especially for radiation mucositis.
   - Use sucralfate to help heal and coat oral mucosa (binds to damaged proteins in mucosal surface); mix 1 tablet in 15 cc water to make a slurry. Swish and spit 3-4 times/day.

• For mucosal bleeding, apply topical thrombin. Remove any dentures or orthodontic retainers. Be aware of secondary infections.

4. **Follow dietary tips.**
   • Avoid foods that are hot, rough, coarse, highly spiced, or acidic.
   • Avoid temperature extremes of food (hot coffee, ice cream).
   • Avoid citrus juices or foods that irritate the mouth.

5. **Control pain.**

16. What agents may be used to treat and relieve pain associated with oral mucositis?

Severe pain associated with stomatitis may require systemic opioids such as intravenous morphine, morphine elixir, or nonsteroidal antiinflammatory drugs (NSAIDS), supplemented with topical anesthetics during more painful times, such as meals or when cleansing the mouth. Mild oral pain may be effectively controlled with local agents in patients with few ulcerations. Mouth care with oral rinsing should be done first to remove excessive debris. Commonly used topical agents include the following:

• Xylocaine viscous 2% solution: 5–15 ml, swish and spit every 2–4 hours as needed
• Diclonine hydrochloride: 5–10 ml, swish and spit every 2–4 hours as needed
• KBX solution (Kaopectate, benadryl, xylocaine viscous in equal parts): 5–15 ml; swish for 1 minute, then spit or swallow, every 2-4 hours as needed. Xylocaine functions as a topical anesthetic, benadryl as a short-acting anesthetic. Mylanta may be substituted for Kaopectate. Both serve as a medium for alkalinizing oral pH, which is usually more acidic in patients with stomatitis.
• Ulcerease: thick gel that coats, protects, and eases pain.
• Zilactin: topical application to oral and lip lesions (burns on application).

BIBLIOGRAPHY

1. Baird S: Decision Making in Oncology. Philadelphia, B. C. Decker, 1988.
2. Bavier AR: Nursing management of acute oral complications of cancer. NCI Monogr 9:123–128, 1990.
3. Beck S: Prevention and management of oral complications in the cancer patient. Curr Issues Cancer Nurs Pract Updates 1(6):1–12, 1992.
4. Dodd MJ, Larson PJ, Dibble SL, et al: Randomized clinical trial of chlorhexidine versus placebo for prevention of oral mucositis in patients receiving chemotherapy. Oncol Nurs Forum 23:921–927, 1996.
5. Eilers J, Berger AM, Peterson MC: Development, testing and application of the oral assessment guide. Oncol Nurs Forum 15:325–330, 1988.
6. Ferretti GA, Raybould T, Brown A, et al: Chlorhexidine prophylaxis for chemotherapy and radiotherapy-induced stomatitis: A randomized double-blind trial. Oral Surg Oral Med Oral Pathol 69:331–338, 1990.
7. Galbraith LK, Bailey D, Kelly L, et al: Treatment for alteration in oral mucosa related to chemotherapy. Pediatr Nurs 17:233–236, 1991.
8. Goodman M, Ladd LA, Purl S: Integumentary and mucous membrane alterations. In Groenwald, SL, Frogge MH, Goodman M, Yarbro C (eds): Cancer Nursing: Principles and Practice, 3rd ed. Boston, Jones & Bartlett, 1993.
9. National Cancer Institute:CancerNet from the National Cancer Institute. PDQ Supportive Care/Screening Information, 1993.
10. Skeel RT, Tipton J: Symptom management. In Brain MC, Carbone PP (eds): Current Therapy in Hematology-Oncology. St. Louis, Mosby, 1995, pp 584–586.
11. Wegs J: Prescriptions for patients with oral complications of cancer chemotherapy. Veteran's Administration Protocol, 1993.

38. NAUSEA AND VOMITING: ARE THEY STILL A PROBLEM?

Rita Wickham, RN, MS, PhD(c), AOCN

1. Are nausea and vomiting (N&V) a big problem in patients with cancer?

N&V are pervasive and significant problems for persons with cancer. It is estimated that 50% or more of patients receiving chemotherapy and a similar number of those with progressive cancer experience nausea and/or vomiting. N&V is most common with chemotherapy but may occur with radiation therapy to some sites as well as postoperatively. Nausea occurs more frequently in the delayed phase after chemotherapy and with progressive disease. Unfortunately, nausea is difficult to manage well in many instances.

2. What are the consequences of poorly managed N&V?

Uncontrolled N&V may have many negative physiologic and psychosocial effects, thus affecting overall quality of life. For instance, severe vomiting may lead to significant fluid and electrolyte imbalance. Rapid weight loss signifies water loss—a liter of fluid weighs 2.2 pounds. Fluid volume deficit (FVD) is characterized as mild, moderate, or severe, with weight loss ranging from 2–8%. Continuing N&V prevent the drinking of oral fluids, which exacerbates FVD and may increase toxicities from certain chemotherapeutic agents (e.g., bladder toxic effects of cyclophosphamide). Sustained nausea also may be associated with anorexia and development of food aversions. Weight loss secondary to depletion of body stores of protein and fat may ultimately render the person less able to tolerate the rigors of cancer therapy.

N&V related to therapy or to progressive disease often interfere with important activities, such as spending time with family and friends, household tasks and outside jobs, leisure activities, and enjoyment of eating and drinking. Patients who experience both uncontrolled vomiting and pain rate vomiting as the worse symptom.

3. Are physiology and pathogenesis the same for all instances of N&V?

Although we have learned a great deal about the physiology of vomiting, all mechanisms are not clearly understood, nor do we have a clear understanding of nausea because of its subjective nature. Vomiting occurs when certain neurons in the brainstem, collectively called the vomiting center (VC), are stimulated. The VC, in turn, is not directly activated by emetogenic stimuli; it is stimulated through several other inputting areas. Afferents implicated in patients with cancer include the vagus and other abdominal visceral nerves; the chemoreceptor trigger zone in the area postrema; and higher brain centers associated with vision, hearing, smell, and memory as well as the limbic region, which is associated with emotion. The vestibular apparatus of the middle ear may play a minor role, and other neural structures and visceral organs may play a yet unidentified role.

The vagus nerve plays a significant role in helping the body rid itself of perceived poisons or noxious agents, including chemotherapy drugs and products of cellular damage from radiation to the abdominal area. The vagus nerve lies in close proximity to enterochromaffin cells within the gastrointestinal (GI) mucosa. These cells release serotonin (5HT) in response to toxins in the GI tract or blood stream. 5HT binds to vagal $5HT_3$ receptors, which transmit the message to vomit, either directly to the vomiting center or indirectly through the chemoreceptor trigger zone. A related neuroreceptor, $5HT_4$, also probably plays some role in N&V, because it plays a role in gastric stasis and transit time through the GI tract. The vagus and/or other visceral nerves also respond to compression and stasis, as occur with obstruction of the GI tract, hepatomegaly, or tumor compression of upper GI structures. The stretch receptors and neurotransmitters involved have not been clearly identified.

The chemoreceptor trigger zone (CTZ) lies at the surface of the fourth ventricle close to the VC. This structure is outside the blood-brain barrier and can detect noxious substances in the bloodstream and cerebral spinal fluid. Numerous receptors for neurotransmitters that may play a role in vomiting are located in and about the CTZ. These include dopamine, serotonin, and histamine.

Higher cortical centers are important in the development of anticipatory nausea and vomiting, the realization of pain-related N&V, and N&V associated with increased intracranial pressure. The cortex and limbic region are responsible for the emotional responses to N&V, such as anxiety and suffering associated with poorly controlled symptoms.

The role of the vestibular apparatus (VA) is clearly evident to anyone who has experienced motion sickness, Menière's syndrome, or viral infection of the inner ear. Dizziness, nausea, and vomiting follow. The VA may play a minor role in N&V from other causes.

Major Afferent Pathways to the Vomiting Center

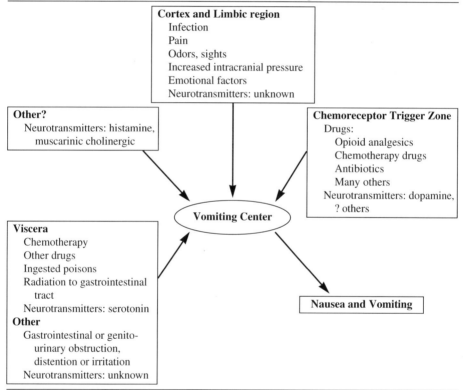

Major afferent pathways for nausea and vomiting in cancer patients include the vagal and visceral nerves, the chemoreceptor trigger zone, and higher brain centers. Neurotransmitters presumed to play the most important role for different pathways are listed, but more than one neurotransmitter may play a role within a given pathway. (From Ettinger DS: Preventing chemotherapy-induced nausea and vomiting: An update and review of emesis. Semin Oncol 22(Suppl 10):9, 1995, with permission.)

4. When are N&V likely to occur after chemotherapy is administered?

Three types of N&V are associated with chemotherapy: acute, delayed, and anticipatory. **Acute** N&V starts within minutes to hours after chemotherapy administration but resolves within 24 hours. **Delayed** N&V begins 16–24 hours after chemotherapy and persists for hours to days. It is probable that different mechanisms are involved in each phase. For instance, the role of serotonin is most important in the acute phase, whereas other mechanisms gain importance in the days after chemotherapy.

In the **delayed** phase, nausea is often worse than vomiting and has a deleterious effect on quality of life. Delayed N&V may persist for one to several days after chemotherapy. In some cases, such as after cisplatin or cyclophosphamide, delayed nausea and/or vomiting may actually worsen for a day or two before they start to subside.

Anticipatory nausea and vomiting (ANV) are thought to result when acute and delayed N&V are not well managed. ANV is thought to be an example of a classic conditioned response. Initially the patient experiences N&V from treatment (an unconditioned response). If N&V are poorly controlled, the events surrounding the treatment (e.g., smells of the treatment site, sights seen at each visit) become the stimulus to feel nauseated (a conditioned response). ANV may persist for years after chemotherapy, especially if N&V were severe. In the past, 25–60% of patients developed ANV within four courses of chemotherapy. Now that serotonin antagonist antiemetics are frequently used, ANV probably occurs less frequently.

5. Which chemotherapy drugs cause N&V?

Chemotherapy has been varyingly classified. Common categories include mildly, moderately, and moderately high or highly emetogenic. In using such categories, several points should be considered:

- Estimates are based on research findings and clinical experience; nurses tend to rate most drugs as more emetogenic than physicians.
- Chemotherapy dose is important. Current strategies often include dose escalations. Therefore, higher-than-standard doses of most chemotherapy drugs should be classified in the next higher stratum.
- Dividing the dose over several days or administering the drug by continuous infusion also changes emetogenicity (e.g., may cause less vomiting but greater nausea).
- The additive effect of two or more chemotherapy drugs that are known to cause N&V has been estimated, and most likely emetogenicity is increased.
- Almost all moderately or severely emetogenic agents cause some degree of delayed N&V.

Emetogenic Potential of Various Chemotherapeutic Agents

MILD (< 30%)	MODERATE (30–60%)	MODERATELY HIGH (60–90%)	HIGH (> 90%)
Bleomycin	Asparaginase	Carmustine	Cisplatin > 75 mg/m^3
Busulfan	Carboplatin	$\geq$ 100 mg/m^2	Cyclophosphamide
Chlorambucil	Carmustine	Cisplatin < 75 mg/m^2	> 1 gm/m^2
Cyclophosphamide (oral)	< 100 mg/m^2	Cyclophosphamide	Cytarabine
Cytarabine $\leq$ 500 mg/m^2	Cyclophosphamide	> 600 mg/m^2	> 500 mg/m^2
Etoposide	< 600 mg/m^2	Dactinomycin	Dacarbazine
Fluorouracil < 1 gm/m^2	Daunorubicin	Daunorubicin	$\geq$ 500 mg/m^2
Fludarabine	< 50 mg/m^2	> 50 mg/m^2	Ifosfamide
Gemcitabine	Doxorubicin	Doxorubicin	> 1.5 gm/m^2
Hydroxyurea	$\leq$ 50 mg/m^2	> 50 mg/m^2	Mechlorethamine
Melphalan	Fluorouracil	Lomustine	Melphalan (high
Methotrexate $\leq$ 500 mg/m^2	$\geq$ 1 gm/m^2	Methotrexate (high	dose)
Mitoxantrone	Hexamethylmelamine	dose)	Stretozocin
Paclitaxel	Idarubicin	Procarbazine	
Pentostatin	Ifosamide $\leq$ 1.5 gm/m^2	Semustine	
Taxotere	Irinotecan		
Thiotepa	Methotrexate		
Topotecan	> 500 mg/m^2		
Vinblastine	Mitomycin		
Vincristine	Teniposide		
Vinorelbine			

Adapted from Ettinger DS: Preventing chemotherapy-induced nausea and vomiting: An update and review of emesis. Semin Oncol 22(Suppl 10):6–18, 1995, with permission.

6. Does radiation therapy cause less N&V than chemotherapy?

Not exactly. Symptoms of radiation therapy are related to the site irradiated. Therefore, patients whose radiation field includes the enterochromaffin cells are at risk for experiencing N&V. Because most of the enterochromaffin cells are in the upper epigastric area, most patients who receive radiation to a large volume of the epigastric area vomit. Sixty to ninety per cent of patients treated to a single large field of the upper abdomen, receiving total body irradiation in preparation for bone marrow transplant, or receiving hemibody irradiation to the upper body for pain control experience N&V. The risk of N&V in patients irradiated to the lower abdomen is lower (20–50%). Patients receiving radiation therapy to the head also may experience N&V, possibly secondary to inflammatory effects leading to increased intracranial pressure. In rare instances, patients radiated to other parts of the body experience N&V. The mechanisms in such cases are unknown but may be related to anxiety and anticipation. Vomiting after radiation occurs within minutes when bone marrow transplantation preparatory doses are given and within a few hours after lower doses. N&V may persist for several hours after each treatment. ANV may occur if symptoms are not well controlled. Premedication with antiemetics may be helpful.

7. How common are postoperative N&V?

Although N&V after surgery are uncommon with the use of newer anesthetic agents, some patients still experience postoperative N&V. Higher risk may be associated with gynecologic or abdominal procedures. A past experience with uncontrolled postoperative N&V, high anxiety, obesity, and childhood also may increase risk. N&V may be caused by opioid analgesics and exacerbated by delayed bowel motility, which may further affect postoperative recovery and delay discharge from the hospital.

8. What other causes should the nurse consider when assessing N&V in patients with cancer?

Because there are multiple causes of N&V in patients with cancer, in-depth nursing assessment is critical. The patient may experience more than one cause. Other possible causes include the effects of gastrointestinal disease (e.g., bowel obstruction, hepatomegaly, stomach cancer, adhesions, ileus, severe constipation) or disease of the central nervous system (meningeal or brain metastases that increase intracranial pressure). Furthermore, some metabolic abnormalities caused by cancer, such as hypercalcemia, hypernatremia, and syndrome of inappropriate secretion of antidiuretic hormone (SIADH), may cause N&V. Unrelieved pain and infection may exacerbate N&V, along with opioid analgesics, antibiotics, and other medications. Antiemetic selection is therefore variable and should be based on presumed causes and involved neurotransmitters.

9. In planning interventions for N&V, what patient-related factors should the nurse consider?

The factors that seem to be most predictive of difficult-to-manage N&V include gender and age. A history of alcohol intake, motion sickness, hyperemesis with pregnancy, and high level of anxiety also may be influencing factors.

Menstruating women experience more N&V than men, whether induced by emetogenic chemotherapy or progressive disease. Even when the best available antiemetic regimens are used, up to 50% of women have inferior control compared with men. The effect of greater N&V in menstruating women is possibly hormone-related; prepubescent girls and post-menopausal women have similar rates of N&V and antiemetic control. Thus the nurse must be extremely diligent in assessing and documenting the patient's subjective satisfaction with control of N&V and must seek different or additional physician orders for antiemetics for select patients.

Age also has an effect. Patients older than 50 years have less N&V than patients younger than 50, and antiemetic control may be better in older persons. Similarly, N&V is often easier to control in patients with a history of regular alcohol use (1–5 alcoholic drinks per day). Inadequate control of N&V with previous chemotherapy increases patient expectation of N&V with new therapy. The effects of anxiety, past motion sickness, and hyperemesis with pregnancy are not as clear but may be important for certain patients.

10. What important questions should the nurse ask when assessing the potential for and evaluating the severity of N&V?

In addition to considering the emetogenicity of the chemotherapy regimen and patient factors, the nurse also should ask how bothersome N&V have been with past chemotherapy and whether the patient has a history of N&V secondary to motion sickness or hyperemesis with pregnancy. Such factors may increase the likelihood of chemotherapy-related N&V. After chemotherapy the nurse should ask the following questions:

- How many times did you vomit?
- How much nausea did you have in the past 24 hours? (Use a 0-to-10 or none-mild-moderate-severe scale.)
- How much did nausea and/or vomiting interfere with activities important to you?
- What, if anything, made the nausea and/or vomiting worse?
- Did you try anything that made the nausea and/or vomiting better?
- Did you have side effects from the antiemetics that you find unacceptable?

11. Which types of antiemetics are useful for cancer- or therapy-related N&V?

Antiemetics may be broadly classified as serotonin ($5HT_3$) antagonists, dopamine D_2 antagonists, and antiemetics with other effects. Most of these drugs also bind with other receptors to cause other effects, which may be therapeutic but more often increase side effects. For instance, chlorpromazine has similar affinity for histamine (H_1) and alpha adrenergic (α_1) receptors as for dopamine receptors. Prochlorperazine, on the other hand, has a high effect at dopamine receptors and a lesser effect at H_1 and α_1 receptors. H_1 and α_1 effects include sedation, anticholinergic effects, dizziness, and orthostasis. Chlorpromazine is therefore most likely to be used in a terminally ill person in whom such side effects are not problematic.

Antiemetics by Classification

CATEGORY	EXAMPLES	DOSES	INDICATIONS/COMMENTS
Serotonin antagonists	Granisetron (Kytril)	10 µg/kg IV within 30 min of chemotherapy	Moderately to highly emetogenic chemotherapy IV: administer undiluted drug IV push over 30 seconds, or dilute in 0.9% saline or 5% dextrose over 5 min
		1 mg PO for 2 doses: first dose up to 1 hr before chemotherapy and second dose 12 hr later	Moderately to highly emetogenic chemotherapy FDA is reviewing data for once-daily dosing of oral granisetron and will probably support use of two 1-mg tablets up to 1 hr before highly emetogenic chemotherapy
	Ondansetron (Zofran)	0.15 mg/kg every 4 hr, or 32 mg IV once; infuse over 15 min starting 30 min before chemotherapy	Highly emetogenic chemotherapy
		8 mg PO for 2 doses: first tablet 30 min before chemotherapy and second 8 hr later	Moderately emetogenic chemotherapy Several studies support that ondansetron is effective when down-dosed for less emetogenic chemotherapy, e.g., to 8–10 mg IV for moderately emetogenic and 20–24 mg for moderately high emetogenic chemotherapy
		8 mg PO every 12 hr for 1-2 days after chemotherapy	Delayed N&V

Table continued on following page.

Antiemetics by Classification (Continued)

CATEGORY	EXAMPLES	DOSES	INDICATIONS/COMMENTS
Serotonin antagonists *(cont.)*	Tropisetron (Navoban)—available in Europe) Dolasetron (in clinical trials in the U.S. and Europe		All 5HT$_3$ antagonists: Should not be administered PRN or by continuous IV infusion May be useful in some instances of delayed N&V but should be used judiciously because of expense and side effects (constipation) Little information on use for disease-related N&V (try if other antiemetics are not effective) If a first 5HT$_3$ antagonist is not sufficiently effective, (1) increase dose (if lower dose ondansetron was used) or (2) try alternate 5HT$_3$ agent
Dopamine antagonists			
Substituted benzamide	Metoclopramide (Reglan)	2–3 mg/kg IV before and repeated every 2–4 hr for 1–4 doses 10–20 mg PO 3–4 times/day 1 mg/hr continuous IV or SQ infusion	Moderately to highly emetogenic chemotherapy Moderately effective at dopamine and 5HT$_3$ receptors For delayed N&V Also has activity at 5HT$_4$ receptors, acts to increase GI motility For N&V of progressive cancer except **contraindicated** for N&V from GI obstruction
Phenothiazines	Prochlorperazine (Compazine) Thiethylperazine (Torecan) Perphenazine (Trilafon) Chlorpromazine (Thorazine)	Doses vary, but available as oral tablets, time-released spansules (Compazine), rectal suppositories, and parenteral formulations	Moderately emetogenic chemotherapy Delayed N&V Radiation-induced N&V Cannot be administered by continuous SQ infusion; irritating Chlorpromazine sedating: use in terminal illness
Butyrophenones	Haloperidol (Haldol)	2–5 mg PO every 4 hr 0.5–2 mg IM/IV every 4–8 hr 0.7–1 mg/hr by continuous IV or SQ infusion	For chemotherapy-induced N&V For N&V of terminal illness Can be administered by continuous SQ infusion for N&V of advanced disease
	Droperidol (Inapsine)	1 mg IV every 2–4 hr as needed	Sometimes used for chemotherapy—highly sedating
Others			
Corticosteroids	Dexamethasone (Decadron)	10–20 mg IV/PO before, 4–8 mg 3 times/day after 4–20 mg IV or PO every 4–6 hr	Additive effect for chemotherapy; useful for acute and delayed N&V Useful for N&V of terminal disease from many causes
Anxiolytics	Lorazepam (Ativan)	0.5–1.5 mg sublingually, PO, IV	Useful for ANV, to counter side effects of phenothiazines, possibly terminal disease
Cannabinoid	Dronabinol (Marinol)	2.5–5 mg PO 3 times/day	May cause dysphoria; start low and increase slowly May enhance appetite

Table continued on following page.

Antiemetics by Classification (Continued)

CATEGORY	EXAMPLES	DOSES	INDICATIONS/COMMENTS
Others *(cont.)*			
Anticholinergics	Scopolamine	0.6 mg SQ/IM every 6 hr	Use for N&V from terminal disease; radiation therapy if other antiemetics not helpful
Others	Benzquinamide (Emete-Con)	50 mg IM every 4 hr	Not usually effective for chemotherapy-induced N&V
	Trimethobenzamide (Tigan)	100–200 mg PO or rectally every 4–6 hr	

12. Which antiemetics should be used for chemotherapy-related N&V?

Selection of antiemetic(s) for chemotherapy is based on the emetogenicity of the specific agent (see question 5); patient-related factors, particularly gender and age; and the time since chemotherapy administration. In choosing antiemetics, knowledge of which receptors they most affect helps to target management. On the day of chemotherapy, $5HT_3$ antagonists are indicated for control of acute N&V caused by highly emetogenic chemotherapy and for many patients receiving moderately to moderately highly emetogenic chemotherapy.

Intravenous metoclopramide or prochlorperazine may be sufficient to control N&V from less emetogenic chemotherapy. These agents are often combined with other drugs (lorazepam, diphenhydramine, or benztropine) to control extrapyramidal side effects that occur in a small proportion of patients who receive dopamine antagonists. Unfortunately, added drugs (particularly diphenhydramine) significantly increase sedation. Many persons hate the sedated feeling because they feel "zoned out" or "lose days" from their lives. Sedation may increase the risk for falls in elderly persons. Thus, added drugs should be considered carefully, and drugs with the least severe side effects should be chosen. In addition, the lowest effective doses of dopamine antagonists should be used.

Different mechanisms play a role in delayed N&V. $5HT_3$ apparently plays much less of a role than in acute N&V. Thus $5HT_3$ antagonists are not first-line antiemetics for delayed N&V. Oral antiemetics, such as prochlorperazine, thiethylperazine, metoclopramide, and dexamethasone (alone or in combination), are used more often. Oral ondansetron is limited to patients whose acute or delayed N&V are not sufficiently controlled with usual antiemetics.

13. What costs are important to consider in the use of antiemetics for chemotherapy?

The cost of antiemetic regimens varies widely. Cost is extremely important, especially in light of decreasing resources for health care. $5HT_3$ antagonists, for instance, are quite expensive, and their use has been curtailed in some institutions. For instance, ondansetron and granisetron may be used only for patients receiving "highly" emetogenic chemotherapy. Institutions may deal with the cost issue by using oral $5HT_3$ antagonists, which may effectively prevent N&V from moderately to highly emetogenic chemotherapy; by limiting use to one $5HT_3$ antagonist; or by down-dosing ondansetron (e.g., to intravenous doses of < 32 mg) to the emetogenicity of the chemotherapy. There is a newly proposed classification system for the emetogenicity of combinations of chemotherapy agents, but it does not take into account patient-related factors.

Nurses are ethically bound to advocate for their patients, particularly because poorly controlled N&V translates into negative quality of life and may increase the risk of N&V with further cycles of chemotherapy. In addition, sedation from some antiemetic regimens, such as metoclopramide plus diphenhydramine, requires that someone accompany the patient to the doctor's office or clinic and may increase the risk of falls. Many regimens are complex and time-consuming, requiring several hours of nursing time and use of treatment facilities. Because these regimens may not control N&V as well as the $5HT_3$ antagonist-containing regimens, patients may need to return to the clinic or hospital for intravenous fluids and antiemetics. All of these considerations are important in the overall calculation of antiemetic costs.

Cost Comparisons of Various Antiemetic Regimens

ANTIEMETIC REGIMEN	DIRECT COSTS (ACQUISITION/AWP 1996*)	INDIRECT COSTS
Granisetron + dexamethasone		
IV granisetron 10 μg/kg (70-kg person)	$116.20‡	Pharmacy may charge for entire 1 mg vial ($166.00) because multidose
IV dexamethasone 20 mg	$2.45‡	vials are not available
Oral granisetron 1 mg before and 1 mg 12 hr after	$78.75	Nursing administration time 1–2 min
Oral dexamethasone 8–12 mg (2–3 tablets) 2 times/day†	$1.28–$1.92	
Ondansetron + dexamethasone		
IV ondansetron		
32 mg	$196.76	Cost for premixed, commercially
20 mg	$116.51‡	available bag
8 mg	$46.60‡	Pharmacy may charge for drug in 10 mg
IV dexamethasone 20 mg	$2.45‡	increments; i.e., if prescription is for
Oral dexamethasone 8 mg (2 tablets) 2 times/day†	$1.28	24 mg, charge is for 30 mg
		Nursing administration time 15–30 min
Metoclopramide + dexamethasone and lorazepam (or diphenhydramine)		
IV metoclopramide 2 mg/kg (70-kg person) before, 2 hr and 4 hr after	$98.70‡	Nursing administration time 45–90 min
IV dexamethasone 20 mg	$2.45‡	
IV lorazepam 1–2 mg before	$4.89‡	
(or IV diphenhydramine 25 mg before)	$1.30‡	
Antiemetics for delayed N&V		
Metoclopramide 10 mg PO 4 times/day†	$1.02	
Compazine spansules 15 mg 2 or 3 times/day†	$3.28–$4.92	
Prochlorperazine 10 mg 3 times/day†	$.52	
Dexamethasone 8 mg PO 3 times/day, then 2 times/day†	$1.92–$1.28	
Ondansetron 8 mg PO 2 times/day†	$37.42	

From Drug Topics Redbook. Montvale, NJ, Medical Economics Co., Inc., 1996, with permission.

* AWP = average wholesale prices. Outpatient pharmacies will mark up price of drug. Markup varies, but inexpensive drugs may be marked up several times, whereas expensive drugs may be marked up < 1–2 times.

† Cost per day. These agents will typically be prescribed for 2–5 days.

‡ Pharmacy costs will vary, but will include not only the antiemetic + markup, but time (pharmacist, technician, and perhaps nursing), IV solution bag, administration set, syringes, etc.

14. Should the same doses of intravenous ondansetron and granisetron be administered to all patients?

Intravenous doses of ondansetron are typically modified according to the emetogenicity of the chemotherapy administered. The empirically selected doses are 8 mg IV for moderately emetogenic chemotherapy, 24 mg IV for moderately high emetogenic chemotherapy, and 32 mg IV for highly emetogenic chemotherapy. These doses are similarly effective; that is, about 70–90% of treated patients have two or fewer emeses. The doses are probably based on the initial use of three doses of ondansetron; that is, 32 mg IV is equivalent to 3 doses of 0.15 mg/kg for a 70-kg person. Therefore rounding doses down slightly (to 10, 20, and 30 mg) simplifies the regimen and results in effective dosing for most people. A few other patients may require larger doses because of their size. Oral ondansetron (8 mg twice daily) controls N&V from moderately to moderately high emetogenic chemotherapy for most patients.

The recommended dose of intravenous granisetron is 10 μg/kg for moderately to severely emetogenic chemotherapy. An alternative to intravenous administration is oral granisetron, 1 mg before chemotherapy and perhaps a second dose 12 hours later. Oral granisetron is similar in efficacy to the intravenous drug because it is rapidly delivered to the vagal terminals, which lie in the crypts of the GI mucosa close to the enterochromaffin cells.

15. The house staff physician has ordered Zofran (ondansetron), 30 mg in 50 ml normal saline, to be infused over 15–30 minutes every 4 hours for 3 days after cisplatin therapy. What is the problem with this order?

$5HT_3$ antagonists act somewhat differently from other antiemetics in that their effectiveness is related to binding a high number of $5HT_3$ receptors. $5HT_3$ antagonists bind with great affinity, and this effect lasts for approximately 16–24 hours. Because of the mechanism of binding, a high initial dose should be administered. Repeated, as-needed, and continuous infusions of $5HT_3$ are not indicated. Tight binding to receptors does not occur with other antiemetics. Therefore, they are scheduled on a regular basis to maintain an adequate serum level of drug.

The second problem with the physician's order is the use of high doses of ondansetron for two additional days after chemotherapy. This is more controversial, because in comparison studies, $5HT_3$ antagonists are no more effective than other antiemetics, such as oral metoclopramide or dexamethasone, for delayed N&V. Furthermore, $5HT_3$ antagonists are considerably more expensive and may cause severe constipation when used for several days. This does not mean, however, that oral ondansetron should never be used for delayed N&V. Rather, smaller oral doses (8 mg twice daily) may be given to patients at high risk for delayed N&V or patients who have had poorly controlled delayed N&V with other antiemetics. Oral ondansetron should be used for only a few days, such as the second and third days after cisplatin therapy and the third and fourth days after high doses of cyclophosphamide.

16. What are the side effects of the $5HT_3$ antagonists?

The most common side effect of ondansetron (Zofran) and granisetron (Kytril) is headache during and after administration, which may be relieved by slowing the rate of intravenous administration. Some patients also may feel dizzy or lightheaded. If the drugs are given for several doses, the risk for constipation increases. The nurse should assess the patient's usual bowel habit, teach the patient to report subjective awareness of constipation, and initiate a bowel program when necessary.

17. What are extrapyramidal effects?

Two types of extrapyramidal symptoms (EPS) may result from administration of dopamine antagonists (metoclopramide, phenothiazines, butyrophenones). EPS may occur immediately after intravenous administration of the antiemetic or minutes to hours after oral administration. In some instances, the symptoms worsen with repeated administration of oral dopamine antagonists. The nurse should carefully review orders for antiemetics, because more than one drug that can cause EPS may be ordered. For instance, a physician may order metoclopramide (Reglan), prochlorperazine (Compazine), and droperidol (Inapsine). If the nurse administers more than one of these agents, the risk of EPS is definitely greater.

The most common EPS is akathisia, which is sometimes called the "dancing feet syndrome." Akathisia has a broad range of presentation. Patients with mild akathisia may feel anxious or jittery; patients with moderate akathisia have a difficult time sitting still; and patients with severe akathisia cannot sit or lie still at all. As one can imagine, akathisia is highly disconcerting and uncomfortable. Dystonia, a less common EPS, involves contraction of muscle groups in the head and neck (torticollis). Dystonia is frightening because patients may feel that they cannot breathe.

18. Can EPS be prevented or reversed?

Akathisia is best prevented or treated with lorazepam, which is sometimes administered prophylactically with dopamine antagonist antiemetics. The recommended drug to prevent or reverse a dystonic reaction is diphenhydramine (Benadryl), but it often is used for any type of

EPS. A small dose (25 mg) is administered prophylactically with metoclopramide, and repeated doses may be given if dystonia or akathisia occurs. Benztropine (Cogentin), 1 or 2 mg IV, also rapidly reverses dystonia; the dose may be repeated if dystonia does not resolve with the first dose.

19. What other drugs are useful to enhance antiemetic regimens?

In many instances, a combination of antiemetics that act at different receptors leads to better control of N&V or counters adverse effects of antiemetics. The best example of a drug that is not typically viewed as an antiemetic but has clear antiemetic efficacy is dexamethasone, which increases the effectiveness of antiemetic regimens by about 20%. Thus, dexamethasone, 10–20 mg (intravenously or orally) is commonly added to regimens of $5HT_3$ (intravenous and oral), metoclopramide, and other agents. Dexamethasone is also effective for delayed N&V and completely controls vomiting in about one-third of such patients (similar to oral ondansetron) and more effectively reduces nausea. Small oral doses, typically 4 mg 2 or 3 times/day, are prescribed for 3–5 days after chemotherapy. Some physicians taper the doses downward, whereas others do not. With short periods of use, the adverse effects of corticosteroids do not occur.

Another drug that may have modest antiemetic activity is lorazepam. Probably the greatest benefit from lorazepam, however, is that it decreases anxiety, offers a sense of control to some persons, and may increase sedation when this effect is desired. Sublingual administration bypasses the GI tract and the first pass effect in the liver, providing rapid transport of drug to the bloodstream. Small doses (e.g., 0.5 mg) may be taken and repeated until the desired effect is reached.

20. What are the benefits of using prochlorperazine sustained-release spansules (Compazine spansules) rather than regular tablets?

Sustained-release spansules are released into the bloodstream over 12 hours, whereas the duration of action for tablets is 4–6 hours. Dosing of each must consider the actual dose to be administered per hour, but an adequate dose administered as a spansule makes regular, scheduled administration easier for the patient. Regular administration of an antiemetic is important for optimal control of N&V in most instances. The nurse must remember that the risk of side effects, such as extrapyramidal symptoms, may increase with repeated administration.

21. Which antiemetics can be administered by continuous subcutaneous infusion? When should this method be considered?

Continuous subcutaneous infusion (CSQI) of metoclopramide or haloperidol may be useful in patients with progressive or terminal cancer. They are especially useful when nausea precludes oral intake or the patient's level of consciousness is deteriorating. Neither drug is irritating to subcutaneous tissues, as are other antiemetics. An added advantage is that both metoclopramide and haloperidol are compatible with morphine, which the patient with progressive cancer may need.

CSQI of antiemetics is started at a low dose, which is then titrated upward to control vomiting. An ambulatory infusion pump is ideal for CSQI. Metoclopramide is concentrated at 1 mg/cc, and the infusion is begun at 0.4–0.5 cc (0.4–0.5 mg) per hour. Similarly, haloperidol is concentrated at 1 mg/cc, and the infusion is begun at about 0.7 or 0.8 cc/hr. The upper chest and abdomen are appropriate sites for CSQI. The site is prepared, and a 25–27-gauge winged needle or small-gauge intravenous catheter is inserted subcutaneously. The needle is changed every 3–7 days, depending on whether the patient is hospitalized or at home. A few patients have subcutaneous reactions of erythema and induration, which preclude use of CSQI.

22. What should be done if the antiemetics fail?

The first step is to make sure that the prescribed doses were administered. In the hospital or clinic the nurse administers the first dose, but the patient or caregiver may be responsible for subsequent doses. Having the patient complete an antiemetic diary or telephone follow-up on the day after treatment may lead to timely changes in antiemetic regimens. An important consideration for self-administration may be the cost of antiemetics, particularly oral $5HT_3$ antagonists. Medicare pays only for prophylactic IV doses of these drugs, and many people do not have prescription plans with their insurance.

In some instances, doses of antiemetics should be escalated, particularly if the patient is not experiencing side effects. For instance, a dose of 8–10 mg of ondansetron may have been ordered because the patient was to receive "moderately" emetogenic chemotherapy. Because of the particular chemotherapy combination and/or patient factors, a particular patient may need 20–32 mg of ondansetron. In addition, if the first $5HT_3$ antagonist is not as effective as the patient desires or causes intolerable side effects, a trial of a second $5HT_3$ may be warranted before switching to another class of antiemetics.

For some patients, addition of other antiemetics may prove useful. The use of dexamethasone and lorazepam has already been mentioned, but a few physicians have added small doses of phenothiazines to $5HT_3$ regimens, which improve the control of N&V.

23. Which antiemetics have a limited role for controlling N&V in patients with cancer?

Trimethobenzamide (Tigan) is considered a generally useless drug. One of its selling points is that it does not cause EPS, probably because it represents such a small dose. Long-term use may cause EPS and opthotonus. Hydroxyzine (Vistaril, Atarax) is an antihistamine and is not very useful as an antiemetic. Repeated parenteral administration may cause pain; Vistaril should be administered by deep intramuscular injection and may cause sedation. Promethazine (Phenergan), like Vistaril, is irritating to tissue and causes dry mouth and other anticholinergic side effects, but it is used as a second-line antiemetic for patients with advanced cancer whose N&V are related to intraabdominal (e.g., hepatomegaly, stomach cancer) or central nervous system disease. The mechanism of antiemetic action of benzquinamide (Emete-Con) is not known, but it does not have dopamine antagonist activity and thus may be useful as a second-line drug when other antiemetics cause side effects or are not effective.

24. How about marijuana for N&V?

Some patients receiving emetogenic chemotherapy smoked marijuana and found that N&V decreased whereas appetite increased. The active ingredient, tetrahydrocannabinol (THC), was subsequently isolated and is now available commercially as dronabinol (Marinol). Marinol is not used often for several reasons. It is not a potent antiemetic; it is available only for oral administration; it is expensive; and it may cause the patient to feel dysphoric or confused. If Marinol is ordered, the nurse should monitor the patient for side effects, especially if the patient is debilitated or elderly. Some people claim that smoking marijuana is more effective than taking a Marinol tablet, but no studies have been done because of the legal status of marijuana. Marinol is not commonly used as first-line therapy for chemoinduced N&V because of the availability of more effective agents.

25. What are BDR suppositories? How useful are they?

Pharmacists can formulate **B**enadryl (25 mg), **D**ecadron (4 mg), and **R**eglan (20 mg) (or Benadryl and Reglan only) into suppositories. They are particularly useful for acute and delayed N&V after chemotherapy and for palliative care if the patient is at home, experiences vomiting, and cannot take oral antiemetics. BDR suppositories are more convenient and less expensive than parenteral medications, and are usually administered every 4–6 hours as needed for N&V.

26. How can a nurse administer a needed antiemetic to a patient who has no venous access and cannot take drugs orally?

Hospice nurses have found that oral tablets can be inserted rectally or vaginally when a patient can no longer swallow. This strategy may be useful if the pharmacist cannot make suppositories. Rectal absorption is probably greater than has been estimated. If two or more tablets are to be administered, they can be placed inside a gel capsule. Diarrhea, bleeding, and infection may limit rectal and vaginal administration.

27. Have any nonpharmacologic measures been shown to be helpful?

A few patients may benefit from nonpharmacologic measures such as relaxation, imagery, or hypnosis. Few scientific data, however, support such measures. Nurses have recommended dietary modifications, such as limiting oral intake of food on the day of chemotherapy. This strategy is probably most useful to avoid the formation of food aversions.

Some nursing studies have shown that regular aerobic exercise decreases the nausea that women with breast cancer experience from chemotherapy. Not all women are able to undertake a regular exercise program, and those who do so require support and encouragement.

Another strategy is to suggest that the patient wear an acupressure band. The band has a small button that is snugly placed over the acupuncture point that corresponds to N&V (about 3 fingerbreadths above the lowest wrist crease between the radial and middle tendons of the dominant arm). Acupressure bands may enhance antiemetic control of N&V from chemotherapy when given with antiemetics and may decrease N&V due to pregnancy and motion sickness. Relief occurs within 1 hour of applying the band and may persist as long as it is worn. Acupressure bands are commercially available.

BIBLIOGRAPHY

1. Bruera E: Ambulatory infusion devices in the continuing care of patients with advanced disease. J Pain Symptom Manage 5:287–296, 1990.
2. Ettinger DS: Preventing chemotherapy-induced nausea and vomiting: An update and review of emesis. Semin Oncol 22 (Suppl 10):6–18, 1995.
3. Grunberg SM: Potential for combination therapy with the new antiserotonergic agents. Eur J Cancer 29A(Suppl 1):S39–S41, 1993.
4. Hesketh P, Beck T, Uhlenhopp M, et al: Adjusting the dose of intravenous ondansetron plus dexamethasone to the emetogenic potential of the chemotherapy regimen. J Clin Oncol 13:2117–2122, 1995.
5. Hesketh PJ, Kris MG, Grunberg SM, et al: Proposal for classifying the acute emetogenicity of cancer chemotherapy. J Clin Oncol 15:103–109, 1997.
6. Lindley CM, Hirsch JD, O'Neill CV, et al: Quality of life consequences of chemotherapy-induced emesis. Qual Life Res 1:331–338, 1992.
7. Wickham R: Nausea and vomiting. In Groenwald S, Frogge MH, Yarbro CH, Goodman M (eds): Cancer Symptom Management. Boston, Jones & Bartlett, 1996, pp 218-251.

39. NUTRITIONAL SUPPORT

Deborah Rust, MSN, CRNP, OCN, and Colleen Gill, MS, RD

> I wish someone had told the secret to me, that I could do anything I wanted to do.
>
> *A patient after diagnosis of cancer*

1. Incidence and significance of malnutrition: why do we care?

From 40–80% of all cancer patients experience some degree of malnutrition, which is a major cause of morbidity and mortality. Severe protein-calorie malnutrition is the single most common paraneoplastic syndrome resulting from cancer and its treatment. Protein-calorie malnutrition occurs when macronutrient intake cannot meet the body's metabolic needs. Consequences include progressive weight loss, muscle wasting, skin breakdown, poor wound healing, potential intolerance to therapy, endocrine abnormalities, electrolyte and fluid imbalances, and inadequate immune function.

2. What causes cancer cachexia?

Cancer cachexia is characterized by inadequate nutritional intake to meet physiologic and metabolic needs. Severe progressive, involuntary weight loss; weakness due to loss of muscle mass; anorexia; early satiety; and serum protein depletion are the result. Primary cachexia is defined as nutritional deterioration with no consistent cause. Secondary cachexia is weight loss and anorexia due to obstruction or malabsorption. The degree and rate at which cachexia develops are determined by a complex mix of tumor, host, and treatment variables that are multifactorial and additive in effect:

- Taste changes: cancer may cause elevated thresholds for sweet and lowered thresholds for bitter tastes; treatment may create mouth blindness and alterations in taste.
- Altered hypothalamic control of appetite with brain metastasis or lesions.
- Abnormal neurotransmitter concentrations, changing levels of tryptophan and serotonin, with profound anorexia.
- Psychological and emotional impact of disease, depression, and anxiety.
- Pain from tumor, surgery, mucositis, or esophagitis.
- Localized mechanical interference from the tumor or treatment side effects may lead to early satiety, nausea and vomiting, diarrhea, malabsorption, and problems with chewing and swallowing.
- Cachectin, or tumor necrosis factor (TNF), is a protein substance or cytokine mediator that creates abnormalities in substrate metabolism and appetite. The only way to reverse TNF production is by removal of the tumor.

3. When should patients begin to get nutrition counseling?

Because malnutrition is a common result of cancer and its treatment, "catch-up" or regaining weight is more difficult than maintaining the status quo. Preventive or early intervention must be the primary goal. Whether in the hospital or clinic setting, nurses are on the front line, spending the most time with patients and thus are essential in identification of patients who develop problems with eating. Even if a full nutrition assessment is needed, nurses should not delay intervention. Written educational materials should be given to patients for reinforcement.

4. How can nurses quickly identify patients at nutritional risk?

The Subjective Global Assessment (SGA) format, developed by Dr. Faith Ottery, has the advantages of being quick (primarily patient-generated), available in Spanish as well as English, and accompanied by an algorithm for determining optimal nutritional intervention. Using the screening tool at every clinic visit for medical oncology and once a week with radiation oncology is the best way to address nutrition proactively.

Patient-generated Subjective Global Assessment (PG-SGA) of Nutritional Status

To the patient: please check the box or fill in the space as indicated in the next four sections.

A. History

1. Weight change:

In summary of my current and recent weight:

I currently weigh about _____ pounds

I am about _____ feet _____ inches tall

A year ago I weighed about _____ pounds

Six months ago I weighed about _____ pounds

During the past two weeks, my weight has

❑ decreased (1)   ❑ not changed (0)   ❑ increased (0)

2. Food intake:

As compared to my normal intake, I would rate my food intake during the past month as either:

❑   unchanged or

❑   changed: ❑ more than usual (1)

                         ❑ less than usual (1)

                         ❑ much less than usual (1)

I am now taking: ❑ little solid food (2)   ❑ only liquids (3)

                         ❑ only nutritional supplements (3)   ❑ very little of anything (4)

3. *During the past two weeks, I have had the following problems that kept me from eating enough (check all that apply):*

❑ no problems eating (0)

❑ no appetite; just did not feel like eating (3)

❑ nausea (1)   ❑ vomiting (3)

❑ constipation (1)   ❑ diarrhea (3)

❑ mouth sores (2)   ❑ dry mouth (1)

❑ pain (where _____?) (3)

❑ Things taste funny or have no taste (1)

❑ Smells bother me (1)

❑ Other (1) _____ depression, money, dental problems, etc.

4. Functional capacity:

Over the past month, I would rate my activity as generally:

❑ normal, with no limitations

❑ not my normal self, but able to be up and about with fairly normal activities

❑ not feeling up to most things, but in bed less than half the day

❑ able to do little activity and spend most of the day in bed or chair

❑ pretty much bedridden, rarely out of bed

The remainder of this form will be completed by your doctor, nurse, or therapist. Thank you.

5. A. History *(continued)*

Disease and its relation to nutritional requirements

Primary diagnosis (specify) _____

(stage, if known) _____

Metabolic demand (stress) ❑ no stress   ❑ low stress   ❑ moderate stress   ❑ high stress

B. Physical *(for each trait specify: 0 = normal, 1 = mild, 2 = moderate, or 3 = severe)*

____ loss of subcutaneous fat (triceps, chest)   ____ muscle wasting (quadriceps, deltoids)

____ ankle edema   ____ sacral edema   ____ ascites

C. SGA rating *(select one)*

❑ A = well nourished

❑ B = moderately (or suspected of being) malnourished

❑ C = severely malnourished

5. Why is weight loss such a critical marker?

Unintentional weight loss represents underlying symptoms that must be addressed to prevent malnutrition. Tumors of the nonvisceral organs usually involve minimal weight changes in contrast to tumors of the upper gastrointestinal (GI) tract, lung, and colon.

$$\text{Percent weight loss} = \frac{\text{Usual weight} - \text{current weight}}{\text{Usual weight}}$$

Weight loss is considered a cause of concern in patients with unintentional weight loss of:
- 5% in 1 month
- 7.5% in 3 months
- 10% in 6 months

6. What laboratory values are helpful in measuring malnutrition?

Unfortunately, no single test can be used to measure wasting or to identify malnutrition. However, helpful laboratory tests and assessment parameters include the following:

Serum proteins are markers of the body's ability to make new proteins. **Albumin** is the most commonly checked; this test is relatively cheap if added to a panel of laboratory values. Its half-life of 20 days reflects only the availability of protein within the past month. Albumin is measured as gm/dl; thus, fluid status must be taken into account during interpretation. The value will be falsely low in patients who retain fluids and falsely elevated in volume-depleted patients. Albumin, like all serum proteins, is manufactured in the liver; any liver dysfunction depresses its level.

Normal	> 3.4
Mild depletion	2.8–3.4
Moderate depletion	2.2–2.7
Severe depletion	< 2.1

Values are laboratory-specific; check the normal range at your institution.

Other serum proteins, **prealbumin** and **transferrin**, provide a more recent snapshot of protein status; however, they are less readily available as part of a lab panel and therefore are much more expensive. These proteins are also affected by fluid status and liver function; transferrin is inversely related to iron reserves and status and thus may be falsely elevated in anemic patients.

Cholesterol levels drop when caloric intake decreases. A low cholesterol value can substantiate suspicions of eating problems and low intake.

Urinary urea nitrogen (UUN) is a 24-hour collection of urine from which the grams of excreted nitrogen from protein are measured, added to normal losses, and subtracted from nitrogen intake. Increasing negative values reflect the breakdown of lean body mass (LBM); in other words, tissue and muscles are being used for calories and needed protein.

Hematocrit and **total lymphocytic count** (TLC) are often not valid because of the effects of cancer and its treatment.

7. How can additional cancer therapies exacerbate current nutritional status?

Chemotherapy regimens have their own unique profiles, but all generally affect rapidly dividing cells of the GI tract, resulting in nausea and vomiting, taste changes, and anorexia. Some have the additional effect of creating severe mucositis, further compromising the ability to eat.

Radiation effects are specific to the region irradiated; radiation to the GI tract is particularly significant. Nausea and vomiting, mucositis, taste changes, swallowing, dry mouth, diarrhea and malabsorption, gastritis, and enteritis are possible side effects. The tissue damage produced by radiation may be severe, with long-lasting sequelae. Early enteral nutrition support by means of percutaneous endoscopic gastrostomy (PEG) should be considered whenever extended mucositis is anticipated. The PEG tube is ideal because it can be concealed, whereas a nasogastric tube cannot.

Side effects of **surgery** depend strictly on the area removed. Potential problems involve surgery to the GI tract and include chewing or swallowing difficulties, aspiration (head and neck), dumping syndrome (gastric), and malabsorption (intestinal tract).

8. **What drugs affect nutrition in patients with cancer?**
   - **Steroids:** sodium retention and hypertension, increased protein and calcium needs, potassium wasting, glucose intolerance or diabetes
   - **Cyclosporine:** renal insufficiency, magnesium and potassium wasting. Grapefruit or grapefruit juice may interfere with its metabolism.
   - **Thiazide and loop diuretics:** loss of electrolytes; potassium replacement needed
   - **Bactrim:** folate deficiency, possible decrease in absorption of vitamin K
   - **Antibiotics:** may increase nausea, creating a baseline "grungy feeling" that is difficult for many patients.
   - **Amphotericin:** may reduce previous food intake by one-half as well as affect renal function.
   - **Opioids:** often sedating and may interfere with normal meal patterns as well as cause constipation, nausea, and vomiting.

9. **What are the most important goals in nutritional management of patients with cancer?**
   Abby Bloch, a dietitian at Memorial Sloan-Kettering Cancer Center, identifies three guiding principles:

   1. **Calories.** The first and foremost requirement of the body is adequate calorie intake. The body has an obligatory requirement for energy and will go to any lengths to meet that need, including autocannibalism (breaking down its own tissue).

   2. **Protein.** After adequate calories, the body must have enough protein for regeneration and synthesis to limit breakdown of muscle mass. Until adequate calories are obtained, however, protein will be burned to meet primary requirements, such as keeping the patient alive, with adequate caloric energy. Excessive protein is not beneficial and may stress the renal and hepatic systems.

   3. **Medications.** Finally, the patient needs adequate medications to support nutrition goals (e.g., antiemetics, antidiarrheals, supplements of pancreatic enzymes, medications for pain control).

10. **What can nurses do when patients complain of eating problems?**
    Triage, or identification of the severity and duration of the patient's problems, entails listening to the patient's concerns and either:
    - Normalizing the recovery process for the patient whose problems are within normal limits and not yet affecting weight status while providing appropriate materials to begin working around the current eating problem
      or
    - Identifying significant problems to the physician, clinical dietitian, and nutritional support team (if available). The use of an assessment tool (SGA) is especially useful in the identification process.

11. **The patient with anorexia often says, "I just don't have an appetite; nothing sounds good." How can you help?**
    The simple loss of hunger or desire to eat takes away the primary incentive that most of us have to eat at regular intervals. Although seemingly more benign than overt nausea and vomiting, it is in fact the most common cause of decreased intake that leads to loss of fat and muscle reserves (weight loss, wasting). Because patients lack an internal clock that reminds them to eat and often have negative experiences related to eating, as well as fatigue and depression, most patients simply eat less often and therefore consume fewer calories.

    If the anorexia is of short duration (e.g., only a few days after chemotherapy cycles), patients can be encouraged to incorporate simple behavior changes. However, the frequency of treatment regimens may be a factor. When weight loss begins or persists despite early interventions, progression through the following options is encouraged (as well as referral to an oncology dietitian):

    1. **Behavioral adaptations.** Positive actions that focus on increased intake and decreased mental stress related to eating commonly include increasing frequency of meals and snacks, taking advantage of the patient's best mealtimes (often earlier in the day), diverting attention with social activity or television during mealtimes, arranging for help with meal preparation as needed, and planning ahead for low-energy days.

2. **Maximizing nutritional intake.** The caloric density of the foods that the patient eats should be increased to provide the most calories in the smallest volume of food. Often one of the key concepts that must be communicated to the patient is a change in priorities. Friends and family may be following a low-fat, high-fiber diet to minimize risk of cancer, but the patient with cancer already has the disease, and by losing weight is compromising immune function with malnutrition. Fat and sugar may be negatives in the well person, but they are critical components in increasing the caloric density of foods for patients with cancer. Patients may be taught strategies to add calories to their favorite foods.

Adding Calories to Foods You Like to Eat

Whether you are losing weight or trying not to lose weight while dealing with problems that make eating difficult, it is always a bonus to pack calories into the smallest volumes possible. Fat and sugar may not seem "healthy", but it is important to see their use as part of a transitional period that requires extraordinary measures. *This is hardly a time you will suddenly learn to like foods you have never liked.* It is possible, however, to add calories to the foods that you do like, even if they are traditionally low in calories.

Milk/dairy
- Good alone, but go up one level in fat content (e.g., from skim to 2%).
- Add Carnation Instant Breakfast (CIB)
- Make milkshakes
  1 cup ice cream (high calorie, of course)
  1 package CIB
  4 oz half and half
  Flavoring:
    ½ tsp almond or peppermint extract
    ½ cup fruit

Eggs
- Mix grated cheese or cream cheese into scrambled eggs; it softens texture, too.
- Melt cheese on fried eggs.
- Eggs Benedict
- Use extra mayonnaise in egg salad or deviled eggs.

Breads/cereals
- Add fruit, raisins, or nuts to cereals.
- Top with sugar, half and half, etc.
- Add CIB to hot cereal, top with syrup.
- Eat croissants, pastries.
- Top pancakes, french toast, or waffles with syrup or fruit and whipped cream.
- Eat fruit and nut breads with cream cheese.
- Top crackers with cheese or nut butters.

Salads/vegetables
- Regular, not low-fat, salad dressings.
- Top with cheese, meat, nuts, avocado, egg.
- Dips or peanut butter on raw vegetables.
- Add margarine/sauces to cooked vegetables.

Meats/main dishes
- Bread and fry meats vs. baked or broiled.
- Add gravies.
- Mix nonfat dry milk into hamburger patties, meatloaf, or casseroles.
- Add extra cheese to pizza, macaroni and cheese, spaghetti, other casseroles.
- Add sour cream.
- Add mayonnaise, cheese, avocado, or bacon to sandwiches.

Soups and stews
- Make soups with milk instead of water.
- Add chopped cooked meats.
- Top with cheese.

Fruits/desserts/snacks
- Add sour or whipped cream or coconut to fruit salads.
- Snack on dried fruits, add to cereals.
- Spread peanut butter on fresh fruit.
- Fruit in heavy syrup has twice the calories.
- Eat dessert with whipped cream or a la mode.
- Eat chips with dip.
- Nuts provide great calories, great snacks.

Extras that count

• Butter	45 cal/tsp
• Sour cream	70 cal/tbsp
• Whipped cream	60 cal/tbsp
• Cheese	100 cal/oz
• Cream cheese	100 cal/oz
• Mayonnaise	100 cal/tbsp
• CIB	130 cal/package
• Avocado	55 cal, ⅙ medium
• Nuts	160–190 cal/oz
• Peanut butter	90 cal/tbsp

3. **Oral supplements.** Start with the higher calorie versions (355 vs. 250/can), which can be diluted if necessary. Most sales representatives are willing to leave trial packs of supplements that allow patients to try several alternatives and decide which they like (or at least tolerate). Consider chilling supplements to enhance flavor. Be positive about supplements; a single negative comment may eliminate the patient's willingness to try.

12. Are any medications useful in increasing appetite?

Anticachectic drugs are used to improve intake or correct metabolic abnormalities that prevent effective utilization of intake. Patients must be counseled that, although the drug may make it easier to increase intake, they must also continue previous efforts.

- **Steroids**, although initially used to enhance appetite, have not been consistently effective in patients with cancer. Of greater significance, their side effects, which include increased muscle breakdown and fluid retention, often reduce intake.
- **Cyproheptadine hydrochloride** (Periactin) is an antihistamine that stimulates appetite as a side effect in cancer-free populations (anorectic and elderly patients); however, studies in patients with cancer at the Mayo Clinic have been inconclusive.
- **Hydrazine sulfate**, a gluconeogenic enzyme inhibitor, decreases futile cycles that waste energy. It is not commonly available in the United States.
- **Dronabinol** (Marinol), a synthetic cannabinoid, increases appetite but usually results in little weight change and may cause dizziness and sedation. Recommended dose: 2.5 mg twice daily.
- **Metoclopramide** (Reglan), although well-known as an antiemetic, may be useful for patients experiencing early satiety because it increases GI transit time, but may have a negative effect if it increases losses with diarrhea. It has been shown to be most useful in patients with GI cancers.
- **Pentoxifylline** (Trentol) suppresses tumor necrosis factor (TNF) in patients whose baseline levels were elevated and thus improves weight gain.
- **Megestrol acetate** (Megace) increases appetite and lean body mass and decreases breakdown of fat reserves. One study found that 65% of patients taking Megace gained an average of 8 pounds compared with 20% of patients receiving placebo + intervention and a 2-pound loss in patients with no intervention. Recommended dose: 20 ml/800mg. The liquid dose is easier than the 20 (40-mg) tablets and has the added benefit of being significantly less expensive ($7–9.00/day vs. $20–40.00/day). The recommended regimen starts at 800 mg/day for 24 days to establish efficacy. If it has not been effective during this time, increased doses will be of little benefit. If it has increased appetite, the dose may be reduced gradually to a lower level that remains therapeutic. Side effects include mild edema and, rarely, deep vein thrombosis.

13. The patient with early satiety often says, "I can only eat a little bit." What can you do?

One of the most commonly reported symptoms is a feeling of early satiety. A family member may notice that meal portions are not quite as large. Physiologically, atrophic changes have been noted in the gut mucosa of patients with cancer. This atrophy and the metabolic abnormalities that cause wasting of muscle in the gut wall may result in increased transit time and delays in digestion. Other metabolic changes related to TNF may cause continuous stimulation of the satiety center in the brain.

- Because patients can tolerate only **small volumes of food**, getting adequate calories requires taking small volumes more frequently. Patients sometimes understand the concept a little better when it is compared to the "preschooler" schedule for children, who also have small stomachs that need to be filled frequently: mid-morning, mid-afternoon, and bedtime snacks.
- **Carbohydrate-containing beverages** are useful as between-meal snacks, because they empty out of the stomach quickly. However, beverages should be discouraged before solids at meals because they occupy volume and reduce the amount of food that the patient can eat.
- **Concentrating caloric density** is also useful, but the patient needs to monitor whether high-fat foods increase early satiety as a result of slower stomach emptying.

• **Metoclopramide** (Reglan) may be helpful in decreasing early satiety when delayed gastric emptying is an issue (and diarrhea is not).

Loss of Appetite and Early Satiety

Plan
- Have small, frequent meals and snacks. Discuss the best times for this with your family, and agree on a schedule. You can set a timer or alarm clock to remind you to eat if others are not around to remind you.
- Drink liquids between meals to avoid getting filled up at mealtimes. Drinking high calorie fluids between meals is an easy way to include snacks.
- Keep a list of ideas for snacks and quick meals on your refrigerator, for the times when you just can't think of anything.
- Keep snacks easily accessible, on the table next to your bed or chair to lessen the work of eating. Using convenience foods makes preparation easier. Let friends bring in a meal.
- Take advantage of your "best" mealtimes, usually earlier in the day.
- When looking at various options, keep your expectations reasonable: "What do I think I can tolerate today?" Don't expect foods to have the same attraction they had prior to treatment.
- Start out with small portions, it will prevent you from being overwhelmed by the task of eating, and make you feel successful when you manage to finish.
- Variety is not important on these days. If only one thing appeals to you, it's okay.
- Food restrictions suggested prior to treatment should not be a priority (for example, low cholesterol). Eliminate them whenever possible.

Concentrate calories
- Eat foods that are calorie-dense, packing the most calories into a small volume. Limit lower calorie foods and fluids like water, tea/coffee, or diet drinks.
- If solid foods are not possible, fluids can often make up for the missing calories. Milkshakes, cocoa, floats, chocolate milk, juices, sodas, and soups can make a meal.
- Limit high-fat foods that delay stomach emptying if they cause you to feel full early; however, it will be difficult to increase your caloric intake with a low-fat diet.

Keep food fun
- Maintain the positive aspects of eating: set your table attractively, and avoid eating out of cans and cartons.
- Social diversion helps take your mind off the difficulties of eating. Eat with friends or family. Whenever possible, watch television, listen to the radio, or read a book while you eat. (Children, however, may be overly absorbed with television and videos and forget to eat.)
- Regular exercise helps stimulate your appetite. Marathons are not necessary; just incorporate walking and activity into your day. It will help prevent muscle loss as well.
- Some patients find that a glass of wine 30 minutes before a meal can help, but check with your doctor first.
- Ask your physician about antidepressants if anxiety or depression is a problem.

14. Patients experiencing nausea and vomiting often say, "What's the use? It just comes back up." What can you do?

A careful history may elicit specific triggers for the patient's nausea. Identifying the underlying cause of nausea and vomiting helps to determine the appropriate intervention and improves treatment of symptoms.

1. **Dietary strategies** (appropriate food choices decrease the likelihood of emesis):
   - Cold clear liquids are often the first foods tolerated. Begin with popsicles, sherbets, sorbets, frozen ices, jello, and beverages; establishment of tolerance before advancing increases the patient's willingness to increase intake slowly. Gradual incorporation of soft, smooth foods such as ice cream, milkshakes, puddings, hot cereals, and soups is usually tolerated next, although some patients best tolerate lower-fat options.

- Vitamin tastes from many supplements may increase nausea, but Scandishakes are usually better tolerated because they can be made with a juice base (the recipe is included in question 23).
- Small, frequent meals reduce distention and reflux.
- Cold or room-temperature foods decrease aroma-related nausea. Nurses should remove the lids to hot foods outside the room to decrease odors for patients.
- Avoid fatty, fried foods that delay stomach emptying if the patient observes increased nausea and vomiting with such foods.

2. **Behavioral strategies** (simple changes around eating times may decrease nausea):
- Rest after eating, avoiding excessive movement and exercise.
- Keep the head elevated to allow gravity to work against reflux. The stomach empties fastest with patient lying on the right side.
- Avoid gagging activities (mouth care, pills) immediately after eating as well as highly textured foods that stimulate gagging.
- Relaxation techniques, including guided imagery, may be beneficial.
- An initial continuous antiemetic dosage plan is best, even after the patient seems to have improved. Doses can be weaned gradually to determine whether the patient is doing well because of the medication or truly no longer needs it. Prevention is crucial. As-needed dosing of secondary antiemetic medications must be thoroughly explained to patients, or they will be unaware of the need to request them.

It is always helpful to teach patients that unless they lose their meals immediately after eating, they are deriving some benefit from them. The stomach empties into the intestinal tract in about 2 hours; thus, even if the food stays down for only 1 hour, approximately one-half of its nutrients have passed through and are available to the body. When initiation of emesis is not meal-related, we can reasonably recommend that the patient keep trying to eat; vomiting occurs independently of intake, and some nutrients will be retained.

15. What do you do for patients who refuse to try foods that previously caused vomiting?

One of the unique experiences in cancer care is watching a patient throw up at the sight of foods (or even people) that she or he associates with chemotherapy and vomiting. Recent clinical trials have indicated that food aversions may develop as early as 48 hours before or after the first treatment. Carried to extremes, this pattern of behavior results in a remarkably short list of options for feeding the patient. The best approach to broadening the menu for such patients is a combination of psychological therapy (relaxation techniques), careful timing of reintroducing foods, and education. The key is rebuilding positive associations: "I was able to eat it, and didn't throw up." Try a three-step process:

1. **Relaxation therapy.** Arrange consultation with a therapist who can teach patients to recognize impending nausea and to calm themselves before vomiting by using relaxation techniques.

2. **Education.** Explain the typical peak nausea times after chemotherapy, and encourage patients to avoid favorite foods during this period in order to limit development of new aversions.

3. **Reintroduction.** Patients should be encouraged to retry foods that previously were associated with nausea and vomiting when the probability of tolerance without nausea is at its highest, thus building positive associations. Often the optimal time is earlier in the day, but most patients can identify "good times" vs. times when they feel more nauseated and need to stay with "safe" foods. Obviously, a key ingredient is adequate antiemetic medication throughout the reintroduction process.

16. Patients often complain, "Nothing tastes good anymore." How does cancer and its treatment affect taste? What can patients do?

Both tumor and treatments commonly cause serious damage to the cells involved in taste and smell. Taste is distinguished by the tongue, buccal cavity, lips, and cheeks. The tongue is most sensitive to salty and sweet tastes; the palate, to sour and bitter tastes. As with most cells of the

GI tract, the cells of the taste bud have a high turnover rate, with an average life span of 10 days. Drug therapy, radiation, and chemotherapy have the potential to affect cell turnover rate. The enteral nervous system also is involved in taste sensation; thus, tumors affecting the cranial nerves also affect taste. Certain chemotherapies (methotrexate, cisplatin, cyclophosphamide, vinca alkaloids) may cause a metallic taste. Decreased saliva production and mucositis, which are common problems, also affect taste.

Patients with cancer often complain that food is absolutely tasteless (ageusia, or mouth blindness) because of widespread damage to tastebuds or has an "off" taste (dysgeusia) due to changes in balance among the taste centers. Our best advice is to encourage foods that have enhanced flavors rather than the bland foods usually suggested to patients. The obvious exception is the patient with mucositis, in whom tart and spicy foods irritate the oral mucosa.

Overcoming Taste Problems

Eliminating problematic tastes
- Practicing good mouth care and rinsing the mouth with a solution of salt, baking soda, and warm water before eating help to eliminate bad tastes.
- Drink fluids with meals to rinse away bad tastes. Fruit-flavored drinks such as Hi-C, Koolaid, or Gatorade are well tolerated; coffee and tea frequently are not.
- Use plastic eating utensils and glass or plastic cooking containers if you notice a metallic taste while eating.
- If red meats seem bitter, substitute chicken, dairy, pork, fish, and eggs as protein sources.
- Minimize odors that can affect taste by drinking fluids cold and with a straw and by choosing cold foods such as cheese, milkshakes, cold cuts, tuna and egg salad.
- Hard candies and fresh fruit eliminate bad tastes in the mouth and leave a more pleasant taste.
- Retry foods; what tastes "off" this week may work next week.
- Eat foods cold or at room temperature.

Enhancing flavors
- Use more strongly seasoned foods, such as Italian, Mexican, curried, or barbequed foods, unless you have mouth sores. These stronger flavors increase the probability you'll sense the taste.
- Tart foods help to overcome metallic tastes. Use lemon, citrus or cranberry juices, and lemon drops.
- Marinate food in wine, fruit juice, soy or teriyaki sauce, Italian dressing, or barbeque sauce.
- Sauces and gravies help to spread taste through the mouth and add calories, too.
- Eat meats with something sweet, such as applesauce, jelly, glazes, or cranberry sauce.
- Salt decreases the excessive sweetness of sugary foods.

Dry mouth
- Choose moist foods, adding sauces, gravies, fat, and other lubricants whenever possible. Dry foods such as breads, crackers, or dry meats are not well tolerated alone.
- Use tart substances such as lemon juice, or suck on hard candies (especially sugarless lemon drops) to stimulate maximal production of saliva.
- Drink lots of fluids (juices, broth soups, and fruit-flavored beverages); switch to liquid diet if necessary.
- Sucking on ice chips keeps the mouth lubricated.
- Rinse your mouth frequently with a saline solution.
- Artificial saliva may be helpful, but some patients complain that such products are thick and have a sticky consistency.
- Regular mouth care is essential with decreased saliva to prevent cavities, gum disease, or mouth ulceration.

17. What can you suggest to patients who are sensitive to smells?

Smells alone can be a primary trigger for nausea, preventing the patient from attempting to eat a meal or snack. Simple management of food choices, preparation, and service can minimize this problem.

- Choose cold foods, which lack the volatile compounds that reach the nose.
- Caretakers can reduce smells in meal preparation using fans, covered pans, microwaves, or outdoor grills.
- Friends may cook meals at their homes and bring them over, reducing the smells of preparation for the patient.
- Take-out foods from restaurants may help.
- Dietary staff and nurses serving meals can reduce odors in patients' rooms by uncovering the trays in the hallway before entering.

18. A patient with mouth or throat sores often says, "It hurts to eat." What can you do?

Mouth and Throat Sores

Whether caused by radiation, chemotherapy, oral infections, or graft vs. host disease, pain is often the final straw when added to the traditional problems associated with eating. Avoidance of foods that increase pain helps to prevent a total breakdown in eating.

Helpful
- When solids are not tolerated, use a liquid diet, including Carnation Instant Breakfast, commercial supplements, pasteurized egg nog, milkshakes, and blenderized foods.
- Cook foods until tender and soft in texture.
- Eat soft foods at room temperature or lukewarm rather than hot (e.g., soups, mashed potatoes, eggs, quiche, cooked cereals).
- Dry foods can be soaked in liquid or covered with gravies or sauces.
- Cold foods are tolerated by many (e.g.,milk shakes, cottage cheese, yogurt, watermelon, jello, soft canned fruits, baby food).
- Try frozen foods, although a few patients cannot tolerate extreme cold temperatures (e.g., popsicles, ice cream, frozen yogurt, slushes/ices).
- Fruit-flavored beverages or nectars are tolerated much better than acidic juices.
- Drink through a straw to bypass mouth sores.
- Tilt your head backward or forward to help with swallowing.
- Small, frequent meals limit the irritation to a sore mouth.
- Maintain good mouth care to prevent infection. Brush and rinse with a salt/baking soda solution several times a day. Avoid commercial mouthwashes that contain alcohol.
- Take pain medications as needed to control pain and make eating possible. Liquid solutions that anesthetize the mouth are helpful to some patients when taken prior to eating.

Harmful
- Tart or acidic foods such as citrus fruits and juices, tomato, or pickles, will burn.
- Salty foods and drinks, including broth, may be irritating.
- Strong flavorings and spices, such as peppers, chili, nutmeg, and cloves, will burn and irritate sensitive tissues. No Italian, Mexican, or other spicy foods. Use seasonings sparingly.
- Rough or coarse foods will scratch (e.g., raw fruits and vegetables, dry breads, cereals, chips).
- Alcohol and tobacco irritate tissues.
- Hot foods or drinks burn already damaged surfaces.

19. A patient with diarrhea often says, "It just goes right through me." What can you recommend to manage diarrhea and identify malabsorption?

Like the tastebuds, the cells of the GI tract turn over rapidly and are more vulnerable to the effects of chemotherapy and radiation. Many health care professionals were trained to "rest the gut" while using oral rehydration solutions (e.g., Pedialyte); recent research, however, has shown that this strategy leads to more weight loss without shortening the duration of diarrhea.

Medications
- Medications that use soluble fiber or clay to absorb water in the stool, such as Kaopectate or Peptobismol, may be helpful. Medications that slow motility (Lomotil, tincture of

opium, Imodium) should not be used until bacterial overgrowth (e.g., *Clostridium difficile*) and infection have been ruled out.

- Stop medications that can exacerbate or cause diarrhea, if possible, including oral magnesium supplementation and metoclopramide (antiemetic).
- Gray or tan, greasy stools that float in the toilet indicate fat malabsorption. Although not common in patients with cancer, this condition may benefit from pancreatic enzyme supplements.

Dietary modifications

- Complex carbohydrates (fruits and starches) are particularly well absorbed and beneficial to gut healing. However, highly insoluble fiber, such as bran, should be limited. Diarrhea is a marker of GI damage, and food safety precautions to limit introduction of pathogenic organisms is recommended.
- Avoid gastric irritants such as caffeine, pepper, and alcohol.
- Absorption of lactose may be impaired by the damage to the GI tract. The lactase enzyme is easily lost and leaves the carbohydrate available for breakdown by normal gut flora. Their metabolic byproduct is gas, which creates the bloating and cramping and, ultimately, the diarrhea associated with lactose intolerance. Alternatives to milk products include soy milk, supplements, sorbet, and tofutti frozen dessert as well as lactose-free milks. Lactase tablets or drops (available over the counter) may be used if milk products are highly desired.
- Fluid replacement is essential, to replace the increased losses in the stool. Nonacidic juices are well tolerated: nectars, fruit-ade drinks, gatorades. Some patients find that it helps to avoid liquids at meal times and to limit liquids with high sugar content.

Total parenteral nutrition

- When diarrhea continues despite diet modifications and appropriate medicines, the gut no longer "works," and the ultimate criteria for the use of total parenteral nutrition are met.

20. How can I help the patient with an overly helpful caregiver?
Often family and friends latch onto feeding the patient, perhaps because it seems to be the one area in which they feel competent to help the person they love. Unfortunately, when the patient is less than cooperative in complying with their direction and help, some caretakers react by exerting increased pressure (or encouragement). This has the predictable result of bringing patients, at least mentally, back to their childhood when they were forced to eat foods that they did not want. In general, patients actually eat less when they are pressured. You can help relationships that are heading for control battles by the following strategies:

- Suggest that the patient and caretakers discuss appropriate meal and snack schedules in advance as well as a list of foods that seems acceptable to the patient. Friends and family can shop for foods, remind the patient at the agreed times, ask the patient what he or she would like to try, and prepare it. The control of what and how much the patient eats must remain with patients, because the consequences are theirs alone.
- Encourage the evaluation of progress over a week's time, not day to day. Remind family that everyone has a variable appetite, but healthy people are not obsessed with the variations. Patients with cancer have "good" and "bad" days as well. If the family expects that every day will be better than the day before, the tendency to push food on "bad" days will increase. This pattern, unfortunately, adds to the patient's list of food aversions, because forced foods are more likely to be associated with feeling badly.
- Discuss the reality of "force feeding": *it never works.* Eating is one area over which the patient exerts total control; others cannot do it in their behalf. In fact, if others attempt to take responsibility for their eating, some patients simply give up the responsibility altogether. The result is a set-up for failure.

21. What other significant psychological issues surround eating?
Weight loss. One of the most frequent comments from patients, especially women in general and men who have had prior weight problems, is that "It doesn't matter. I can afford to lose a

few pounds." Although some are open enough to joke about their "cancer diet," others are affected on a more subliminal level. For most of their life they have tried to avoid eating too much or to lose a few pounds. Changing engrained thoughts requires education about changing priorities and the affect of weight loss on strength and muscle mass.

Expectations from food. Of necessity, food has been part of our life since birth. Simple observation of the various ethnic preferences shows that the foods to which we are exposed determine what we eventually like or dislike, what "sounds good" to us. Globally, eating has always been a self-reinforcing activity: food tastes good, so we want more of it. For patients with cancer, such expectations are no longer fulfilled. **It is important to help patients to realize that eating is part of their treatment.** Re-keying expectations to "What do I think I can tolerate?" may help significantly.

22. What additional considerations are necessary for pediatric patients?

Although most issues apply equally to adult and pediatric patients, three areas of difference warrant special attention:

- The child is still growing. Optimizing nutrition is even more critical to ensure that body and brain growth are not significantly impaired during the treatment process.
- Getting more calories into children is complicated by their increased sensitivity to nausea and vomiting and taste changes due to the youthfulness of their sensory receptors.
- Depending on age and maturity, many children cannot conceive of delayed gratification. This difference is crucial, because we often ask patients with cancer to eat without incentives—and often despite significant disincentives. Working closely with the family to establish a reward system for eating helps to address this issue. In working with adolescents, control issues can be especially important to review with parents and patient.

23. When are commercial supplements helpful? How do I decide which is best?

Many patients with cancer find it easier to drink their calories, because fluids do not require the energy of chewing, rarely stimulate the gag reflex, and generally empty out of the stomach more quickly with fewer complaints of early satiety. Most fluids are relatively low in protein, however, and therefore are not complete nutritional sources. Various complete nutritional products are now on the market, but cost containment generally restricts hospitals to one option within a category. Some formulas are meant for oral intake and others solely for tube feeding (unflavored). Specific contents are detailed in information provided by the manufacturer.

When a patient is no longer able to eat an adequate amount of calories, tube feedings are preferred over total parenteral nutrition (TPN). Tube feedings have a lower risk of infection, require less medical assistance, create less disruption of normal eating patterns, and are significantly less expensive. The classic phrase, "When the gut works, use it!," is based on these advantages as well as the knowledge that the GI tract nourishes itself from the inside as nutrients travel through it. GI health is therefore maintained far better with enteral feedings than with TPN, even when calories are equal. A nighttime tube feeding may improve the patient's quality of life by allowing a more normal lifestyle during the day and by lessening the pressure on the patient to "force feed" the total requirement of calories.

Lactose-containing supplements. Benefits include decreased cost, improved taste for many patients more familiar with milk products, and somewhat less of a vitamin aftertaste. The major risk is lactose intolerance.

- Flavored packets of Carnation Instant Breakfast, generally found in the cereal aisle, provide 250–280 calories added to 8 oz milk (2% or whole) and 12 gm of protein.
- Scandishake (Scandipharm) initially was used for patients with cystic fibrosis, whose calorie needs are increased. It is now popular among patients with AIDS or cancer and is available in sugar free, and lactose free formulas as well. Scandishake provides 440 calories and may be added to 8 oz milk (total of 600 calories) or 6 ounces of juice and ice (total of 500 calories). The juice version is particularly well tolerated by patients with cancer, because tart juices counteract the sweet taste that many do not tolerate.

Standard lactose-free supplements.
- Containing intact proteins from soy isolates or calcium caseinate, lactose-free supplements provide 9–11 gm of protein and 250 calories per 8 oz. Examples: Ensure, Sustacal, Osmolite, Resource, Nutren.
- Also available in higher calorie versions (355/8 oz), with increased protein. Examples: Ensure Plus, Resource Plus, Nutren 1.5 or 2.0, Deliver 2.0, Magnacal. The 2 cal/cc options are generally not as well tolerated. All options require additional fluids to meet hydration needs.
- Higher protein versions with standard 250 calories for patients with increased protein needs include Osmolite HN, Sustacal HN, and Ensure HN.
- Fiber-containing versions for use in decreasing diarrhea include Jevity, Nutren with Fiber, and Fibersource HN. Sustacal with Fiber is an oral supplement that is often preferred by patients because it tastes less sweet.

Predigested supplements provide a peptide-based diet that can be beneficial for patients with impaired GI function. Examples: Peptamen, Peptamen VHP. They contain more fat than the truly elemental formulas, although primarily in the form of medium-chain triglycerides, which are more easily absorbed.

Elemental supplements. All of the protein is hydrolyzed to free amino acid form for absorption with minimal digestion. Fat is provided at very low levels that nonetheless meet the need for essential fatty acids. Vivonex Plus is occasionally associated with increased diarrhea. Current research indicates that peptide-based formulas may be better absorbed than strictly elemental formulations.

24. How can nutrition be reinstated after the gut has not been used?

The mucosal lining of the small bowel requires nutritional support, and the lack of enteral intake results in significant mucosal atrophy within days. The villi decrease in height and number, and the rate of mucosal cell turnover also decreases. In this setting, instituting enteral intake too rapidly may result in diarrhea and abdominal cramping. This problem is best overcome by slowly reinstituting feeding, titrating upward the rate of feeding over days at a pace determined by the patient's tolerance. The diarrhea and cramps are not dangerous, and if you are trying to maximize caloric intake, antidiarrheals such as Imodium may be tried if the diarrhea is not severe. In any case, the problem of mucosal malnutrition and diarrhea should be temporary.

If the gut is functional, enteral tube feedings should be used. The nasogastric or nasoduodenal (Dobbhoff) tube is most often used if the feeding time frame is short, but for long-term feeding, especially in patients who cannot take food orally for more than 1 month, a tube placed directly into the stomach (via percutaneous endoscopic gastrostomy [PEG]) or small bowel may be used. In considering the type of enteral solutions, several factors should be kept in mind: functional capacity of the gut, tube size, patient's metabolic status, and cost. The primary food of enterocytes is the amino acid glutamine, which is supplied by most nutritional supplements. Blenderized formulas have the advantage of lower cost; however, they are mainly suitable only for large-diameter tubes, such as the PEG tube. Commercial milk-based products such as Carnation Instant Breakfast may serve most patients' needs, but if mucosal malnutrition is severe, a lactose-free formula is better.

25. When is TPN appropriate?

TPN may be used when the gut is not functional because of cancer or its treatment. Common reasons for implementation include extensive GI surgery, bowel obstruction, or severe malabsorption. Prolonged oral or esophageal mucositis may be an indication for short-term TPN, but if long-term support is needed, physicians should consider placement of a gastrostomy-tube. TPN involves much higher costs ($300–500/day) and increased risk of infection, especially in patients with high blood sugar levels. Without insurance, TPN is usually not financially feasible at home; TPN for > 3 months may exceed the patient's lifetime insurance benefits. One study showed a 5-fold increase in infection if blood sugars were above 200. TPN has not been shown to be beneficial for patients with cancer unless they are severely malnourished or the gut is not functional. It should be initiated only when problems prevent adequate oral intake for > 10 days, the patient has a life expectancy of at least 40 days, and central line access can be established.

26. What are appropriate nutrition goals in the outpatient setting?

With the increase in outpatient therapy, many patients with nutritional problems are not identified until weight loss and loss of muscle mass are extensive. Screening is equally important in the outpatient environment, and the SGA format may be used to identify developing eating problems. Goals include:

- Weight maintenance or maximal weight loss within ½–1 pound/week to minimize loss of lean body mass, and to spare dietary protein for needed tissue repairs.
- Adequate hydration; approximately 1 cc/calorie needed = 30 cc/kg ideal weight.

27. What should I say to patients who ask about using nutrition and vitamins as adjuvant therapy?

Nutritional management should include the use of vitamin and mineral supplementation. Vitamin deficiencies commonly result from decreased caloric intake, tumor effects, gastrointestinal losses, vomiting, and vitamin/mineral deficiencies due to tumor lysis. General recommendations for nutrition and vitamin therapy include:

- Ideal body weight. Overweight patients may have increased cholesterol and ½ survival time; each 1% increase in body fat = 13% increased risk of recurrence.
- Low fat. Each 1,000 gm of additional fat intake/month =1½ times risk of death; the 10-year survival rate is twice as high among Japanese compared with Americans.

Recommended dietary intake must be modified depending on patient status:

1. Well, in remission, or well with active disease = A or B
2. Well, active disease with therapy or early malnutrition = B or B+ (20/50/30)
3. Malnourished, active disease with or without therapy = B+ or C (whatever works)

A	10–15% fat	70–75% carbohydrates	15% protein
B	10–20% fat	60% carbohydrates	20% protein
C	20–30% fat	40–50% carbohydrates	30% protein

- High fiber
- Limit sugar and alcohol
- Increase omega 3 (fish/marine) and omega 9 fatty acids (monounsaturated: canola oil, olive oil)
- Active conditioning to regain or maintain muscle mass
- Stress modification and relaxation
- Vitamin recommendations:

Beta carotene, 20 mg	Selenium, 100–200 µg
Vitamin E, 400 IU (twice-daily dose)	Vitamin C, 350 mg–2 gm
Multivitamin without iron (unless anemia is documented)	

28. Where can professionals find educational materials or answers to nutrition questions?

1. American Institute for Cancer Research
   1759 R. Street N.W.
   Washington, DC 20069
   Hotline: 800-843-8114 (9 AM–5 PM EST). A registered dietitian is available to answer questions. Free materials offering practical information about how to lower cancer risk. Pamphlets include recipes "From Around the World," information about vitamins, AICR Vitamin and Mineral Guide, Nutrition and the Cancer Patient, and other resource booklets. The booklet "Cancer Information: Where to Find Help" includes nonnutrition resources as well.

2. National Cancer Institute
   9000 Rockville Pike
   Building 31, Room 10A18
   Bethesda, MD 20892
   Hotline: 800-4-CANCER (422-6237) (9 AM–7 PM EST). Spanish-speaking assistance is available. Free single copy of "Eating Hints: Recipes and Tips for Better Nutrition during Cancer Treatment." Additional information is included in booklets about chemotherapy and radiation treatment.
3. Nutritional Oncology (NOAT)
   PO Box 7805
   Philadelphia, PA 19101
   (215-351-4050).
   Quarterly newsletter with information for professionals, annual conferences, cancernet bulletin board.

From the Internet
   1. U.S. Food and Drug Administration (FDA): http://www.fda.gov.
   2. National Health Information Center (NHIC): provides information to put professionals and consumers in touch with the organizations best able to provide answers. http://nhic-nt.health.org.
   3. American Institute for Cancer Research: updates on nutrition and cancer research, answers to common cancer-related questions, and recipes. http://www.aicr.org/aicr.
   4. Oncolink: sponsored by the University of Pennsylvania Cancer Center. http://www.oncolink.upenn.edu.
   5. International Cancer Information Center: sponsored by the National Cancer Institute. http://wwwicic.nci.nih.gov.

BIBLIOGRAPHY

1. Block AS: Defining and applying supportive nutrition. Nutr Oncol 2:5–6, 1995.
2. Block AS: Nutrition and cancer: The paradox. Diet Curr 23(2):1–4, 1996.
3. Cunningham R: The Anorectic–Cachetic Syndrome in Cancer. Bristol-Myers Squibb Oncology/Immunology Monograph, 1997.
4. Frankmann CB: Nutritional care in neoplastic disease. In Mahan LK, Arlin M (eds): Food, Nutrition and Diet, 9th ed. Philadelphia, W.B. Saunders, 1996, pp 805–828.
5. Guidelines on Diet, Nutrition, and Cancer Prevention: Reducing the risk of cancer with healthy food choices and physical activity. CA Cancer J Clin 46:325–341, 1996.
6. Nahikan-Nelms ML: General feeding problems. In Shils ME, Olson JA, Shike M (eds): Modern Nutrition in Health and Disease, 8th ed. Philadelphia, Lea & Febiger, 1994.
7. NCI/PDQ Supportive Care/Screening. Nutrition 6/96 (http://oncolink.upenn.edu/pdg/304467.html)
8. Ottery FD: Rethinking nutritional support of the cancer patient: The new field of nutritional oncology. Semin Oncol 21:770–778, 1994.
9. Ottery F: Scored Patient Generated Subjective Global Assessment. Nutr Oncol 2(8):3–5, 1995.
10. Rust DM, Shuster MH: Anorexia and protein calorie malnutrition. In Yasko JM (ed): Nursing Management of Symptoms Associated with Chemotherapy, 2nd ed. Philadelphia, Meniscus Health Care Communications, 1993.
11. Shils ME: Nutrition and diet in cancer management. In Shils ME, Olson J, Shike M (eds): Modern Nutrition in Health and Disease, 8th ed. Philadelphia, Lea & Febiger, 1994, pp 1317–1348.

40. ORGAN TOXICITIES AND LATE EFFECTS: RISKS OF TREATMENT

Brenda Ronk, RN, MS, OCN

1. Define late effects of therapy.

Late effects are toxicities caused by cancer therapy that appear months to years after treatment. They may be mild, severe, or life-threatening.

2. How do late effects differ from acute toxicities?

Late effects often occur in tissues with slowly proliferating cells, such as the heart. Acute toxicities tend to occur in tissues with rapidly proliferating cells, such as bone marrow and mucous membranes of the gastrointestinal tract. They occur during or shortly after treatment. Some drugs cause specific toxicities only when given in high doses or in combination with other chemotherapy agents or radiation therapy.

Some acute and late toxicities are well-defined and predictable, whereas others are unpredictable and vary with dose, duration of treatment, method of administration, and the status of the patient. (Refer to Chapter 7 for common toxicities of chemotherapy.)

3. What is the most common dose-limiting toxicity of chemotherapy?

Depression of bone marrow stem cells or peripheral blood cell lines is caused to some degree by almost all chemotherapy agents. The acceptable degree of myelosuppression depends on the type of cancer, the duration of myelosuppression, treatment goals, and patient status. Neutropenia occurs before thrombocytopenia and anemia because the half-life of granulocytes is much shorter (6–8 hours) than the half-lives of platelets (5–7 days) and red cells (approximately 120 days). The nadir of myelosuppression for most chemotherapy drugs generally is between 7 and 14 days. The nitrosureas cause a late thrombocytopenia 4 to 6 weeks after administration, and drugs such as ifosfamide and mitoxantrone are relatively platelet sparing. Drugs that usually do not cause bone marrow depression include steroidal hormones, bleomycin, vincristine, and L-asparaginase.

4. What are the most common late effects of cancer treatment on the major organ systems? How are they managed or prevented?

Selected Late Effects of Therapy

ORGAN SYSTEM	LATE EFFECT	CAUSATIVE TREATMENT	MANAGEMENT
Cardiovascular	Cardiomyopathy	Anthracycline chemo-therapy; risk increases with mediastinal irradiation	Prevention by limiting dosage to lifetime maximum Treatment of congestive failure (diuretics, digitalis, diet modifications)
	Pericarditis	Mediastinal irradiation	Treat pericardial effusion if necessary
Pulmonary	Pulmonary fibrosis	Lung irradiation Some chemotherapeutic agents, especially in high doses	Avoid other respiratory irritants Corticosteroids may be beneficial For drug-induced toxicity, avoid high concentrations of oxygen

Table continued on following page.

Selected Late Effects of Therapy (Continued)

ORGAN SYSTEM	LATE EFFECT	CAUSATIVE TREATMENT	MANAGEMENT
Musculoskeletal	Kyphosis, scoliosis	Radiation therapy in childhood	Orthopedic rehabilitation
	Fibrosis, joint immobility	Radiation therapy for head and neck cancers, sarcoma	Physical therapy
	Shortening of a growing bone	Radiation to long bones in childhood	Counseling about unequal length of limbs
Gastrointestinal	Chronic enteritis	Radiation therapy to pelvis	Symptomatic treatment with antidiarrheals, low residue diet
Neurologic	Peripheral neuropathy	Cisplatin (usually higher doses), vinca alkaloids	Effect may be permanent
	Orthostatic hypotension due to autonomic nervous system defects	Vinca alkaloids	Teach patient to change positions slowly
	Cataracts	Cranial irradiation High-dose corticosteroids	Surgical correction
	Hearing loss (high-frequency range)	Cisplatin	Audiology consultation Fit with hearing aid

5. Which chemotherapeutic agents are cardiotoxic?

Doxorubicin, daunorubicin, and, to a lesser degree, idarubicin, epirubicin, and mitoxantrone may cause cardiac damage, commonly manifested as myocardial depression or congestive heart failure (CHF). At a cumulative dose of 450–550 mg/m^2, the incidence of CHF related to doxorubicin is only 0.1 to 0.2%, whereas it increases to 30% for doses above 550 mg/m^2.

5-FU has been implicated as causing myocardial ischemia, particularly when given as a continuous infusion or in combination with cisplatin. Cyclophosphamide normally has no cardiac effects at standard doses but can be cardiotoxic at high doses. Paclitaxel causes asymptomatic bradycardia, and its safety in patients with significant preexisting cardiac problems is still being defined.

6. How can cardiac toxicity be prevented?

Numerous studies have documented that lifetime doses of anthracyclines (daunorubicin, doxorubicin) above 450–550 mg/m^2 are likely to produce cardiac symptoms. Generally, total lifetime doses of anthracycline are maintained at these limits. Dosing depends on current cardiac status, age of the patient, and amount of chest irradiation. Often left ventricular ejection fraction (LVEF), which is the portion of blood in the ventricle that is ejected during systole, is measured in patients before therapy with high doses of anthracyclines. LVEF can be measured by performing a multigated acquisition (MUGA) blood pool scan, a radionuclide imaging study of ventricular function. Normal LVEF is > 50%. Measurement of LVEF before treatment assists in making decisions about chemotherapeutic agent and dosage for persons with impaired cardiac function.

Because of the importance of dose-intensive therapy in prolonging disease-free survival, alternatives and modifications for current therapy have been developed. One such alternative is mitoxantrone, an anthracycline analog, which may produce less cardiotoxicity than doxorubicin. Mitoxantrone may be substituted for doxorubicin for patients at risk of cardiac compromise. A second method of reducing cardiac toxicity is use of dexrazoxane, a cardioprotective agent that is given intravenously 30 minutes before administration of an anthracycline. Dexrazoxane (Zinecard) is currently used in patients who have already received some doxorubicin, and need to continue therapy. Varied administration schedules of doxorubicin have also been used to prevent cardiac toxicity. Doxorubicin by continuous infusion or on a weekly schedule in lower doses produces less toxicity than the traditional higher dose given every 21 days. Cardiotoxicity can also be reduced by administering doxorubicin over 30 to 45 minutes instead of as a bolus infusion.

7. What is radiation recall?

Radiation recall is severe erythema, pain, blistering, or ulceration in areas previously irradiated. Radiation recall occurs 3 to 7 days most commonly after infusion of dactinomycin, doxorubicin, daunorubicin, or bleomycin. Other agents include mitoxantrone, idarubicin, mitomycin, 5-FU, methotrexate, cyclophosphamide, and paclitaxel. Dry or moist desquamation is another common cutaneous toxicity experienced by patients receiving chemotherapy agents before, concurrently, or after radiation.

8. A 26-year-old woman who has undergone autologous bone marrow transplant for Hodgkin's disease presents with dyspnea and dry cough 4 months after discharge from the transplant unit. Which long-term effect is likely to produce these symptoms?

A frequent effect of high-dose chemotherapy is pulmonary toxicity. In treatment regimens for bone marrow or peripheral stem cell transplant, cyclophosphamide, carmustine (BCNU), and busulfan are commonly responsible. Bleomycin and methotrexate also may produce acute or chronic pulmonary toxicity. Dyspnea that worsens with exercise, dry cough, and decreased diffusion capacity on pulmonary function testing are hallmark signs. Often open lung biopsy is necessary to distinguish pulmonary toxicity from metastatic disease or an infectious process.

9. What is the treatment for pulmonary toxicity?

Corticosteroids may be of some benefit in many cases of pulmonary toxicity. Often after an aggressive course of gradually tapered steroids, pulmonary symptoms resolve. However, severe cases may be disabling or life-threatening.

10. Why are patients with pulmonary toxicity cautioned about using oxygen?

Oxygen must be used judiciously in patients with pulmonary toxicity, especially if the toxicity is produced by bleomycin or BCNU. In such patients, high-concentration oxygen may cause acute respiratory failure that requires mechanical ventilation and exacerbates lung injury. Oxygen may be used during anesthesia as long as the patient receives the least amount needed to produce an oxygen saturation of > 90%. Patients who have received high doses of chemotherapeutic agents or who have experienced pulmonary toxicity should carry identification describing their pulmonary condition and the risk of oxygen administration.

11. In what ways may cancer therapies affect the sexual and reproductive functions of men and women?

Chemotherapy, radiation therapy, and hormonal therapy may have permanent and significant effects on sexual and reproductive functioning, which are summarized in the table.

Changes in Sexual and Reproductive Function after Cancer Treatment

TREATMENT	EFFECT
Chemotherapy Busulfan Chlorambucil Cyclophosphamide Nitrogen mustard Nitrosureas Procarbazine	Amenorrhea, ovarian failure, decreased or absent production of sperm, decreased libido

Table continued on following page.

Changes in Sexual and Reproductive Function after Cancer Treatment (Continued)

TREATMENT	EFFECT
Radiation therapy	
External beam	Ovarian failure, decreased or absent production of sperm, impotence, erectile dysfunction, decreased libido
Brachytherapy	Vaginal stenosis
Hormonal therapy	
Estrogens	Gynecomastia
Androgens	Masculinization (in women)
Antiandrogens	Decreased libido, impotence, erectile dysfunction

12. What are some dermatologic toxicities caused by chemotherapy?

Dermatologic effects include rashes (docetaxel, idarubicin), hyperpigmentation (hydroxyurea, methotrexate), nail thickening or banding, acral erythema, phlebitis, chemical cellulitis, radiation recall and enhancement, photosensitivity, reactivation of UV light-induced erythema (methotrexate), seborrheic inflammation or actinic keratoses (dacarbazine, dactinomycin, doxorubicin, cisplatin, cytarabine), scleroderma-like changes, and vasculitis (cytarabine, hydroxyurea, methotrexate).

13. Do hyperpigmentation and photosensitivity induced by 5-FU, bleomycin, or methotrexate ever resolve?

Hyperpigmentation, photosensitivity, generalized skin darkening, dermatitis, and nail changes are usually of short duration (during the course of treatment) and diminish gradually once therapy has stopped.

14. What is "hand-foot syndrome"?

Palmar–plantar erythrodysesthesia (acral erythema) syndrome, referred to as hand–foot syndrome, is a painful erythema of the palms, fingers, and soles of the feet that may progress to bullae or vesicular formation and desquamation before healing spontaneously within a week. Patients with this condition frequently require opioids for pain relief. The condition may respond to pyridoxine treatment and cooling. Acral erythema is induced by standard and high-dose cytarabine, hydroxyurea, continuous infusion 5-FU, bleomycin, doxorubicin, methotrexate, high-dose etoposide, thiotepa, and docetaxel.

15. What are some hepatoxic effects of chemotherapy and which drugs usually require dose modification with hepatic dysfunction?

Hepatoxic effects of chemotherapy agents include hepatocellular injury, necrosis, veno-occlusive disease, and reactivation of chronic hepatitis B virus infection. Combination chemotherapy and high-dose regimens used for autologous bone marrow transplantations have enhanced the potential for hepatoxicity, particularly hepatic venoocclusive disease. At conventional doses, venoocclusive disease has been associated with cytarabine, dacarbazine, 6-mercaptopurine, and 6-thioguanine. If there is evidence of hepatic impairment or abnormal liver function tests (e.g., bilirubin > 1.5 mg/dl), the following agents should be held or reduced: doxorubicin, daunorubicin, vinblastine, vincristine, cyclophosphamide, methotrexate, 5-FU, and paclitaxel.

16. Can chemotherapy affect vision or cause other ocular complications?

Although relatively uncommon, the incidence of ocular complications has increased in accordance with increased patient survival and high-dose chemotherapy regimens. Ophthalmologic side effects include decreased or blurred vision (cisplatin, cyclophosphamide, cytarabine, mitomycin C, methotrexate); eye pain (busulfan, cytarabine, methotrexate); papilledema (cisplatin);

altered color vision (cisplatin); conjunctivitis (cytarabine, 5-FU, methotrexate); tear duct stenosis and increased lacrimation (5-FU, doxorubicin, methotrexate); photophobia (cytarabine, methotrexate); optic neuropathy or blindness (vincristine); photopsia (paclitaxel); and cataracts (busulfan). Conjunctivitis related to high-dose cytarabine may be reduced effectively with prophylactic glucocorticoid eye drops, as well as artificial tears, which probably decrease toxicity by diluting intraocular drug concentrations.

17. How can sexual and reproductive changes be prevented or managed?

In chemotherapy and radiation therapy, older age at time of treatment is more likely to cause permanent infertility. Sperm banking and in vitro fertilization may make conception possible in some patients. In women receiving pelvic irradiation, the ovaries may be surgically moved behind the uterus (oophoropexy) to shield them from the beam. Changes in sexual functioning require open and sensitive discussion of the issue, with exploration of possible solutions or modifications in activity.

18. What is the most frequent long-term effect of radiation therapy to the head and neck?

Xerostomia (dryness of the mouth) is the most frequent chronic effect of radiation to the oral cavity. Radiation, both external beam and implanted, may produce permanent injury to the acinar cells of the salivary glands. The small amount of saliva that is produced is thick and ineffective at performing the normal salivary functions: lubricating the mouth, providing a buffer for acids, and washing food and organisms from the teeth and gums. Chronic xerostomia is a highly distressing condition. Swallowing dry foods and taking pills become difficult, and the patient frequently awakens at night with dry mouth. Artificial saliva products are available. Some patients may find relief with pilocarpine hydrochloride. Many patients find that water, hard candies, or lozenges are equally effective in relieving the sensation of dryness.

19. How is dental caries related to radiation therapy? How can it be prevented?

Inadequate production of saliva increases the risk of dental caries, because there is too little saliva to clear bacteria from the mouth. In addition, patients undergoing radiation therapy may also have poor oral hygiene if they experience mucositis. Despite instructions to perform meticulous mouth care, patients may not be compliant if pain due to mucositis is poorly controlled. These factors contribute to the development of dental caries, which may create a problem for several years. Dental caries is prevented by the following methods:

1. A thorough dental evaluation before the start of therapy, with diseased teeth repaired or extracted
2. Meticulous oral hygiene with frequent saline rinses, gentle toothbrushing, and fluoride application
3. Provision of adequate analgesia for oral care to be performed
4. Prompt treatment of any infection in the oral mucosa
5. Prevention of further irritation to the oral mucosa by avoiding the use of alcohol and tobacco.

20. A 10-year-old girl who underwent total body irradiation during a bone marrow transplant for acute lymphoblastic leukemia developed a cataract 3 years later. How does her cataract compare with a cataract in an elderly person?

Physiologically, the girl's cataract is exactly the same as a non–radiation-related cataract and should be surgically removed in the same manner. The lens of the eye is sensitive to radiation, more so in children than in older persons. Cataracts may result from cranial or ocular radiation therapy, especially at higher doses. They often present several years after treatment.

21. How is the gastrointestinal tract affected by radiation therapy to the pelvis?

Proctitis and enteritis, which may be acute effects of radiation therapy, also may become chronic effects if the mucosa is permanently damaged. Radiation may produce shortening of the intestinal villi and thus prevent adequate absorption. Acutely injured mucosa may become atrophied, thickened, or ulcerated. Proctitis or small bowel enteritis results, causing diarrhea with cramping. This chronic condition is physically and psychologically debilitating. A few individuals also experience fecal incontinence. Nurses may assist patients to cope with this problem by instructing them about low residue diets and use of antidiarrheals. Steroid enemas are sometimes used. If conservative measures fail, a colostomy may be required.

22. How are the late effects of therapy different in children?
Because children undergo such rapid growth and development, effects on their developing tissues are different from those seen in mature tissues. Children often receive treatment to the central nervous system (total body irradiation, brain irradiation, intrathecal chemotherapy) for leukemia or brain tumors. The most serious long-term effects are seen in children under the age of 3 years, when brain development is rapid. Such patients may later manifest intellectual deficits, as well as attention and memory problems. CNS treatment also may affect endocrine function because of damage to the hypothalamic–pituitary axis. Frequently seen are growth impairment with growth hormone deficiency and delayed or arrested development of secondary sexual characteristics. Children may need exogenous hormones to produce normal growth and maturation.

Common Late Effects of Treatment of Childhood Cancer

Short stature	Dental caries
Intellectual deficits	Cataracts
Delayed sexual development	Kyphoscoliosis
Secondary malignancies	Skeletal growth retardation

23. What are secondary malignancies?
Secondary malignancies are cancers caused by damage to the DNA of normal cells exposed to chemotherapy and radiation therapy. The most common secondary malignancy is acute myeloid leukemia due to therapy with an alkylating agent for Hodgkin's disease, non-Hodgkin's lymphoma, and multiple myeloma. Agents that may cause secondary malignancies include nitrogen mustard, procarbazine, melphalan, cyclophosphamide, busulfan, chlorambucil, and thiotepa. Radiation-induced sarcomas have been known to occur in patients treated for Hodgkin's disease and non-Hodgkin's lymphoma. The period of highest risk for developing secondary leukemia is 2–10 years after treatment. Secondary leukemia is one of the most serious long-term effects of therapy, because it generally has a poor prognosis.

24. What late psychosocial effects may be seen in patients after treatment for cancer?
Numerous psychosocial changes may be experienced by patients who have received cancer treatment. Often they live with the fear of recurrence of cancer and death. Any change in health status may produce worry about cancer recurrence. Changes may occur in relationships with family, friends, coworkers, and sexual partners. Persons who are healthy after recovering from cancer and its treatment may still be perceived as ill or disabled, creating relationship stress and feelings of isolation. Disabilities and physical changes may require adjustment in lifestyle, employment, or family role.

BIBLIOGRAPHY

1. Coia LR, Moylan DJ III: Introduction to Clinical Radiation Oncology. Madison, WI, Medical Physics Publishing, 1991.
2. DeVita VT Jr, Hellman S, Rosenberg SA (eds): Cancer: Principles and Practices of Oncology, 5th ed. Philadelphia, Lippincott-Raven, 1997.
3. Green DM: Effects of treatment for childhood cancer on vital organ systems. Cancer 71 (Suppl 10):3299–3305, 1993.

4. Groenwald SL, Frogge MH, Goodman M, Yarbro CH (eds):Cancer Nursing: Principles and Practice, 2nd ed. Boston, Jones & Bartlett, 1992.
5. Neglia JP, Nesbit ME Jr: Care and treatment of long-term survivors of childhood cancer. Cancer 71(Suppl 10): 3386–3391, 1993.
6. Perry MC (ed): The Chemotherapy Source Book, 2nd ed. Baltimore, Williams & Wilkins, 1996.
7. Ruccione K, Weinberg K: Late effects in multiple body systems. Semin Oncol Nurs 5:4–13, 1989.

41. PAIN MANAGEMENT

Diana Ruzicka, RN, MSN, MAJ, AN, *Rose A. Gates*, RN, MSN,
and Regina M. Fink, RN, PhD(c), AOCN

1. What is cancer pain?

As defined by McCaffery, "Pain is whatever the experiencing person says it is, existing whenever the experiencing person says it does" (McCaffery and Beebe, 1989). It is an unpleasant sensory and emotional experience associated with actual or potential tissue damage or described in terms of such damage (IASP, 1980).

Unrelieved pain affects quality of life in all dimensions, including physical, psychological, and spiritual well-being, and social concerns (Ferrell et al., 1991). Cancer patients have multiple sources and sites of pain due to:
- Direct tumor involvement and related pathology (65–80% of patients)
- Anticancer therapy and invasive diagnostic or therapeutic procedures (25% of patients)
- Unrelated to cancer or therapy; prior or concurrent painful conditions (3–10% of patients)

2. Can cancer pain be controlled?

Pain is well controlled by oral analgesics in 90% of patients with cancer. Unfortunately, about 25% of all patients with cancer die with unrelieved pain because of patient, provider, and family misconceptions, and fears. Adequate pain control is further complicated by regulatory agencies that scrutinize professional licensure and restrictively regulate controlled substances. To address issues related to the undertreatment of cancer pain, position papers, educational materials, and guidelines have been developed by the Oncology Nursing Society, American Society of Clinical Oncology, American Pain Society, and the Agency for Health Care Policy and Research (AHCPR).

Management of cancer pain requires a multidisciplinary approach. As with other symptoms, the best way to treat pain is to treat the cause. Surgery, radiation and chemotherapy may be used to control the pain by removing or shrinking the tumor. Drugs (nonopioids and opioids) remain the mainstay of pain treatment.

3. How do the types of pain differ?

Pain is classified as nociceptive (traveling along normal nerve conduction pathways) or neuropathic (caused by damage to the central or peripheral nervous system). Nociceptive pain may be further divided into somatic and visceral.

Type of Pain	Descriptors	Etiology	Treatment
Somatic (well localized)	Achy Throbbing Dull	Originates at peripheral nerve endings Bone and spine metastases Cutaneous or deep tissue inflammation or injury	Opioids ± nonsteroidal antiinflammatory drug Muscle relaxants Pamidronate Strontium 89
Visceral (poorly localized)	Squeezing Pressure Cramping Distention	Originates in deep organ; often referred to dermatomes innervated by same fibers Bowel obstruction, stretching, or infection Blood flow occlusion	Opioids (caution with bowel-obstructed patients)
Neuropathic	Burning, "fire" Shooting Numbness Radiation "Electrical sensation"	Nerve damage by tumor or fibrosis of nerve plexus Postherpetic neuralgia Peripheral neuropathies secondary to tumor, radiation fibrosis, or chemotherapy	Antidepressants Anticonvulsants Benzodiazepines

4. How is pain assessed?

Patient assessment needs to be ongoing, individualized, and documented so that everyone involved has an understanding of the problem. Pain should be reassessed during each follow-up visit, by every shift during hospitalization, or after every intervention. Recent studies of health care professionals identified poor pain assessment, lack of knowledge, and insufficient time as the greatest barriers to adequate pain treatment. The American Pain Society currently has a campaign to make pain assessment the fifth vital sign. (*Note:* Vital signs are neither sensitive nor specific indicators of chronic pain.) In addition to assessment of pain characteristics, psychosocial and thorough physical and neurologic evaluations are necessary, as is a review of other symptoms (e.g., anxiety, nausea, insomnia, constipation, anorexia). Cultural and ethnic backgrounds also may influence pain expression and behavior; however, patients should not be stereotyped. An easy way to assess pain is to incorporate the **WILDA** strategy:

Pain Assessment Guide

Words to describe pain

aching	throbbing	shooting
stabbing	gnawing	sharp
tender	burning	exhausting
tiring	penetrating	nagging
numb	miserable	unbearable
dull	radiating	squeezing
crampy	deep	pressure

Pain in other languages

itami	Japanese
tong	Chinese
dau	Vietnamese
dolor	Spanish
doleur	French
bolno	Russian

Intensity (0–10)

If 0 is no pain and 10 is the worst pain imaginable, what is your pain now? . . . in the last 24 hours?

Location

Where is your pain?

Duration

Is the pain always there?
Does the pain come and go?

Aggravating and alleviating factors

What makes the pain better?
What makes the pain worse?

How does pain affect

sleep	energy	relationships
appetite	activity	mood

Are you experiencing any other symptoms?

nausea/vomiting	itching	urinary retention
constipation	sleepiness/confusion	weakness

Things to check

vital signs, past medication history, knowledge of pain, and use of noninvasive techniques

---

Two commonly used assessment scales are shown below. The Numeric Pain Intensity (0–10) Scale is very useful in the clinical setting for patients older than 5 years. For example, ask the patient, "If 0 is no pain and 10 is the worst pain imaginable, what is your pain right now?" The Faces Pain Rating Scale is appropriate for children older than 3 years and for patients with language barriers.

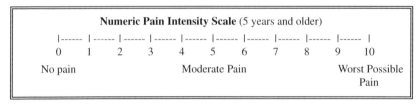

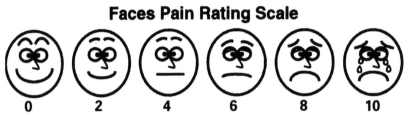

Explain to the child/adult that each face is for a person who feels happy because he has no pain (hurt) or sad because he has some or a lot of pain.
Face 0 is very happy because he doesn't hurt at all;
Face 2 hurts just a little bit;
Face 4 hurts a little more;
Face 6 hurts even more;
Face 8 hurts a whole lot;
Face 10 hurts as much as you can imagine, although you don't have to be crying to feel this bad.
Ask the child/adult to choose the face that best describes how he is feeling. **Recommended for persons aged 3 or older.**

(From Wong D, Whaley L: Clinical Handbook of Pediatric Nursing, 2nd ed. St. Louis, Mosby, 1986, p. 373, with permission.)

5. Should placebos be used to assess pain?

No. According to the Oncology Nursing Society's Position Statement on the Use of Placebos, "Placebos should not be used (a) to assess or manage cancer pain, (b) to determine if the pain is "real," or (c) to diagnose psychological symptoms, such as anxiety associated with pain. Nurses should not administer placebos in these circumstances even if there is a medical order." Placebos are appropriate in the context of controlled studies when patients have given informed consent. Because placebos involve secrecy, ethical tenets of truth-telling and patient autonomy are violated. Use of placebos can potentially destroy a therapeutic relationship if the patient becomes aware of their use. Placebos may mimic drug effects, make symptoms worse, produce side effects and directly affect body organ functions. Placebos may be highly effective, as demonstrated by studies in patients with postoperative pain. About 30–35% of patients in control groups reported pain relief from placebos. Instead of labeling patients who respond to placebos as "fakers" or "addicted," the mechanism of the placebo response should be examined (McCaffery et al., 1996).

6. What are the common patient and family concerns about pain medications?

During the assessment of pain, it is important to solicit patients' and families' worries about pain control and medications to legitimize and clarify their concerns. Patients may fail to report pain in the desire to be "good" patients or because of the following common myths about opioids:

- If I take pain medicine (opioids) regularly, I will get hooked or addicted.
- Pain is inevitable with cancer. I just need to bear it or hang in there.
- If the pain is worse, it must mean that the cancer is spreading, and nothing can be done.
- I had better wait to take my pain medication until I really need it, or else it won't work later.
- I'd rather have my bowel movement than take the pain medication and become constipated.
- My family thinks I'm getting too spacy or I'm taking too much medicine. I'd better hold back.

7. How do you deal with physicians, nurses, or patients who are afraid of addiction?

First, describe the difference between physical dependence, tolerance, and addiction (psychological dependence). Then quote studies reporting the low incidence of addiction among patients taking opioids to relieve pain. Emphasize that the incidence of addiction is less than 1% in patients without a previous history of addiction. For patients afraid of addiction, ask whether they would take the drug if they were not having pain. If they say "no," then reassure them that they are not going to become addicted if they use pain medications for the right reason.

8. Are patients with cancer addicted when they keep asking for more pain medicine?

No. They are probably exhibiting signs of **tolerance**, a normal pharmacologic effect in which the patient requires higher doses to provide adequate pain relief. Physiologically, the body requires more opioid to provide the same analgesic effect. Signs of tolerance should be treated by increasing the drug dose, decreasing the interval between doses, or switching to another drug. It is important, however, to determine whether treatable disease progression is responsible for the increased opioid requirement.

9. Do signs of withdrawal mean the patient is addicted?

No. The patient is probably showing signs of **physical dependence**, which develops when patients take opioids for an extended period (usually 1 week or more). Like tolerance, physical dependence is a normal body response. If an opioid is abruptly stopped, the patient may experience withdrawal symptoms: nervousness, sweating, anxiety, chills alternating with hot flashes, salivation, lacrimation, rhinorrhea, diaphoresis, piloerection, nausea, vomiting, abdominal cramps, or insomnia. Reassure patients that physical dependence is not unique to opioids. For example, an abstinence syndrome occurs when patients abruptly stop taking long-term steroids. Opioids should be tapered gradually, like steroids.

In contrast, **addiction** or **psychological dependence** is an abnormal behavior involving an overwhelming desire to obtain the medication for its psychological effects. Addiction rarely occurs in patients with cancer. Most patients would prefer not to take the medication and not to have the pain.

10. How should opioids be tapered to prevent an abstinence or withdrawal syndrome when they are no longer needed?

The rate of tapering may vary with individual patients; however, the following approach is often used:

- Decrease the 24-hr total dose by 50%, and administer as divided doses on schedule for 2 days.
- Decrease the dose by 25% every 2 days thereafter until the total daily dose is equivalent to 30 mg of oral morphine/day or 0.6 mg/kg/day in a child.
- After 2 days on this final dose, stop the medication. If the patient is anxious or nervous, a clonidine patch (changed every seven days), 0.1–0.2 mg/day, may be used to lessen or prevent anxiety, tachycardia, sweating, and other autonomic symptoms.

11. What nondrug modalities are used to control pain?

Nondrug modalities include physical and psychosocial interventions, which should be introduced early to augment, not replace, pharmacologic therapy for pain management. The success of several of these modalities requires an understanding of the mind/body connection and depends on a therapeutic relationship between the nurse or health care provider and patient. Physical modalities used to reduce pain in cancer patients include cutaneous stimulation (heat, cold, massage, vibration), exercise, immobilization, transcutaneous nerve stimulation (TENS), reflexology, therapeutic touch, and acupressure or acupuncture. Psychosocial interventions help patients to gain a sense of control by using cognitive techniques that affect how pain is interpreted and behavioral techniques that provide the patient with skills to cope with and modify responses to pain. Examples of psychosocial interventions include relaxation and imagery, meditation and deep breathing, distraction and reframing (replacing negative thoughts with more positive ones), music therapy, humor therapy, psychotherapy, biofeedback, peer support groups, hypnosis, and pastoral counseling. For further information about nondrug modalities, refer to the *Clinical Practice Guideline on Management of Cancer Pain* (1994) and McCaffery and Beebe's book, *Pain: Clinical Manual for Nursing Practice* (1989).

12. Is heat or cold better in relieving pain?
    The use of heat or cold is an individual preference, so use what is most effective for the patient, unless it is contraindicated. Cold may relieve more pain than heat for some conditions, such as painful muscles, because it works faster and the relief lasts longer after the cold is removed. Either heat or cold may be used for aching muscles or spasms, joint stiffness, and back pain. Heat is particularly useful for abdominal cramps, and cold may be more effective for pruritus, muscle spasms, and acute, but not severe, injuries (e.g., minor sports injuries or sprains). Severe pain is best treated by intermittent heat applications or by alternating applications of heat and cold. Cold or heat packs should be sealed, flexible to conform to body contours, and wrapped with a dry or moist cloth. Moist cloths should be used with caution because water permits faster cooling or greater heat intensity. Commercially available (dual controlled heat/cold) or homemade packs (e.g., 1-lb bag of frozen green peas or corn kernels) can be used. (**Note:** Heat should not be used over skin exposed to radiation therapy, and ice should not be used over skin that has been damaged from radiation therapy.)

13. What can be done if a patient feels that the painful site is too tender to tolerate a heat or cold application?
    By an unknown mechanism, the benefits of heat and cold are not limited to the direct sites of application and may have distant effects. Thus, cold or heat applications can be effective over an opposite site, or the patient can experiment using the cold or heat at various sites distant from the painful area (e.g., between pain and the brain, acupuncture or trigger points). For example, ice over the unaffected side may be used to reduce pain during a bone marrow biopsy.

14. Is pain treated in comatose or verbally unresponsive patients?
    Yes. Comatose or verbally unresponsive patients should be placed minimally on baseline level of analgesia. Some patients in whom opioids were stopped during a comatose period have reported severe pain after recovering from the coma. They also may experience withdrawal but be unable to express it. The family or significant others should be queried about their assessment of the patient's level of pain. Health care providers should pay attention to nonverbal cues and other signs or symptoms and be prepared to increase the dose as needed.

15. How do you know which analgesic to use?
    The analgesic must be selected according to the patient's type and severity of pain as well as the appropriate route of administration. (**Note:** The intramuscular route is not recommended for management of cancer pain.) Successful relief of cancer pain requires around-the-clock dosing with as-needed doses for breakthrough pain. The choice of drug also should be based on the patient's previous experience with the medication, age, physical condition (e.g., renal and hepatic function), response to the prescribed regimen, provider recommendations, and possible interactions with current therapies.

A step-wise approach, as suggested by The World Health Organization (WHO) analgesic ladder, provides a convenient method for starting analgesics. Each step describes analgesic interventions appropriate to pain intensity (0 = no pain to 10 = worst pain imaginable).

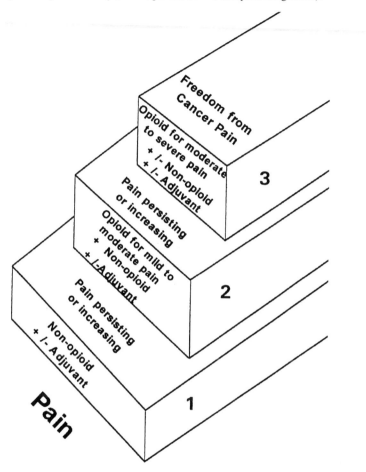

The World Health Organization (WHO) analgesic ladder:

Step 1   For mild pain (intensity = 1–3), start with nonopioid drugs such as acetaminophen or nonsteroidal antiinflammatory drugs (NSAIDs) such as ibuprofen. Add adjuvant drugs if indicated (e.g., tricyclic antidepressant, anticonvulsant).

Step 2   If pain persists, add an opioid for mild-to-moderate pain (intensity = 4–6), such as hydrocodone or low-dose oxycodone (5 mg) plus aspirin or acetaminophen with or without adjuvant drugs.

Step 3   If pain persists or increases, switch to an opioid for moderate-to-severe pain (intensity = 7–10), such as oxycodone, morphine, hydromorphone, fentanyl (transdermal), levorphanol, or methadone with or without a nonopioid and with or without an adjuvant drug.

The ladder was originally proposed with three steps as depicted; however, a 2-step approach is currently considered more appropriate for patients with cancer. The first step includes NSAIDs, and the second step combines step 2 and 3 from the previous ladder with emphasis on use of non-compounded opioids (e.g., analgesics not combined with acetaminophen or aspirin). Compounded opioids are limited by the analgesic ceiling effect of acetaminophen (doses > 1000 mg add minimal analgesia) and its ceiling for toxicity (dose should not exceed 4–6 gm/day because of potential liver necrosis or toxicity). Chronic use of 5–8 gm/day for several weeks or 3–4 gm/day for a year has resulted in liver damage. There is also a risk of renal tubular damage and myocardial damage.

16. Explain the use of NSAIDs in controlling pain.

NSAIDs may relieve bone pain or generalized musculoskeletal pain by decreasing subperiosteal swelling around nerve endings and inhibiting prostaglandin synthesis. Research has been inconclusive about the efficacy of NSAIDs as a primary treatment of bone pain. Although NSAIDs may be given in higher than recommended doses, they have a ceiling effect; that is, increases above a certain dose do not provide additional analgesia.

The selection of NSAIDs is influenced by side-effect profile, patient preference, and cost (over the counter NSAIDs, such as ibuprofen, are the cheapest). The use of NSAIDs in patients with cancer is limited by concerns about side effects, such as platelet dysfunction, nephritis, fluid retention, and gastrointestinal tract bleeding or ulceration. NSAIDs must be used with extreme caution in patients with thrombocytopenia or poor renal function. Patients should be assessed for potential hypersensitivity reactions; patients with a history of aspirin or NSAID allergy, rhinitis, nasal polyps, or asthma are susceptible to development of severe respiratory reactions. (**Note:** Monitor serum levels of blood urea nitrogen [BUN] and creatinine. Instruct patients not to take on an empty stomach.)

Nonacetylated salicylates are often recommended because they do not affect platelet aggregation profoundly or clinically alter bleeding time; however, their analgesic effect may not be strong enough for patients with more intense pain. NSAIDs such as nabumetone (Relafen) cause less gastric distress. For chronic use of NSAIDs, histamine-2 blockers or prostaglandin analogs may be used to decrease the potential for gastric ulceration.

Nonopioid Analgesics	*Dose*
Acetaminophen (Tylenol) or acetylsalicylic acid (aspirin)	325–1000 mg every 4–6 hr (maximal daily dose: 4 gm)
Choline magnesium trisalicylate (Trilisate)	1000–1500 mg 3 times/day (maximal daily dose: 4500 mg)
Salsalate (Disalcid)	1000–1500 mg every 8–12 hr (maximal daily dose: 4000 mg)
Ibuprofen (Motrin)	200–800 mg every 4–6 hr (maximal daily dose: 3200 mg)
Naproxen (Naprosyn)	375–500 mg every 8–12 hr (maximal daily dose: 1500 mg)
Nabumetone (Relafen)	1000 mg in 1 dose or 2 divided doses; may increase up to 2000 mg/day

17. What other agents are used for metastatic bone pain?

- **Radiation therapy** is the mainstay for palliation of localized bony metastases. Wide-field and hemibody irradiation has been used for diffuse bony metastasis.
- **Strontium 89**, a radioisotope that follows the same biochemical pathways as calcium, has been used for pain due to diffuse bony metastasis from breast or prostate cancer. Patients need to be warned about possibility of flare pain for a few days after administration (see chapter 30).
- **Biphosphates** may be helpful in bone pain associated with hypercalcemia. Pamidronate (Aredia) inhibits accelerated bone resorption, and etidronate (Didronel) retards mineralization, growth of heterotropic ossification, and possibly bone resorption. Pamidronate is given in doses of 60–90 mg over 24 hours. Etidronate is given initially in intravenous doses of 7.5 mg/kg/day for 3 days, then in oral doses of 20 mg/kg/day for 30–90 days (beginning on the day after the last infusion).
- **Calcitonin** inhibits osteoclastic bone resorption by the tumor and has also been reported to be effective for bone pain and phantom limb sensation. It is given in doses of 4 IU/kg every 12 hours. The dose may be increased to 8 IU/kg every 12 hours if no response is seen in 2 days. If this regimen produces no response in 2 days, the dose may be increased to 8 IU/kg every 6 hours.

18. How are tricyclic antidepressants used to control pain?

Tricyclic antidepressants relieve neuropathic pain by blocking the reuptake of the neurotransmitter serotonin, which is released by the pain-modulatory systems that descend from the brainstem to the spinal cord. Accumulation of serotonin and norepinephrine at the synapse inhibits transmission of pain impulses. Amitriptyline also has morphine-sparing effects by increasing the plasma concentration or morphine. Dose-related side effects of the tricyclics include sedation, orthostatic hypotension, and anticholinergic effects, particularly dry mouth. Uncommon, serious side effects include cardiac arrhythmias, obstipation, and urinary retention. Desipramine and imipramine are less sedating and may produce insomnia; they can be given during the day. Amitriptyline and doxepin are sedating and should be given at bedtime. Nortriptyline produces intermediate sedation and has little anticholinergic effects. Trazodone is not anticholinergic, but is sedating and can cause priapism. Dosages to control pain are much lower (e.g., 10–50 mg/day) than needed to treat depression (e.g., 100–150 mg). Although it takes weeks for a therapeutic antidepressant effect with tricyclics, the onset of analgesia is much sooner (usually a week). Pain can be reduced by the next morning after taking one dose of amitriptyline. To increase patient compliance and decrease side effects, start with low doses (10 mg in elderly or frail patients) and gradually titrate up. (**Note:** To prevent confusion in patients, avoid increasing at the same time that opioids are increased.) After symptoms are controlled, titrate dosage downward to the lowest level that maintains pain relief.

Antidepressants	Dose
Amitriptyline (Elavil)	Start 10–25 mg at bedtime; increase gradually to 50–150 mg
Doxepin (Sinequan)	Start 10–25 mg at bedtime; increase gradually to 75–150 mg
Desipramine (Norpramin, Pertrofrane)	Start 25 mg; increase by 25–50 mg every 3–4 weeks; maintenance dose: 25–150 mg/day
Nortriptyline (Aventyl, Pamelor)	Start 10–50 mg; increase by 10–25 mg every 3–4 weeks; maintenance dose: 10–150 mg/day
Imipramine (Tofranil)	Start 10–25 mg; maintenance dose: 20–150 mg/day
Trazodone (Desyrel)	Start 50 mg; maintenance dose 50–200 mg/day

19. How are anticonvulsants used to control pain?

Anticonvulsants (e.g., phenytoin, carbamazepine, clonazepam) stabilize the nerve membrane, prevent depolarization. and block transmission of pain impulses. They are indicated for trigeminal and postherpetic neuralgias, lancinating pains, and nerve injury caused by cancer or cancer treatment. (**Note:** Phenytoin and carbamazepine should be initiated at low doses and titrated upward according to patient response and plasma levels. Dosing follows antiseizure guidelines.)

- **Phenytoin** and **valproic acid** are best for continuous neuropathic pain. Plasma levels of phenytoin should be monitored for therapeutic and toxic concentrations. Side effects include skin rash, ataxia, and liver function abnormalities. (**Note:** Be aware of drug interactions; e.g., phenothiazines and trazodone increase phenytoin levels, whereas phenytoin increases the metabolism of meperidine and methadone).
- **Carbamazepine** is best for lancinating or shooting pain. Because carbamazepine may cause bone marrow depression (e.g., aplastic anemia), continuous hematologic monitoring is necessary (e.g., baseline and follow-up complete blood counts). Plasma drug levels also should be monitored for therapeutic and toxicity concentrations. Other common side effects include sedation, vertigo, or confusion. (**Note:** Like phenytoin, carbamazepine is metabolized by the liver and associated with multiple drug interactions; e.g., carbamazepine levels are increased with propoxyphene and decreased with doxorubicin and cisplatin).
- **Gabapentin** is a new amino acid anticonvulsant that may increase the rate of synthesis and accumulation of gamma-amino-butyric acid (GABA) or its binding to an unknown receptor in brain tissue. GABA is the main inhibitory pathway in the body. The two types of receptors,

GABA-A and GABA-B, are equally distributed throughout the central nervous system. Because gabapentin has relatively mild side effects and has been highly effective, it is probably preferred for use in patients with cancer. Dosing should start at 100 mg/day and be titrated upward according to patient tolerance. Common side effects include blurred vision, dizziness, and mild generalized edema.

- **Clonazepam**, which binds to GABA-A, is effective in controlling neuropathic pain. It is also excellent for use in patients with cancer as an antianxiety agent with the added benefit of reducing pain.

Anticonvulsant	Dose
Carbamazepine (Tegretol)	Start with 100 mg/day; increase by 100 mg every 4 days to 500–800 mg/day.
Phenytoin (Dilantin)	Start with 100 mg/day; increase by 25–50 mg every 4 days to 250–300 mg/day
Clonazepam (Klonopin)	0.5–6 mg/day in 2 or 3 divided doses.
Valproic acid (Depakote)	250–2000 mg/day at bedtime or in 3 divided doses; titrate upward by 5–10 mg/kg; maximal dose: 40 mg/kg/day.
Gabapentin (Neurontin)	300–2400 mg/day in divided doses; mean dose: 1000 mg/day.

20. When are local anesthetics indicated?

Local anesthetics may produce analgesia by stabilizing the nerve cell membrane and inhibiting depolarization and transmission. They also may inhibit the release of neurotransmitters centrally. They are effective for lancinating neuropathic pain and various neuralgias. Patients may be given an IV trial of lidocaine. If the IV lidocaine is effective, the patient may respond to mexiletine (oral form of lidocaine) or other oral neuropathic agents. During IV administration, the patient should be observed for slurred speech (a sign of toxicity) and the dose adjusted accordingly.

Local Anesthetic	Dose
Lidocaine	1–5 mg/kg of 0.1% solution by slow IV infusion over 10–60 minutes; total dose of 50–300 mg.
Mexiletine	150–200 mg (2–3 mg/kg) 2 or 3 times/day; increase by 50 mg every 2 weeks as needed. Maintenance dose: 150–400 mg 3 or 4 times/day. Maximal dose: 1200 mg/day.

21. How do corticosteroids decrease pain?

Corticosteroids help to reduce pain due to perineural edema, visceral organ distention, infiltration of soft tissues, and bone pain in advanced disease. They are part of the emergency management of spinal cord compression and increased intracranial pressure.

Corticosteroid	Dose
Decadron	4 mg orally 3–4 times/day
Prednisone	10 mg orally 3 times/day; maximal dose: 20–80 mg/day

22. What is capsaicin and how is it used?

Capsaicin (Zostrix), a cream made from cayenne pepper, depletes and prevents reaccumulation of substance P in peripheral sensory neurons. Capsaicin (0.025%) has been reported to be effective in some patients with chronic postherpetic neuralgia, but it should not be applied to open lesions. It has also been of benefit to patients with postmastectomy pain. A thin film is applied to the affected area of intact skin 3–5 times/day. Fewer applications per day may decrease efficacy. Onset of action may take 14–28 days. Treatment should be continued to provide an adequate trial and to achieve optimal clinical response. Patients need to be warned about transient burning that occurs with application but decreases within several days. To ease or prevent the burning sensation, opioids should be administered during this initial period. Investigators at Yale University have made a candy containing cayenne pepper that reduces the pain of oral mucositis in patients undergoing chemotherapy.

Cayenne Candy for Oral Mucositis

Place in a heavy pan large enough to allow for foaming:

2 cups brown sugar	2 tbsp water
¼ cup molasses	2 tbsp vinegar
½ cup butter	½ tsp cayenne pepper (McCormick brand)

Stir mixture except for pepper over low heat until sugar is dissolved. Boil gently, stirring frequently until the hard crack stage (300° F, the temperature at which a spoonful of candy separates into hard and brittle threads when dropped into cold water). Add the cayenne pepper toward the end of the boiling process. Drop candy from a teaspoon onto a buttered slab or foil to form patties. Makes about 1 pound. For additional recipes, contact Ann Berger, M.D., Supportive Care Services, PO Box 20851, New Haven, CT 06520-8050.

23. How is pain due to muscle spasms treated?

Baclofen, cyclobenzaprine, and methocarbamol are skeletal muscle relaxants. Common side effects are sedation, confusion, or muscle weakness. These drugs are often used in combination with rest or physical therapy. Of these, baclofen is used most often as an adjuvant analgesic for management of cancer pain. Other useful agents include quinine sulfate, dicyclomine, oxybutynin chloride, and diazepam. Calcium supplementation is effective when crampy pain is due to calcium deficiency.

- **Baclofen**, which binds to GABA B receptors, is primarily indicated for spasticity but is also effective for neuropathic pain, organic headache, trigeminal and postherpetic neuralgias, and fibromyalgias. Baclofen is comparable to diazepam but less sedating.
- **Quinine sulfate** is effective for nocturnal leg cramps. It increases the refractory period of skeletal muscles by direct action on muscle fiber, decreases excitability of the motor endplate, and affects distribution of calcium within the muscle fiber.
- **Dicyclomine** acts on smooth muscles of the gastrointestinal tract. It is effective for abdominal cramps (colorectal cancer) and irritable bowel syndrome.
- **Oxybutynin chloride** has direct effects on the bladder. Belladonna and opium suppositories (B&O Supprettes) are also effective for bladder spasms.
- **Diazepam** is used as an acute antianxiety agent but is also an excellent antispasmodic. Side effects include sedation, decreased muscle tone, and hypotension.

Relaxant/Antispasmodic	Dose
Baclofen (Lioresal)	5 mg 2 times/day to 20 mg 3 times/day; increase by 5 mg every 3 days to maximum of 80 mg/day
Cyclobenzaprine (Flexeril)	10 mg 3 times/day; range: 20–40 mg/day in 2–4 divided doses; maximal dose: 60 mg/day
Methocarbamol (Robaxin)	Initially 1500 mg 4 times/day for 2–3 days; maintenance dose: 4–4.5 gm/day in 3–6 divided doses
Quinine sulfate	260–300 mg at bedtime
Dicyclomine (Bentyl)	10–20 mg 3 or 4 times/day to maximum of 40 mg 4 times/day orally or 20 mg every 4–6 hr intramuscularly
Calcium	500 mg/day
Oxybutynin chloride (Ditropan)	5 mg 2 or 3 times/day; maximal dose of 5 mg 4 times/day
Diazepam (Valium)	2–10 mg orally or intravenously 2 or 3 times/day

24. How do you switch from one opioid to another?

An equianalgesic chart is used to help convert medication dosages from one route to another and from one drug to another with morphine as the prototype opioid. Doses should be adjusted to the patient's age, condition, and pain intensity. In patients with hepatic or renal impairment, opioids should be initiated at $\frac{1}{3}$ to $\frac{1}{4}$ of the usual dose and slowly titrated upward. There is no maximum tolerated dose or ceiling effect for opioids. The correct dose is whatever dose it takes to relieve the patient's pain without adverse side effects. (**Note:** Equianalgesic doses are approximate conversions of one drug to another, and doses may need to be decreased to allow for incomplete cross-tolerance. Decreasing the dose may not be as applicable to patients with cancer who experience increasing pain).

Equianalgesic Chart: Approximate Parenteral and Oral Doses (mg)*

OPIOID AGONISTS (MORPHINE-LIKE, MU AGONISTS)	PARENTERAL (IM, SQ, IV)	ORAL	COMMENTS
Morphine	10	30	Active metabolite: morphine 6 glucuronide. Available as twice-daily (every 8–12 hr) MS Contin, 15, 30, 60, 100, and 200 mg, or Oramorph SR, 30, 60, and 100 mg, and as once-daily (every 24 hr) Kadian, 20, 50, and 100 mg controlled-release tablets, sublingual soluble crystal (30 mg), immediate-release tablets (10, 15, 30 mg) and rectal suppositories (5, 10, 20, 30 mg). Morphine solution contains 10 or 20 mg/5 ml; morphine concentrate contains 20 mg/ml. Single oral dose may require conversion of 6:1.
Codeine	130	200 NR	Doses over 65 mg may produce diminishing incremental analgesia. Oral tablets usually compounded with nonopioid. Tylenol # 3 = 30 mg codeine + 300 mg acetaminophen; Tylenol # 4 = 60 mg codeine + 300 mg acetaminophen. Tylenol-codeine elixir contains 120 mg acetaminophen + 12.5 mg codeine/5 ml. Some clinicians recommend not exceeding 1.5 mg/kg codeine because of increased incidence of side effects with higher doses.
Fentanyl	100 µg	—	Transdermal (Duragesic) patches available in 25, 50, 75, and 100 µg/hr. Equianalgesic conversion: divide total 24-hr oral morphine dose (mg) by 2 to get fentanyl dose in µg/hr. Reaches therapeutic serum level 12–24 hr after initial application. Change patch every 48–72 hr. Serum concentration decreases 50% approx. 17 hr after discontinued. Pending FDA approval, Fentanyl Oralet, 200, 300, or 400 µg; onset, 15 min; duration, 1.5–2 hr.
Hydrocodone (Vicodin, Lortab)	—	30? NR	Equianalgesic data not available. Vicodin = 5 mg hydrocodone + 500 mg acetaminophen; Vicodin ES = 7.5 mg Vicodin + 750 mg acetaminophen.
Hydromorphone (Dilaudid)	1.5	7.5	Available as 2, 4, 8 mg tablets; liquid, 1 mg/ml; 3-mg rectal suppository; and high-potency injectable solution, 10 mg/ml.
Levorphanol (Levo-Dromoran)	2	4	Half-life = 12–15 hr; accumulates on days 2–3. Available as 2-mg tablets, 2 mg/ml injection.

Table continued on following page.

Equianalgesic Chart: Approximate Parenteral and Oral Doses (mg)* (Continued)

OPIOID AGONISTS (MORPHINE-LIKE, MU AGONISTS)	PARENTERAL (IM, SQ, IV)	ORAL	COMMENTS
Methadone (Dolophine)	10	20	Half-life = 12–190 hr; accumulates on days 2–5. To convert opioid-tolerant patient from current opioid to methadone, reduce equianalgesic dose of methadone by 50–75%. Available as 5 or 10 mg tablets; oral solution (5 or 10 mg/5 ml) or (10 mg/ml) and injectable solution.
Meperidine (Demerol)	75	300 NR	Normeperidine (toxic metabolite) accumulates with repetitive doses, causing CNS excitation. Avoid high frequent doses, chronic use, and use in patients with impaired renal function.
Oxycodone (Percocet, Tylox, Roxicet, Percodan)	—	30	Available as twice-daily (every 12 hr) 10, 20, 40, and 80 mg controlled-release tablets; immediate-release tablets, 5 mg; elixir, 5 mg/5 ml; and concentrate, 20 mg/ml. Often compounded with nonopioid. Tylox = 5 mg oxycodone + 500 mg acetaminophen; Percodan, Percocet, Roxicet = 5 mg oxycodone + 325 mg aspirin/acetaminophen.
Propoxyphene (Darvon)	—	? NR	Half-life = 12 hr. Propoxyphene (P) and toxic metabolite norpropoxyphene accumulate with repetitive dosing. Darvon = 32 mg P; Darvon compound = 65 mg P, 389 mg aspirin, + 32.4 mg caffeine; Darvocet N50 = 50 mg P + 325 mg acetaminophen; Darvocet N100 = 100 mg P + 650 mg acetaminophen.
Oxymorphone (Numorphan)	1	10 rectal	Available in 5-mg suppositories.

* Equianalgesic doses are approximate. All doses must be titrated to individual response. Rescue dose for breakthrough pain is calculated as 10–20% of the 24-hr dose. For single IV bolus, use half the intramuscular dose. NR = not recommended at that dose. Unless otherwise stated, half-life of opioids ranges from 2–3 hr. Adapted from McCaffery M: Pain Assessment and Intervention in Clinical Practice Course Syllabus. Los Angeles, 1995 (phone 310-649-2219). E-mail comments to dianaruz@aol.com.

25. Give an example of switching from one opioid to another, using an equianalgesic chart.

To convert 6 mg of oral hydromorphone every 3 hr to oral, continuous-release morphine:

1. Calculate the 24-hr dose of medication that the patient currently receives:

   6 mg × 8 (every 3 hr) = 48 mg hydromorphone/24 hr

2. Review the equianalgesic chart for equivalence guidelines:

   7.5 mg oral hydromorphone is equivalent to 30 mg oral morphine.

3. Equation: $\dfrac{30 \text{ mg oral morphine}}{7.5 \text{ mg hydromorphone}} = \dfrac{X \text{ mg morphine}}{48 \text{ mg hydromorphone}}$

4. Cross-multiply to solve for X:

   48 mg hydromorphone × 30 mg morphine = 7.5 mg hydromorphone × X mg morphine
   1440 mg = 7.5X   1440/7.5 = X   X = 192 mg oral morphine

5. Divide the dose by the number of administration times per day to obtain the interval dose.

   Continuous release morphine is dosed every 12 hr.
   192 mg/2 = 96 mg orally 2 times/day (100-mg tablet or three 30-mg tablets)

6. In addition to the scheduled dose, order as-needed doses for breakthrough pain; for example, morphine elixir (20 mg/ml), 20–40 mg orally every 2–4 hr as needed.

26. How do you calculate the dose of medication for breakthrough pain?

Breakthrough pain refers to an exacerbation or transitory flare of pain, which occurs in about 65% of patients who take regularly scheduled analgesics for stable or baseline pain (Portenoy, 1990). The recommended breakthrough dose should be 10–20% of the 24-hr dose.

27. What is important to know about controlling pain in elderly patients?

In addition to other pain relief barriers, elderly patients fail to report pain because they believe pain is expected with aging. Furthermore, health professionals may believe that elderly patients experience a lower pain level or that they are unable to tolerate high doses of opioids. Assessment is further complicated by sensory or cognitive impairments. The patient should be assessed frequently, and the dosage should be adjusted based on the patient's response. A thorough medication history is essential. Tips in administering or selecting analgesics include:

- Avoid opioids with long half-lives, such as methadone, propoxyphene (Darvon), or levorphanol. Drugs may have longer half-lives in elderly patients because of decreased renal clearance, decreased hepatic function, and decrease in lean body mass to fat ratio.
- Avoid meperidine because accumulation of its metabolite, normeperidine, is associated with confusion and seizures.
- Be aware that morphine also has active metabolites (morphine 6 glucuronide) that may accumulate, resulting in nausea, confusion, and sedation.
- Avoid long-term use of NSAIDs.
- Use steroids cautiously because they aggravate osteoporosis.
- For a tricyclic antidepressant, consider nortriptyline over amitriptyline because of its lower anticholinergic effects.
- With both opioids and adjuvant medications, the recommendation is to "start low and go slow." When the equianalgesic chart is used to convert from one agent to another, the dose of the new analgesic should be decreased by 25% to account for incomplete cross-tolerance.
- Start one medication at a time, and give it a thorough trial before changing or adding a new medication.
- Keep it simple. Avoid high-technology pumps, especially if the patient lives alone.
- Provide medication instructions to the patient and a responsible family member verbally and in writing (large print).
- Assess and treat constipation vigilantly because of elderly patients' decreased mobility, decreased fluid intake and concomitant use of other medications.

28. How is pain treated in a patient with cancer and a history of substance abuse?

In patients with cancer and a history of substance abuse pain still should be treated with opioids as indicated. If they are actively abusing opioid drugs or on a methadone maintenance program, they may require substantially higher starting doses to provide adequate analgesia because of drug tolerance. The dosing interval also may need to be shortened. Morphine, which has a usual duration of action of 3–4 hr, may need to be dosed every 1–2 hr in persons with opioid addiction and a large degree of pharmacologic tolerance.

The use of opioids should be openly discussed with the patient. Patients may fear repeat addiction and should be encouraged to express concerns and fears. Patients and health care providers should contact the recovery program for advice and collaboration. A patient's wish to decline opioids should be honored.

Explicit rules should be established to guide behavior: (1) prescription renewals, (2) procedure to be followed with lost or stolen prescriptions or medications, and (3) procedure to ensure that only one clinician is prescribing analgesic medication. Consequences of failure to conform with rules should be delineated: (1) if drugs are "lost," patient may be readmitted to the hospital for pain control; (2) the patient may be required to come to the treatment facility to obtain daily doses; and (3) if the source of pain is gone, opioids may no longer be prescribed and the patient is referred to a drug treatment program. Patients should be assessed frequently and prescribed a set amount of opioids. Nonopioid or adjuvant drugs may be helpful in decreasing opioid requirements.

29. How do you start a patient-controlled analgesia pump?

An intravenous patient-controlled analgesia (PCA) pump allows the patient to self-administer a predetermined dose of analgesics at a specified time interval. In addition, a basal infusion can be programmed into most pumps.

1. Calculate the equianalgesic IV dose of agent that the patient currently receives.
2. Divide the 24 hr dose by 24 to obtain the hourly or basal dose.
3. Set the hourly rate (mg/hr), PCA or bolus dose, and interval.
4. If the patient has uncontrolled or increased pain, be sure to administer a loading dose to control the pain before starting the PCA. Loading doses should be individualized. A good starting loading dose is equal to one-third, one-half, or one full hour total of the patient's normal maintenance (hourly plus PCA or as-needed doses).

In contrast to patients with acute postoperative pain, patients with chronic cancer pain require that most of the analgesic dose be programmed into the hourly PCA infusion so that pain is prevented (similar to around-the-clock oral dosing). The PCA (breakthrough) dose is usually one-half of the hourly infusion rate set at every 6–15 minutes. Thus, if the equianalgesic dose of IV morphine was 6 mg/hr, the pump may be set at the following values: continuous infusion, 3–6 mg/hr, and 1–3 mg PCA dose with a 15-minute lockout. However, if the patient's pain was not well controlled on the oral dose, the hourly and PCA dose may be set higher. The patient should be reassessed frequently, and the continuous rate should be increased based on the patient's response. The table below lists starting dosages for commonly used PCA opioids; after the initial setting, however, the dose should be titrated to effect.

Drug	Concentration	PCA Dose	Continuous Infusion	Onset (min)	Peak (min)
Hydromorphone (Dilaudid) (Adult)	0.2 mg/cc	0.2 mg	0.2–0.4 mg/hr	5	10–20
Hydromorphone (Dilaudid) (Pediatric)	0.2 mg/cc	0.003–0.0045 mg/kg	0.0015–0.003 mg/kg/hr	5	10–20
Morphine (Adult)	1 mg/cc	1 mg	1–2 mg/hr	10–20	15–30
Morphine (Pediatric)	1 mg/cc	0.02–0.03 mg/kg	0.01–0.02 mg/kg/hr	10–20	15–30
Fentanyl	10 μg/cc	10–25 μg	10–25 μg/hr	1	1–5

30. Can a PCA pump be used in patients without venous access?

A PCA pump can also be used to deliver analgesics subcutaneously. Hydromorphone (Dilaudid) is ideal for this purpose because it provides a high concentration of medication (high-potency preparation, 10 mg/cc) in a low volume. Butterfly (25–27 gauge) or special needles for subcutaneous administration may be used (e.g,. Baxter 27-gauge, ¼-inch needle with extension tubing). The site is covered with a transparent dressing, and the needle needs to be changed every 3–7 days with routine inspection of the site for erythema, swelling, or tenderness.

31. What is the relevance of plasma half-lives and steady states in opioid dosing?

The half-life is the time taken for a drug to reach half of its plasma concentration. For all drugs and routes of administration, usually 4 to 5 half-lives are necessary to reach steady state; therefore, dose changes should not be made until steady state is achieved. This is often not possible in patients with increasing levels of pain. In such patients, it is more advantageous to use opioids with short half-lives for breakthrough pain. Drugs with long half-lives may result in delayed or prolonged side effects, particularly in elderly patients or patients with liver or renal impairment. Half-lives for commonly used opioids are listed below:

Opioids with short half-life	Opioids with long half-life
Morphine (2–3.5 hr)	Methadone (12–190 hr)
Hydromorphone (2–3 hr)	Levorphanol (12–15 hr)
Oxycodone (2–3 hr)	Propoxyphene (12 hr)

32. How effective is sublingual morphine?

For patients who cannot swallow, morphine concentrate (20 mg/cc) is ideal for sublingual administration. Drug bioavailability is estimated at 20–30%. Problems with sublingual morphine include sour taste, dry mouth, and bitter taste. Also available are 30-mg soluble sublingual morphine crystals.

33. What opioids are available in rectal suppositories?

Morphine, hydromorphone, and oxymorphone are available in rectal preparation. Several of the immediate-release oral preparations can be crushed and diluted or crushed and placed in a gel suppository shell and administered rectally. Although sustained-release compounds are not to be crushed, rectal administration in whole form has been reported.

34. Does methadone or levorphanol have a place in the management of cancer pain?

Methadone (Dolophine) and levorphanol (Levo-Dromoran) are synthetic opioids indicated for moderate-to-severe pain; their side effects are similar to those of morphine. Before the availability of continuous-release morphine formulas, they were the mainstay of oral analgesic therapy. Both have long half-lives and are difficult to titrate; therefore, caution is necessary in elderly patients and patients with major hepatic or renal failure or dementia. If their long half-lives are taken into consideration, both drugs are highly effective analgesics for cancer pain. They are also good alternatives if the patient is allergic to morphine. The normal dosing schedule is every 6 hours around the clock. Methadone is quite cost-effective ($0.05/tablet).

35. Why is meperidine not recommended for use in patients with cancer?

Meperidine (Demerol) is not indicated for treatment of cancer pain because of its toxic metabolite, normeperidine, which has a 15-hour half-life. Normeperidine accumulation causes CNS excitability and seizures.

36. How do you switch to a fentanyl patch?

A fentanyl patch is a transdermal system that delivers fentanyl over 72 hours. Patches deliver 25, 50, 75, and 100 µg/hr. Equianalgesic charts are available with ranges of oral morphine equivalent to fentanyl patches of various strengths; however, the following formula is a simple method of calculating equivalent doses:

1. Convert the 24-hour dose of current opioid to the equianalgesic dose of oral morphine, using an equianalgesic chart.

2. Divide the result by 2 to equal the dose of fentanyl in µg/hr. For example, an opioid converted to 180 mg of oral morphine/24 hr is divided by 2 to equal 90 µg or a 100-µg patch.

3. Because the patch takes approximately 9–16 hours to provide analgesia, an additional analgesic is needed. If the patient is being converted from continuous-release morphine, the last 12-hr dose may be administered at the same time as the patch is applied. If the patient was receiving a short-acting analgesic, continue this medication for the next 12 hours.

4. Calculate an appropriate dose of oral medication for breakthrough pain. This dose may be 10–20% of the 24-hr equivalent of continuous-release oral morphine. For example, the breakthrough dose for a 50-µg fentanyl patch should be 10–20 mg of immediate-release morphine (50 µg = 90–100 mg of oral morphine/24 hr).

37. What are special considerations for using fentanyl patches?

- Patients must have adequate fat stores to absorb and retain the medication to enable the patch to last 72 hr. In emaciated patients, the patch may need to be changed more frequently because of more rapid absorption.
- Increased absorption in febrile patients may result in oversedation.
- To secure the patch in place for diaphoretic patients, apply a transparent dressing over the patch.

38. What is Brompton's cocktail?

Brompton's cocktail, devised at Brompton's Hospital, was used in early hospices in England for cancer pain. The cocktail consists of the following: morphine hydrochloride 15 mg; cocaine l0 mg; alcohol 90% 2 ml; chloroform water 15 ml; and syrup 4 ml (Twycross, 1984). Before World War II, the alcohol and syrup were replaced by gin and honey. A solution allows easier titration of the analgesic; however, if side effects develop or increase, it is difficult to determine which component is responsible. Brompton's cocktail has been replaced with other liquid preparations (morphine sulfate elixir). No evidence suggests that Brompton's cocktail has an analgesic advantage over single opioids.

39. When should tramadol be used for cancer pain?

Tramadol (Ultram), an opioid for mild-to-moderate pain, is comparable to codeine, hydrocodone, or oxycodone. Normal doses are 50–100 mg, administered orally every 6 hours, not to exceed 400 mg/24 hours. Tramadol seems to be effective for patients with early bone or neuropathic pain and for that reason is used primarily to treat chronic pain. In patients with cancer, it may be appropriate as an early opioid substitute for analgesics such as Tylenol #3 (tylenol and codeine). It is not a good choice for breakthrough pain because it may compete for the same binding site and act as a significantly weaker mu agonist. **Note:** Usually Tylenol 500 mg is given with each dose of tramadol.

40. What interactions of opioids with other drugs are causes of concern?

Because patients with cancer experience multiple symptoms and receive numerous drugs, nurses need to be constantly aware of potential clinical and physical interactions and incompatibilities. Fortunately, opioids such as morphine are physically compatible with many supportive care drugs.

- Any medication that causes sedation must be used cautiously with opioids. The phenothiazine antiemetics (promethazine, droperidol, prochlorperazine), muscle relaxants (baclofen, cyclobenzaprine), benzodiazepines (diazepam, midazolam), alcohol, clonazepam, and phenytoin also cause sedation. When such drugs are given with opioids the patient should be monitored closely and the opioid dose may need to be decreased to prevent oversedation and respiratory depression. **Note:** It is safe for patients in pain to take an opioid dose along with a regularly scheduled sleeping pill.
- Monoamine oxidase (MAO) inhibitors (e.g., phenelzine [Nardil], tranylcypromine [Parnate]) may produce severe, fatal reactions when given in combination with opioids. In addition, concomitant use of MAO inhibitors and tricyclic antidepressants may result in death.
- Phenytoin sodium is physically incompatible with the following opioids: fentanyl citrate, hydromorphone hydrochloride, methadone hydrochloride, and morphine sulfate.

41. What are the possible complications or side effects of drugs used to treat pain? How do you avoid or treat side effects?

Sedation. Tolerance to sedation usually develops within 3–5 days with repeated doses of opioids. In addition to caffeine drinks (tea, coffee, coke), antisedatives such as dextroamphetamine and methylphenidate are helpful. Antisedatives should be given in the morning or early afternoon. Dextroamphetamine and caffeine also increase analgesia when combined with other opioid or nonopioid analgesics. Doses of remedies for sedation include the following:

Caffeine	100–200 mg/day (1.0–1.5 mg/kg in children)
Dextroamphetamine (Dexedrine)	2.5–10 mg orally (0.05–0.1 mg/kg in children)
Methylphenidate (Ritalin)	5–10 mg orally (0.1–0.2 mg/kg in children)

Respiratory depression. High-dose opioids given to an opioid-naive patient may cause respiratory depression; however, tolerance to respiratory depression develops with repeated doses over several weeks. Pain acts as an antagonist to respiratory depression. It is not unusual for a patient to take 1600 mg of morphine/day. Doses as high as 10,000 mg/day have been reported. The risk of respiratory depression in a patient receiving chronic opioid therapy is less than 1%. Oversedation can usually be managed by holding or not giving the opioid dose and stimulating the patient. Naloxone (Narcan), an opioid antagonist, should be administered only to patients with significant respiratory depression or apnea. In the rare instance that naloxone is indicated, the following regimen is appropriate: (1) dilute 1 ampule (0.4 mg/cc) with 9 cc of normal saline, and (2) administer 20 µg (0.02 mg or 0.5 cc) every 3 minutes to desired effects. The goal is to reverse the respiratory depression or sedation without reversing the analgesia.

Nausea and vomiting. Nausea and vomiting due to stimulation of the chemoreceptor trigger zone usually resolve in 48–72 hr. Antiemetics, such as oral Compazine spansules, 15–30 mg every 12 hours for the first 3–5 days, help to prevent nausea and improve patient acceptance (see chapter 38).

Constipation. Unfortunately, tolerance to constipation does not develop. All patients receiving opioids should be placed on a prophylactic bowel regimen consisting of both stool softener (e.g., Colace, 100–300 mg/day) and laxative (e.g., senna, 2–6 tablets twice daily) (see chapter 33).

Ileus. Ileus induced by opioids has been reversed with continuous infusion of metoclopramide and oral naltrexone.

Pruritus. Pruritus due to IV or oral opioids is associated with histamine release and may be treated with Benadryl. Pruritus from epidural opioids is not due to histamine release but may result from binding of the opioid to the trigeminal nerve as it spreads rostrally (e.g., facial itching); it is also treated in many institutions with Benadryl, 25–50 mg IV. Mild pruritus may be treated with cool compresses or lotion. Narcan and Nubain (mixed agonist/antagonists) have been used to reverse pruritus due to spinal opioids; however, analgesia also may be reversed. Recently, naltrexone (a long-acting formulation of Narcan) has been recommended with an epidural morphine bolus to prevent pruritus. Other causes of pruritus (e.g., drug allergy) should be ruled out. Doses for treatment of pruritus are listed below:

Benadryl	25–50 mg IV, orally every 6 hr
Narcan	20 µg IV, may repeat to desired effect
Nubain	2.5–5 mg IV every 4–6 hr
Naltrexone	5 mg, orally

42. What is the difference between intrathecal and epidural administration?

Intrathecal administration. The subarachnoid fluid is bounded by the dural ligament (ligamentum flavum). Intrathecal or subarachnoid catheters are placed into the subarachnoid space, and medications are delivered directly into the spinal fluid. Because medication delivered intrathecally does not have to diffuse across the dural ligament, smaller doses are required.

Epidural administration. Epidural catheters go just outside the dural ligament. Medication is delivered into the epidural space, which is a potential space located below the ligament of flavum and above the dura mater. The medication diffuses across the dura mater and arachnoid mater into the cerebrospinal fluid, where it binds with opiate receptors to block pain transmission. Epidural catheters are at greater risk for compression of flow due to tumor growth than intrathecal catheters.

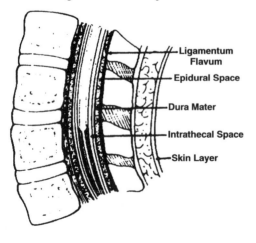

Lateral Section of the spine. (From St. Marie B: Management of Cancer Pain with Epidural Morphine. St. Paul, MN, Pharmacia Deltec, 1994, with permission.)

43. When should epidurals be considered for cancer pain?
- When the dose of oral or intravenous opioids reaches a point at which side effects become a significant issue. Epidural analgesics are associated with fewer side effects (e.g., sedation) because the IV dose of morphine may be reduced by 1/10 and the oral dose by 1/30. When the intrathecal route is used, the amount of morphine is even less: the IV dose is reduced by 1/100 and oral dose by 1/300.
- For neuropathic pain, such as tumor invasion of a nerve plexus or nerve root and scarring from radiation therapy. Neuropathic pain is effectively treated with epidural or intrathecal placement of local anesthetics and clonidine.

44. What are the advantages and disadvantages of the spinal delivery of pain medications?
Advantages
- Direct delivery to involved receptors (allows use of less medication and effective control of intractable pain)
- Less sedation
- Ability to use a combination of agents with minimal side effects
- Effective control of neuropathic pain

Disadvantages
- Initial high cost if a completely implantable system is used
- Risk of infection leading to epidural abscess with risk of nerve damage and paraplegia
- Risk of meningitis with intrathecal catheters
- Greater incidence of pruritus

45. Are there any new drugs to treat pain? What kinds of drugs are planned for the future?
- Oxycontin is a twice-daily (every 12 hr), continuous-release form of oxycodone.
- Kadian is a recently marketed, 24-hr preparation of morphine.
- Oral transmucosal fentanyl citrate lozenges, which can be used as breakthrough medication for patients currently on fentanyl patches, are available in clinical trials and are awaiting FDA approval.
- An intermittent-delivery fentanyl patch that acts like PCA device is currently in clinical trials. The patient applies the patch on the skin but receives a dose only when pushing the patch.
- Rhenium-186 and samarium-153 phosphonate chelates are awaiting FDA approval. Both have demonstrated 65–80% efficacy in international clinical trials for management of metastatic bone pain.
- Clonidine, an alpha$_2$ agonist, has recently been approved by the FDA for epidural administration. When used with opioids, clonidine helps to decrease neuropathic pain. Intrathecal approval is currently before the FDA. (**Editor's note:** A combination of intrathecal clonidine, midazolam [Versed], and dilaudid has proved highly effective in a patient with pancreatic cancer).
- Inhaled morphine has been used as a treatment for terminal patients with pulmonary metastases to decrease air hunger. One-third to one-half of the inhaled morphine gets into the bloodstream.
- Dexmedetomdine, an investigational clonidine-like drug (alpha$_2$ agonist), and cone's snail venom, a calcium channel blocker, show promise for neuropathic pain.

46. What are some key resources or organizations available to assist with pain management?
Organizations
   American Pain Society
      4700 W. Lake Ave.
      Glenview, IL 60025
      (847) 375-4715
      http://www.ampainsoc.org/; e-mail: info@ampainsoc.org

American Society of Pain Management Nurses
1550 South Coast Highway
Suite 201
Laguna Beach, CA 92651
(888) 34-ASPMN
City of Hope MAYDAY Pain Resource Center
1500 East Duarte Road
Duarte, CA 91010
(818) 301-8111 ext. 3829
International Association for the Study of Pain
909 NE 43rd St., Suite 306
Seattle, WA 98105-6020
(206) 547-6409; e-mail: IASP@locke.hs.washington.edu
http://weber.u.washington.edu/~CRC/IASP.html
Resource Center for State Cancer Pain Initiatives
1300 University Avenue
Madison, WI 53706
(608) 265-4013

Publications

Journal of Pain and Symptom Management (quarterly)
Elsevier Publishing Co., Inc.
655 Avenue of the Americas
New York, NY 10010
(212) 633-3650
Clinical Journal of Pain (quarterly)
Raven Press Books, Ltd.
1185 Avenue of the Americas
New York, NY 10036
(212) 930-9500
Principles of Analgesic Use in the Treatment of Acute Pain and Cancer Pain (41-pages)
4700 W. Lake Ave.
Glenview, IL 60025
(847) 375-4715
http://www.ampainsoc.org/
e-mail: info@ampain.soc.org
Handbook of Cancer Pain Management, 1996 (36-pages)
1300 University Avenue, Rm 4715
Madison, WI 53706
(608) 262-0978
e-mail: wcpi@facstaff.wisc.edu
http://www.wise.edu/molphorm/wcpi/
   index.html

AHCPR Clinical Practice Guidelines: Acute Pain Management: Operative or Medical Procedures and Trauma; Management of Cancer Pain
AHCPR Clearinghouse
P.O. Box 8547
Silver Spring, MD 20907
(800) 358-9295
http://text.nlm.nih.gov/
Pain Digest
Springer-Verlag New York, Inc.
P.O. Box 2485
Secaucus, NJ 07094
Topics in Pain Management
Williams & Wilkins
P.O. Box 23291
Baltimore, MD 21203-9990
American Journal of Hospice and Palliative Care
Circulation Department
470 Boston Post Road
Weston, MA 02193
Pain (free to IASP members)
Elsevier Science Publishers
P.O. Box 211, 1000 AE
Amsterdam, The Netherlands

Complimentary Publications

Analgesia
Abbott Laboratories
Medical Department, AP30
1 Abbott Park Road
Abbott Park, IL 60064

Palliative Care Letter
Roxane Laboratories, Inc.
P.O. Box 16532
Columbus, OH 43216

The views expressed in this manuscript are those of the author and do not reflect the official policy or position of the Department of the Army, Department of Defense, or the U.S. Government.

ACKNOWLEDGMENT

The author thanks Robin Slover, MD, for her review and contributions to this chapter.

BIBLIOGRAPHY

1. Bruera E, Brenneis C, MacDonald RN: Continuous Sc infusion of narcotics for the treatment of cancer pain: An update. Cancer Treat Rep 71:953–958, 1987.
2. Chandler SW, Trissel LA, Weinstein SM: Combined administration of opioids with selected drugs to manage pain and other cancer symptoms: Initial safety screening for compatibility. J Pain Sympt Manage 12(3):168–171, 1996.
3. Coluzzi PH: Effective strategies for managing cancer pain with opioid pharmacotherapy. In Miaskowski C (ed): Helping Patients Manage Cancer Pain: Challenges and Opportunities. Deerfield, IL: Discovery International, 1997.
4. Coyle N, Cherny N, Portenoy RK: Pharmacologic management of cancer pain. In McGuire DB, Yarbro CH, Ferrell BR: Cancer Pain Management, 2nd ed. Boston, Jones & Bartlett, 1995, pp 89–130.
5. Eisenberg E, Berkey CS, Carr DB, et al: Efficacy and safety of nonsteroidal anti-inflammatory drugs for cancer pain: A meta analysis. J Clin Oncol 12:2756–2765, 1994.
6. Ferrell BR, Dean GE, Grant M, Coluzzi T: An institutional commitment to pain management. J Clin Oncol 13:2158–2165, 1995.
7. Ferrell BR, Rhiner M, Cohen MZ, Grant M: Pain as a metaphor for illness. Part I: Impact of cancer pain on family caregivers. Oncol Nurs Forum 18:1303–1309, 1991.
8. Hodgson BB, Kizior RJ, Kingdon RT: Nurse's Drug Handbook 1996. Philadelphia, W.B. Saunders, 1996.
9. IASP Subcommittee on Taxonomy: Pain terms: A list with definitions and notes on usage. Pain 8:249–252, 1980.
10. Jacox A, Carr DB, Payne R, et al: Management of Cancer Pain. Clinical Practice Guideline No.9. AHCPR Publication No.94-0592. Rockville, MD, Agency for Health Care Policy and Research, U.S. Department of Health and Human Service, Public Health Service, 1994.
11. Max M, Payne R: Principles of Analgesic Use in the Treatment of Acute Pain and Cancer Pain, 3rd ed. Glenview, IL, American Pain Society, 1992.
12. McCaffery M, Beebe A: Pain: Clinical Manual for Nursing Practice. St. Louis, Mosby, 1989.
13. McCaffery M, Ferrell BR, Turner M: Ethical issues in the use of placebos in cancer pain management. Oncol Nurs Forum 23:1587–1593, 1996.
14. Omoigui S: The Pain Drugs Handbook. St. Louis, Mosby, 1995.
15. Portenoy RK: Management of cancer pain: Opioid and adjuvant pharmacotherapy. In Portenoy RK (ed): Real Patients, Real Problems: Optimal Assessment and Management of Cancer Pain. Glenview, IL, American Pain Society, 1997, pp 5–13.
16. Portenoy RK, Hagen NA: Breakthrough pain: Definition, prevalence and characteristics. Pain 41:273–281, 1990.
17. Porter J, Jick H: Addiction rare in patients treated with narcotics. N Engl J Med 302:123, 1980.
18. Skobel SW: Epidural narcotic administration: What nurses should know. Oncol Nurs Forum 23:1555–1562, 1996.
19. Stein WM: Cancer Pain in the Elderly. In Ferrell BR, Ferrel BA (eds): Pain in the Elderly. IASP Press, Seattle, 1996.
20. Twycross RG: Strong narcotic analgesics. In Twycross RG (ed): Pain Relief in Cancer. Philadelphia, W.B. Saunders, 1984, pp 109–133.
21. Watson CPN, Evan RJ, Watt VR: Postherpetic neuralgia and topical capsaicin. Pain 38:177–186, 1989.
22. Weissman DE, Dahl JL, Dinndorf PA: Handbook of Cancer Pain Management, 5th ed. Madison, WI, Wisconsin Cancer Pain Initiative, 1996.
23. Wong D, Whaley L: Clinical Handbook of Pediatric Nursing, 2nd ed. St. Louis, Mosby, 1986, p 373.
24. World Health Organization: Cancer pain relief and palliative care. Report of a WHO Expert Committee. WHO Technical Report Series 804. Geneva, Switzerland, World Health Organization, 1990, pp 1–75.

42. PALLIATIVE CARE

Karyn P. Prochoda, RN, MD, and Paul A. Seligman, MD

1. What is palliative care?

Palliative care as defined by the World Health Organization (WHO) is "the active total care of patients whose disease is not responsive to curative treatment. Control of pain, of other symptoms, and of psychological, social, and spiritual problems, is paramount." Symptoms are controlled with a variety of medical and non-medical interventions. The goal of palliative care is to promote comfort and quality of life without prolonging or hastening death. Palliative care can be delivered in a hospital setting (dedicated beds or wards), the home, or a single-purpose facility or hospice.

2. Why is palliative care usually provided in a hospice?

Hospice is derived from the Latin words, *hospes* (guest) and *hospitum* (hospitality). A hospice was a place of rest and entertainment for traveling pilgrims. This meaning changed in the 11th century when the Knights of Hospitallers of the Order of Saint John established hospices along the routes of the crusades for the ill and dying. During the reign of Henry the VIII in the 16th century, a hospice was a shelter for the sick, dying, and poor. In the 1800s the Sisters of Charity in Dublin established a home for the incurably ill. This idea traveled to England, where St. Joseph's Hospice was founded in 1905. Dame Cicely Saunders worked here as a nurse in the early days of her career. Dame Saunders later became a physician and was instrumental in promoting hospice as a philosophy of care for the terminally ill. Under her guidance a hospice was no longer merely a place to go to die; it became a program of care focused on relieving the symptoms and suffering of the dying.

In 1974 the hospice movement came to the United States and expanded rapidly as a reaction to experiences of isolation, abandonment, and poor symptom control encountered by dying patients under the care of conventional medicine. Hospice care in the United States became focused on providing comfort for the terminally ill in the home.

3. When should a palliative approach to care be considered?

The decision to shift care to a palliative mode is not always an easy decision to make and is individualized with input from the patient, family, and formal caregivers (medical and nursing staff). Palliative care is considered when all agree that curative therapies are no longer working and new goals of care are needed.

Cancer patients are traditionally considered in discussions of palliative care. In a 1992 survey by the Centers for Disease Control (CDC), 65% of people in a hospice program had a primary diagnosis of cancer. A 1994 follow-up survey by the National Hospice Organization found the same percentage of primary cancer diagnoses among its membership. Other diagnoses considered appropriate for palliative care include end-stage cardiovascular disease, end-stage lung disease, end-stage renal disease, and AIDS.

4. Who is involved in the care of an individual in a palliative care program?

The skills of a multidisciplinary team are required for controlling symptoms and providing comfort, palliation, and support for patients in a palliative care program. Nonphysician members are essential to the team; nursing care is the keystone. Because nursing provides day-to-day care, nurses are in the best position to alert team members to changing patient care issues. A pharmacist evaluates the medication regimen and offers suggestions for alternatives when needed. Physical and occupational therapists assist in maintaining the patient's comfort by minimizing the effects of immobility and inactivity. Social workers aid the family and patient by counseling during the dying process and locating resources in the community for supportive as well as financial services. Pastoral counselors help the patient and family with spiritual issues, and bereavement counselors support the family during the grieving process. Ideally the team meets weekly to discuss the plan of care and makes changes as needed.

5. What is the most common symptom treated in a palliative care program?

Pain affects more than 80% of terminally ill cancer patients; the prevalence increases toward the very end of life. At most, 17% of pain is not related to the terminal illness. Assessment of a pain complaint should include type of pain, location, and exacerbating or alleviating factors. Solid tumors most commonly cause pain through (1) organ infiltration, (2) tumor infiltration of nervous tissue, and (3) compression of organs, vasculature, and nerves. Other sources of pain related to a cancer diagnosis include (1) pathologic fractures and (2) disease-modifying treatments (surgery, chemotherapy, radiation therapy). Nonmalignant sources of pain result from exacerbation of other disease processes, including heart failure, arthritis, osteoporosis, venous and arterial insufficiency, chronic constipation, and diabetes mellitus, all of which are worsened when immobility, deconditioning, and additional medications result from treating pain and other symptoms caused by the terminal illness.

6. What are the two most common side effects of analgesics used for treatment of pain complaints?

Constipation is the most frequent side effect of opioid or narcotic analgesics and can evolve into an uncomfortable, painful paralysis of the gut. No opioid regimen is complete without the addition of a laxative. Opioids act to slow the forward movement of the gut while promoting an increase in fluid absorption in the colon, forming hard, firm, difficult to pass stools. The approach to management includes both pharmacologic and nonpharmacologic measures. The frequency of bowel movements needs to be closely monitored. A natural elimination pattern is provided by having the patient participate in a bowel program and maintain an adequate fluid intake. The use of stimulant laxatives, such as a senna derivative, is indicated to promote the forward movement of fecal matter for elimination. Having a patient sit on the commode for 10–15 minutes after meals uses the natural urge for defecation and promotes the correct anatomic position for defecation.

Nausea occurs during the initiation of most opioids but becomes less problematic as opioid tolerance develops. Nausea also may be a lingering side effect of some chemotherapy regimens. Intestinal obstruction due to severe constipation or tumor blockage may result in nausea. Treatment of nausea varies with the cause. Antiemetics taken for the first 5–7 days of starting an opioid will minimize nausea. Nonpharmacologic means of controlling nausea include offering foods in small portions served at room temperature to minimize noxious odors; offering a liquid diet, especially clear liquids; and minimizing odors in the surrounding environment. Intestinal obstructions resulting from the use of opioids may be resolved by a good bowel program. Blockages resulting from tumor bulk and spread are more difficult to treat. Occasionally a nasogastric tube with suction provides the most comfort, but often a surgical procedure is the only means to relieve the obstruction.

7. Mrs. K is an 80-year-old woman with congestive heart failure and metastatic colon cancer. She was admitted to the hospital for intractable pain. After being on the ward for two days, she is noted to be intermittently confused and combative. What has happened?

Delirium is a waxing and waning of mental status. Periods of agitation and confusion are coupled with periods of somnolence or lucidity. Delirium frequently occurs among elders with a history of dementia. The causes for delirium are multifactorial but most often relate to medications, especially opioids. With the onset of delirium a review of medications is needed, and all nonindicated medications should be stopped. Examples include heart medications, such as digoxin, that may no longer be needed for heart failure or antihypertensives that may be eliminated or reduced if blood pressure is controlled by a decline in activity and physical functioning. If an opioid is the cause, adjusting the dose, substituting another equianalgesic opioid, or switching to a nonopioid analgesic may be required. For example, the study by Maddocks et al. showed an attenuation of morphine-induced delirium when patients were switched to a subcutaneous infusion of oxycodone.

Other causes of delirium and agitation include poorly controlled pain, dehydration, and electrolyte imbalances. Not all causes are easily treated. An attempt should be made to determine a reversible cause whenever possible. After careful assessment of reversible causes, occasionally a low-dose neuroleptic (e.g., haloperidol, 0.5 mg orally or intramuscularly every 6 hr) may be indicated to relieve the distressing symptom of confusion.

8. Mr. M is a 75-year-old man with severe lung disease and a new diagnosis of lung cancer. The nursing staff has noted that he is very demanding and always on the call light. Why?

Mr. M may be depressed or anxious. The prevalence rate for depression and anxiety among patients with cancer is reported to vary from 23–58%, with approximately 5–15% of patients developing severe depression. Symptoms of depression, such as anxiety, insomnia, weight loss, anorexia, and fatigue, also may be symptoms of the underlying disease.

Anxiety and depression can be situational or related to a variety of causes, including drugs (e.g., steroids, bronchodilators, anticholinergics, stimulants) and other diseases or physical conditions (e.g., hyperthyroidism, hypoglycemia, neurologic conditions, psychiatric disorders). A recent diagnosis of cancer with an immediate recommendation for palliative care can be frightening; the unknown is odious. Uncontrolled or poorly controlled symptoms at the end of life are feared. When symptoms are poorly controlled, a patient may withdraw, stop eating, become angry, or wish for an early end to suffering. Suffering may be related not only to physical symptoms but also to unresolved family and spiritual conflicts.

9. What are nonpharmacologic ways of treating anxiety and depression?

Nonpharmacologic means of treating anxiety and depression include relaxation techniques and allowing the patient to verbalize fears and concerns, exploring sources of anxiety, and offering explanations and reassurance. Psychological counseling for both patient and family may help to resolve troublesome conflicts. A patient's sense of autonomy can be promoted by allowing control in the environment and treating bothersome physical symptoms that interfere with daily functioning.

10. Which medications are useful in treating anxiety?

Pharmacologic treatment of anxiety requires that nonpharmacologic methods have failed. Nonpharmacologic methods should include a review of medications and discontinuance of drugs no longer required. Anxiolytics consist of benzodiazepines and nonbenzodiazepine tranquilizers. Anxiolytics should be used with caution because they increase sedation and may cause confusion, especially in elderly patients.

The agents of choice in treating anxiety are the benzodiazepines. Most drugs in this class share similar efficacy and side effects. Drugs with short-to-intermediate half lives and inactive metabolites, such as lorazepam (elimination half life = 10–20 hr) and oxazepam (elimination half life = 5–20 hr), are tolerated better in elderly and debilitated patients than drugs with long half-lives and active metabolites, such as diazepam (elimination half life = 20–80 hr). In addition to reducing anxiety, alprazolam (elimination half life = 12–15 hr) has antidepressant and antipanic effects in doses of 0.25–0.5 mg 2 or 3 times/day. Clonazepam in doses of 0.5 mg twice daily (elimination half life = 18–50 hr) is useful in treating anxiety and has the added benefit of reducing neuropathic pain. Nonbenzodiazepines, such as buspirone, have fewer sedating side effects but may not be as effective as benzodiazepines for controlling anxiety.

11. Which drugs are commonly used to treat depression in patients with cancer?

For short-term situational depression related to changes in circumstances (e.g., new diagnosis of terminal illness, move to a new environment), methylphenidate is a good first-line agent. It is started in doses of 2.5 mg twice daily (morning and noon); the dose can be rapidly escalated to a total dose of 20 mg twice daily. An effect will be seen in the first few days of therapy once an adequate dose is established. Methylphenidate can be used for up to 6 weeks. It is an excellent agent to be used while titrating longer-acting agents that require weeks to produce an effect.

Traditionally tricyclics have been used to treat depression. Although tricyclics are usually effective, the delay from onset of treatment until therapeutic effect (up to 3 weeks) and anticholinergic and sedative side effects may be unacceptable in some terminally ill patients. Of the tricyclics, desipramine is the least sedating and has moderate anticholinergic effects. Nortriptyline has few anticholinergic or orthostatic effects and intermediate sedation. A more rapid therapeutic effect can be achieved with a selective serotonin reuptake inhibitor (SSRI), such as fluoxetine (Prozac), sertraline (Zoloft), or paroxetine (Paxil). SSRIs have the advantage of no anticholinergic or cardiovascular side effects.

12. What factors influence the choice of antidepressant?

The desired time until onset of action and consideration of side effects are important in choosing an antidepressant (see table below). Patients who have difficulty falling asleep or who experience agitation may benefit from an antidepressant with sedating side effects, such as trazodone. Psychomotor retardation or excessive fatigue is treated with an antidepressant with stimulating qualities, such as sertraline or methylphenidate. For patients experiencing pain, the use of a tricyclic antidepressant is recommended for augmenting pain control.

Medication	Dosage	Onset of Action	Common Side Effects
Sertraline (Zoloft)	Start 25 mg, increase to 50–100 mg for therapeutic effect (morning dosing)	5–7 days	Anorexia, diarrhea, restlessness
Nortriptyline (Pamelor)	Start 10–25 mg, increase to 50–100 mg for therapeutic effect (bedtime dosing)	7–14 days	Dry mouth, constipation, sedation, orthostasis, cardiac arrhythmias
Methylphenidate (Ritalin)	Start 2.5 mg twice daily, may increase to 20 mg twice daily; titrate to therapeutic effect (morning and noon dosing)	1–2 days	Insomnia, agitation, restlessness, psychosis
Desipramine (Norpramin, Pertofrane)	Start 10–25 mg, increase to 100 mg for therapeutic effect	7–14 days	At higher doses: dry mouth, orthostatic hypotension
Trazodone (Desyrel)	Start 25–50 mg, increase to 100–150 mg for therapeutic effect (bedtime dosing)	7–14 days	Somnolence, not anticholinergic, priapism

13. Do dosages of antidepressants need to be lowered in patients with cancer?

Dosages of antidepressants should be lowered in patients debilitated by age or disease or patients with compromised hepatic metabolism or impaired renal excretion. All too often this description fits the patient with cancer. Generally medications should be started at low doses and increased slowly to achieve therapeutic effect. Most of the antidepressants are increased on a weekly basis, with the exception of methylphenidate, which can be increased every 2–3 days. Targeted behaviors should be monitored for desired changes. For example, in using trazodone to assist a patient who has difficulty with sleeping, sleep can be used as the target behavior. If increasing the dose of trazodone from 50 to 100 mg helps the patient to fall asleep, 100 mg of trazodone may be considered the therapeutic dose for this patient.

14. Is depression undertreated in patients with cancer?

In general, depression is underdiagnosed and therefore undertreated. The diagnostic difficulty may be increased in patients with cancer. The signs and symptoms of depression may be confused with the side effects of cancer therapies and medications. Examples include fatigue, loss of appetite, and weight loss. Loss of interest in usual activities and feelings of hopelessness or helplessness should be considered as symptoms of depression, especially if they are prolonged and interfere with the patient's relationships with loved ones and caregivers.

15. How common is dyspnea in the terminally ill?

Dyspnea, an unpleasant awareness of the action of breathing, occurs in over 70% of terminally ill patients. It is most common in patients with lung cancer and patients who have received chemotherapy with pulmonary toxicity. Radiation to more than 25% of the lung predisposes to the development of dyspnea.

16. What assessment is required to determine the cause of dyspnea?

In addition to the causes listed in question 15, there are non–cancer-related causes for dyspnea. Anxiety can both be cause and result of dyspnea. Assessment should include determination of the events that trigger the dyspneic spell. Vital signs are important; a fever may cause tachycardia and increased respiratory rate, resulting in dyspnea. The volume load from a recent blood transfusion may trigger congestive heart failure with pulmonary edema. Chest pain may signal myocardial ischemia, compromising the heart's ability to pump blood and thus leading to pulmonary edema. Dyspnea after the placement of a central venous catheter may signal incorrect placement or pneumothorax. Cardiac arrhythmia may cause the patient to feel short of breath. A respiratory assessment is indicated to rule out alterations in gas exchange due to collapsed lung, effusion, pneumonia, pulmonary edema, or bronchospasm.

17. How is dyspnea treated?

Treatment depends on the underlying cause. Nonpharmacologic treatment should be tried. For example, a patient with chronic obstructive pulmonary disease may become less dyspneic by simply removing clutter from the room or by placing a table fan by the bedside. If anxiety is the cause of the dyspnea, spending time with the patient and offering reassurance may be comforting.

If the dyspnea is related to a collapsed lung or effusion, it is reasonable to place a chest tube or drain the excessive fluid to increase lung expansion. These procedures are not without discomfort, and the health care worker must work with the patient to determine if there will be a benefit.

Pharmacologic methods of treating dyspnea most often are directed at relieving the unpleasant sensation of not being able to breathe. Morphine sulfate acts centrally by reducing ventilatory responses to carbon dioxide and hypoxia. Morphine can be given parenterally, orally, or via nebulizer. A usual starting dose of morphine is 5–10 mg of oral immediate-release preparation every 2 hours. The dose can be titrated to meet the patient's need. Anxiety contributes to the sensation of inadequate ventilation and may be relieved with a combination of morphine and anxiolytic agents.

18. Mrs. C is a 78-year-old woman with metastatic colon cancer. On her abdominal wall is a large fungating mass. Mrs. C is distressed by the odor from this mass. What can be done?

Odors from wounds can cause discomfort for both patients and caregivers. Odors result from an overgrowth of bacteria on necrotic and dying tissue. Frequent dressing changes to remove drainage may decrease odors. In addition, the use of local antiseptic and astringent solutions such as Domeboro may lessen odors. Buttermilk and yogurt with active cultures may influence the bacteria colonizing a wound by promoting lactobacilli colonization, which reduces the number of odor-causing anaerobic organisms. When these measures fail, a short course of oral antibiotics, such as clindamycin or metronidazole, may be used to reduce the anaerobic bacterial burden within the wound. In addition, a recent study by Finlay et al. showed the benefit of topical 0.75% metronidazole gel in decreasing odor and eliminating infection from malodorous cutaneous ulcers.

19. Mr. G is a 50-year-old man with jaundice due to biliary obstruction from pancreatic carcinoma. Recently he has been complaining of intense itching. Why is he itching? What can be done?

Pruritus or itching in patients with cancer may result from many factors. Drugs may cause itching either as an allergic or idiosyncratic reaction. In allergic reactions the itch can occur without the presence of a rash. Opioids may cause pruritus as a result of drug-induced histamine release from skin mast cells. Opioid-induced pruritus can be treated by changing the opioid or adding an antihistamine.

Jaundice results from a build-up of bilirubin, a breakdown product from destruction of red cells in the blood, because of the inability of the liver to conjugate for excretion or (as in this patient) the inability to excrete conjugated bilirubin. Some patients develop pruritus as a result of jaundice. More commonly, patients with renal failure develop pruritus because of uremia. Pruritus associated with these conditions responds best to topical measures, lukewarm baths with either oatmeal additives or oiled additives, or mentholated lotions. Antihistamines such as hydroxyzine (Atarax) and diphenhydramine (Benadryl) also may help. Hot baths and showers worsen itching.

20. Mrs. T. is an 80-year-old woman with metastatic breast cancer. She lives in a nursing home and is incontinent. Recently moving her has become quite painful as a result of bony metastasis. Is it appropriate to place a Foley catheter?

Yes. In general, there are four reasons to place a urinary catheter in any patient: (1) urinary obstruction, (2) need for accurate output in incontinence, (3) skin breakdown exacerbated by incontinence, and (4) terminal condition. Placing a Foley catheter in this patient will help to promote comfort by allowing her to be dry and minimizing the amount of turning required for changing wet linen or diapers.

21. A 65-year-old man with metastatic prostate cancer is admitted from home for evaluation of leg weakness and back pain. The family is concerned that he is not eating or drinking and requests that he be force-fed by the nursing staff if he refuses to eat. Is the patient suffering without food or fluids?

No. Physiologically anorexia has been described as an adaptive, protective mechanism that leads to a gentler death; death from dehydration and starvation is not painful. Anorexia is most difficult for family members to accept because culturally food and drink are considered nurturing and life-sustaining.

Anorexia is multifactorial and commonly found in hospice patients. It may result from persistent nausea, medication side effects, cancer effects, or depression. An assessment is required to determine the more easily treated causes, such as controlling nausea or eliminating unnecessary medications. A recent prospective study evaluated the need for food and fluid at the end of life. Thirty-two patients were followed from the time they entered a hospice program until their death. Of the 32 patients, only one maintained an appetite. Others felt no hunger or desire for food. If hunger or thirst was felt, small sips of fluid or moistening the mouth with a swab satisfied the sensation.

Forced feeding is not recommended, including enteral and parenteral nutrition. Artificial nutrition and hydration may lead to such symptoms as congestive heart failure, increase in tracheal and bronchial secretions, nausea and vomiting, painful edema, and diarrhea. Family members need support, education, and reassurance that dehydration does not mean a decrease in comfort and that forced feeding of a dying patient may only aggravate some symptoms and increase anxiety, leading to worsened quality of life.

22. Miss V is actively dying from metastatic lung cancer. Her sister comes to the desk crying that Miss V is struggling to breathe. On entering the room you hear Miss V breathing a coarse, rattling sound. She appears to be struggling but is unresponsive to her surroundings. Should Miss V be suctioned? What is "death rattle"?

Death rattle is noisy breathing in terminally ill patients shortly before death as a result of upper airway or pulmonary secretions that they are unable to clear. Generally the patient is unresponsive at this point. This situation is often more distressing for family and caregivers than patients themselves. However, accumulated secretions may lead to dyspnea and restlessness in some patients. Prevention of the death rattle is one argument for not forcing hydration as death approaches because build-up of pulmonary secretions is less likely in dehydrated patients. This claim, however, has not been supported by recent evidence.

Whether to suction the patient is determined by the level of comfort that the family and care-takers perceive in the dying patient. A family member who is distraught by apprehension that their loved one is suffering may be comforted by the results of suctioning. However, suctioning can also cause trauma, bleeding, and shortness of breath. Turning the patient to a lateral position to facilitate drainage of secretions may be helpful. Other authors have suggested the use of scopo-lamine or intramuscular atropine to minimize pulmonary secretions. Hyoscine hydrobromide (scopolamine) has often been used with variable results as a subcutaneous continuous infusion in doses ranging from 0.8–2.4 mg over 24 hours or as an injection of 0.4–0.6 mg. A study by Bennett suggested that scopolamine was more effective in death rattle due to salivary secretions rather than bronchial secretions. Alternatively, morphine sulfate can be used to relax respiratory efforts. Nursing judgment is important in determining how the comfort of the patient nearing death is affected by the proposed interventions.

23. What are intractable hiccups?

Hiccups, properly called singultus, have no useful function and are common in dying pa-tients. Intractable hiccups last longer than 1 month, whereas persistent hiccups last longer than 48 hours but less than 1 month. Adverse effects of persistent or intractable hiccups include fa-tigue and exhaustion, wound dehiscence, dehydration, severe reflux esophagitis, malnutrition, and even death.

Hiccups are commonly related to upper gastrointestinal disease and other conditions irritat-ing the vagus or phrenic nerves. Other etiologic factors include gastric distention (possibly most common cause in terminal cancer patients), central nervous system disorders (intracranial tumors, subdural hematomas), metabolic (renal insufficiency, hypocalcemia) and drug-induced disorders (barbiturates, diazepam, midazolam, intravenous dexamethasone), infectious disease (meningitis, herpes zoster, tuberculosis), psychogenic factors (anxiety, hysteria), and idiopathic causes.

24. How are hiccups treated?

As with other symptoms, treatment should be directed at the underlying cause; however, be-cause an extensive medical work-up is generally not practical in palliative care, treatment is em-piric. Stimulation of the pharynx or interruption of the vagal and/or phrenic nerve limbs of the hiccup reflex arc usually leads to cessation of hiccups.

Nondrug methods include gargling ice water, rapid swallowing of dry granulated sugar, drinking from the far side of a glass, having someone scare the person by shouting "boo," palatal massage, and pharyngeal stimulation with a cotton swab or insertion of a rubber nasal catheter followed by back-and-forth movements (not recommended because of discomfort and possible retching and vomiting). Maneuvers that involve vagal stimulation (e.g., Valsalva maneuver, carotid or ocular massage) also have worked. Home remedies, breath-holding, or breathing into a paper bag interfere with normal respiratory function and may work by pro-ducing a mild respiratory acidosis that exerts a central effect and suppresses diaphragmatic action.

Drugs with reported efficacy in treating persistent and intractable hiccups include:
Chlorpromazine (25–50 mg intravenously, intramuscularly, orally, or rectally 3 or 4
   times/day)
Metoclopramide (10–20 mg intravenously, intramuscularly, or orally 4 times/day)
Carbamazepine (200 mg 3 times/day)
Cisapride (10–20 mg 4 times/day)
Amitriptyline (10 mg 3 times/day)
Baclofen (10–20 mg 3 times/day)
Metoclopramide is particularly useful in hiccups due to gastric stasis or distention and gas-troesophageal reflux; however, it is contraindicated in patients with bowel obstruction.

25. Mr. S is a 76-year-old man so debilitated by end-stage metastatic lung cancer that he is bed-bound and able to take only small sips of liquid several times during the day. He was previously energetic and active. His family is worried that he is having a miserable existence in the last days of his life. On the other hand, Mr. S states that he feels that "in some ways the past month has been the best of my life" and that he "enjoys having his family around." Is Mr. S just trying to make his family feel better by putting on his "best face"?

Although the interpretation is subjective, Mr. S's answer indicates that he is satisfied. Quality of life is the individual's own evaluation of satisfaction with important areas of life and functioning. Only recently have various quality-of-life issues been included in the care of dying patients. Quality-of-life questionnaires make it clear that some patients can be quite comfortable with support from their families. In some ways, they may feel more support than they have ever before.

It is important for all caregivers to value and facilitate improvements in nonphysical well-being. The best quality-of-life questionnaires generally include questions related to various domains, including physical, psychological, emotional, spiritual, and existential aspects of the patient's life. For example, some patients with a high degree of physical symptoms, including weakness and residual pain, may have a sense of psychological well-being because they are no longer encumbered with some of the aggravations that they experienced in their professional lives. Such patients may be emotionally comforted by their families. Some patients even find comfort in what might be termed existential values, knowing that the end is near but seeing added importance in each day because family is present. Such patients often remark that "each day is a gift." It is important to realize that each individual defines his or her quality of life. Placement of value on nonphysical well-being, in particular, is one of the most satisfying aspects of palliative care.

BIBLIOGRAPHY

1. Bennett MI: An audit of hyoscine (scopolamine) use and review of management. J Pain Symptom Manage 12:229–233, 1996.
2. Centers for Disease Control: Home health and hospice care—United States, 1992. MMWR 42:820–823, 1993.
3. Drug Facts and Comparisons, 50th ed. St. Louis, J.B. Lippincott, 1996.
4. Enck RE: The Medical Care of Terminally Ill Patients. Baltimore, John Hopkins Press, 1994.
5. Finlay IG, Bowszyc J, Ramlau C, Gwiezdzinski Z: The effect of topical 0.75% metronidazole gel on malodorous cutaneous ulcers. J Pain Symptom Manage 11:158–162, 1996.
6. Maddocks I, Somogyi A, Abbott F, et al: Attenuation of morphine-induced delirium in palliative care by substitution with infusion of oxycodone. J Pain Symptom Manage 12:182–189, 1996.
7. McCann RM, Hall WJ, Groth-Juncker A: Comfort care for the terminally ill patient: The appropriate use of nutrition and hydration. JAMA 272:1263–1266, 1994.
8. Miller RJ: Force feeding the dying: An act of kindness or cruelty. Am J Hospice Care Nov/Dec:13–14, 1989.
9. Payne R: Cancer pain: Anatomy, physiology, and pharmacology. Cancer 63:2298S–2307S, 1989.
10. Rousseau P: Hospice techniques: Hiccups in terminal disease. Am J Hospice Palliat Care 11(6):7–10, 1994.
11. Rousseau P: Review article: Hiccups. South Med J 88(2):175–179, 1995.
12. Smith SA: Patient-induced dehydration—can it ever be therapeutic? Oncol Nurs Forum 22:1487–1491, 1995.
13. Twycross RG: Dysphagia, dyspepsia, and hiccup. In Doyle D, Hanks GWC, MacDonald (eds): Oxford Textbook of Palliative Medicine. Oxford, Oxford University Press, 1993, pp 291–299.
14. Walsh TD (ed): Symptom Control. Boston, Blackwell Scientific Publications, 1989.
15. World Health Organization: Cancer Pain Relief and Palliative Care. Geneva, World Health Organization, 1990.

43. SEXUALITY

Patricia W. Nishimoto, RN, MPH, DNS, LTC, AN, USAR

1. Why bother with sexuality in cancer nursing?

Sexuality is an integral part of well-being that is important throughout an individual's life span. In 1975 the World Health Organization stated that "Sexual health is the integration of the somatic, emotional, intellectual, and social aspects of sexual being in ways that are positively enriching and that enhance personality, communication, and love." The Oncology Nursing Society's standard on sexuality supports interventions for the purpose of identifying alterations in client sexuality and maintaining sexual identity. To meet this standard, the oncology nurse must recognize that a patient's sexual health is influenced by sexual function before diagnosis, past sexual experiences, other illnesses, medications, stage of disease, religious and cultural background, emotional and psychological status, and relationships with other people. It most definitely will be affected by a diagnosis of cancer, cancer therapies, and life as a cancer survivor.

Too often, nurses avoid the topic of sexuality in the mistaken belief that sexuality refers only to the act of intercourse. In fact, sexuality must be considered in a much broader context, encompassing feelings, insights, motivations, thoughts, or behaviors related to gender, sexual identity, and sexual activity. Sexuality becomes a broad-spectrum rainbow, ranging from intimate touching, verbal communication, and outward appearances to kissing, masturbation, and intercourse.

When nurses are silent and do not discuss sexuality, patients are given the message that sexuality is not appropriate; as a result, holistic patient care suffers. Waiting until the patient asks about sexuality is not realistic, because multiple studies have found that patients are hesitant to ask health care providers about sexuality. Some patients may choose not to engage in sexual activity during or after treatment. The decision not to become sexually active should be respected. However, if the patient desires to continue sexual activity, the role of the nurse is to provide helpful information.

2. What should nurses know before discussing sexuality?

First, nurses must believe that helping patients to deal with changes in sexuality is a part of nursing care. Second, they must want to provide holistic care and understand that treating a patient's sexuality is part of such care. Third, before discussing sexuality, nurses should have a basic knowledge of sexuality and how cancer and its treatment may affect sexual functioning. Fourth, nurses should be aware of their own attitudes toward their own sexuality and sexual issues and put aside personal opinions and biases. Nurses may gain greater confidence and comfort by attending conferences, reading, role playing, or mentoring with an expert.

When counseling patients about sexuality, nurses should have an open, accepting attitude; respect the patient's beliefs and practices; avoid making assumptions; and keep in mind that sexuality is very personal and defined by each individual. Nurses should be careful not to impose their own biases and should be aware of myths; they do not have to be experts in sexual therapy. Many sexual problems require sensitive listening, explanations, and reassurance—the same skills that nurses use daily in clinical practice. Nurses who are uncomfortable about discussing sexual issues can still be helpful by making appropriate referrals or providing written information about available resources. Knowing what, when, and how to inquire about patients' sexual concerns requires awareness, knowledge, skills, and practice.

3. Why do some nurses hesitate to include sexuality counseling as part of their holistic care?

Although all members of the health care team need to be prepared to address sexuality in their teaching and counseling, it is often the nurse who is the first to become aware of sexual concerns. Why nurses fail to address the sexuality standard of care is unclear and complex; it may be a reflection of their upbringing or cultural background. Many nurses feel "too busy" and unqualified or believe that sexual counseling is someone else's job. Other nurses are uncomfortable discussing sex and believe that sex is too private a topic to discuss with patients.

Some nurses wait for the patient to bring up the issue of sexuality, concerned that if they initiate the conversation, they will offend or distress patients. This is especially true if the nurse believes that "cancer ends sexuality" or that "focus needs to be on life-or-death issues." Other myths, such as "they're too old, too ugly, or too fat," can stop the nurse from initiating discussion. Finally, in the current atmosphere of health care reform, sexual concerns are given a low priority because they are "not part of the critical pathway," "not a requirement," or "not reimbursable."

4. How can I provide sexual counseling?

Robinson and Annon developed the **PLISSIT** model, which is based on four levels of intervention: permission, limited information, specific suggestions, and intensive therapy.

Permission to express sexual concerns or questions. An example is the 16-year-old boy with osteosarcoma who asks if it is "normal" to masturbate or if masturbation caused the cancer. The nurse should give the patient permission to ask further questions by responding that masturbation did not cause the cancer and that it is normal to masturbate. At this level, the nurse needs to know basic physiology, normal cultural beliefs about sexuality, and developmental issues—in other words, information that nurses already have because of their training.

Limited information related to the concern, such as common sexual changes that may occur during or after cancer treatment. When a 36-year-old mother with three children who is receiving chemotherapy after mastectomy comments that she does not "get turned on as often," the nurse should first confirm that she is referring to decreased vaginal lubrication. The nurse then gives the patient "limited information" that chemotherapy decreases lubrication and causes fatigue, which affects libido. This information is all that some patients need: "Oh, it is normal for this to happen. Nothing is wrong with me after all." Others may want to know what to do, and the nurse either should proceed to the next level or refer the patient to someone who can. At this level, the nurse needs to know how cancer or its treatments can affect sexual functioning.

Specific suggestions to deal with changes in sexuality. For example, the patient may say, "I'm glad to find out that decreased lubrication is normal when you're on chemo. I was worried something was wrong with our marriage." But if she also asks what to do, the nurse can give a specific suggestion (after assessing the patient's cultural and religious beliefs and current sexual practice), such as using a water-soluble lubricant during intercourse. At this level, the nurse needs a solid knowledge of sexual behaviors and alternatives.

Intensive therapy usually involves more than four sessions and referral to an advanced practice nurse, psychologist, social worker, or other health care provider who specializes in sexual counseling. For example, intensive therapy is needed for a 42-year-old woman diagnosed with cervical cancer who, after repeated gynecologic examinations, begins to relive her rape experiences when she was only 17 years old. At this level, formal advance practice training and clinical work experience are required.

5. How do I give the patient permission to talk about sexual concerns?

Nurses can let patients know that it is all right to talk about sexuality in many ways, but none will work if the nurse giggles, turns red, or tries to rush out of the room when patients begin to talk about sexuality. In other words, as the first requirement, the nurse must be comfortable with the topic of sexuality and prepared to use his or her nursing communication skills. If the nurse perceives that a comment about sexuality has been taken in the wrong way, the appropriate response is the usual one in situations of misunderstanding (which occur in every nurse's career): expression of regret, reassurance that no offense was intended, and expression of hope that the patient understands. The initial communication about sexuality may be difficult because of its emotionally charged and private nature. The nurse needs to establish a level of rapport, comfort, and trust before openly discussing sexuality.

Using the **3 L's and 1 P** may help: language, labeling, listening, and privacy. Some patients may use **language** that is "raw or earthy" and causes a few blushes, whereas others may use euphemisms or oblique sexual references. For example, a patient may ask what to do for the pain she feels when "we do it." But the problems of language and miscommunications are not one-sided. The nurse who responds to the euphemistic question with a long monologue about "strategies to prevent dyspareunia" may get a polite nod followed by the question, "But what do I do so it doesn't hurt?" Nurses need to use appropriate language understood by the patient and not hide behind professional jargon. **Labeling** means that neither nurses nor patients should label themselves with words such as "impotent" or "weird." **Listening** is a basic nursing skill, but it may be uncomfortable to listen about sex at first. Nurses must give themselves time to learn. **Privacy** is having the common sense not to shout in the busy treatment room, "Hey, Mrs. S., did the lubricant help you and your husband?"

6. What guidelines may help the patient to feel more comfortable about expressing sexual concerns?

Once you have mastered the 3 L's and 1 P, the following guidelines help to increase the patient's comfort about discussing sexual concerns:

1. Do not wait for patients to bring up sexuality. When the opportunity to discuss sexuality arises or the patient provides an opportunity, follow through and be flexible. Do not avoid direct questions, such as "After my laryngectomy, can I still have oral sex?" When discussing sexuality, use language and terms appropriate to the patient. For example, if the patient asks, "When we fuck, it really hurts. Is there anything that can be done?," you may reply: "What kind of pain do you have when you fuck or have sexual intercourse?" Even if you are uncomfortable using the patient's term, do not embarrass the patient. Repeat the patient's term, and then use the term you prefer.

2. Provide a relaxed, private place for discussions. When possible and if desired by the patient, include the significant other in discussions.

3. Give patients permission and opportunity to bring up sexual problems or to ask questions by including open-ended questions or statements about sexuality as part of your routine nursing history. Point out to the patient that you routinely ask questions about sexuality of all your patients to help promote overall health and well-being and to prevent problems. Open the door for discussions about sexuality by prefacing your questions with a comment about a sexual concern. For example, if you ask "Are you having any sexual problems?," the patient is likely to answer yes or no. It is better to make a statement such as, "Many of our patients who are taking chemotherapy lose their desire for sex," "many women experience vaginal dryness," or "many men have difficulty having an erection," and then to ask, "Are you having the same problem?," or simply to say, "if you are having this problem, our advice is to...." You may be pleasantly surprised by the response.

4. Keep brochures or books about sex prominently displayed on your desk or in your book case. Seeing such brochures and books helps to reassure patients that sexuality is a topic of health care concern and that you are open to discussing the issues. Having anatomic models or sketches readily available is also helpful for discussions.

5. Include sexuality-related topics in your teaching handouts about chemotherapy or radiation therapy. This legitimizes the topic of sexuality and gives patients implied permission to ask questions at a later time.

6. Initiate discussions of sexual concerns at various stages of illness, i.e., before, during, and after treatment. Recognize that discussions of sexuality are not necessarily a one-time event but rather a series of conversations over an extended period and may involve a variety of changing situations and conditions. Discuss sexuality when you have time to listen, not when the clinic is packed with patients and you are trying to do twenty things.

7. Consider altering hospital policies to include private time for patients and their significant other or to establish conjugal visiting rooms, that is, initiate changes that move sexuality beyond the mere discussion phase to tangible practice.

7. What questions about sex are most commonly asked by patients with cancer?

Certain basic questions may seem to have obvious answers, but they are important and would not be asked if the patient knew the answer:

1. Will my partner "catch cancer from me" if we have sex?
2. Will my partner leave me because I have cancer?
3. Will my partner think my [ostomy, mastectomy, surgical incision] is disgusting and be "turned off"?
4. Is _____ normal?
5. Will my partner still love me?
6. Will anyone ever want to date me?

Nurses should remember three basic principles: (1) they do not have to know all of the answers; (2) seldom is sexuality an emergency; and (3) it is all right to tell your patient, "That is a good question, and I've never really thought about it. Let me do some reading and talking with our consultant. I can either call you at home with the answer or give you the information at your next appointment."

8. How does cancer affect phases of the sexual response cycle?

Cancer or its treatment affects sexual functioning, fertility, and body image. Virtually any symptom or side effect of treatment can potentially affect sexuality. Stress alone can decrease androgen, resulting in decreased desire. Cancer and its treatment affect the first three phases of the sexual response cycle in the following ways :

1. **Excitement** is influenced by physical state, emotions, body image, anxiety, hormonal functioning, and other physical factors. In patients with cancer, other significant factors include drugs, surgery, and radiation therapy, which may interfere with the vasocongestion or muscle tension. Even if a patient with cancer has undergone mastectomy, she still may have the phantom sensation of the nipple erection during excitement. Often people become more attentive or hypervigilant of their body and changes to their body after a diagnosis of cancer. For example, before diagnosis a patient may not have noticed the body rash that accompanies excitement. In the hypervigilant condition that may arise after diagnosis, the patient may notice a body rash and stop sexual activity because of concern that the rash is a reaction to chemotherapy.

2. During **plateau**, which is characterized by continued vasocongestion and myotonia, the pulse may increase to 100–175 beats per minute, blood pressure may rise, and the labia may change color. The hypervigilant cancer patient may misinterpret these changes as symptoms of cancer or treatment and cease sexual activity.

3. **Orgasm** is associated with a sense of warmth in the pelvis and muscle contractions that last 3–15 seconds. Respirations may increase to 40 per minute, depending on the patient's age. In patients who take tranquilizers as part of treatment, muscle contractions may not be as strong because the drug relaxes pelvic muscles.

9. What are some specific examples of how symptoms of cancer and its treatment might affect sexuality?

Symptom	Effect on Sexuality
Nausea/vomiting	Patient may not want to go out to restaurants or on a date. Use of antiemetic may decrease sexual desire.
Skin and nail changes	Body image and self-image may be affected. For example, dry, less pliable skin from x-ray treatment may make the patient feel less attractive. If toe sucking is part of usual sexual practice, change in toenails may affect frequency or enjoyment.
Stomatitis	May make kissing painful. If painful to talk, intimate communications with significant other may be difficult. Lesions also may occur on vaginal mucosa.
Diarrhea	May affect patient's body and self-image in terms of loss of control. Patients may avoid social situations because of concern about closeness to bathroom. Rectum may become uncomfortable so that anal stimulation is no longer pleasurable.

Continued on following page.

Symptom	Effect on Sexuality
Neutropenia	Risk of vaginal infections may increase, especially if vaginal lubrication is decreased. Anal stimulation may be too risky because of potential for infection. In neutropenic patients, safer sex needs to be discussed because of increased risk of sexually transmitted diseases.
Fatigue	May need to discuss changes in sexual activity or positions during sex to conserve energy.
Decreased platelets	Patient may bruise more easily during oral sex or nipple stimulation. Stimulation with nipple or penile rings may damage platelets. If a patient engages in bondage and discipline, it may be necessary to change to soft restraints.
Changes in sense of smell	Body smells that used to have an aphrodisiac effect may become too strong or unpleasant.
Neuropathy	Loss of sensation may decrease enjoyment of toe and finger sexual play.
Ototoxicity	Hearing the intimate whispers of a significant other may become more difficult and make aural sexual arousal more difficult.
Inability to return to school or work	Loss of mobility and diminished activity may decrease opportunities to meet potential partner and lower self-esteem or cause depression, thus decreasing libido.
Change in weight	Partner may be reminded of life-threatening diagnosis; examples: discomfort when pelvic bones hit during coitus, clothes that no longer fit.
Decreased hormone levels	Orchiectomy or hormone treatment to decrease testosterone levels for metastatic prostate cancer may affect libido. Chemotherapy that decreases estrogen in women may decrease vaginal lubrication and cause dyspareunia.
Cardiac/pulmonary toxicity	May affect libido and ability to engage in strenuous sexual activity. Patients may need to change positions or use pillows to conserve energy. Advise patient about what to do if chest pain or shortness of breath occurs.
Alopecia	Single patients may be reluctant to date because of effect of hair loss on body image. Patient's partner may not want sexual contact because alopecia is daily reminder of patient's cancer. Loss of pubic hair may be sexually exciting (increased genital sensation), or it may remind patient or partner of being a child so that sex is avoided because it feels like incest. If eyelashes are lost, patient's constant blinking may "turn off" partner.
Lymphedema	Body image may be affected. Affected limb may become so heavy or so large that it needs to be supported with pillows. Patients may have pain or decreased strength. Joint complications may affect range of motion, which in turn affects position during sexual play. Edema may compress nerves so that tactile sensations and pleasure are decreased. Skin may become fragile.
Pain	In anticipation of pain, a "plan for sex" (e.g., taking a pain pill 30 minutes before sexual activity) may become necessary. Because many people enjoy spontaneous sex, this "plan" may interfere with desire or excitement. Orgasm releases endorphins and provides pain relief for up to 6 hours.

10. What chemotherapy drugs impair fertility? Are such effects permanent?

Although reproductive ability is not specifically a sexual function, the meaning of fertility can affect a patient's perception of sexual well-being. Changes in fertility, whether temporary or permanent, may have positive, negative, or no effects on the patient's perception of his or her sexuality. Therefore, it should not be assumed that infertility will have a negative effect for every patient; the topic needs to be addressed during sexual counseling.

Studies of elderly men after prostate surgery indicate that fertility is not of importance to men in their 70s or 80s. In the author's study, loss of fertility due to retrograde ejaculation was not a concern for many men, but each man commented on it. Surprisingly, 20% of the men, whether heterosexual or homosexual, voiced regret about perceived loss of fertility even though they had no desire to father children. Thus, fertility may be of concern to male patients, no matter what their age or sexual orientation.

The effects of chemotherapy are many and varied. How chemotherapy affects fertility depends on the age of the patient receiving chemotherapy (50% of women over the age of 35 who receive a single alkylating agent experience permanent infertility); total amount of chemotherapy received (combination chemotherapy is more likely than single-agent treatment to cause dysfunction); and whether any other treatment (e.g., radiation therapy, surgery) also affects fertility. Drugs that affect testicular and ovarian function include cyclophosphamide, Busulfan, and nitrogen mustard. Chlorambucil, procarbazine, and nitrosoureas affect men, whereas L-phenylalanine affects women. Drugs with probable risk to testicular epithelium but unknown risk to ovaries include doxorubicin, vinblastine, cytosine arabinoside, and cisplatin. Drugs with unlikely risk to fertility for men or women include methotrexate, 5-fluorouracil, and 6-mercaptopurine. Vincristine is also unlikely to affect male fertility.

Although the primary focus is adult patients, children also are affected by chemotherapy. For example, chemotherapy seems to affect boys more when it is given during puberty than when it is given before puberty. Chemotherapy does not seem to affect many prepubertal and pubertal girls because the immature ovary is relatively insensitive to chemotherapy.

11. What are the most common drugs that cause sexual dysfunction? What are their effects?

Drug	Effect on Sexuality
Antihypertensive medications	Erection dysfunction, decreased vaginal lubrication. Retarded ejaculation, especially with monoamine oxidase (MAO) inhibitors.
Antidepressants	May temporarily decrease erections or vaginal lubrication.
Tranquilizers	May decrease anxiety and improve sexual functioning. Retard ejaculation. Large dose may decrease erection and vaginal lubrication. Relax pelvic muscles and affect orgasm (i.e., loss of muscle tension decreases pleasure of orgasm)
Recreational drugs (e.g., cocaine, marijuana)	May cause euphoria and increase self-confidence. May increase tactile pleasure or may block sexual arousal and pleasure. May cause extended, painful erections or painful ejaculations.
Anitcholinergics	Affect arousal (decreased erection and vaginal lubrication).
Opioids	Less pain increases enjoyment of sex. Side effect of constipation may interfere with sexual activity. Long-term opioids may retard ejaculation.
Hormones	May decrease serum testosterone and thus sexual desire. Secondary sex changes (deepening of voice, increased facial hair) may affect body image.
Alcohol	Decreases libido. Decreased inhibitions may interfere with use of safer sex and thus increase risk for infection. Decreased vaginal lubrication and erection.
Antiadrenergics	Decrease libido, vaginal lubrication, and erection. May cause retrograde ejaculation.
Endocrine drugs	Hot flashes, dyspareunia due to decreased vaginal lubrication. Mood swings.
Chemotherapy drugs	Alopecia, stomatitis, fatigue, anorexia, decreased immunity.

12. What effect does radiation therapy have on sexuality?

Radiation therapy affects patients in different ways, depending on the site of the radiation field, amount of rads delivered, previous level of health, and beliefs about radiation. Patients may have many misperceptions that need to be addressed. A patient may believe that radiation therapy is a "last-ditch effort" and therefore avoid sexual activity because of the belief that "terminally ill people shouldn't do that." Patients may have a total misunderstanding of how radiation works; they may worry that they are "radioactive" and so avoid contact of any kind. Other patients may understand how radiation therapy works, but their partner, who did not come to the clinic appointment, may worry his "penis will glow in the dark" if they have sex. Below are some of the side effects of radiation therapy that a nurse may need to address during discussions of sexuality.

- Decreased blood flow to genitals from vascular scarring (erection dysfunction, decreased vaginal lubrication)
- Skin changes (skin becomes too tender for partner to touch; skin texture or color changes)
- Fatigue (possible loss of libido)
- Shortening of vaginal vault
- Vaginal stenosis
- Decreased vaginal sensation
- Alteration in sexual patterns
- Concern about bleeding
- Concern about possible recurrence
- Decreased skin sensitivity due to nerve damage
- Pelvic radiation may cause urethral irritation (women may experience pain with penetration or men with ejaculation)

13. How does a laryngectomy affect sexuality?

Frequently nurses forget to address sexuality when the site of the cancer or treatment does not directly affect a "sexual organ," such as the breast or testicle. Yet a sexually neutral site may have even more effect on sexual functioning. In dealing with the many aspects of treatment for patients with a head or neck tumor that requires laryngectomy, nurses may overlook sexual functioning. The following are but a few of the potential effects:

- Patients cannot whisper intimately into partner's ear.
- Partners may find it discomforting to feel the patient's breath on their neck. Wearing a T-shirt or stoma shield may help.
- During oral sex, pubic hairs may get caught in stoma and cause the patient to cough.
- Patient may have increased incidence of halitosis, which may be sexually unattractive.
- Coughing up a "gumba" (increased secretions) can be a turn-off.
- Increased respirations after orgasm may stimulate coughing.
- If patient and partner make love in the shower or hot tub, water may get in stoma.
- Limited neck mobility after radical neck dissection affects positioning during sexual activity.
- Visual appearance may affect ability to attract new partner.
- Body image is radically changed.
- Decreased range of motion of shoulder may affect positions.
- Patients cannot hold their breath at moment of orgasm.
- Patients and partners may be reminded of diagnosis of cancer whenever they see the incision site.

14. What are the special concerns of patients with same-sex partners?

Patients with same-sex partners experience the same physiologic changes from cancer and therapy, but they may be even more hesitant to ask questions. Thus, the challenge to the health care provider is not to learn unique facts about same-sex partners but instead to learn to be open and nonjudgmental so that patients can confide their concerns.

This is not simple when most books and pamphlets about cancer and sexuality have a heterosexual bias (male and female partners on the covers) and the text refers primarily to "married couples." Opening up is even more difficult when professional or military/legal consequences must be considered.

In the nursing or sexuality assessment, nurses may ask, "Do you have a partner? Is your partner male or female, or do you have both?" Nurses should practice this routine so that they feel comfortable. Nurses who are comfortable with same-sex issues will be surprised at the information they receive. Visiting policies should be expanded to include nonspouses. Nurses with strong feelings against same-sex partners should use the PLISSIT model (see question 4) and make the appropriate referral.

As with all patients, cancer and its therapy can suppress bone marrow and compromise the immune system. Thus, nurses must assess specific sexual practices to make suggestions for decreasing the risk of infection or bleeding. If sex toys are used, advise the patient to avoid sharing the toy or to wash the toy carefully with soap and water to decrease the risk of infection. If the patient enjoys anal stimulation (no matter what their sexual orientation), caution the patient about how easily rectal tissue can be torn. Tears may result in bleeding and infection (when the patient is myelosuppressed). Although it is best to refrain from anal stimulation during therapy, the patient may choose to continue; in this case, nurses need to help the patient rethink risk-reduction strategies. Examples include liberal use of lubricant and keeping fingernails very short. Nurses who are uncomfortable with this issue should refer the patient.

15. What practical suggestions can nurses make to a patient with a new ostomy before their first postoperative sexual encounter?

- Crotchless panties
- Picture-frame appliance with tape
- Sexy cloth bag to cover appliance
- Use vaginal lubricant
- Empty appliance before activity
- Avoid "gassy" food
- Role play what to do if appliance "slips"

Keep in mind that ostomy surgery affects body image. How much of an impact it will have depends on the patient's developmental stage, how their partner reacts, and how the patient and partner usually cope with change or crisis. Help patients to communicate their concerns to their partner, or refer them for couple counseling if they so desire.

Physiologic changes are inevitable. Decreased blood flow may affect vaginal lubrication or penile erection. After bladder surgery, it is not uncommon for the vagina to become shorter or narrower, which affects the comfort of normally used positions. Possible odor from the appliance may be a real concern. Tell patients about helpful strategies, and encourage them to attend ostomy support groups so that they can discuss their concerns with others. Belonging to a support group gives patients the opportunity to hear guest speakers discuss sexual issues and to receive ostomy literature with information about sexuality.

16. How should I counsel patients who want to resume sexual activity?

Many nurses avoid this question, because they are concerned that answering it may require a lengthy session. If a patient asks the question, the nurse's job is already half done, because the nurse has earned the patient's trust. If time is a factor, the nurse should find out what specifically concerns the patient and address that concern. The PLISSIT model is a sound guide. Patients may need only permission to have sexual contact or limited information or specific suggestions about what positions they can use. Most patients do not need intensive therapy, but they may appreciate being told how to obtain a pamphlet or book about sexuality after a diagnosis of cancer.

Below is a checklist of factors that nurses may want to consider in answering questions about sexuality:

- Body image
- Partner's reactions
- Fear of abandonment
- Performance anxiety ("spectator droop" may occur if patients concentrate only on physiologic response)
- Worry about pain. Patients should stop if they have pain. If they do so, their partners will then trust them and not refrain from touching them for fear of causing pain.
- Worry that sexual activity may cause recurrence
- Nurses and patients alike should expect the unexpected.
- "Use it or lose it." If patients are older, the longer they do not engage in sexual activities, the more difficult—but *not impossible*— it may be to restart sexual play.
- Let patients role-play communication skills.
- Patients should set aside plenty of time to explore; they should not rush. It may be wise to make a date for sex.

- Appropriate timing of activity (after nap, after pain medication, after bath) may increase enjoyment of sex.
- Patients should learn to rest during sexual activity. Sex does not have to be a "marathon" or a "race."
- Inform patients about available resources, including counseling services, books, pamphlets, and support groups.
- Patience (taking one day at a time) and sense of humor will help patients in their exploration of new sexual expressions.
- Skin is the largest sex organ, and the brain is the most important sex organ. Possibilities are limitless.
- Neither the diagnosis of cancer nor treatment side effects dictate what patients can or cannot do. They should use creativity and a sense of play.

17. What is sperm banking? What instructions should be provided to patients?

When cancer treatment may affect future fertility, men may choose the option of storing sperm in a sperm bank for later use in artificial insemination or in vitro fertilization. Sperm banking has had growing success for over 40 years. To be eligible for this option, men must be able to provide adequate semen for storage. If they have a diagnosis of Hodgkin's disease, non-Hodgkin's lymphoma, or testicular cancer, the sperm count may be too low to bank. It is unclear why these particular diseases seem to cause low counts at diagnosis. Sometimes medications and anesthesia may contribute to the problem. Usually, the average ejaculation consists of 2.5–3.5 cc of fluid with 50–80 million motile sperm in each cc. Ideally, the greater the number of specimens, the better. It is preferable for specimens to be given every 3 days. Because of need for immediate treatment, often men have time for only one or two specimens over a period of 2 days.

The following steps usually occur before sperm banking is done: (1) tests are conducted for sexually transmitted diseases (including HIV and hepatitis); (2) a trial freeze is done on a sperm sample to assess the effects of cryoinjury; (3) an initial sperm analysis is done to determine percent of sperm with normal motility and shape; and (4) informed consent is secured after discussion of possible risks, costs, and benefits. If the patient has a rapidly growing tumor and treatment must be started immediately, sperm banking may be precluded as a reasonable alternative. Before banking is done, the nurse needs to talk with the patient about religious or cultural beliefs about self-stimulation. If the patient believes that masturbation is "wrong," sperm banking may not be an option. Some banks allow the man to have intercourse with his partner and use sperm collected in a condom, but this technique reduces the amount of sperm collected.

The potential sperm donor should be made aware of the personal financial obligation and legal implications. Sperm banking can be costly, if not covered by insurance. The patient needs to be aware of the costs of the required tests, storage, and artificial insemination. Besides the procedural complications, legal issues have emerged. For example, if the patient dies and the partner uses the sperm for impregnation, questions arise to whether the child is eligible for inheritance, father's military benefits, or other benefits. The patient should be informed of all of these implications in order to make a informed decision.

Sperm banking is a common option for men whose fertility may be affected by treatments for cancer. Unfortunately, ovum banking for women is still in the experimental stage and not widely used. As a result, fertility issues for women have more to do with prevention by use of drugs less toxic to the gonads or shielding the ovaries during radiation therapy.

18. What advice should be given to patients about sexuality after mastectomy?

Discharge teaching should include information about the effect of surgery on everyday activities, such as how to wear a seat belt if the belt touches the surgical site. Incorporation into discharge teaching makes sexuality a part of the patient's life without isolating it as a taboo subject. Patients may be asked if they have thought about how they are going to sleep with their partner when they get home. Nurses may find it helpful to share their own experiences in order to promote the patient's comfort. For example, I note that my husband and I often sleep spoon-fashion, with him holding my breast, and that I have trouble sleeping without him. I comment that if I had a mastectomy, I would wonder where he was going to put his hand as we slept. It is not appropriate to tell the patient about your entire sex life, but you may try to put them at ease without embarrassing them. You are asking intimate questions that they may not have discussed with anyone in the past.

I offer to share the many practical suggestions gleaned over the years from my patients so that the woman can choose the ones she wants to use. If she is going home with a drain in place, I remark that many women do not choose to have intercourse but do want to be held. Whether or not she chooses to have intercourse, she or her partner may worry about bumping or pulling the drain. Application of extra tape ensures that it is not pulled by mistake. If the woman does not want her husband to look "at such a horrible scar," I discuss body image and mention research with women who had mastectomies. Nurses found that if women hid in the bathroom or closet to dress and undress, it sometimes took months or years before they felt comfortable enough to let their partner see the scar. I comment on the wasted anxiety and energy and suggest that it may be better to use the energy to heal themselves and fight the cancer.

Regardless of gender, age, or cultural background, body image after diagnosis with cancer can be a major concern. Loss of a breast can affect posture and result in back pain or clothes that do not fit "right." Weight gain, which is common after a diagnosis of breast cancer, further affects body image and emotional well-being.

Chemotherapy and hormone therapy may cause premature menopause. Menopausal symptoms may have a negative impact on sexual well-being, resulting in decreased vaginal lubrication, vaginal atrophy, or decreased androgen (which may decrease libido). In Europe, many women who have menopausal symptoms with breast cancer are allowed to take estrogen. In the United States, concern that use of estrogen may trigger tumor growth, especially if the tumor is hormone-dependent, has discouraged this strategy. A clinical trial to investigate this issue is currently proposed.

Patients who are single and without a steady partner may have many questions about if and when to tell a new partner. Encouraging patients to attend a support group or talk with a "Reach for Recovery" volunteer may help them to decide how to answer such questions. Whether single or in a relationship, patients often have concerns about abandonment.

19. How should the nurse counsel a patient who is unable to achieve an erection?

The first step is to determine whether the patient wants to have an erection. Reassure the patient that touching will continue to bring pleasure and that an erection or intercourse is not necessary to maintain intimacy. Some men are so focused on the penis and whether it goes up or stays down that they forget about the other 90% of sexuality. This is not to say that concerns about erectile dysfunction are to be ridiculed, but it is good to remind male patients that erection does not equal intimacy. Find out what the patient has already tried to achieve an erection in order to assess for unsafe practices (e.g., using a vacuum cleaner to suck blood into his penis, using tongue blades taped to his penis, or "magic" potions that may interact with other medications). Appropriate interventions should be initiated if unsafe practices are discovered.

Provide anticipatory guidance of what to expect if the patient wants to pursue work-up and treatment options. The work-up includes laboratory work, a thorough physical examination (including neurologic, peripheral vascular, and pelvic examinations), evaluation of erectile function to assess firmness achieved at night, and psychological examination that includes a history of sexual practices. Treatment options are varied and depend on patient's desires and physical condition. Examples include vacuum constriction devices (which draw blood into the penis to make it erect), intracavernous injections (vasoactive drugs such as papaverine, prostaglandin E, and phentolamine), cockrings, combined injection and vacuum constriction, counseling, penile arterial reconstruction, and penile prosthesis (malleable rods, hinged prostheses, inflatable prostheses; one-piece, two-piece, three-piece prostheses). If erection dysfunction is caused or compounded by the use of alcohol or smoking (both of which constrict the vascular system), the patient needs to be informed so that he can make an appropriate decision.

20. What is retrograde ejaculation?

Retrograde ejaculation occurs when ejaculate goes into the bladder instead of out the penis. It can be a consequence of external radiation therapy as well as retroperitoneal or pelvic surgery that affects the bladder neck. Retrograde ejaculation can affect sexual satisfaction of both partners. Many men are visually oriented. Although they are still able to have orgasm, they do not enjoy it as much when they cannot observe the ejaculation. Their partner may miss the sensation of ejaculate during orgasm.

Treatment strategies are varied. The patient and partner can discuss with the nurse practitioner or physician the use of sympathomimetic drugs, such as ephedrine, that close the bladder neck and allow the ejaculate to go out the penis. These drugs also may be used by the man who desires to regain fertility. If the drug is not effective and he continues to have retrograde ejaculation, sperm sometimes can be retrieved from the bladder. When fertility is an objective, the man may be asked to void immediately after ejaculation, or a catheter may be used to obtain fluid from the bladder. The specimen is then spun down to extract the sperm. Be sure to discuss whether religious or cultural beliefs prevent use of this strategy.

21. How can a nurse deal with religious or cultural taboos about discussing sexuality?

No nurse can learn every single religious or cultural taboo, although it is helpful to learn about taboos in certain groups. For example, during the nursing assessment the patient may say that he is Buddhist but grew up in the Catholic religion; thus, his personal beliefs may be a mixture of both. Or the patient may be an Irish-American living in a rural environment, but if his wife is Japanese-American and he grew up in a Polish-American neighborhood, he may have his own unique mixture of beliefs.

Let patients know that sexuality is unique for each person. Acknowledge that you may say something that is either embarrassing or against their beliefs. Remind patients that your comments are not intended to offend, and ask them to let you know if you say or do anything that is offensive. Make it clear that as a nurse you are not embarrassed to ask patients if they have had a bowel movement or what size it was because that is part of nursing care. Therefore, you feel just as comfortable talking about a penis or a clitoris. Probably neither bowel movements nor sexual organs are topics of discussion at church or with friends, but they need to be discussed to give good nursing care.

22. How do you counsel a patient who experiences painful intercourse?

Determine when the patient began to have dyspareunia and its cause. If she had a vaginal hysterectomy, she may have increased sensitivity to vaginal barrel distention, especially if she had a postoperative infection. Conversely, the patient may have a loss of vaginal sensation for several months. If she had an abdominal hysterectomy, the small nerves may have been severed, resulting in numbness in the mons for up to 12 months. If the pain is due to a shortened vagina or stenosis from either bladder surgery or radiation, the patient may need to stretch the vagina with dilators.

If the pain is due to decreased vaginal lubrication from treatments, suggest the use of lubricants. Often nurses and physicians offer a sterile lubricant because it is available in the hospital or clinic; I consider this a "male, communist plot" against women. After several strokes, the jelly "balls" up, just as it would on a t-shirt. Thus the woman has not only a dry vagina but also little balls rolling up and down in her vagina.

When discussing possible lubricants, keep safety in mind, but remember that the lubricant does not need to be equivalent to a hospital sterile field. Saliva and whipped cream are both fine, but they dry quickly and are not really effective. If the couple uses condoms for birth control, it is important to suggest water-soluble lubricants. Many lubricants can be bought in a drug store so that they do not need to go to a "sex shop." It may be embarrassing for patients to buy such products in the drugstore, especially if they know the clerk. Appropriate lubricants include Astroglide, Replens, Gyne-moistren, or Lubrin (Kenwood Laboratories, Fairfield, NJ). Nurses may want to keep samples in the clinic so that patients can take them home and try them. Not all lubricants may be comfortable to use. For example, one type of body lotion feels warm when light air touches it. This sensation may be exciting and pleasurable on external skin but not on mucosa. If patients are not using condoms, they can even use a light vegetable oil for lubrication. It is inexpensive, easily obtained at any grocery store, not embarrassing to buy, edible, and light enough that, even with decreased vaginal lubrication, it flushes out and does not cause infection. Many women taking tamoxifen find this option helpful.

23. What positions are most comfortable or best to conserve energy?

To conserve energy, patients may want to consider having sexual activity in the morning when they are the least tired. (This is a problem if the couple has children who need help getting up for school or breakfast). To enhance comfort during sex, the patient may want to consider taking a pain medication 30 minutes before having sex, taking a warm bath to loosen tight muscles, using pillows for support, or trying new sexual activities that are less tiring. If a hot tub is available, the water is a good place for sexual play and supports the patient while trying different positions for comfort. There are alternative forms of sexual stimulation, but before extolling the joy of toe sucking, make sure that the patient is interested in discussing options.

When making suggestions, think of how each activity that you suggest can be made safe for patients with specific conditions, such as neutropenia or thrombocytopenia. For example, if a neutropenic patient wishes to suck a partner's toe, you may want to remind the couple to trim the toenail so that it does not accidentally tear oral mucosa and put the patient at risk of infection.

Patients may fatigue easily but miss sexual play and want to explore new options. If their partner is male, patients can use pillows to get comfortable, rest their head on the partner's belly, and chew or mouth gently the partner's penis while listening to music or watching television. If the patient is male and his partner wants to chew on his penis, remind him/her not to do so if platelet counts are low.

Often we forget to talk about the use of fantasy. Remind patients of the times when they were separated because of work or school and only talked on the telephone. Phone sex is not only fun but expends little energy.

If a limb was amputated because of cancer, discuss different positions that the patient may use. If patients used to feel muscle tension in the amputated limb during orgasm, they may still have phantom sensation. Multiple books are available with pictures demonstrating the use of pillows and different positions. Visit the library and bookstore so that you can make good recommendations.

If the woman had an abdominoperineal resection, talk with her about positions in which her partner's penis does not hit the posterior vaginal wall. Sitting or lying on top may let her feel even more control and pleasure.

24. What resources are available for learning more about sexuality?

American Association of Sex Educators,
  Counselors, and Therapists (AASECT)
11 Dupont Circle, N.W., Suite 220
Washington, DC 20036

American Cancer Society
(800)-ACS-2345 or contact your
local chapter

Mary-Helen Mautner Project
  for Lesbians with Cancer
1707 L Street, NW, Suite 1060
Washington, DC 20036
(202) 332-5536

Planned Parenthood Organization
810 7th Avenue
New York, NY 10019

Sex Information Education Council
  of the U.S. (SEICUS)
130 West 42nd St, Suite 2500
New York, NY 10036

Society for Scientific Study of Sexuality
P.O. Box 29795
Philadelphia, PA 19117

United Ostomy Association, Inc.
36 Executive Park, Suite 120
Irvine, CA 92714
(800)-826-0826

The views expressed in this chapter are those of the author and do not reflect the official policy or position of the Department of the Army, Department of Defense, or the United States Government.

BIBLIOGRAPHY

1. Annon JS: Behavioral Treatment of Sexual Problems: Brief Therapy. Hagerstown, MD, Harper & Row, 1976.
2. Cartwright-Alcarese F: Addressing sexual dysfunction following radiation therapy for a gynecologic malignancy. Oncol Nurs Forum 22:1227–1232, 1995.
3. Ferrell BR, Dow KH, Leigh S, Gulasekaram P: Quality of life in long-term cancer survivors. Oncol Nurs Forum 22:915–922, 1995.
4. Hughes MK: Sexuality issues: Keeping your cool. Oncol Nurs Forum 23:1597–1600, 1996.
5. Shell JA, Smith CK: Sexuality and the older person with cancer. Oncol Nurs Forum 21:553–558, 1994.
6. Smith DB: Sexuality and the patient with cancer: What nurses need to know. Oncol Pat Care 4:1–3, 15, 1994.
7. Smith DB, Babian RJ: The effects of treatment for cancer on male fertility and sexuality. Cancer Nurs 15:271–275, 1992.
8. Young-McCaughan S: Sexual functioning in women with breast cancer after treatment with adjuvant therapy. Cancer Nurs 19:308–319, 1996.
9. Zarcone J, Smithline L, Koopman C, et al: Sexuality and spousal support among women with advanced breast cancer. Breast J 1:52–57, 1995.

44. SKIN BREAKDOWN: PREVENTION AND TREATMENT

Marion Tolch, RN, BSN, CETN

1. Why are patients with cancer more at risk for skin breakdown?

Any patient who, because of pain or extensive disease, becomes increasingly chair- or bedbound is at risk for skin breakdown due to pressure. Additional risk factors include malnutrition and moisture due to incontinence or wound drainage. Because pressure is not the only cause for skin breakdown, it is important not to label all skin breakdown as "pressure ulcers" or "bedsores."

2. Are there standardized protocols for prevention of skin breakdown?

In 1992, the U.S. Agency for Health Care Policy and Research (AHCPR) published clinical practice guidelines for prevention and treatment of skin breakdown (pressure ulcers). The prevention guidelines focus on four goals: (1) identifying at-risk patients who need prevention and their specific risk factors; (2) maintaining and improving tissue tolerance to pressure to prevent injury; (3) protecting against the adverse effects of pressure, friction, and shear; and (4) reducing the incidence of pressure ulcers through educational programs. These guidelines are available through the AHCPR Publications Clearinghouse at 800-358-9295.

3. What specific interventions help to maintain and improve tissue tolerance to pressure?

Caregivers should include the following as part of daily care:
- Inspect skin thoroughly, with particular attention to bony prominences and creases prone to moisture.
- Clean skin at the time of soiling and at appropriate intervals based on patient's needs.
- Minimize environmental factors leading to dry skin; use moisturizers if necessary.
- Minimize skin exposure to moisture, using topical moisture skin barriers and absorbent moisture pads.
- Use proper positioning, transfer, and turning techniques to prevent friction and shearing damage. Examples include maintaining the head of the bed at the lowest degree possible based on patient needs and using devices such as trapezes, transfer boards, and turn/lift sheets to avoid dragging patients over bed or chair surfaces.
- Identify factors influencing nutritional intake, and offer support and supplements as needed.

4. Pressure seems to be the major cause of skin breakdown. What interventions help to prevent damage due to pressure?

Pillows should be used generously to keep bony prominences (e.g., ankles, knees) from direct contact with one another. Avoid positioning the patient directly on the trochanter; even the smallest degree of turning may reduce surface pressure. Although heels usually sustain higher surface pressures than other bony prominences, heel pressures can be easily reduced by use of pillows or several thicknesses of flannel blankets under the calves. Uninterrupted periods of sitting should be avoided. When possible, patients should be taught to shift their weight frequently when sitting for extended periods.

5. Can "donuts" be used to prevent pressure ulcers?

Ring cushion donuts are not recommended because they increase venous congestion to the area and are more likely to *cause* than to prevent breakdown. Soft pillows, foam, or gel pads may be used to reduce pressure for chairbound patients.

6. Discuss options for reducing surface pressures.

A wide variety of products is available. Options range from gel, air, or water mattress replacements or overlays to electric air flotation or air-fluidized beds. To date, research has not demonstrated that one approach is statistically more effective than another. Product selection, therefore, should be based on patient needs. For example, because pressure reduction for patients with cancer is frequently a long-term need, it may be more cost-effective to consider purchasing a 5-inch foam mattress replacement than renting an air mattress for months at a time. The Health Care Financing Administration (HCFA), which administers Medicare, has developed coverage criteria for reimbursement of support surfaces. Many health maintenance organizations (HMOs) and insurance carriers also require prior authorization for reimbursement of pressure-reducing surfaces.

7. How can family caregivers help to prevent skin breakdown?

For continuity of care, it is important that home caregivers understand the causes of skin breakdown and the importance of their role in prevention. They should be taught the potential causes of skin breakdown; how to do a thorough skin assessment; proper positioning to decrease risk of pressure breakdown; and the importance of good hygiene in maintaining skin integrity.

As part of the skin assessment, caregivers may be taught how to evaluate an area of reddened skin for blanching. Blanching redness describes an area that becomes white when compressed by a fingertip. Nonblanching redness remains red after finger compression and is usually indicative of impaired circulation or already existing tissue damage.

8. How do I determine the most appropriate treatment for skin breakdown?

Treatment should be based on cause, size, condition, and location of breakdown. For example, treatment of breakdown due to moisture should focus on elimination or reduction of moisture, use of moisture barrier products, and absorbent linen or pads. Treatment of redness due to friction may include use of a protective dressing, such as a transparent dressing or a protective wafer barrier. Friction damage to heels can be alleviated with use of socks. Treatment of larger wounds that involve necrotic tissue (due to pressure) should include elimination of causative factors; debridement of necrotic tissue, if appropriate; cost-effective management of drainage; and protection of the wound base. Many of the occlusive dressing or hydrophilic wound products may not be absorbent enough to be cost-effective for larger wounds.

9. Despite vigilant care, a bedbound patient may still develop a pressure ulcer over the coccyx. What is the appropriate treatment?

The AHCPR guidelines recommend three components for an effective pressure ulcer treatment plan, which should be addressed simultaneously:
1. **Nutritional assessment and support**
   - Low serum albumin (< 3.5) and less than ideal body weight in patients with cancer frequently contribute to skin breakdown.
   - If compatible with patient wishes and overall goal of care, adequate intake and supplements should be encouraged to maintain a positive nitrogen balance (approximately 30–35 calories/kg/day and 1.25–1.50 gm of protein/kg/day).
2. **Management of tissue loads**
   - Use positioning techniques, and avoid pressure to existing ulcer areas and other high-risk bony prominences.
   - Provide pressure-reducing support surfaces such as a mattress replacement or chair cushion, taking into consideration ease of use, maintenance requirements, and costs and reimbursement.
3. **Ulcer care**
   - Debride necrotic tissue as necessary, selecting the method most appropriate to the patient's condition and goals. Methods include sharp (scalpel), mechanical (wet to dry dressings), enzymatic (ointments), and autolytic (body's own immune system) debridement.

- For wound cleansing in areas where healthy tissue is present, avoid use of cytotoxic agents such as hydrogen peroxide, Betadine, or Dakin's solution. Normal saline adequately cleans most wounds.
- Use cost-effective dressings that protect, provide a moist environment, manage exudate, and maintain integrity of surrounding skin.

10. Are any dressings better than others?

Because no one product is appropriate for all wounds, selection should be based on size, condition, and location of wound. For example, a transparent dressing or hydrocolloid wafer (e.g., Stomahesive) may be inappropriate for a heavily exudating wound near the rectum but highly appropriate for small superficial breakdown on the outlying buttocks. Dressings that initially seem to be expensive may actually be cost-effective because they decrease frequency of dressing changes.

11. How are pressure ulcers staged?

Staging of pressure ulcers classifies the degree of tissue damage *observed*. Wounds with necrotic surface cannot be staged until the necrotic tissue is debrided and the wound base is visible.

Stage I	Nonblanchable erythema of intact skin.
Stage II	Partial-thickness skin loss involving epidermis and/or dermis. The ulcer is superficial and presents clinically as an abrasion, blister, or shallow crater.
Stage III	Full-thickness skin loss involving damage or necrosis of subcutaneous tissue that may extend down to, but not through, underlying fascia. The ulcer presents clinically as a deep crater with or without undermining adjacent tissue.
Stage IV	Full-thickness skin loss with extensive destruction, tissue necrosis, or damage to muscle, bone, or support structures.

12. Does massage have a role in preventing skin breakdown?

AHCPR guidelines recommend that massage be avoided over bony prominences because of preliminary evidence that it may lead to deep tissue trauma. There is inadequate scientific evidence to support the theory that massage stimulates circulation.

13. Are Maalox and heat lamps still used?

The old Maalox and heat lamp recipe for treatment of open wounds is not appropriate. After positive initial findings by Winter in 1962, subsequent studies have confirmed that the rate of healing is better in a moist environment. Conversely, healing is delayed when the wound bed is allowed to dry. Maalox and heat lamps have been replaced by multiple wound care products that provide a moist environment for wound healing.

14. What can be done to secure dressings for patients with tape allergies?

- Many of the newer tape products are hypoallergenic and less likely to cause skin problems.
- A liquid skin sealant on the skin to be taped serves as a barrier to prevent allergies.
- Pieces of ostomy barrier wafer may be applied to surrounding skin; then tape is applied to the wafer pieces instead of the skin.
- Tubular stretch net dressing, which comes in many sizes, holds dressings in place and alleviates the need for tape.

15. Are any over-the-counter ointments or creams better than others?

There are many good ointments and creams on the market. The first step in choosing an appropriate product is to determine whether one needs a moisture barrier product or a skin moisturizer to maintain skin integrity and reduce friction damage. Label information usually identifies whether a product is a barrier, moisturizer, or both.

16. What are helpful hints for dealing with skin irritation around an ostomy?

The first step is to determine the cause of the irritation; the second step is to deal with the cause. Current ostomy products rarely cause skin allergies; however, an area of irritation that conforms to the outline of the wafer or tape may indicate an allergy. Irritation of the immediate peristomal area may be caused by infrequent pouch changes or too large of a stoma opening in the wafer barrier. In the immunosuppressed patient, a red rash with satellite lesions is suspicious of candidiasis, which is best treated with an antifungal powder (oil-based antifungals interfere with adherence of the pouch to the skin).

17. How is odor managed for a patient with a fungating wound due to necrotic tumor?

Daily wound cleansing is the best way to prevent and manage odor and should be emphasized. Many patients avoid this aspect of care because of inadequate pain control or tumor appearance. Cleansing options include a gentle hand-held shower or deodorizing wound cleansers. To keep dressings from sticking to the tumor surface (which causes bleeding and pain on removal), nonadherent dressings or wound gels may be used. Dressings should be adequately secured to keep odorous drainage from seeping through to clothing.

BIBLIOGRAPHY

1. Bryant R: Acute and Chronic wounds—Nursing Management, St. Louis, Mosby, 1992.
2. Panel for the Prediction and Prevention of Pressure Ulcers in Adults. Pressure Ulcers in Adults: Prediction and Prevention. Clinical Practice Guideline, Number 3. AHCPR Publication No. 92-0047. Rockville, MD: Agency for Health Care Policy and Research, Public Health Service, U.S. Department of Health and Human Services. May 1992.
3. Treatment of Pressure Ulcers. Clinical Practice Guideline, Number 15. AHCPR Publication No. 95-0652. Rockville, MD: Agency for Health Care Policy and Research, Public Health Service, U.S. Department of Health and Human Services, December 1994.

VI. Oncologic Emergencies and Complications

45. CARDIAC TAMPONADE

Dawn Camp-Sorrell, RN, MSN, FNP, AOCN

1. What is cardiac tamponade?

Cardiac tamponade is a life-threatening emergency in which excessive accumulation of fluid or blood between the pericardium and heart prevents an adequate amount of blood from flowing into the heart to fill the ventricles. This excessive volume is usually between 200 and 1200 ml with a median volume of 500 ml. The rate of fluid accumulation, as well as the volume, is important in causing tamponade. Cardiac tamponade results from increased intrapericardial pressure, which leads to impaired diastolic filling and low cardiac output (the amount of blood ejected by the ventricle). As blood is increasingly unable to flow into the heart, the patient exhibits the signs and symptoms of systemic venous congestion.

2. How much fluid does the pericardial sac usually hold?

Under normal conditions the pericardium is a thin, tough, double-layered sac that encloses the heart with two distinct components: (1) visceral pericardium (covers the heart) and (2) parietal pericardium. Approximately 15–20 ml of pericardial fluid is located between the layers to prevent friction between the membranes during contraction and relaxation of the heart.

3. What is pericardial pressure?

Pericardial pressure is a reflection of the ability of the two membranes to adapt to changes in the fluid volume. An increase in the volume within the sac increases pericardial pressure.

4. What are the common signs and symptoms of cardiac tamponade?

Small effusions usually do not cause symptoms. Larger or rapid accumulation of fluid may cause epigastric or retrosternal chest pain that is relieved by sitting up or leaning forward (pain is more severe when the patient is supine); dysphagia; cough; dyspnea; hoarseness; increased jugular vein distention; muffled heart sounds (pericardial effusion); pericardial friction rub (when tumor is present); tachycardia; and pulsus paradoxus.

5. Why do some patients present with symptoms whereas others are asymptomatic?

Symptoms depend on how the condition develops. As small effusions begin, the pericardium stretches gradually to accommodate the fluid pressure within the sac and the patient is asymptomatic. When the effusion progresses, causing an increase in pericardial pressure and a resultant decrease in ventricular expansion and diastolic filling, cardiac output drops and the patient becomes symptomatic. Rapid accumulation causes a rapid decrease in cardiac output and acute symptoms.

6. List the common causes of cardiac tamponade.

Infection	Heart failure
Primary cancer	Myocardial infarction
Cancer metastasis	Trauma
Central vascular catheter perforation	Drugs (e.g., anthracyclines, anticoagulants,
Autoimmune diseases	hydralazine, procainamide)
Renal failure	Dissecting aortic aneurysm

7. What types of cancer can cause cardiac tamponade?

Autopsies have proved that up to 21% of all patients with cancer have metastatic disease to the heart or pericardium. Although all cancer types can affect the heart, specific cancers with higher incidence include lung cancer, breast cancer, leukemia, lymphoma, mesothelioma, sarcoma, and melanoma.

8. Can pleural effusions lead to cardiac tamponade?

Yes. Cardiac tamponade may result from an increase in intrapleural pressure, which may be transmitted to the pericardial space.

9. Can cancer treatments cause cardiac tamponade?

Yes. Radiation affects the fine capillary stroma of the myocardium. Pericardial effusion may occur when up to 45 Gy is administered to the mediastinum. Chemotherapy, especially antitumor antibiotics, may affect the myocardial fibers and thus lead to pericardial effusion.

10. What is pulsus paradoxus?

Pulsus paradoxus results from an increase in intrathoracic pressure and is characterized by an exaggerated inspiratory fall in systolic blood pressure > 10 mmHg or > 10%. Pulsus paradoxus is measured by inflating the blood pressure cuff until no sounds are audible. The patient is asked to breathe in and out normally. During expiration, the cuff is gradually deflated until sounds are audible, at which point the pressure is recorded. The cuff is further deflated until sounds are audible during inspiration, at which point the pressure is again recorded. The difference between the two recorded pressures should be 5–10 mmHg.

11. Can pulsus paradoxus be present in other conditions?

Yes. Pulsus paradoxus may be present in chronic obstructive pulmonary disease, bronchospasm, or marked shifts in intrapleural pressure. Arrhythmias may hamper the measurement.

12. Which tests are used to diagnose a pericardial effusion?

A chest radiograph reveals only an enlarged heart shadow. An echocardiogram, computed tomography (CT), or magnetic resonance imaging (MRI) reveals a large pericardial chest effusion and can be used to estimate the volume of the effusion. The electrocardiogram (EKG) provides limited information, as results can be used to diagnose other cardiac abnormalities. Elevated ST segments, nonspecific T wave changes, decreased QRS voltage, and sinus tachycardia may be seen. A common EKG abnormality is the alternation of amplitude and direction of the P wave and QRS complexes on every other beat (electrical alternans). This abnormal finding is thought to result from variations in the position of the heart at the time of electrical depolarization.

13. Describe the treatment of a pericardial effusion.

In an emergency, cardiac tamponade is usually relieved by pericardiocentesis; a 16–18-gauge needle is placed into the pericardial sac to withdraw fluid. Surgical intervention depends on the cause of tamponade and the patient's overall condition. An indwelling pericardial catheter may be inserted to withdraw fluid or to instill medications. A pericardial window may be made to allow drainage of fluid into the surrounding tissue. A total pericardiectomy may be used if the window is not effective in relieving the tamponade and is indicated if the patient has constriction secondary to radiation therapy.

14. What are the complications of surgical intervention?

Potential complications include puncture of the right atrium, right ventricle, or coronary arteries; infection; dysrhythmia; and pneumothorax. Indwelling catheters may cause infection, catheter blockage, dysrhythmias, and pericarditis.

15. What does sclerosing mean? How is it used to relieve cardiac tamponade?

Sclerosing is a method used to produce an inflammatory response that eventually obliterates the pericardial space. The intent is to prevent reaccumulation of fluid. Several sclerosing agents have been used, including tetracycline, bleomycin, nitrogen mustard, 5-fluorouracil, doxorubicin, and thiotepa. The patient must be premedicated before the procedure, which is very painful.

16. Is balloon angioplasty also used to treat cardiac tamponade?

Percutaneous balloon pericardiotomy may be used. A balloon is placed across the parietal pericardium. Inflation of the balloon creates an opening into the pericardium that allows internal drainage of the effusion into the pleural space for reabsorption.

17. Should the pericardial fluid be assayed?

To establish the diagnosis of malignancy and to rule out preexisting infection, the fluid should be assayed for lactate dehydrogenase (LDH), protein, specific gravity, glucose, cell count, cytology, and pH; it also should be cultured for bacteria and fungi. Most malignant effusions are serosanguineous or bloody and have malignant cells, alkaline pH, glucose, and increased LDH.

18. What assessment parameters must be included in the care of patients with cardiac effusion?

The assessment should include frequent auscultation of heart sounds and blood pressure; palpation of the apical pulse and peripheral pulses; observation for jugular venous distention; and checking the extremities for cyanosis, coolness, and edema.

19. What is the prognosis for a patient with cardiac tamponade?

Prognosis depends on rapidity of fluid accumulation, stage of disease at time of diagnosis, presence of metastatic disease, performance status of the patient, and effectiveness of treatment. Life expectancy ranges from a few hours to years; the average duration of remission is 4–6 months.

20. Can radiation therapy be used to treat cardiac tamponade?

If cardiac tamponade is of gradual onset and caused by a radiosensitive tumor such as lung or breast cancer or lymphoma, radiation therapy may be the treatment of choice. Usually 200–400 Gy of external radiation is delivered to the heart, pericardial structures, and lower mediastinum. In most patients who have received previous mediastinum radiation (e.g., for Hodgkin's disease), the maximal dose to the pericardial region has already been used.

21. What supportive care strategies can be used?

To ease the patient's suffering, the nurse can administer oxygen, reposition the patient to enhance circulation, assist with all activities, administer analgesics, encourage relaxation techniques, and administer antianxiety or other medications as prescribed.

BIBLIOGRAPHY

1. Chong HH, Plotnick GD: Pericardial effusion and tamponade: Evaluation, imaging modalities, and management. Comprehen Ther 21(7):378–385, 1995.
2. Collier PE, Goodman GB: Cardiac tamponade caused by central venous catheter perforation of the heart: A preventable complication. J Am College Surg 181:459–463, 1995.
3. Markman M: Common complications and emergencies associated with cancer and its therapy. Cleve J Med 61 (2):105–114, 1994.
4. Shuey KM: Heart, lung, and endocrine complications of solid tumors. Semin Oncol Nurs 10(3):177–188, 1994.
5. Vassilopoulos PP, Nikolaidis K, Filopoulos E, et al: Subxiphoidal pericardial window in the management of malignant pericardial effusion. Eur J Surg Oncol 21:545–547, 1995.

46. DISSEMINATED INTRAVASCULAR COAGULATION

Carol S. Viele, RN, MS

1. What is disseminated intravascular coagulation?

Disseminated intravascular coagulation (DIC) is a process that occurs with generalized activation of the hemostatic system, which results in widespread fibrin formation followed by lysis within the vascular system. DIC may result in consumption of both platelets and clotting factors as well as formation of microthrombi.

2. What causes DIC?

DIC does not occur in isolation; it is always a symptom of underlying disease. Of the many disease processes that can cause DIC, one of the most important is cancer. DIC is the direct response to the presence of specific proteins or procoagulants, which may be secreted by malignant cells. Tissue factor, tumor necrosis factor (TNF), and cell proteases are among the proteins responsible for initiating DIC.

3. What is the mechanism of bleeding in DIC?

Fibrin degradation products and D-dimers are almost always abundant in DIC and frequently clump together. These fragments or clumps, particularly D-dimers, competitively inhibit the formation and action of thrombin by binding to thrombin at its fibrinogen receptor site. These fragment complexes, if soluble, may deposit indiscriminately throughout the vasculature. Others bind abnormally to preexisting, growing microthrombi, weakening clot structure. This is the clotting mechanism of DIC.

The mechanism of bleeding comes from the failure of the clotting cascade, which results in systemic release of fibrinogen, fibrin degradation products, or D-dimers. This release creates a host of circulatory disturbances, including the formation of small fragments that inhibit platelet function, large fragments that induce platelet clumping, and mixtures of soluble fragments that may increase capillary permeability, cause extravascular coagulation, and disturb endothelial activity. The result is significant bleeding throughout the vascular system. Both thrombosis and bleeding occur from many areas at the same time.

4. What types of malignancies are associated with DIC?

Both solid tumors and leukemia have been reported to cause DIC. Patients with mucin-secreting adenocarcinomas, prostatic carcinoma, or disseminated carcinomas are at highest risk for developing DIC. In addition, all leukemias, to various extents, may induce DIC. However, promyelocytic leukemia (M_3) is almost universally associated with the development of some degree of DIC.

5. What are some other causes of DIC in cancer?

Infection is the most common cause of DIC. Gram-negative organisms triggering sepsis may be the culprit. DIC is also seen in gram-positive bacterial sepsis and viremias, most often involving varicella, hepatitis, and cytomegalovirus (CMV). Patients also may develop DIC from intravascular hemolysis secondary to multiple transfusions of whole blood and transfusion reactions. At times, the administration of chemotherapy may cause destruction of blast cells, releasing substances with procoagulation properties.

6. What are the types of DIC?

DIC can be divided into acute and chronic forms. Acute DIC develops rapidly over a period of hours. The patient presents with sudden bleeding from multiple sites. It must be treated as a medical emergency. Chronic DIC may be subclinical and develop over a period of months. Eventually, however, it evolves into an acute DIC pattern with hemorrhage or thromboembolic episodes.

7. What are the symptoms of DIC?

The most common sign of DIC is bleeding, usually manifested by ecchymosis, petechiae, and purpura. The patient usually presents with bleeding from multiple sites, including skin, nose, gums, lungs, and central nervous system. This bleeding may range from the continuous oozing of venipuncture sites or wounds to uncontrollable hemorrhage that will lead to shock and death unless intervention is swift and effective. If DIC persists for more than a few hours, hemorrhages may be extensive and involve the pleura and pericardium. When this occurs, patients may complain of dyspnea and chest pain.

8. How is DIC diagnosed?

DIC is diagnosed on the basis of clinical presentation plus laboratory evidence of abnormalities. The activated partial thromboplastin time is a less helpful test for diagnosing DIC except in severe cases because it may be physiologically prolonged in children and masked by elevated factor VIII in adults.

Laboratory Abnormalities Associated with DIC

TEST	ABNORMALITY
Platelet count	Decreased
Fibrin degradation products	Increased
Prothrombin time	Prolonged
Activated partial thromboplastin time	Prolonged
Thrombin time	Prolonged
Fibrinogen	Decreased

9. How is DIC managed?

The overall management of DIC is highly controversial because of the lack of controlled studies. The immediate goal of therapy is to stop the patient from actively bleeding and clotting. However, the most important component in the management of DIC is to treat the underlying disorder. Management of DIC can be divided into two categories: use of blood component therapy and use of medications.

10. Describe the use of blood component therapy.

Platelet concentrates, cryoprecipitate, and fresh frozen plasma are frequently used to attempt to control the bleeding associated with DIC. Patients should not be automatically transfused; transfusion is appropriate only when the diagnosis is well established with documented depletion of factors. The exception, of course, is a life-threatening situation in which there is no time to establish a diagnosis. Replacements for thrombocytopenia include 6–10 units of random donor platelets or a single unit of donor hemapheresed platelets. Hypofibrinogenemia (i.e., fibrinogen level < 100 mg/dl) may be treated with 8 units of cryoprecipitate. A prolonged prothrombin time due to a factor deficiency may be corrected by administering two units of fresh frozen plasma. Depending on the severity of DIC, replacement therapy may need to be given and repeated every 8 hours, with adjustments for platelet count, prothrombin time, activated partial thromboplastin time, fibrinogen level, and volume status. Replacements are discontinued when levels are normal or near normal.

11. Which medications may be used to treat DIC?

Heparin. Because the patient with DIC has evidence of clotting in addition to bleeding, heparin is used to prevent further clotting. It is indicated as a treatment for DIC in acute promyelocytic and acute monocytic leukemia during induction therapy. Heparin is also used for DIC-induced thromboembolic complications in large vessels and prior to surgery in patients with metastatic carcinoma.

Antithrombin III (AT III). AT III concentrate has been used as treatment for patients with DIC, either alone or in combination with heparin. To date, no definitive studies have shown a decrease in mortality with use of AT III.

Fibrinolytic inhibitors. Fibrinolytic inhibitors are used only in the setting of an undeniable threat to hemostasis—that is, bleeding that has not responded to any other measures. The two agents currently available are **epsilon aminocaproic acid** (Amicar) and **tranexamic acid** (Cyklokapron). Epsilon aminocaproic acid (EACA) is a protease inhibitor that is uniquely reactive with plasminogen activators. It inhibits spontaneous fibrinolytic activity. A standard loading dose of 4 gm followed by 6–12 gm/day in divided doses provides sufficient plasma concentration to preserve the fibrin of a hemostatic vascular plug. The adverse effects are gastrointestinal disturbances, muscle necrosis, impotence, and the risk of creating clots in the urinary tract and bladder in patients with renal bleeding and hemorrhagic cystitis. Tranexamic acid is approximately 100 times more potent than EACA in inhibiting plasminogen activation. Tranexamic acid has a greater specificity of action and fewer side effects. The current recommended dosage for managing systemic fibrinolysis is 30–50 mg/kg orally or 10 mg/kg intravenously every 12 hours. Tranexamic acid should be avoided in patients with suspected renal bleeding or evidence of intravascular clotting to prevent clotting of the blood supply to the kidneys.

12. What is the controversy over the use of heparin for DIC?

Heparin may be given to inhibit factors IX and X, enhancing the neutralization of thrombin and halting the clotting cascade. However, hemorrhage is one of the main causes of death in patients with DIC, and heparin may induce bleeding. Heparin therapy is not indicated in patients who bleed in areas that compromise important functions (e.g., intracranial or intraspinal hemorrhage). Heparin therapy should be stopped if the patient has any life-threatening bleeding episode. Sometimes physicians think it is safer to use factor replacement therapy, especially if the underlying cause, such as infection, can be treated successfully.

13. What is the prognosis of DIC?

Both DIC and underlying disorders contribute to the high mortality rate. Mortality is correlated independently with the extent of organ or system involvement. It is also correlated with the degree of hemostatic failure and increasing age of patient at onset. Mortality rates in various studies have been reported to range from 42–86%, whether or not heparin was used to treat DIC.

14. What nursing interventions are important to patients with DIC?

Bleeding is the major symptom associated with DIC. Nurses should assess the patient for any signs or symptoms of bleeding. It is essential that the nurse use a thorough and organized approach when assessing the patient suspected of having DIC and that the physical assessment be performed at least every 4 hours. Starting with the skin, the nurse inspects the patient from head to toe, including palms of the hands and soles of the feet, looking for petechiae or bruising. Particular attention should be paid to the sclera and buccal mucosa. The patient should also be asked about vision. Blurred, cloudy, or diminished vision may indicate retinal hemorrhage and should be reported to the physician immediately. The nurse also should inspect the oral cavity, evaluating for bleeding, ulcers, or hematomas. A mouth care regimen is imperative for patients with DIC because oral cavity bleeding may be significant. Both nares should be inspected for signs of bleeding; epistaxis may be a significant source of blood loss. The inspection proceeds to the chest, back, abdomen, groin area, and lower extremities. Pressure areas should be inspected closely because they are common sites of petechiae, hematomas, and ecchymoses.

15. What can be done to stop bleeding from a central line site?

If a patient has a central line, bleeding from the site is common until DIC is under control. Many leukemic patients with DIC require central line dressing changes every 2 hours because of bleeding. Pressure should be applied during each dressing change for at least 5–10 minutes to reduce oozing. If pressure is not sufficient, Gelfoam sponges may be used at the exit site to enhance hemostasis. An alternative method is to apply topical thrombin to the Gelfoam sponges in an effort to control bleeding. Once the bleeding has stopped, do not remove the topical thrombin-soaked sponge until it falls off, or the site may again begin to bleed. The Gelfoam sponge will fall off when clotting conditions have returned to normal. A patient may lose units of blood from the central line site; up to 100 cc of blood may be contained within each hematoma.

16. What other key areas should the nurse assess?

After a thorough inspection of the skin, the nurse should assess the chest cavity, including the heart and lungs, and the abdominal cavity, including the liver, spleen, and bowels. To assess the chest cavity, the nurse should auscultate the patient's lungs. Because patients with DIC may develop diffuse alveolar hemorrhage, listening for rales, rhonchi, or areas of decreased breath sounds is important. Any positive finding should be reported, in addition to signs or symptoms of respiratory distress such as dyspnea, shortness of breath, nasal flaring, and increased respiratory rate.

17. What other medical emergencies may occur with DIC?

In a few patients, cardiac tamponade may result from DIC and thrombocytopenia. This is an obvious medical emergency. Signs of tamponade may be acute in onset and include chest pain and shortness of breath. An electrocardiogram should be done at once, along with medical interventions as appropriate.

Patients with DIC may have symptoms of abdominal pain due to ischemic bowel. Abdominal examination should include listening for bowel sounds in all four quadrants; any areas of decreased or absent bowel sounds should be noted. Evaluation also should include palpation and observing for peritoneal signs, indication of rebound tenderness, or a fluid wave due to bleeding in the abdominal cavity. The liver and spleen should be palpated and percussed to determine size and degree of tenderness. Any abnormal findings should be noted and reported to the physician. Urine and stool should be inspected for any sign of blood.

18. How else can the nurse offer support to patients with DIC?

The nurse's role in the care of patients with DIC also includes both patient and family education. Explaining the syndrome, along with the expected treatment, whether it be blood components, heparin, and/or an antifibrinolytic, is important. Patients and families are especially anxious because of the symptoms of DIC. Every effort should be made to explain the cause, treatment, side effects, and goals in the simplest way possible. Explanations should be repeated as often as necessary to reduce anxiety and increase patient understanding. Fear is prevalent because the patient looks quite different from normal and bleeding is a scary symptom. Many people ask how long the bleeding will last; it is important to be honest and to let them know that bleeding time varies with each individual. The most important nursing intervention is to provide safe care during this stressful time.

BIBLIOGRAPHY

1. Gobel B: Bleeding disorders. In Groenwald S, Frogge M, Goodman M, Yarbro C (eds): Cancer Nursing: Principles and Practice. Boston, Jones & Bartlett, 1993, pp 575–607.
2. Hathaway W, Goodnight S: Disorders of Hemostasis and Thrombosis: A Clinical Guide. New York, McGraw-Hill, 1993, pp 219–229.
3. Jandl J: Disseminated intravascular coagulation. In Blood: Textbook of Hematology. Boston, Little, Brown, 1996, pp 1440–1447, 1996.
4. Kurtz A: Disseminated intravascular coagulation with leukemia patients. Canc Nurs 16:456–463, 1993.
5. Linker C: Blood. In Tiernery L Jr, McPhee S, Papadakis M (eds): Current Medical Diagnosis and Treatment. Norwalk, CT, Appleton & Lange, 1994, pp 415–466.
6. Schafer S: Oncologic complications. In Otto S (ed): Oncology Nursing, 2nd ed. St. Louis, Mosby, 1993, pp 376–440.
7. Seligsohn U: Disseminated intravascular coagulation. In Beutler E, Lichtman M, Coller B, Kipps T(eds): New York, McGraw-Hill, 1995, pp 1497–1516.
8. Siegrist C, Jones J: Disseminated intravascular coagulopathy and nursing implications. Semin Oncol Nurs 1:237–243, 1985.

47. HYPERCALCEMIA OF MALIGNANCY

Gari Jensen, RN, BSN, OCN

1. What is hypercalcemia?

Hypercalcemia is a common oncologic emergency in which the serum calcium level is above normal parameters. Although there may be variations among institutions, normal serum calcium is generally considered to be 8.5–11 mg/dl of blood. Hypercalcemia occurs when serum calcium levels exceed 11.0 mg/dl. A serum calcium level between 12–14 mg/dl is considered to be moderate hypercalcemia and may or may not be associated with symptoms. Severe hypercalcemia is present with levels over 14 mg/dl and is always symptomatic.

In the general population, hyperparathyroidism is the most common cause of hypercalcemia. Hypercalcemia caused by cancer is called hypercalcemia of malignancy (HCM).

2. Is HCM common in patients with cancer?

HCM is the most common syndrome associated with cancer and occurs in 10–20% of patients with cancer. The highest incidence is in patients with breast cancer (40–50%) or multiple myeloma (20–50%). HCM is also associated with squamous cell and large cell carcinoma of the lung, squamous cell carcinoma of the head and neck, renal carcinoma, lymphomas, leukemias, and prostate, ovarian, and gastric cancers, but it may be found in any cancer. HCM is usually seen in advanced cancer when tumor burden is heavy.

3. How do patients with HCM usually present?

Because it frequently presents with nonspecific symptoms commonly associated with cancer and its treatment, HCM may be overlooked. The usual clinical picture includes fatigue, lethargy, weakness, nausea and anorexia, constipation, dehydrated appearance, decreased mental functioning, thirst, and polyuria. Patients with mild-to-moderate HCM may be asymptomatic.

4. Why is HCM considered an oncologic emergency?

If HCM goes undiagnosed and untreated, about 50% of cases rapidly progress to renal failure, hypotension, severe dehydration, coma, and death. In cases of chronic HCM, the patient is at risk for serious complications from hypercoagulative states and widespread calcifications.

5. How is HCM diagnosed?

Hypercalcemia can be diagnosed through simple blood tests—either a calcium and albumin level or an ionized calcium level. Ionized or free calcium is the physiologically active form of calcium circulated in the blood. Of the total serum calcium, only about 50% is ionized; 40% is bound to plasma proteins (primarily albumin); and 10% is bound in complexes with substances such as citrate, phosphate, and sulfate.

After a state of hypercalcemia is determined, it must be differentiated by etiology. In patients with cancer this is usually done by history because of the dramatic onset and strong association of HCM with advanced cancer. In hyperparathyroidism the onset is usually gradual and less severe. Assessment of parathyroid hormone level is also useful; the level is elevated in hyperparathyroidism but normal or depressed in HCM.

6. How is ionized calcium calculated?

Ionized calcium can be measured directly, but at many institutions this test is not used because of greater expense, lack of availability, or habit. Traditionally, the serum calcium level is assessed and corrected on the basis of the serum albumin level. The corrected serum calcium is obtained by adjusting the calcium level upward by 0.8 mg for every gram of albumin under 4 gm/dl or downward by 0.8 mg for every gram of albumin over 4 gm/dl:

1. Subtract the albumin level from 4.0.
2. Multiply the difference by 0.8.
3. If the result is a positive number, add it to the serum calcium; if it is a negative number, subtract it.
4. The answer is the corrected calcium.

For example, R.G., a 76-year-old black man with a history of multiple myeloma, presents with mild confusion and disorientation, lethargy, and decreased appetite. His wife states that his mental status has steadily declined over the past week. Serum calcium level is 11.4 mg/dl, and albumin level is 1.9 gm/dl:

1. $4.0 - 1.9 = 2.1$
2. $2.1 \times 0.8 = 1.7$
3. $11.4 + 1.7 = 13.1$

The ionized calcium level, 13.1 mg/dl, indicates moderate HCM; it is significantly higher than the uncorrected serum calcium level of 11.4 mg/dl.

7. What are the functions of calcium in the body?

Calcium is essential in the formation and maintenance of bones and teeth, contractility of muscle cells, transmission of nerve impulses, and normal clotting mechanisms. It is also involved in cardiac automaticity, many enzyme reactions, white blood cell chemotaxis, and cell-membrane permeability.

Excessive calcium depresses neuromuscular function, causes increased contractility and irritability in the heart, interferes with antidiuretic hormone (ADH), promotes blood clotting, and may result in deposition of calcium outside the skeletal system, especially in the kidneys.

8. Describe the mechanisms for regulating calcium.

Calcium is regulated through bone formation and resorption, gastrointestinal absorption, and urinary excretion. Controlling these mechanisms are three hormones: parathyroid hormone, vitamin D (cholecalciferol), and calcitonin.

The **bones of the skeletal system** are the major repository of calcium stores. Depending on need, osteocytes differentiate into osteoblasts or osteoclasts. When serum calcium is elevated, osteoblasts secrete collagen to form a bone matrix in which calcium can be deposited. When serum calcium is low, osteoclasts erode existing bone, resulting in calcium resorption (release) into the serum.

The **intestinal tract**, through the mediation of vitamin D, can increase calcium levels by increasing absorption of calcium ingested through diet.

The **kidneys** are able both to conserve and to eliminate calcium. They also play an indirect role in intestinal absorption by converting vitamin D to its active form.

9. How do the three hormones control calcium regulation?

Parathyroid hormone (PTH) has an integral role in calcium regulation through effects on all three of the above mechanisms. PTH is released from the parathyroid gland in response to a drop in serum calcium. It directly acts on bone by stimulating increased osteoclast formation and activity and by inhibiting osteoblasts. PTH also has a direct effect on the kidneys by stimulating increased reabsorption of calcium while inhibiting reabsorption of phosphorus. Limiting phosphorus minimizes the formation of hydroxyapatite crystals, the form in which calcium is deposited into bone. PTH indirectly stimulates the gastrointestinal tract to increase calcium absorption by causing the kidneys to convert vitamin D (cholecalciferol) to its active form, 1,25-dihydroxycholecalciferol.

Vitamin D (cholecalciferol) has a paradoxical role in calcium regulation. After conversion to its active form, 1,25-dihydroxycholecalciferol, its primary effect is to increase calcium and phosphorus absorption from the intestinal mucosa. It also stimulates reabsorption of calcium and phosphorus by the kidneys. Bone formation is promoted by the abundance of both calcium and phosphorus. When calcium levels are inadequate, vitamin D stimulates bone resorption and release of calcium into the serum.

Calcitonin is released by the thyroid gland in response to high serum calcium levels. It has an antagonistic relationship with PTH but is of short duration. By inhibiting osteoclast formation and activity, it reduces calcium release into circulation as a result of bone resorption. It also causes increased osteoblast activity and thereby promotes calcium deposition. In addition to its effect on bone, calcitonin also works through the kidneys by inhibiting calcium and phosphorus reabsorption.

10. What are the causes of HCM?

It was once thought that HCM resulted from release of calcium by bone after its invasion and destruction by cancer cells. A troubling aspect of this theory was that no reliable correlation could be found between amount of bone destruction and level of serum calcium. In fact, hypercalcemia may be present without bone metastases. Understanding is limited, but researchers have identified a number of substances secreted or mediated by cancer cells that cause or have some association with HCM.

One of the most significant substances, **parathyroid hormone–related protein** (PTH-rP), closely resembles PTH. It exerts the same effects in the regulation of calcium but is not regulated by the normal feedback mechanisms that suppress PTH. Whereas in response to hypercalcemia PTH levels decrease, PTH-rP is unaffected and continues to stimulate osteoclast activity and increased calcium reabsorption by the kidneys. By stimulating the breakdown of bone, it also may enhance the opportunity for cancer cells to attach and invade bone. Spectrum immunoradiologic assays have detected PTH-rP in 80–90% of patients with HCM. It is associated with cancer of the kidney, lung, head and neck, gastrointestinal tract, and genitourinary system as well as with hematologic cancers. Other substances implicated in HCM are osteoclast-activating factors (OAFs), transforming growth factors (TGFs), and prostaglandins of the E class (PGEs).

11. What other factors contribute to the development of HCM?

1. Immobilization results in increased resorption (release) of calcium from bone.
2. Thiazide diuretics decrease renal excretion of calcium.
3. Patients may continue to take calcium supplements and vitamin D without realizing that they are contributing to the development of HCM.
4. Androgens, estrogens, and antiestrogens have precipitated HCM in some cases. The onset is usually dramatic, within the first 2 weeks of therapy.
5. Some breast cancers and lymphomas have been shown to convert vitamin D to its active state.
6. Granulocyte-macrophage colony-stimulating factor (GM-CSF) may stimulate osteoclast formation after interleukin-1 (IL-1) stimulation.

12. Is dietary restriction of calcium necessary?

Dietary restriction of calcium is usually not necessary because calcium absorption from the gastrointestinal tract is already decreased by negative feedback mechanisms and frequently by anorexia, nausea, and vomiting.

13. What is the pathologic process in HCM?

Tumor secretion of PTH-rP and other tumor-derived or tumor-mediated substances causes calcium release from bone secondary to osteoclast activity and increased reabsorption of calcium from the renal tubules. As the calcium load increases, it interferes with the ability of the kidneys to reabsorb sodium, which leads to sodium and water loss through polyuria. Common symptoms of cancer and cancer therapy—nausea, vomiting, and anorexia—contribute to the developing dehydration and are worsened by the effects of rising calcium levels on the gastrointestinal tract. The dehydrated state becomes self-perpetuating. Immobilization from weakness, fatigue, and bone pain caused by hypercalcemia further increases resorption of bone.

14. What are the signs and symptoms of HCM?

Mental status and vision

Fatigue	Lethargy
Weakness	Apathy
Hyporeflexia	Restlessness
Visual disturbances	Somnolence
Confusion	Stupor
Depression	Coma

Cardiovascular system

Hypertension	Digitalis sensitivity
Bradycardia	Hypotension
Electrocardiographic	Heart block
abnormalities	Cardiac arrest

Gastrointestinal tract

Anorexia	Constipation
Nausea and vomiting	Adynamic ileus
Pain and distention	

Skeletal system

Bone pain	Pathologic fractures

Kidneys

Polyuria/nocturia	Nephrocalcinosis
Polydipsia	Nephrolithiasis
Dehydration	Renal failure
Azotemia and proteinuria	

Systemic symptoms

Ectopic calcification	Metabolic alkalosis
Pruritus	Hypercoagulopathy

15. What are the three major considerations in planning treatment?

1. **Prognosis.** Controlling the malignancy is the most effective treatment for HCM. When the cancer is treatment-sensitive, aggressive treatment of both cancer and HCM is appropriate. In patients whose disease is refractory to treatment, interventions may be focused more on palliation and enhancing quality of life.

2. **Patient's overall condition.** Treatment for cancer and HCM must be modified for patients with underlying medical conditions such as renal and cardiac disease.

3. **Severity of HCM.** The urgency and aggressiveness of treatment should correlate with the severity of HCM and its symptoms to prevent mortality and alleviate suffering.

16. What is the usual treatment for HCM?

1. **Hydration** is fundamental to treatment, both to correct the inherent dehydration and its sequelae and to promote calcium excretion. In mild cases, forcing oral fluids (3–4 L/day) may be adequate to lower calcium levels. Interventions for nausea may be required to facilitate this goal. Generally, intravenous hydration with normal saline is required. Based on the severity of the hypercalcemia and dehydration as well as the patient's cardiovascular status, 2.5–6 L are given over 24 hours. Because calcium is excreted in parallel with sodium chloride, use of saline promotes calcium excretion in the renal tubules. It is essential to monitor electrolytes carefully, especially magnesium and potassium, because imbalances may lead to cardiac dysrhythmias. A urinary output of 100 cc/hr is desirable after euvolemia has been restored.

2. **Elimination of drugs that worsen hypercalcemia**, such as calcium and vitamin D supplements, calcium-based antacids, thiazide diuretics (which decrease renal excretion of calcium), and hormonal therapy.

3. **Loop diuretics** (e.g., furosemide) are initiated after intravascular volume has been rstored. They accelerate the elimination of calcium by blocking reabsorption in the loop of

Henle and also serve to prevent volume overload from the vigorous hydration. Hydration and diuresis eliminate excessive calcium but do not alleviate the cause of the condition—bone resorption.

    4. **Intravenous biphosphonate therapy** (see question below)

17. What are the key agents used to treat HCM?

    The biphosphates are highly effective inhibitors of bone resorption and lower serum calcium in 70–100% of cases. It is thought that they bind to bone matrix and prevent release of calcium. **Etidronate** must be given with normal saline hydration and requires 3–7 days of therapy. **Pamidronate** (a second-generation biphosphate) may be given in a single dose and has become the biphosphate of choice. Both lower calcium in 3–5 days and last 2–4 weeks. Etidronate has three disadvantages: it must be given with vigorous hydration, it must be given over multiple days, and it prevents bone mineralization. Usual dosing for etidronate is 7.5 mg/kg over 4 hours for 3–7 days. Pamidronate is dosed at 60–90 mg and also may be given over 4 hours. Because of their effectiveness and relatively minor side effects, biphosphates have become the mainstays of therapy. Other agents useful as adjuncts are outlined in the table below.

Other Agents Used in the Treatment of HCM

AGENT	DOSE	ACTION	ADVANTAGES	DISADVANTAGES
Calcitonin	4–8 U/kg every 6–12 hr	Inhibits osteoclasts Increases renal excretion	4–6 hr onset Well-tolerated May decrease pain	1–2 days' duration Relatively weak Rare allergic reactions (1 unit skin test recommended)
Plicamycin (mithramycin)	25 μg/kg	Toxic to osteoclasts	Effective Onset in 1–2 days Up to 2 weeks' duration	Thrombocytopenia Nausea and vomiting Vesicant Renal and hepatic toxicities
Glucocorticoids	200–500 mg for 3–5 days	Inhibit resorption Increase excretion Decrease GI absorption	Selectively effective	Side effects of steroids
Gallium nitrate	200 mg/m^2 over 24 hr for 5 days	Decreases resorption	Effective	5-day dosing Renal toxicity Anemia

18. What specific measures should patients and families be taught to help themselves?

    1. Report early signs and symptoms, such as decreased or absent appetite, nausea, vomiting, constipation, increased fatigue, weakness, excessive thirst, frequent voiding, dry mouth and skin, and dizziness with position changes.

    2. Promote hydration by monitoring intake, encouraging patient to drink 2–3 L (quarts)/day, keeping favorite fluids handy, and reminding the patient to sip. Give antinausea medications as ordered.

    3. Help the patient to stay mobile by encouraging standing or walking several times a day or isometric exercises if the patient is unable to bear weight. Support the patient in performing self-care activities as much as possible. Monitor pain medications, and inform the nurse or physician if pain control is not adequate.

    4. Promote safety by keeping the environment uncluttered and well-lit and encouraging the patient to use safety aids such as a walker or cane to prevent falls. Do not allow the patient to overstress bones, and educate others to be gentle when helping. They should not pull on arms or legs or squeeze ribs. Report bone pain and have it evaluated.

BIBLIOGRAPHY

1. Bilezikian JP: Management of acute hypercalcemia. N Engl J Med 326:1196–1203, 1992.
2. Kaplan M: Hypercalcemia of malignancy: A review of advances in pathophysiology. Oncol Nurs Forum 21:1039–1056, 1994.
3. Miaskowski C: Oncologic emergencies. In Baird SB, McCorkle R (eds): Cancer Nursing: A Comprehensive Textbook. Philadelphia, W.B. Saunders, 1991, pp 888–889.
4. Schmitt R: Quality of life issues in lung cancer—New symptom management strategies. Chest 103(Suppl): 51S–55S, 1993.
5. Taylor BM, Weller LA: Hypercalcemia. In Groenwald SL, Frogge MH, Goodman M, Yarbro CH (eds): Cancer Nursing—Principles and Practice. Boston, Jones & Bartlett, 1991, pp 291–297.
6. Wall J, Bundred N, Howell A: Hypercalcemia and bone resorption in malignancy. Clin Orthop Rel Res 312:51–63, 1995.
7. Waters HF, Stuckey PA: Oncology alert for the home care nurse: Hypercalcemia. Home Healthcare Nurse 6:32–36, 1988.

48. INFECTIONS IN IMMUNOSUPPRESSED PATIENTS

Robert H. Gates, MD

1. Are infections an important cause of mortality in cancer patients?

Yes. Infections are the major cause of mortality in many cancers. Infection has replaced bleeding as the major cause of mortality in leukemia. Data about mortality causes from cancer center statistics vary; however, about 75% of deaths in patients with acute leukemia and 50% of deaths in patients with lymphoma result from infection.

2. What factors place a cancer patient at risk for infection?

Factor Promoting Infection	Examples of Associated Organisms	Examples of Disease States
Diminished antibody response	Encapsulated organisms: Pneumococci *Hemophilus influenzae* *Neisseriae* sp. Staphylococci Streptococci	Multiple myeloma Poor nutrition B-cell lymphoma After splenectomy (Hodgkin's disease) Myelophthisis
Poor white blood cell function or decreased number	Aerobic gram-positive organisms Staphylococci Enterococci Aerobic gram-negative organisms *Pseudomonas aeruginosa* *Enterobacter* sp. Fungi *Candida* sp. *Aspergillus* sp.	Leukemias Lymphomas Myelophthisis Chemotherapy
Poor cellular immunity	*Listeria* sp. Herpes Mycobacteria Cryptococci *Legionella* sp. *Pneumocystis* sp.	Hodgkin's disease Non-Hodgkin's lymphoma Poor nutrition Chronic leukemias Chemotherapy, esp. fludarabine Steroids
Skin and mucosal defects	Staphylococci *Candida* sp. Herpes Aerobic gram-negative organisms	Chemotherapy *Pneumocystis carinii* infection Radiation therapy Vascular access devices
Environmental problems: Construction, poor airflow, contaminated water supply, raw foods	*Aspergillus* sp. Tuberculosis *Legionella* sp. Aerobic gram-negative organisms	Organ transplants Neutropenia
Anatomic mechanical problems	Anaerobes Staphylococci Aerobic gram-negative organisms	Lung cancer (airway blockage) Skin or mucosal disruption Bowel obstruction Urinary tract obstruction
Prior infection with organism that has propensity to recur	*Aspergillus* or *Candida* sp. Herpes group virus	Not disease-specific

3. What is the most significant predisposing factor for infection in patients with cancer?

Neutropenia is the single most important factor in determining whether a cancer patient will become infected. Neutrophils are mature white cells that attack and destroy invading bacteria, viruses, and fungi (particularly *Aspergillus* and *Candida* spp.). The absolute neutrophil count (ANC) is calculated by multiplying the percentage of granulocytes (neutrophils or segments + bands) by the total white blood cell (WBC) count. The risk of infection rises as the WBC count falls, with the greatest risk at neutrophil counts less than 500/mm³. Most serious infections occur with neutrophil counts below 100/mm³. In addition to presence and degree, duration of the neutropenia is also important. As the duration of neutropenia increases, the risk of infection increases, ultimately reaching 100%. A duration of 3–7 days is much less of a risk than a duration beyond 14 days. Currently, about one-third of neutropenic patients with fever have a microbiologically proven infection (positive cultures), whereas about one-fifth have clinically apparent infection with negative cultures.

4. What are neutropenic precautions?

1. Strict handwashing is the most important precaution.

2. Routinely, it is not necessary for health care providers to wear masks. Providers with a transmissible respiratory disease should not care for the patient. The practice of requiring the patient to wear a mask when leaving the room varies by institution.

3. Ideally, the airflow in the patient's room should be positive compared with the hall. The intent is to avoid exposure to airborne pathogens such as *Aspergillus*.

4. The patient's room should not be cleaned in a manner that causes dust to be shed (e.g., from drapes).

5. Sources of gram-negative organisms should be avoided (e.g., live flowers in water, raw food, fresh fruits and vegetables).

5. What else can be done to prevent infections in neutropenic patients?

High-efficiency particulate air (HEPA) filtration is used by many centers for patients who undergo organ transplantation or who are expected to have prolonged neutropenia from therapy. The intent is to remove airborne pathogens such as *Aspergillus*.

Immunizations should be up to date, including pneumococcal and *Hemophilus* vaccines. Special consideration should be given to the patient about to undergo an elective splenectomy. Such patients should receive the above vaccines as well as meningococcal vaccine.

The use of **prophylactic antibiotics** often depends on institutional practice. Experience with prophylactic agents has been mixed, ranging from spectacular success with acyclovir and ganciclovir in bone marrow transplant recipients to failure with nystatin. Major problems of prophylactic agents are that they promote resistant bacteria and are partially responsible for the emergence of *Staphylococcus epidermidis* and enterococci as significant pathogens in neutropenic patients. To prevent or delay infection in patients undergoing chemotherapy, several different prophylactic agents have been used:

1. Antibiotics: quinolones, trimethoprim-sulfamethoxazole, oral aminoglycosides, and oral amphotericin B for selective bowel decontamination. The use of trimethoprim-sulfamethoxazole is well established in bone marrow transplant recipients to prevent development of *Pneumocystis carinii* pneumonia.

2. Antifungal agents: nystatin, clotrimazole, and the imidazoles.

3. Antiviral agents: acyclovir and ganciclovir.

4. Isoniazid to prevent reactivation of tuberculosis in patients with a positive tuberculosis skin test, particularly patients with lymphoreticular cancer.

6. What is the source of most bacteria that infect patients with cancer?

Although some infections are acquired from the environment, about 50% of infections in neutropenic cancer patients result from bacteria that make up the patient's own endogenous flora (e.g., *Escherichia coli, Enterobacter* sp., *Klebsiella* sp., other gram-negative bacteria, yeast, and anaerobes). A patient's flora may change rapidly upon admission to the hospital. In the immuno-suppressed patient, the bacterial flora can change in a matter of hours, quickly resembling the bacteria found in the hospital setting.

7. When is fever in neutropenic patients significant?

Fever in the presence of neutropenia is always significant and should be treated as a medical emergency. A patient may die within hours if prompt and effective therapy is not begun. In neu-tropenic patients fever is usually regarded and treated as indicating the presence of bacteria in the blood (bacteremia). Clinical evidence of infection and systemic response are usually equated with sepsis; evidence of organ dysfunction (oliguria, altered mentation) indicates sepsis syn-drome. If hypotension is added to the list, the result is severe sepsis. If the hypotension does not respond to fluid resuscitation, septic shock is present. This spectrum of response to infection in-volves a complex and incompletely understood cascade of events triggered by the presence of bacteria, fungi, or viruses.

Although there is no universal agreement, most authorities agree that significant fever in the neutropenic patient is a single oral temperature greater than 38.3° C (101° F) in the absence of a clear cause, (e.g., administration of blood products) or the presence of a temperature greater than 38° C (100.4° F) for 1 hour or more. In certain situations the febrile response may be greatly blunted, absent, or less than expected. Steroid therapy is the most common culprit. Nonsteroidal antiinflammatory drugs (NSAIDs), old age, renal failure, and overwhelming infection also may blunt the normal fever response. Unfortunately, the absence of fever does not mean that the pa-tient does not have a potentially serious infection.

8. Are all fevers due to infections?

No. Fevers in patients with cancer are commonly drug-induced or related to the cancer itself (e.g., leukemias, lymphomas, renal cell cancer, liver cancer).

9. What is drug-induced fever?

Drug-induced fever is caused by the drug itself. Drugs that induce fevers include antibiotics, antifungals (e.g., amphotericin B), allopurinol, biologic response modifiers, and chemotherapy agents (e.g., bleomycin, dactinomycin, and gemcitabine). The usual mechanism is production of antibody by the patient's immune system that reacts with the drug to cause fever. The diagnosis of drug-induced fever may be relatively easy or obscure and challenging. Clues to the presence of drug-induced fever include:

1. Timing of the fever is often a clue. Drug-induced fever may occur with each administra-tion of the drug or after 10–14 days of treatment (a typical time frame for the patient's immune system to develop antibodies to the drug). The time to development of drug fever may be acceler-ated if the patient has received the drug before and already has developed antibodies.

2. The patient often appears well. The pulse may not be elevated in proportion to the fever. Patients also may appear quite ill, with shaking chills (as in reactions to quinidine).

3. The patient may have a rash (not due to infection) and/or other evidence of drug-induced end-organ dysfunction (e.g., interstitial nephritis or hepatitis).

4. Thorough investigation reveals no other reason for fever.

10. What should be done when the neutropenic patient becomes febrile?

After appropriate cultures are obtained, antibiotic therapy should be promptly ordered and ad-ministered, ideally within 1 hour of recognizing the fever. The assessment and evaluation should proceed without delay. Obtain cultures of blood, urine (even with no signs or symptoms), throat (in presence of abnormal findings), stool (in presence of diarrhea), stool for *Clostridium difficile* toxin assay (with current or recent antibiotics), and cultures of intravenous (IV) line sites with evi-dence of inflammation. For new skin findings, consider immediate evaluation with biopsy and cul-ture. It is mandatory to obtain a baseline chest radiograph in the presence of signs or symptoms attributable to the lungs. A question of sinus disease should prompt an early CT scan of the si-nuses; plain radiographs are often not sensitive enough to pick up early evidence of infection.

Brilliant diagnoses are usually made by ordinary people being dull and methodical. Keep in mind that without neutrophils, many of the expected signs and symptoms of inflammation may be minimal or absent. Assess vital signs, and look for early signs and symptoms of serious infection:

- a decrease in mentation
- a decrease in urine output
- a decrease in platelet count

- a *decrease* or *increase* in temperature
- an increase in glucose
- an increase in heart rate or respiration

In the physical assessment, pay particular attention to the following areas:

1. Skin: Check all current and previous IV sites

New rashes: consider drug reaction, blood-borne spread of bacteria or fungi

Perianal pain or inflammation: consider hemorrhoids, fissure, phlegmon (inflammation of soft tissue due to infection)

2. Head and neck:

Headache, sinus, or jaw pain: consider sinusitis

Nasal ulcers or mucosal necrosis: consider fungal involvement

Cotton wool spots in front of retina: consider candida

Oral mucosal white patches that rub off and bleed: consider candida

Oral ulcers—consider herpes, gram-negative bacteria, chemotherapy

Odynophagia (pain when swallowing): with oral ulcers, consider herpes; with thrush, consider candida esophagitis

3. Lungs: Findings on exam may be minimal; may precede x-ray abnormalities

4. Abdomen: Tenderness, rebound especially involving the right lower quadrant, consider typhlitis

11. How many blood cultures should be done? How much blood per culture? How far apart should the blood cultures be done? Should blood cultures be obtained from venous access devices?

Two pairs of aerobic and anaerobic blood cultures are usually enough to obtain a positive result. More than two contributes little to the statistical likelihood of a positive culture but may contribute to anemia. It is important to obtain the amount of blood required by the hospital laboratory. Many culture systems are optimized for a given amount of blood; indeed, the blood itself may help to provide the nutrients that the bacteria need to grow. Too little blood may decrease the yield from the culture. The interval between cultures need be only as long as it takes to prepare the second site after the first culture is obtained. Delaying therapy so that a second blood culture can be done in 30 or 60 minutes places the patient at needless risk. Whether to draw blood through a vascular access device (VAD) is controversial but usually done. The advantage is that a positive culture from the VAD may suggest the catheter as the source of infection. The bad news is that it may be a contaminant from the hardware of the VAD.

12. What is a Gram stain?

The Gram stain allows bacteria to be picked out from cellular material and debris under a microscope. It is a basic test that can be done in a few minutes with little cost. This valuable tool was developed over 100 years ago by Dr. Hans Gram and is still relevant today in directing initial antibiotic selection. The technique consists of several sequential steps with a different staining solution (crystal violet, iodine, acetone-alcohol, and safranin) in each step. It takes advantage of the differences in the way the staining solutions are retained within bacteria. Bacteria that retain the crystal violet-iodine complex appear dark blue or violet. Bacteria that cannot retain this complex are stained by the safranin and appear pink under the microscope. Organisms that retain the stain and appear blue are said to be gram-positive, whereas organisms that do not retain the stain are said to be gram-negative. Examples of gram-positive organisms include staphylococci, streptococci, enterococci, *Listeria* sp., and bacilli. Examples of gram-negative organisms include *Escherichia coli, Klebsiella* sp., *Enterobacter* sp., *Pseudomonas aeruginosa*, and *Bacteroides* sp.

By making the organism visible, the Gram stain makes it possible to determine the morphology of the bacteria; that is, whether it is a coccus or rodlike.

13. What empirical antibiotics should be prescribed to neutropenic febrile patients?

In the absence of findings that may direct therapy (e.g., pus from a VAD exit site with gram-positive cocci in clusters, which suggests a staphylococcal species), all broad-spectrum regimens (regimens containing antibiotics that are anticipated to be effective against the commonly found gram-negative bacteria) appear to work well. Initial clinical responses vary from 60–80%. This variation is probably due to differences in study design, patient populations in different centers, antibiotic use, and antibiotic susceptibility, according to the institution. Broad-spectrum combination antibiotic regimens may include an extended-spectrum penicillin (e.g. ticarcillin or piperacillin) plus an aminoglycoside (e.g., gentamicin or amikacin) or a third-generation cephalosporin (e.g., ceftazidime). Factors to consider in choosing an antibiotic regimen include:

- Patient drug allergies
- Route of administration
- Concomitant drugs
- Suspected organism
- Antibiotic resistance patterns
- Previous antibiotic therapy
- Previous infecting organisms
- Duration of neutropenia
- Patient exposure to pathogens

Most authorities believe that two antibiotics with activity against *Pseudomonas aeruginosa* should be given initially. Clinical trials and experience also support the use of broad-spectrum monotherapy with agents that have antipseudomonal activity (e.g, ceftazidime or imipenem). Some physicians prefer two antibiotics when the patient exhibits altered vital signs from infection. The decision is usually determined by the institution's antibiotic susceptibilities. For example, if a patient is on a medical or surgical ward with infection problems from a resistant strain of *Enterobacter*, initial therapy should cover the possibility that the patient is infected with this organism. Coverage for staphylococci is not given initially unless there is a reason to suspect a source for staphylococci. Other agents may be added as necessary for special circumstances (e.g., to cover for anaerobes in the case of suspected typhlitis).

Commonly Used Antibiotics

ANTIBIOTIC CLASS	EXAMPLES	SPECTRUM/ACTIVITY	CAUTIONS
Penicillins	Ticarcillin Piperacillin	Streptococci Gram-negative anaerobes	Allergic reactions Potassium loss Rash with allopurinol Drug-induced neutropenia
Cephalosporins	Ceftazidime	Streptococci Gram-negative organisms	Allergic reactions Drug-induced neutropenia
Quinolones	Ciprofloxacin Ofloxacin	Gram-negative organisms *Legionella* sp.	GI absorption decreased by aluminum, magnesium, iron, zinc, sucralfate Red neck, red man syndrome
Aminoglycosides	Gentamicin Tobramycin Amikacin	Gram-negative organisms	Avoid with cisplatin Avoid with cyclosporine Ototoxicity Nephrotoxicity Avoid with amphotericin B
Sulfonamides	Sulfamethoxazole (with trimethoprim)	Gram-negative organisms *Pneumocystis carinii*	Allergic reactions Marrow suppression
Vancomycin	Vancomycin Teicoplanin	Gram-positive organisms	Red neck, red man Drug-induced neutropenia
Imidazoles	Ketoconazole	*Candida* sp.	Antacids decrease GI absorption

14. Why is it necessary to review the patient's previous antibiotic regimens?

Prior antibiotics can greatly affect the likely organisms currently infecting a neutropenic patient. If an antibiotic that kills or suppresses one kind of bacteria is given, other bacteria or fungi that are resistant to the agent will try to take over the niche left by the killed bacteria. In treating a patient with a quinolone antibiotic, beware of anaerobic bacteria and yeast. Vancomycin therapy leaves gram-negative organisms without the usual competition from gram-positive organisms. Broad-spectrum antibiotics permit the fungi a free hand. Even the imidazole class of antifungal agents (ketoconazole, fluconazole, itraconazole) may allow growth of fungi that are resistant to the imidazoles.

15. How long should antibiotics be continued?

In general antibiotics are continued for the duration of the neutropenia. Guidelines to consider include the following:

No fever and ≥ 500 neutrophils
- No source of infection → stop antibiotics
- Known source of infection → give course appropriate for source

No fever and < 500 neutrophils → continue antibiotics for up to 14 days

Fever and ≥ 500 neutrophils → Consider changing or stopping therapy after evaluation for:
- Hidden site of infection
- Abscess or catheter-related infection
- Resistant bacteria, fungi, virus
- Drug fever
- Tumor fever

Fever and < 500 neutrophils → Continue antibiotics and consider:
- Fungal superinfection
- Inadequate antibiotic dosing
- Resistant bacteria
- Viral infection
- Abscess or catheter-related infection

16. What is meant by a third-generation antibiotic?

The habit of referring to cephalosporins by generation was popularized by pharmaceutical companies and tacitly approved by general use. The habit has evolved into calling an antibiotic with expanded activity the product of a new generation. The generation refers roughly to the order in which the drug was introduced and the range of bacteria against which the antibiotic is active. The first-generation cephalosporins (e.g., cephalothin, cefazolin) had good activity against *Staphylococcus aureus*. The following generations tend to have less activity against staphylococci. The second- and third-generation cephalosporins (e.g., cefamandole and ceftriaxone, respectively) tend to have increased activity against gram-negative aerobic bacteria.

17. What is antibiotic lock therapy?

Antibiotic lock therapy is a relatively new approach to the management of an infected catheter line. A small volume of concentrated antibiotic solution is placed in the lumen of the catheter and allowed to remain for hours. The approach is said to work poorly for candidal infections.

18. What about the colony-stimulating factors?

Granulocyte colony-stimulating factor (G-CSF) and granulocyte-macrophage colony-stimulating factor (GM-CSF) shorten the duration of chemotherapy-induced neutropenia and may enhance the function of neutrophils. These agents are glycopeptides that stimulate the bone marrow to speed the production and maturation of neutrophils. They are expensive and may cause symptoms such as myalgias. The cost-benefit ratio is best in patients with an expected prolonged duration of neutropenia (> 7–10 days) and high risk of infection with agents such as *Aspergillus* sp. G-CSF is started after chemotherapy and continued until the neutrophil count recovers.

19. Amphotericin B has a bad reputation for side effects and for causing problems with kidney and bone marrow function. Is there any truth to this reputation? What can be done to lessen the problems?

Considerable folklore surrounds the administration of amphotericin B ("ampho-terrible"). Common signs and symptoms include chills and fever, phlebitis, and nausea and vomiting. Renal problems include tubular dysfunction leading to loss of electrolytes (particularly potassium and bicarbonate) and suppression of erythropoietin production by the kidney.

Fiction: Heparin in the amphotericin B solution decreases the risk of phlebitis.

Fact: Heparin is not proved to prevent phlebitis. It is not needed when amphotericin B is given through a central line. Indeed, even small amounts of heparin may lead to immune-mediated platelet destruction.

Fiction: A test dose of amphotericin B is required to avoid anaphylaxis.

Fact: The "test-dose" practice was adapted as a result of side effects seen with the administration of early, relatively impure preparations of amphotericin B. In patients who have not received Amphotericin B before, the test dose may be safely omitted.

Fiction: Steroids should be added to the amphotericin B infusion to decrease the occurrence of febrile reactions.

Fact: Although steroids are often used, there is little scientific evidence of their efficacy. Some authorities advocate against the routine use of steroids because of the theoretical concern of increasing immunosuppression. If steroids are used, they should be the shortest-lived preparations available (e.g., hydrocortisone succinate). Methylprednisolone should not be used.

Fiction: Amphotericin B is better tolerated if the infusion is given over at least 4–6 hours.

Fact: Although bolus therapy is dangerous, amphotericin B is tolerated by most patients when given over 1–2 hours.

20. What should done to assist in the administration of amphotericin B?
- Individualize the symptomatic medications to the patient's needs.
- Reassure the patient that administration of the drug usually is better tolerated with time.
- Use meperidine, 25–50 mg intravenously, to terminate chills and fever. Rare intractable chills and fever may be treated with dantrolene.
- To help avoid renal toxicity, maintain adequate volume status. Saline boluses given with the infusions are often used for this purpose.
- Consider using the newer lipid-complexed and liposomal preparations of amphotericin B, which may be better tolerated and have less renal and bone marrow toxicity. Thus larger doses may be given.

21. True or false: A patient who receives vancomycin and experiences flushing, wheezing, and hypotension is most likely allergic to the vancomycin.

False. The so-called red neck or red man syndrome (from the flushed appearance of the face, neck, and upper torso) is not, strictly speaking, an allergy. Classic allergic reactions are defined by the presence of an antibody that reacts with the patient's immune system to produce the allergic response. With vancomycin, the drug itself interacts with mast cells (antibodies have no role) and directly causes release of histamine from the mast cells. The histamine causes the vasodilation, flushing, and wheezing. As histamine release from mast cells is also important in anaphylactic reactions (IgE-mediated mast cell degranulation), it is not difficult to understand how the patient's clinical appearance suggests an allergic reaction. The patient is not allergic to vancomycin in this setting.

Tolerance to infusions tends to improve with time. Do not infuse vancomycin rapidly unless you have never seen the red neck syndrome and would like to do so. Infusion over 60–90 minutes is recommended.

22. What is typhlitis?

Typhlitis or neutropenic enterocolitis is a necrotizing infection of the bowel secondary to a combination of factors toxic to the intestinal mucosa. The resulting mucosal damage allows bacterial invasion. The infection, usually involving the large bowel (especially the cecum), results in bowel wall edema, thinning, and perforation. The situation is a set-up for bacterial translocation in a big way. Patients may present with symptoms suggesting appendicitis, such as abdominal pain, nausea and vomiting, and fever. Typhlitis is particularly common in children. Blood cultures may be positive despite administration of effective antibiotic therapy. In the proper clinical setting, the diagnosis may be made by CT scan, which shows a thickened bowel wall. Peritoneal lavage with a positive culture for the same organisms as the blood cultures is confirmatory. Medical therapy includes antibiotics to cover the gram-negative organisms, Candida sp., and anaerobic organisms. Laxatives and enemas should be avoided. Surgical intervention may be indicated. Unfortunately, surgery is usually difficult because the patients are critically ill and poor surgical risks.

23. What is ecthyma gangrenosum?

Ecthyma gangrenosum is a skin manifestation of the vascular spread of bacteria, usually gram-negative. *Pseudomonas aeruginosa* is the most commonly involved organism. Other organisms include staphylococci and fungi such as *Aspergillus* and *Alternaria* spp. Blood cultures are often positive for the causative bacteria. Lesions begin as nodular papules that quickly progress to central blebs, then ulcerate with underlying induration and central necrosis. The lesions are usually erythematous, often with a violaceous hue. Not unlike petechiae, they may be somewhat hidden in skin folds, buttocks, and the perineum.

24. What are MRSA and MRSE? What is their significance?

MRSA is methicillin-resistant *Staphylococcus aureus*. MRSE is methicillin-resistant *Staphylococcus epidermidis*.

Penicillins and cephalosporins belong to the beta-lactam class of antibiotics. The beta-lactam antibiotics bind to a receptor in bacteria and interrupt the synthesis of the bacterial cell wall, leading to cell death. Shortly after the introduction of penicillin, many bacteria developed resistance by producing a beta-lactamase enzyme that destroyed a portion of the penicillin molecule (the beta-lactam ring), rendering the antibiotic inactive. Biochemists retaliated by making penicillins that were resistant to the destructive action of this enzyme (e.g., nafcillin and methicillin). In recent years staphylococci have evolved that are resistant to all antibiotics of the beta lactamase-resistant class. These staphylococci have a receptor that is much more difficult for the antibiotics to bind. MRSAs are resistant to all beta-lactam antibiotics (e.g., penicillins, cephalosporins, and carbapenems). They are sometimes susceptible to trimethoprim-sulfamethoxazole but are usually treated with vancomycin. Infection with MRSA can be deadly, and the necessity of using more vancomycin has lead to increased resistance of other bacteria to vancomycin. A good example of this resistance development is the vancomycin-resistant enterococci, which have become a problem in many medical centers.

25. What is bacterial translocation?

Bacterial translocation is the movement of living bacteria from the gastrointestinal tract to the mesenteric lymph nodes and blood stream and thus to other organs. Every moment of our lives, bowel flora are prevented from translocating or quickly cleared when they try to move across the bowel wall. In the presence of neutropenia and other immunosuppression, life-threatening infections can result from mucosal disruption of the bowel wall caused by chemotherapy, invading organisms, or antibiotic suppression of normal bowel anaerobic bacteria (the predominant normal bowel flora that help to prevent translocation). Gram-negative organisms most likely to translocate include *E. coli, Klebsiella* sp., and *Pseudomonas aeruginosa*. Nutritional counseling may be important. Many authorities believe that fiber ingestion assists in mucosal preservation, thus decreasing the rate at which bacterial translocation occurs.

26. What is low-risk neutropenia?

Low-risk neutropenia is a relative term used to describe neutrophil counts less than $500/mm^3$ but greater than $100/mm^3$ with an expected duration of less than 7–10 days. Such neutropenias are often seen during chemotherapy for solid tumors (as opposed to the neutropenia that follows therapy for leukemias or bone marrow transplant). Patients are considered at low risk because they usually respond well to initial antibiotic therapy.

Some centers have initiated outpatient therapy for patients with low-risk neutropenia who respond well to initial inpatient treatment. Outpatient management should be done only by clinicians experienced in the management of neutropenic fevers. Candidates for outpatient therapy should have no comorbid conditions (e.g., no heart or kidney failure), a responsive tumor, good outpatient support systems, and easy access for follow-up and readmission.

27. What are the indications to remove an infected VAD?
- Nonresponse to appropriate antibiotic therapy after 48–72 hours
- Persistent positive blood cultures
- Deteriorating patient
- Line malfunction
- Infection with organisms poorly responsive to antimicrobial therapy (e.g., bacillus, *Corynebacterium* sp., or fungal species)

28. What strategies are used to guide therapy for infected VADs?
Therapeutic strategies are guided by infecting organism and location of infection:
- *Staphylococcus epidermidis*
  Exit site—medical therapy
  Tunnel—consider removal
  Port—remove Huber needle and give antibiotic at remote IV site
- *Staphylococcus aureus*
  Exit site—medical therapy
  Line or tunnel—remove line
  Port—consider removal
- *Candida* sp.
  Exit site—remove line
  Tunnel—remove line
  Port—remove line
- Gram-negative organisms
  Exit site—try medical therapy
  Line—remove line
  Tunnel—50% failure rate with medical therapy

29. Allogeneic bone marrow transplants by their nature result in severe immunosuppression in recipients. When and what infections are patients prone to develop?
The time of greatest risk for infection in bone marrow recipients can be roughly divided into 3 phases:

1. The first 30 days after transplant involve the immunosuppressant effects following a pretransplant bone marrow-eradicating regimen of irradiation and chemotherapy. After transplant, immunosuppressive medication such as cyclosporine is also used. Profound, prolonged neutropenia is present with the possibility of gram-negative and gram-positive infections. Antibiotic treatment promotes candidal infection. A striking concern is the risk for herpes simplex virus in patients who are seropositive before transplant.

2. After this 30-day period, initial engraftment of the transplanted marrow begins. Cytomegalovirus infections replace herpes simplex as the major viral concern, with the potential for severe involvement of multiple organ systems. *Aspergillus* sp. replaces *Candida* sp. as the major fungal pathogen.

3. In the third time period, after 90–100 days, bone marrow engraftment is completed. Unfortunately, the immune system does not completely recover for up to 1–2 years. The patient remains at increased risk for infections with organisms that take advantage of poor immunoglobulin

function, particularly the pneumococci. Varicella zoster replaces cytomegalovirus as the principal viral pathogen. Another major problem is graft vs. host disease, which can begin during the time of bone marrow engraftment. Graft vs. host disease may require immunosuppressive therapy, which further increases the risk of infection.

30. Why should patients have a dental consultation before they begin chemotherapy?

Before administering myelosuppressive chemotherapy, it is good practice to take care of sites that are actively infected and to consider preventive care for potential sources of infection. A dental site that is a minor problem in normal hosts may become a life-threatening source in neutropenic patients.

31. Does it matter what type of dressing is placed on the exit site of a central VAD?

After reviewing the data from clinical trials, noting the good results from institutions with catheter care teams, and discussing the pros and cons with nurses and physicians, my recommendation is to pay meticulous attention to protocol in caring for dressings on the exit site of a central VAD. The kind of dressing is not as important as the attention the provider and patient give to the care of the access line. A reasonable strategy is to use a gauze dressing immediately after line placement and during drainage. After the site is healed or drainage has stopped, a transparent, semipermeable occlusive dressing can be used alone or with gauze. It is also appropriate to use no dressing for tunneled catheters.

The views and opinions in this chapter are solely the author's and do not reflect the views or the policies of Tripler Regional Medical Command, the Department of Defense, or the United States Government.

BIBLIOGRAPHY

1. Brandt B, DePalma J, Irwin M, et al: Comparison of central venous catheter dressings in bone marrow transplant recipients. Oncol Nurs Forum 23:829–836, 1996.
2. Chanock SJ, Pizzo PA: Fever in the neutropenic patient. Infect Dis Clin North Am 10:777–796, 1996.
3. Giamarellou H: Empiric therapy for infections in the febrile, neutropenic, compromised host. Med Clin North Am 79:559–580, 1995.
4. Hoeprich PD: Clinical use of amphotericin B and derivatives: Lore, mystique, and fact. Clin Infect Dis 14(Suppl 1):S114–S119, 1992.
5. Wujcik D: Infection control in oncology patients. Nurs Clin North Am 28:639–650, 1993.

49. SPINAL CORD COMPRESSION

Linda Petersen-Rivera, RN, MSN, OCN, and Michael R. Watters, MD

1. Why is spinal cord compression an oncologic emergency?

Spinal cord compression is a true neurologic emergency that develops in up to 10% of cancer patients. Without prompt treatment, the patient may become partially or completely paralyzed. Spinal cord compression is sometimes the first presentation of undiagnosed cancer. The neurologic outcome depends on how rapidly the symptoms are manifested and the neurologic status of the patient at the start of treatment. The more rapid the development of symptoms and the more advanced the neurologic deterioration, the worse the prognosis for recovery. The key to good patient outcome is quick recognition of signs and symptoms of spinal cord compression and prompt therapy.

2. What are the most common malignancies associated with spinal cord compression?

The most common malignancies are carcinomas of the lung, breast, or prostate and multiple myeloma. Less common sources include lymphomas, melanomas, renal cell cancers, gastrointestinal adenocarcinomas, and sarcomas. In children, be aware of sarcomas, neuroblastomas, and lymphomas.

3. What levels of the spine are most frequently involved?

Spinal Level	Involvement (%)	Associated Cancers
Cervical	10	Lung, breast, kidney, lymphoma, myeloma, melanoma
Thoracic	70	Lung, breast, kidney, lymphoma, myeloma, prostate
Lumbosacral	20	Lung, breast, kidney, lymphoma, myeloma, melanoma, prostate, gastrointestinal

4. How does spinal cord compression occur?

The most common source of spinal cord compression in patients with cancer is metastasis to the epidural space with or without bony involvement. Tumors may also reach the epidural space by direct extension through the intravertebral formation, particularly lymphomas and nerve sheath tumors. Some primary cancers may occur within the cord itself and may not be associated with pain. Regardless of the route of access, the mass effect of the tumor with associated edema compresses the cord, resulting in ischemia and neural damage. The degree of involvement and speed of compression of the cord explain the wide range of signs and symptoms.

5. What is the first symptom of spinal cord compression?

Because the dura is pain-sensitive, over 95% of patients with spinal cord compression report back pain as the first symptom, preceding other symptoms by weeks to months. The areas most commonly involved are the thoracic, lumbosacral, and cervical spine.

6. How is back pain caused by spinal cord compression characterized?

The pain may be localized or radicular. Local pain usually occurs at the level of the lesion and is said to be dull and constant. The pain is more severe with recumbency and when a patient coughs, bears weight, or uses the Valsalva maneuver. Ideally the diagnosis will be made while the patient is having only spinal axis pain—before neurologic deficits develop.

7. How does dural pain from tumor compression differ from referred pain of visceral origin or musculoskeletal back pain?

Patients with cancer also have other sources of back pain. Musculoskeletal pain, by far the more common, is accentuated by movement and improved with rest; it is not associated with imaging changes of spinal metastasis.

Visceral tumor pain may refer to the back, with a constant boring quality that worsens at rest. The pain may have fleeting sharp qualities, cause sleeplessness, and even be improved with activity. This type of pain may be seen in patients with intraabdominal tumors (pancreatic cancer, lymphoma, or sarcoma). Abdominal computed tomography (CT) scan may be diagnostic.

8. What other signs and symptoms are associated with spinal cord compression?

If the epidural lesion is not detected at the painful phase, ischemic and compressive damage to neurons may follow, often initially manifested as weakness (75–85% of cases). Weakness may progress rapidly, adding to the clinical urgency of making a diagnosis. The weakness is typically bilateral and corresponds to the level of spinal cord involvement. Cervical lesions cause quadriparesis, whereas thoracic or lumbosacral lesions cause paraparesis. Other motor signs include spasticity, hyperreflexia, abnormal stretch reflexes, and extensor plantar responses. Sensory loss below the level of cord compression and autonomic dysfunction with impotency and bladder or bowel retention (or incontinence) may result. These deficits may occur in any sequence and progress rapidly.

9. How long is the interval from diagnosis of cancer to presentation with symptoms of spinal cord compression?

The interval from diagnosis to presentation depends on the biologic rate of growth of the cancer and varies from the initial presentation to decades later.

10. How is spinal cord compression diagnosed?

1. **Physical examination.** Back pain in any cancer patient should prompt a rapid evaluation. Palpation with gentle percussion over the vertebral spinous processes will often reveal tenderness at the site of involvement. The neurologic findings follow logically from the extent of compromise of cord function. Weakness, as noted above, is often found associated with signs of upper motor neuron involvement (spasticity, hyperreflexia). A change in the patient's sensory exam is usually seen below the level of cord involvement. Decreased rectal tone and a distended bladder signal autonomic dysfunction.

2. **Laboratory results.** In adults, an elevated alkaline phosphatase may suggest bony involvement by the cancer.

3. **Complete spinal images.** *Radiographs* of the spine may reveal erosion of a pedicle, lytic lesions of the vertebral body, or collapse of a vertebral body. Most patients with spinal cord compression eventually have an abnormal radiograph; however, normal spine films do not exclude the possibility of an epidural metastasis, and radiographic changes may not be evident for several months after the presence of a tumor.

Bone scans can be helpful in locating metastasis to the vertebrae but do not differentiate cancer from benign processes such as vertebral collapse or osteoporosis and do not visualize the epidural space or neural elements. Twenty percent of scans reveal lesions missed on plain films.

Myelogram metrizamide CT scans are more sensitive for determining the extent of tumor involvement, particularly in the axial plane. The risks of myelography include neurologic deterioration after lumbar puncture (rare in patients with complete myelographic block) and adverse reactions to contrast agent.

Magnetic resonance imaging (MRI) is currently the imaging modality of choice. Its advantages over myelography include its noninvasive nature and the ability to distinguish prevertebral, vertebral, extradural, intradural, extramedullary, and intramedullary lesions. MRI provides better anatomic visualization with sagittal and axial images of the spinal cord than CT scans. MRI contrast agents are less likely to produce neurologic or systemic adverse reactions and are administered parenterally rather than intrathecally.

4. **Fine-needle aspiration** (FNA) may provide tissue confirmation, especially in patients with metastatic involvement of the dorsal bony elements.

11. How is treatment of spinal cord compression determined?

Once the diagnosis of spinal cord compression is made, the patient is started on corticosteroids, regardless of further immediate therapy. The type of therapy depends on :
- Primary tumor type and prior treatment
- Level of the myelopathy
- Degree of the spinal block
- Potential for neurologic reversibility

Consider surgery for:
- Radiation therapy failure
- Relapse in area of prior radiation therapy
- Complete block
- Unstable spine
- Single lesion when complete removal may be possible
- Diagnosis is uncertain
- Mild deficits

Consider chemotherapy for:
- Cancers that are highly sensitive to chemotherapy or hormones; always give with other modalities

Consider radiation therapy for:
- Early diagnosis
- Incomplete block
- Severe deficits

12. What brings radiation oncologists to work on weekends and at night?

Emergency radiation therapy for spinal cord compression. Expedient treatment is just as important as timely diagnosis. The mainstay of treatment is radiation therapy with the field extending 1–2 vertebral bodies above and below the compression. The usual dose is 3000–4000 cGy, given in fractionated doses over 2–4 weeks. Patients tolerate the treatment well when pretreated with corticosteroids. Eighty-five percent of patients obtain pain relief; neurologic deficits are stabilized in about 50% of patients.

13. Are surgery and radiation equal in treating spinal cord compression?

In the past, surgical decompression with laminectomy via a posterior approach or vertebral body resection was done for quick relief of compression. In clinical trials, radiation and surgery together were no better than radiation alone. Thus, most patients are treated with radiation without surgery. The recent development of an anterior approach has allowed surgery to be an option for patients with pathologic fractures, radiation-resistant tumors, or areas of prior radiation therapy.

14. Why are corticosteroids given to patients with spinal cord compression?

Corticosteroids are used in conjunction with all of the treatment options. They are begun as soon as spinal cord compression is suspected to reduce edema and mass effect, which may lessen pain. The appropriate dose recommendations are largely empirical. An intravenous bolus of dexamethasone, 10 mg, is commonly followed by 4–6 mg orally every 6 hours for 2 days; then a slow taper is begun. If a high degree of compression is diagnosed, some providers recommend larger doses with an initial intravenous bolus of 100 mg of dexamethasone, followed by 24 mg orally every 6 hours for 2 days, with a rapid taper. Although there is reason to believe that large doses of corticosteroids may assist in pain relief, no convincing evidence shows an improvement in patient outcome. Steroid-related side effects are common (e.g., hyperglycemia, gastrointestinal bleeding, psychosis) and require specific monitoring.

15. What percentage of patients with spinal cord compression are able to ambulate after pretreatment motor dysfunction?

Of patients who were ambulatory before treatment, 80% remain so; of patients who were paraplegic before treatment, 10% regain ambulation. This is why treatment must be instituted immediately!

16. What is the nurse's role in caring for patients with a diagnosis of spinal cord compression?

The major role of the oncology nurse is continual assessment of the patient and prompt notification of changes in pain, sensory, motor, urinary, or bowel function. Because 95% of patients report back pain as their first symptom, pain assessment and treatment are crucial.

Another important nursing role is to preserve and maximize the patient's functional status. A bowel and bladder program may be required. It also may be necessary to provide skin care, wound care, and rehabilitation services. The nurse needs to instruct the patient about treatment and possible side effects and complications (e.g., corticosteroids, radiation therapy), diagnostic tests, and general care. Emotional support for patient and family must be a major focus of care, particularly if spinal cord compression is the presenting sign of a cancer diagnosis.

The views contained in this manuscript are solely those of the authors and do not reflect the views or policies of Tripler Army Medical Command, the Department of Defense, or the U.S. Government.

BIBLIOGRAPHY

1. Boogerd W, van der Sande JJ: Diagnosis and treatment of spinal cord compression in malignant disease. Cancer Treat Rev 19:129, 1993.
2. Dyck S: Surgical instrumentation as a palliative treatment for spinal cord compression. Oncol Nurs Forum 18:515–521, 1991.
3. Flynn DF, Shipley WV: Management of spinal cord compression secondary to metastatic prostatic carcinoma. Urol Clin North Am 18:145–152, 1991.
4. Krecker E, Muggia FM: Oncologic emergencies. In Brain MC, Carbone PP (eds): Current Therapy in Hematology-Oncology. St. Louis, Mosby, 1995, pp 606–608.
5. Miaskowski C: Oncologic emergencies. In Baird SB, McCorkle R, Grant M (eds): Cancer Nursing: A Comprehensive Textbook. Philadelphia, W.B. Saunders, 1991, pp 885–893.
6. Sorensen PS, Borgesen SE, Rohe K: Metastatic epidural spinal cord compression: Results of treatment and survival. Cancer 65:1502, 1990.

50. SUPERIOR VENA CAVA SYNDROME

Kelly C. Mack, RN, MSN, OCN

1. What is superior vena cava syndrome?

Superior vena cava syndrome (SVCS) is a clinical diagnosis that describes a pattern of physical findings resulting from obstruction of blood flow through the superior vena cava. The resulting engorgement of collateral veins of the thorax, head, and neck produces the classic symptoms.

2. What causes SVCS?

Obstruction of blood flow can be caused by any of the following three factors:

1. **Compression.** Extrinsic pressure on the blood vessel as a result of tumor or enlarged lymph nodes is the most common mechanism of superior vena cava obstruction.

2. **Thrombosis.** Thrombosis, usually caused by compression by a tumor or central venous catheter or pacemaker wire, is becoming an increasingly common cause of superior vena cava obstruction.

3. **Invasion.** Invasion within the superior vena cava by tumor is an unusual cause.

3. What anatomic mechanism underlies SVCS?

The superior vena cava is the major vessel for drainage of venous blood from the head, neck, upper extremities, and upper thorax. It is located in the right anterior superior mediastinum and is surrounded by rigid structures: sternum, trachea, right bronchus, aorta, pulmonary artery, perihilar and paratracheal lymph nodes, and vertebral bodies. The superior vena cava is a low-pressure, large but thin-walled, easily compressible structure. It is vulnerable to any space-occupying process in its vicinity.

When the superior vena cava is fully or partially obstructed, venous return to the right atrium is diminished, resulting in increased venous pressure behind the obstruction. This increase in venous pressure (venous hypertension) causes venous stasis in the head, arms, and upper chest. Engorgement and dilation of superficial veins result, and extensive venous collateral circulation in the neck and thorax develops in an effort to bypass the obstruction. Other mediastinal structures, such as the bronchi, esophagus, and spinal cord, may be threatened as a result of an enlarging mass within the mediastinum. The symptoms depend on the rate, degree, and location of obstruction; the aggressiveness of the tumor; and the competency of collateral circulation.

4. What are the classic signs and symptoms?

The most common **early** symptoms include dyspnea, orthopnea (ability to breathe easily only in the upright position), and a sensation of fullness in the head, face, and upper extremities. A "tight-collar" feeling is characteristic. Less frequently, chest pain and dysphagia are experienced.

The physical findings are classic and unmistakable. Venous distention of neck, scalp, anterior and posterior chest wall, and shoulders is the hallmark of SVCS. The veins become prominent, dilated, tortuous, and palpable. This sign is more evident with the patient prone. Veins often run a vertical or nearly vertical course. They can be distinguished from the telangiectasias of the elderly in that they are more numerous, widespread, and enlarged.

Other features of SVCS include facial and periorbital edema and swelling of the upper extremities, in particular the right arm. Plethora (ruddy, purple-red complexion), cyanosis, and cough are less common but still considered classic features.

Symptoms of **advanced** disease are rare. Examples include hoarseness, stridor, engorged conjunctiva, and symptoms of increased intracranial pressure, such as headache, dizziness, visual changes, changes in mental status, and respiratory distress (respiratory rate > 30/min).

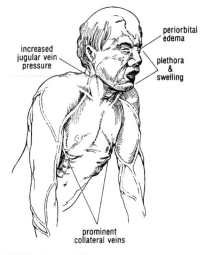

Classic clinical symptoms of SVCS. (From Miller SE: Superior vena cava syndrome. In Polomano RC, Miller SE (eds): Understanding and Managing Oncologic Emergencies. Columbus, OH, Adria Laboratories, 1987, with permission.)

5. What determines the severity of symptoms?

The severity of symptoms is determined by how rapidly the obstruction develops. A slowly developing obstruction allows time for collateral circulation to develop, and the severity of symptoms is lessened. Conversely, rapid onset of symptoms precludes development of collateral circulation and therefore increases circulatory compromise. Regardless of rapidity of onset, all symptoms and physical findings are aggravated by bending forward, stooping, or lying down—anything that increases intrathoracic or intracranial pressure.

6. Who is at risk for developing SVCS?

Up to 97% of all cases of SVCS are caused by cancer. Nonmalignant causes are responsible for only 3–10% of cases. Although these numbers suggest that SVCS is a common disorder, in fact it is relatively uncommon. Only 3–4% of oncologic patients develop SVCS, usually in later stages of disease.

7. Are certain types of malignancies associated with SVCS, or are all patients with cancer at risk?

Lung cancer is responsible for 70% of all cases of SVCS. Small cell carcinoma is the most common histologic type, followed by squamous cell carcinoma of the lung. Cancers arising in the right lung are four times more likely to cause SVCS because the superior vena cava is located in the right lung. Nonetheless, only 6–7% of patients with lung cancer develop SVCS.

Non-Hodgkin's lymphoma is the second most common malignancy to cause SVCS. Although Hodgkin's disease commonly involves the mediastinum, it is an uncommon cause of SVCS.

Breast cancer is the most common metastatic disease causing SVCS. Rarely, thymoma, germ cell tumors and Kaposi's sarcoma also may cause SVCS.

8. What are the nonmalignant causes of SVCS?

Traditionally, nonmalignant cases of SVCS have been caused by infectious agents. The first described case of SVCS was caused by a syphilitic aortic aneurysm, reported in 1757. Historically, tuberculosis mediastinitis was a common cause of SVCS, accounting for up to 45% of cases before the development of effective antiinfective agents. With the increasing incidence of AIDS and the corresponding increasing incidence of tuberculosis and syphilis, some clinicians warn that infectious etiologies must again be considered in the differential diagnosis.

Currently the most common nonmalignant cause of superior vena cava syndrome is thrombosis. This iatrogenic complication is seen most commonly in the presence of central venous catheters or pacemakers. Mediastinal fibrosis, a narrowing or stricture of the superior vena cava, may be caused by radiation therapy to the mediastinum or histoplasmosis. This cause is exceedingly rare.

9. How is the diagnosis of SVCS made?

Clinical identification of SVCS is simple. The signs and symptoms are typical and unmistakable. Imaging studies alone are insufficient to make the diagnosis. Current practice demands a tissue diagnosis before instituting treatment unless the patient has a malignancy known to cause SVCS. The only exception to this dictum is when respiratory and neurologic status are so compromised that a delay in treatment would pose a threat to life; this situation is rare.

Imaging Study	Comments
Chest radiograph	Shows a right superior mediastinal mass (widening) and mediastinal and paratracheal lymphadenopathy. May be normal despite obstruction.
Computed tomography of chest	Gives more detail about superior vena cava, its tributaries, and other critical structures (bronchi and spinal cord). Can identify intrinsic vs. extrinsic causes of obstruction. May guide attempts at biopsy.
Contrast venography	Controversial because of invasive nature and use of contrast. Carries risk of thrombosis. Can confirm clinical diagnosis, outline anatomy, and define pattern of collateral flow. Has largely been replaced by radionuclide studies (SPECT scan or technetium-99 scan) but is useful if surgery is contemplated.*
Magnetic resonance imaging	Because of multiplane capabilities, better than CT to show relationship of nodes, vessels, and other mediastinal structures and to demonstrate vessel patency. Chest wall collaterals easier to see on CT scan.

* Concern that interrupting the integrity of a vessel wall in the presence of increased intraluminal pressure may lead to excessive bleeding has been refuted by clinical experience.

10. What procedures are used to obtain tissue for diagnosis?

As a general rule, the least invasive method of obtaining tissue is used first. The likelihood of getting a diagnostic sample must be factored into this decision.

Diagnostic Procedure	Comments
Sputum cytology	For patients with suspected lung carcinoma; approximately 50% chance of diagnostic success.
Thoracentesis	Indicated if pleural effusion present.
Bone marrow biopsy	Rarely done; only if bone marrow involvement suspected.
Lymph node biopsy	If suspicious lymph node available.
Bronchoscopy	Useful if small cell lung cancer is suspected.
CT-guided needle biopsy	Effective and safe alternative to open biopsy or mediastinoscopy.
Mediastinoscopy	If all other procedures fail; carries some risk because of difficulty with hemostasis in presence of large, dilated veins.
Thoracotomy	If all other procedures fail; again, risk of hemorrhage because of dilated veins in the operative field; parasternal approach is known as the Chamberlain procedure.

11. SVCS is listed among oncologic emergencies. Is there an urgency to begin treatment?

SVCS has long been considered a potentially life-threatening medical emergency. However, in the absence of tracheal obstruction, it is unlikely to prove life-threatening. Historically it was common practice to give emergent radiotherapy with initial high-dose fractions, sometimes even before histologic diagnosis was established. Invasive diagnostic procedures were avoided because they were considered to be dangerous because of the high intraluminal pressure and the presumed increased risk of hemorrhage. In fact, a study done by Ahmann revealed an approximate 1% complication rate with invasive procedures, none of them life-threatening. Biopsy does not carry an excessive risk in patients with SVCS. Concern about exposure to anesthesia in patients with SVCS was also allayed. Whenever possible, the standard of care demands that time be taken to establish a histologic diagnosis so that proper treatment may be initiated.

12. What is the goal of treatment?

The goal of treatment is to decrease the size of the tumor, thereby relieving the obstruction and restoring normal venous drainage. This strategy brings rapid resolution of symptoms. Secondarily and simultaneously, the goal is to attempt a cure of the primary malignant process. Small cell lung carcinoma, non-Hodgkin's lymphoma, and germ cell tumors constitute 50% of the malignant causes of SVCS and are potentially curable.

13. What is the prognosis?

Prognosis of SVCS strongly correlates with prognosis of underlying disease. Important prognostic variables include underlying malignancy (histology), extent of the primary tumor (stage), responsiveness of the tumor to radiation therapy or chemotherapy, patient's performance status at the time of diagnosis, treatment history, and availability of remaining treatment options.

14. Once the diagnosis is made, how is SVCS treated?

Treatment of SVCS varies, depending on the underlying cause.

Small cell lung cancer. Small cell lung cancer is a chemosensitive tumor and, therefore, is treated initially with combination chemotherapy alone. If there is no response or if disease progresses, radiation therapy is used. The mean time to resolution of symptoms for small cell carcinoma treated with combination chemotherapy is 7 days (range: 7–10 days). The presence of SVCS is not an adverse prognostic factor for small cell lung cancer. In this setting, onset of SVCS develops quickly because of the characteristic rapid doubling time of small cell lung cancers.

Non-small cell lung cancer. Non-small cell lung cancer is not considered chemosensitive. The initial treatment is radiation therapy. The likelihood of relieving symptoms is high, but overall prognosis is poor.

Non-Hodgkin's lymphoma. The most common subtypes are diffuse large cell and lymphoblastic lymphoma. Both are high-grade lymphomas and are considered chemosensitive and curable in the earlier stages. Patients should undergo a complete staging work-up before treatment is initiated if time permits, which is usually the case. For patients with lymphoma, chemotherapy is the treatment of choice. It provides both local and systemic therapeutic activity. Local consolidation with radiotherapy may be beneficial in patients with bulky mediastinal disease (> 10 cm or > one-third the diameter of the chest on chest radiograph). In this setting, radiation is used to treat the obstruction of the superior vena cava; chemotherapy follows and is used to treat systemic disease. Chemotherapy alone is mandated if the patient has already undergone previous mediastinal radiation. Most patients achieve complete relief of symptoms within 2 weeks after beginning treatment.

Thrombus. If obstruction is caused by a thrombus, fibrinolytic therapy with urokinase, streptokinase, or recombinant tissue-type plasminogen activator (tPA, a highly selective fibrinolytic agent) is a common intervention. Another alternative is to remove the catheter that induced thrombus formation with simultaneous anticoagulant therapy to prevent embolization. Surgical removal of a thrombus (mechanical thrombectomy) is rare.

Thrombolytic therapy is limited to catheter-induced SVCS. Urokinase is administered as a continuous infusion, with a bolus dose of 4400 U/kg followed by 4400 U/kg/hr directly into the thrombosis. A mean of 26 hours is required to dissolve a clot. A response rate of 73% is reported if the urokinase infusion is started within 5 days of clot formation. It is important to begin thrombolytic therapy early in the obstructive process. A delay in administering therapy beyond 5 days of symptom onset is associated with treatment failure. Urokinase is more effective than streptokinase without the pyrogenic and allergic reactions of the latter. Tissue-type plasminogen activator (alteplase, Activase) has been used recently with great success. It has selective action on a clot and can be used safely when thrombolytic therapy is administered systemically. tPA is administered as a continuous infusion. The total dose (1.25 mg/kg) is administered over 3 hours; 60% is given in the first hour and the remaining 40% over 2 hours. Compared with urokinase, tPA is less likely to cause hemorrhagic complications, has a shorter time to clot lysis, and is more likely to dissolve a clot formed more than 5 days before the start of the infusion. These advantages must be balanced against the added cost of tPA.

Patients receiving either urokinase or tPA are monitored closely for bleeding complications. Vital signs are monitored every 15 minutes for the first hour, then every 30–60 minutes for the duration of the infusion, depending on the clinical situation. Monitoring for bleeding complications should continue beyond the discontinuation of thrombolytic therapy because the effects of these agents last for several hours. Any thrombolytic agent must be administered with an infusion pump. No other invasive monitoring is necessary.

In addition to the thrombolytic agent, patients also receive a heparin infusion and are converted to an oral anticoagulant before discharge. The patient must be educated about discharge medications and periodic laboratory studies (protime measurement). As always, thrombolytic therapy is contraindicated in patients with cerebral metastases or those at risk for intracranial hemorrhage. Compression of the superior vena cava by tumor or adenopathy can be complicated by a secondary thrombosis. Venous stasis distal to the obstruction may allow a clot to form. For this reason, heparin or oral anticoagulants may be used to reduce the extent of thrombus formation and prevent progression.

15. What is the role of surgery in the treatment of SVCS?

Surgery is rarely needed for malignant SVCS. It is considered when the obstructive process progresses rapidly. In general, surgery is reserved for patients with chronic or recurrent SVCS who have a good prognosis and in whom all other treatment options have been exhausted. There are two types of surgical procedures:

1. Superior vena cava bypass graft—creates a new vessel that circumvents the obstruction.

2. Stent placement—inserted into the superior vena cava to dilate and expand the narrowed lumen of vessel; provides immediate relief of symptoms for both malignant and benign causes. Complications include stent migration, misplacement, and occlusion.

16. Discuss the morbidity and mortality associated with surgery for SVCS.

Surgical intervention has been shown to be an effective technique for the handful of patients reported in the literature. All patients had immediate relief of symptoms. At long-term follow-up, 80% of bypass grafts remained patent up to 15 years, and the majority of patients were symptom-free. There were no reports of operative mortality. It must be remembered that surgery is a rare intervention done only in highly selective situations.

17. Are there alternatives to surgery in these select situations?

The most effective alternative is transluminal angioplasty using a balloon technique similar to that used for cardiac vessel disease, with insertion of expandable wire stents through the angioplasty device. If a thrombus is causing the obstruction, thrombolytic therapy may be administered directly to the clot via the angioplasty device.

18. What are the major differences in presentation and behavior between superior vena cava caused by benign and malignant causes?

Patients who present with a benign obstruction of the superior vena cava often have symptoms long before seeking medical advice. Short duration of symptoms (3–4 weeks) usually indicates malignancy. It often takes more time to establish the diagnosis of benign SVCS, but survival is markedly longer for a nonmalignant etiology.

19. Do steroids have a role in the treatment of SVCS?
The role of steroids is controversial. An inflammatory reaction is usually not associated with SVCS. Steroids are probably indicated when respiratory distress is present.

20. What is the role of radiation therapy?
Radiation therapy is the initial treatment of choice when the histologic diagnosis cannot be established and the patient's clinical status is deteriorating. This situation, however, is exceedingly rare. In a true emergency, the bronchus is likely to be obstructed. Other critical structures, including the esophagus, trachea, vocal cords, and pericardium, may be involved. The total dose of radiation ranges from 3,000–5,000 cGy, depending on the underlying malignancy. Initially, 2–4 large daily fractions (300–400 cGy) are followed by conventional fractionation (180–200 cG/day). The radiation field includes gross tumor with appropriate margins plus mediastinal, hilar, and supraclavicular lymph nodes. Usually improvement is seen within a week or sooner. More rapid responses are seen with non-Hodgkin's lymphoma than with small cell carcinoma. Clinical improvement may be due to development of collateral circulation in addition to decreased obstruction of the superior vena cava by a smaller tumor mass.

21. What important nursing interventions are involved in the care of patients with SVCS?
1. **Maintain airway patency.** Bedrest with the head of the bed elevated (Fowler's position) plus use of supplemental oxygen may temporarily relieve dyspnea and other symptoms caused by decreased cardiac output and increased venous pressure. Assistance with activities of daily living is also recommended to decrease energy expenditure.

2. **Monitor fluid and electrolyte balance.** Overhydration may exacerbate symptoms of SVCS. Although diuretic therapy and reduced salt diets have been used to decrease edema, their efficacy has not been demonstrated. Conversely, dehydration and the associated increased risk of thrombosis should not be ignored.

3. **Monitor vital signs and level of consciousness.** The patient should be observed for respiratory stridor and changes in mental status. Respiratory and neurologic changes may signal onset of a true emergency (from extension of thromboses to cerebral veins).

4. **Avoid accessing veins of involved extremity** (usually the right arm) because of the risk of poor circulation, venous stasis, phlebitis, thrombosis, and hemorrhage. Postprocedural bleeding as a result of venous engorgement is a major concern. If chemotherapy is administered, decreased circulation may result in local accumulation of drug with poor absorption into the systemic circulation. This tendency is of particular concern when vesicant or irritant drugs are used. The safety of administering chemotherapy into the peripheral veins of lower extremities is controversial. Therefore, surgical cannulation of the femoral vein with a Broviac or Hickman-type catheter is recommended.

5. **Avoid invasive or constrictive procedures of the involved extremity.** Rings and restrictive clothing should be removed. Blood pressure measurement can be done on the thigh. Venipunctures can be done on the lower extremities.

6. **Reduce anxiety.** A calm, restful environment with visible support is helpful. Analgesics and tranquilizers may be administered for discomfort and anxiety. Interventions to avoid the Valsalva maneuver (e.g., stool softeners, cough suppressants) may be indicated to keep intrathoracic pressure as low as possible.

7. **Assist with medical intervention.** Coagulation profiles should be monitored if anticoagulants are used. Emergent treatment must be instituted for symptoms of cerebral edema, decreased cardiac output, or airway obstruction.

8. **Assess teaching needs.** For some patients, malignancy is diagnosed after the onset and diagnosis of SVCS. Such patients must deal with the emergency of SVCS as well as the unexpected diagnosis of malignancy and need teaching related to the disease process, treatment of

SVCS, treatment of the malignancy, and body image changes. The nurse should stress that changes in physical appearance are temporary; body image changes secondary to facial edema and plethora subside with successful treatment.

9. **Treat side effects related to therapy.** For most patients with SVCS, chemotherapy or radiation therapy is used to treat the underlying malignancy. Radiation side effects may include skin reactions, dysphagia, esophagitis, dry cough, nausea, vomiting, and fatigue. Chemotherapy has its own set of side effects and toxicities, depending on the specific agents used.

22. What is the overall prognosis?

For untreated malignant SVCS, survival is often less than 6 weeks. With treatment, survival depends on responsiveness of the underlying malignancy to treatment. The prognosis for lymphoma is better than that for lung cancer.

23. What is the risk of recurrence after successful treatment of SVCS?

Recurrence is rare in patients with non-Hodgkin's lymphoma; unfortunately, it is more common with small cell carcinoma of the lung.

24. What follow-up care is required after resolution of SVCS?

Routine follow-up care provided for the oncology patient is sufficient. No long-term special care is needed after resolution of symptoms.

ACKNOWLEDGMENT

The author acknowledges with thanks the contributions of David H. Garfield, MD, and Jeanne Currey, RN, MS, in their review of this manuscript.

BIBLIOGRAPHY

1. Abner A: Approach to the patient who presents with superior vena cava obstruction. Chest 103:394S–397S, 1993.
2. Ahmann FR: A reassessment of the clinical implications of the superior vena cava syndrome. J Clin Oncol 2:961–969, 1984.
3. Baker GL, Barnes HJ: Superior vena cava syndrome: Etiology, diagnosis, and treatment. Am J Crit Care 1:54–64, 1992.
4. Dietz KA, Flaherty AM: Oncologic emergencies. In Groenwald SL, Frogge MH, Goodman M, Yarbro CH (eds): Cancer Nursing Principles and Practice, 3rd ed. Boston, Jones & Bartlett, 1993.
5. Escalante CP: Causes and management of superior vena cava syndrome. Oncology 7(6):61–68; discussion, 71–72, 75–77, 1993.
6. Gray BH, Olin JW, Graor RA, et al: Safety and efficacy of thrombolytic therapy for superior vena cava syndrome. Chest 99:54–59, 1991.
7. Greenberg S, Kosinski R, Daniels J: Treatment of superior vena cava thrombosis with recombinant tissue type plasminogen activator. Chest 99:1298–1301, 1991.
8. Rantis PC, Littooy FN: Successful treatment of prolonged superior vena cava syndrome with thrombolytic therapy: A case report. J Vasc Surg 20:108–113, 1994.
9. Yahalom J: Oncologic emergencies: Superior vena cava syndrome. In DeVita V, et. al. (eds): Cancer: Principles & Practice of Oncology, 4th ed. Philadelphia, J.B. Lippincott, 1993.

51. SYNDROME OF INAPPROPRIATE ANTIDIURETIC HORMONE

Leigh K. Kaszyk, RN, MS

1. What is the syndrome of inappropriate antidiuretic hormone (SIADH)?

SIADH is a syndrome of hyponatremia due to abnormal secretion or production of antidiuretic hormone (ADH). ADH levels are inappropriate for the osmotic or volume stimuli that normally cause release of ADH. Despite a normal intravascular volume, the urine osmolality is inappropriately high (concentrated) compared to the plasma osmolality. ADH causes water retention, which leads to decreased sodium and inability to excrete dilute urine. Cancers, particularly small-cell lung cancer, are the most common causes of SIADH.

2. What pathophysiologic mechanisms maintain normal plasma osmolality and plasma sodium concentrations?

1. Antidiuretic hormone (ADH), also known as vasopressin, helps to conserve water. ADH is secreted by the posterior pituitary in response to hypotension, decreased fluid intake, and blood loss.

2. Thirst mechanism is activated by osmoreceptors located in the hypothalamus in response to dry mouth, hyperosmolality, and plasma volume depletion. A water loss of 2% of body weight or increase in osmolality results in thirst mechanism activation.

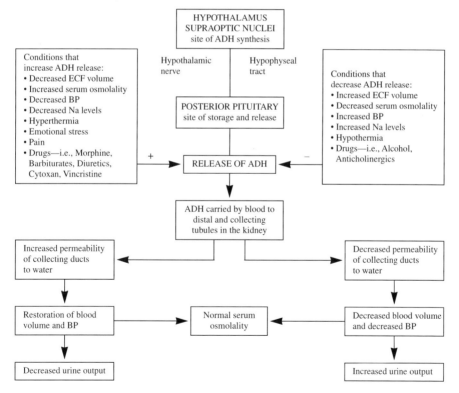

Mechanisms of ADH release. (From Poe CM, Taylor LM: Syndrome of inappropriate antidiuretic hormone: Assessment and nursing implications. Oncol Nurs Forum 16:373–381, 1989, with permission.)

3. How does ADH affect the body?

When blood levels of ADH increase, the epithelium of the cortical collecting ducts of the kidneys becomes water-permeable. As a result, water enters the extracellular fluid through osmosis, less water is excreted, and urine osmolality increases.

4. What are the causes of SIADH?

Any patient presenting with symptoms of SIADH without a known cause should have a complete malignancy work-up; 60% of patients with SIADH are diagnosed with cancer. Only 1–2% of patients with cancer, however, develop SIADH. The most common malignancy causing SIADH is lung cancer. Up to 15% of patients with small cell lung cancer have SIADH at presentation, and ADH levels are increased in 50% of the cases.

Causes of SIADH

Malignant tumors	Central nervous system disorders
Lung cancer	Trauma
Thymoma	Stroke
Mesothelioma	Infection
Prostate cancer	**General surgery**
Lymphomas	**Pharmaceutical agents**
Hodgkin's disease	Cytotoxic agents
Gastrointestinal cancers	Vinca alkaloids
Pulmonary disease	Cisplatin
Acute respiratory failure	Cylcophosphamide
Tuberculosis	Tricyclic antidepressants
Positive pressure ventilation	Morphine

5. Why do people with cancer develop SIADH?

SIADH most often results from ectopic production of ADH by the tumor. People with cancer often receive drugs such as cytotoxic agents, morphine, and tricyclic antidepressants, which release or potentiate the action of ADH. In addition, certain lung conditions that patients with cancer often develop (e.g., pneumonia, empyema) may result in SIADH.

6. What other pathophysiologic mechanisms are responsible for SIADH?

One pathologic mechanism is inappropriate secretion of ADH from the supraoptic hypophyseal system. This mechanism is seen in postoperative patients and patients with central nervous system disorders, shock, positive pressure ventilation, or other conditions that increase intrathoracic pressure or decrease venous return (e.g., intrathoracic tumors).

7. What is the cause of SIADH in patients infected with the human immunodeficiency virus (HIV)?

The majority of HIV-infected patients with SIADH have *Pneumocystis carinii* or bacterial pneumonia. Other diagnoses include central nervous system infections or malignant disorders.

8. What other factors contribute to the development of SIADH in patients with cancer?

- Chemotherapy with or without hydration due to water-retaining properties of agents (e.g, cisplatin) in combination with vigorous hydration.
- Nausea (common side effect of chemotherapy) stimulates ADH release.
- Tricyclic antidepressants may potentiate the action of ADH.
- Narcotics for pain relief may enhance ADH secretion or its effect on the distal nephron.

9. How is SIADH diagnosed?

First the patient must be assessed clinically (history and physical exam) to determine whether the patient's intravascular volume status is normal, low, or expanded. If low, the patient's volume status must be corrected. Then blood and urine specimens for sodium and osmolality are obtained. The patient has SIADH if the intravascular volume is normal or increased; urine osmolality is high compared with plasma osmolality; and renal, thyroid, and adrenal function are normal.

10. Which laboratory values should the nurse be concerned about in patients with SIADH?

SIADH levels	Normal levels
Hyponatremia (< 130 mEq/L)	135–145 mEq/L
Low serum osmolality (< 280 mOsm/kg)	280–300 mOsm/kg
High urine sodium level (> 20 mEq/L)	40–220 mmol/d
High urine osmolality (> 1000 mOsm/kg)	200–800 mOsm/kg
Low blood urea nitrogen (BUN)	6–23 mg/dl

11. What are the clinical symptoms of SIADH?

Signs and symptoms are a reflection of water intoxication.

Mild hyponatremia	Fatigue
(sodium level: 115–130 mEq/L)	Anorexia
	Nausea/vomiting
	Thirst
	Diarrhea
	Headaches
Severe hyponatremia	Altered mental status
(sodium level: 100–110 mEq/L)	Confusion, personality changes
	Lethargy, weakness
	Psychosis
	Seizures
	Coma

12. What are the goals of treatment of SIADH?

Primary treatment of SIADH in patients with cancer is treatment of the underlying tumor with systemic chemotherapy. Initial interventions are aimed at correcting the sodium–water imbalance.

13. How are symptomatic patients treated until the tumor is affected by chemotherapy?

Symptomatic treatment consists of restriction of fluids to 500–1,000 ml/day. In the presence of life-threatening hyponatremia, an intravenous solution of 3% hypertonic saline and furosemide is administered. Care must be taken not to increase the serum sodium level too quickly, or neuronal damage may result, causing cerebral edema and seizures.

14. What fluids with a high sodium concentration may be offered to a patient with SIADH?

Tomato juice, V-8 juice, beef or chicken broth, Gatorade.

15. What is done for patients with chronic or recurrent SIADH despite chemotherapy?

Chronic or recurrent SIADH is treated with drugs that inhibit secretion of renal effects of ADH. Demeclocycline is most widely used. It may take 5–7 days after initiation of treatment for symptoms to decrease. Demeclocycline is given orally in a dose of 900–1200 mg/day. This tetracycline derivative interferes with ADH action, causing isotonic or hypotonic urine and an increase in serum sodium. Absorption may be impaired if the drug is taken with milk or milk products. Side effects include photosensitivity, hematologic changes, azotemia, super infection, and mild nephrotoxicity.

16. Does recurrent SIADH mean that the cancer is returning?

Not always. SIADH usually resolves once the cancer is treated. However, it may return during stable disease while the patient is receiving maintenance chemotherapy. Nurses need to be aware of the patient population at risk for developing SIADH. Involving patients in the management of SIADH is critical in reversing symptoms.

BIBLIOGRAPHY

1. Glover DJ, Glick JH: Metabolic Oncologic Emergencies. Cancer J Clin 37:302–317, 1987.
2. Groenwald SL, Frogge HH, Goodman H, Yarbro CH (eds): Cancer Nursing: Principles and Practice, 3rd ed. Boston, Jones & Barlett, 1995.
3. Kovacs L, Robertson GL: Syndrome of inappropriate antidiuresis. Endocrinol Metab Clin North Am 21:859–875, 1992.
4. Moses AM, Streeter DHP: Disorders of the neurophysis. In Isselbacker KJ, Breunwold E, Wilson JD, et al (eds): Harrison's Principles of Internal Medicine, 13th ed., vol. 2. New York, McGraw-Hill, 1994.
5. Otto S: Oncology Nursing. St. Louis, Mosby, 1991.
6. Poe CM, Taylor LM: Syndrome of inappropriate antidiuretic hormone: Assessment and nursing implications. Oncol Nurs Forum 16:373–381, 1989.
7. Sorensen JD, Andersen MK, Hansen HH: Syndrome of inappropriate secretion of antidiuretic hormone (SIADH) in malignant disease. J Intern Med 238: 97–110, 1995.
8. Tank WW, Kaptien EM, Feinstein EI, Massry SG: Hyponatremia in hospitalized patients with the acquired immunodeficiency syndrome (AIDS) and the AIDS-related complex. Am J Med 94:169–174, 1993.
9. Wallach PM, Flannery MT, Stewart JM: Paraneoplastic syndromes for the primary care physicians. Prim Care 19: 727–745, 1992.

52. TUMOR LYSIS SYNDROME

Anne Zobec, MS, RN, CS, ANP, AOCN

1. What is tumor lysis syndrome?

Tumor lysis syndrome (TLS) is usually a complication of cancer therapy that occurs when a large number of tumor cells are destroyed. It occurs during aggressive treatment of large, rapidly dividing tumors.

2. Describe what happens in TLS.

Chemotherapy given to fast-growing tumors causes massive necrosis of cancer cells. As tumor cells die, they release cellular contents into the bloodstream. When the cell membrane is ruptured, nucleic acids that form DNA and RNA are released along with potassium and phosphorus. The nucleic acids are converted by the liver into uric acid. Abnormally high levels of uric acid, potassium, and phosphorus cause a host of metabolic alterations.

3. What are the harmful effects of TLS?

The high levels of intracellular contents that are liberated from the tumor cells overwhelm the kidneys. High levels of uric acid may crystallize in the distal tubules and collecting ducts, leading to obstructions and eventually acute renal failure. Increased levels of potassium and phosphorus may cause cardiac, neurologic, and gastrointestinal toxicities.

Clinical Manifestations of Tumor Lysis Syndrome

Renal problems	Neuromuscular irritability	
Decreased urine output	Tetany	
Elevated BUN and serum creatinine	Carpopedal spasm	
Elevated serum uric acid	Muscle cramps	
Uric acid crystallization in renal tubules	Confusion, delirium, or hallucination	
Acute renal failure	Seizures	
	Digital and perioral paresthesias	
Cardiac arrhythmias	**Gastrointestinal effects**	
AV blocks	Nausea and	Anorexia
Ventricular tachycardia	vomiting	Intestinal colic
Cardiac arrest	Diarrhea	Hyperphosphatemia

4. Are there certain kinds of cancers in which TLS is more common?

TLS is seen most often in patients with high-grade lymphoma or acute lymphoblastic leukemia. It also occurs in patients with acute myelogenous leukemia, chronic myelogenous leukemia in blastic transformation, Burkitt's lymphoma, and non-Hodgkin's lymphoma. These kinds of cancers have a high growth fraction; that is, they multiply and grow very quickly. Tumors with rapid growth rates are highly sensitive to the effects of chemotherapy drugs. When treatment begins, the tumor cells are rapidly destroyed.

5. Does TLS present in patients with solid tumors?

TLS is rare in patients with solid tumors because they respond more slowly to chemotherapy. It has been seen in small cell lung cancer, metastatic breast cancer, and metastatic medulloblastoma.

6. Can TLS occur in patients who are not treated with chemotherapy?

TLS occasionally occurs with radiation therapy. In untreated patients with cancer, TLS may develop if a rapidly growing large tumor mass undergoes profound cell destruction. This syndrome has also been reported in patients receiving corticosteroids and alpha-interferon.

7. What are the identifying laboratory features of patients at risk for TLS?

Patients with elevated levels of blood urea nitrogen (BUN), creatinine, uric acid, and electrolytes before treatment are at a greater risk of developing TLS. These abnormal laboratory studies indicate that the patient may have problems with renal function or dehydration. Patients with increased levels of lactate dehydrogenase (LDH) are also at a greater risk for TLS. LDH levels are correlated with large tumor masses.

8. What are the most common metabolic abnormalities in TLS?

The four hallmark signs of TLS are hyperuricemia, hyperphosphatemia, hyperkalemia, and hypocalcemia. These abnormalities result when the kidneys are unable to process and excrete the huge amount of intracellular products and metabolites that are released when the tumor cells are destroyed.

9. What contributes to a decrease in uric acid excretion?

Uric acid is not excreted well in the following situations: low urinary flow rate in the 24 hours before treatment, history of hyperuricemia or renal failure, renal insufficiency, dehydration, and acidic urine.

10. When does TLS occur?

TLS develops within hours to a few days after treatment. It most often occurs within the first 24–72 hours after chemotherapy is initiated. TLS may persist for 5–7 days after therapy; this is the period when the most significant tumor cell destruction occurs.

11. What are the goals of treatment of TLS?

The primary goal of TLS management is prevention of renal failure and severe electrolyte imbalances. This goal is accomplished by increasing urine production, decreasing uric acid concentrations, and increasing the solubility of uric acid in urine.

12. Can TLS be prevented?

Yes. When patients are identified as being at high risk for developing TLS, special treatments can be initiated to prevent its development. Preventive measures should be started before chemotherapy is initiated and continued for at least 7 days after chemotherapy. Being alert for early symptoms and close monitoring of laboratory values can reduce the risk of TLS.

13. Describe the important treatment strategies.

Prevention is the best strategy. The medical management of TLS includes adequate hydration, forced diuresis, alkalinization of urine, administration of allopurinol, and treatment of metabolic alterations. Dialysis may be necessary in severe cases.

14. What is the role of allopurinol in TLS?

All patients at risk for TLS are treated with allopurinol before and during initial chemotherapy. Allopurinol decreases uric acid concentration; it inhibits the enzyme xanthine oxidase, which, in turn, blocks the conversion of uric acid precursors into uric acid and prevents uric acid nephropathy. Allopurinol reduces both serum and urine levels of uric acid. Remember to stop allopurinol when it is no longer needed because it can sometimes cause drug fever.

15. Why is alkalinization of the urine important?

Uric acid is only slightly soluble in acid urine, but it is much more soluble (> 10 times) in alkaline urine. When the urine is acidic, high levels of uric acid form crystals in the tubules of the kidneys. To prevent crystallization, intravenous fluids are given to hydrate the patient and to increase the amount of fluids flowing through the kidneys. Sodium bicarbonate is frequently added to the intravenous fluids to create alkaline urine (50 mEq sodium bicarbonate to each liter of intravenous fluid). Urine pH values are obtained and should be kept at a level > 7.0.

16. Describe the most important nursing interventions.

Nursing care should focus on prevention and management of symptoms that are caused by metabolic disturbances. Nursing assessment should center on the symptoms of hyperkalemia, hypocalcemia, and hyperphosphatemia. Hyperkalemia results in cardiovascular change that may lead to atrioventricular block, ventricular tachycardia, ventricular fibrillation, or asystole. Neuromuscular effects of hyperkalemia include muscle weakness and paresthesia. Gastrointestinal effects are nausea, diarrhea, and intestinal colic. Symptoms of hypocalcemia include ventricular arrhythmias, 2:1 heart block, and cardiac arrest. Neurologic symptoms include muscle cramping and twitching, carpedal spasms, tetany, laryngospasm, paresthesia, confusion, delirium, and convulsions. Hyperphosphatemia primarily causes renal problems: anuria, oliguria, and azotemia.

17. What simple assessment tests can be done to detect a low calcium level?

Low levels of serum calcium cause neuromuscular irritability. A low calcium level can be detected by Chvostek's and Trousseau's signs. Chvostek's sign is tested by lightly tapping the facial nerve area below the zygomatic process in front of the ear. A positive response (low calcium level) is indicated if the facial muscles and upper lip contract or twitch. Trousseau's sign is tested by inflating a blood pressure cuff to a level slightly above the patient's systolic blood pressure for 1–3 minutes. The sign is considered positive if contractions of the hand result.

18. How is hyperkalemia treated?

Hyperkalemia can be treated with oral Kayexalate, 15–30 gm, with 50 ml of 20% sorbitol given 2–4 times daily. Kayexalate also can be given rectally in enema form, if the patient cannot take oral medications. Fifty grams of Kayexalate in 200 ml of 20% sorbitol is given as a retention enema and held for 30–60 minutes.

19. What is significant about the patient's fluid level?

Maintaining optimal fluid balance is crucial to the patient's recovery. Intravenous fluids are frequently given at rates of 150–300 cc/hr to ensure that the patient is well hydrated. Hourly assessments of urine output are essential in evaluating kidney function. Nurses should be aware that fluid volume overload may occur. Monitoring the blood pressure and pulse at least every 4 hours, auscultating lung sounds, watching for signs of edema and cough, and checking the patient's weight every 12–24 hours can demonstrate early signs of fluid overload.

20. What is the treatment for an elevated phosphate level?

Phosphate-binding antacids, such as Amphojel or Basaljel given orally in doses of 30–60 ml every 4–6 hours, reduce the serum phosphate level. These antacids may cause constipation, however; thus, stool softeners may be advised.

21. Which medicines should be avoided in patients at risk of TLS?

Aspirin, radiographic contrast, probenecid, and thiazide diuretics should be avoided because they block tubular reabsorption of uric acid. Phosphate and potassium-containing medications also should be avoided.

BIBLIOGRAPHY

1. Groenwald D, Frogge M, Goodman M, Yarbro CH: Cancer Nursing: Principles and Practice, 4th ed. Boston, Jones & Bartlett, 1997.
2. Hussein AM, Feun LG: Tumor lysis syndrome after induction chemotherapy in small cell lung carcinoma. Am J Clin Oncol 13:10–13, 1990.
3. Nance CS, Nance GS: Acute tumor lysis syndrome: Pathophysiology and nursing management. Crit Care Nurs 5(3):26–34, 1985.
4. Sparano J, Ramirez M, Wiernik P: Increasing recognition of corticosteroid-induced tumor lysis syndrome in non-Hodgkin's lymphoma. Cancer 65:1072–1073, 1990.
5. Stucky LA: Acute Tumor lysis syndrome: Assessment and nursing implications. Oncol Nurs Forum 20:49–59, 1993.

VII. Caring for the Person with Cancer

53. VASCULAR ACCESS DEVICES

Charlene Berlam, RN, MS, ANP, OCN

1. What is a central line?

A central line, commonly called a vascular access device (VAD) or central venous catheter (CVC), is a temporary or long-term intravenous catheter inserted into one of the major veins of the neck or chest (subclavian, internal or external jugular) or peripherally through the brachial or cephalic vein. The distal tip of a central line terminates in or near the superior vena cava, just above the right atrium. The femoral venous system (leading to the proximal inferior vena cava) may be used if the superior vena cava cannot be catheterized.

2. How soon can a CVC be used after placement?

The central line may be used after the position of the catheter in the superior vena cava is confirmed by fluoroscopy or radiography. Ports may be used immediately after placement, perhaps even accessed during surgery. Some surgeons may request that the port not be accessed until postoperative swelling has decreased.

3. What is the advantage of a central line?

- The high blood flow of the vena cava promotes rapid dilution of intravenous (IV) fluids and concentrated solutions, thereby preventing an inflammatory response and the rapid thrombosis that occurs in smaller peripheral veins.
- A central line provides more stable access to the venous system, decreasing the risk of infiltration and tissue damage when irritating agents are administered.
- Central lines are capable of infusing incompatible solutions at the same time, through two or more separate lumens.
- CVCs shorten hospital stays by providing access for therapy in an outpatient setting.
- Central venous access also may be used to overcome physical or psychological factors associated with repeated venipuncture.

4. What are central lines used for?

CVCs can be used for administration of intravenous drug solutions, blood products, and total parenteral nutrition as well as for blood sampling. They also can be used for measurement of central venous or pulmonary capillary wedge pressure and determination of cardiac output. Central lines are commonly inserted in patients with human immunodeficiency virus (HIV), cancer, sickle cell disease, burns, Crohn's disease, endocarditis, osteomyelitis, or any illness requiring intensive care.

5. What materials are used to make central lines?

Central lines are made of several different materials, including polyethylene, polyvinyl chloride, polyurethane, and silicone. The stiffer nature of polyethylene and polyvinyl chloride catheters allows easier insertion but also may damage the tunica intima, leading to platelet aggregation and thrombus formation. Silicone is biocompatible, extremely soft and pliable, inexpensive, and hydrophobic (offers protection from bacterial growth). Silicone, however, is associated with a high degree of thrombogenicity. Polyurethane catheters are indicated for short-term use and placed percutaneously; they are stronger than silicone but become softer and longer after insertion when warmed by blood.

Newer catheters, such as hydromer-coated polyurethane, have higher success rates on insertion and are designed to prevent bacterial growth and adherence (more common on rougher surfaces) as well as platelet deposition and aggregation.

6. What are the different types of central lines?

Nontunneled catheters, available with 1–3 lumens, are easily placed, with an insertion cost of roughly $500. They are the most commonly used central line but are associated with the highest incidence of catheter-related infections. Disadvantages include daily flushing, routine sterile dressing changes, and restrictions on activities such as swimming, contact sports, and rough play for adolescents or children. Optional features include heparin, antibiotic, or antiseptic coatings along the catheter and addition of a Dacron cuff.

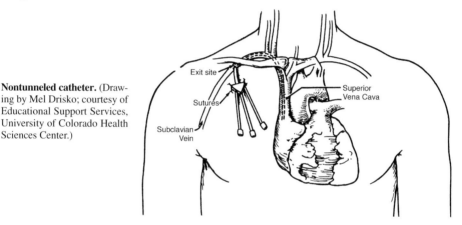

Nontunneled catheter. (Drawing by Mel Drisko; courtesy of Educational Support Services, University of Colorado Health Sciences Center.)

Tunneled catheters (Hickman, Broviac, Leonard, and Groshong) are indicated for long-term therapy (more than several months). Single-, double-, and triple-lumen catheters are available. Insertion costs are high (approximately $2500–3000) if anesthesia and the operating room are used; however, most tunneled catheters can be placed safely under fluoroscopy in the radiology department or other clinical areas. CVCs may be placed with minimal risk of catheter infections

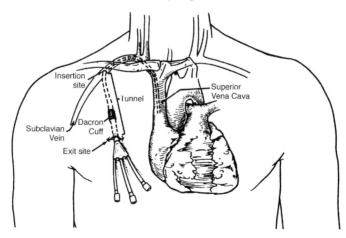

Tunneled catheter. (Drawing by Mel Drisko; courtesy of Educational Support Services, University of Colorado Health Sciences Center.)

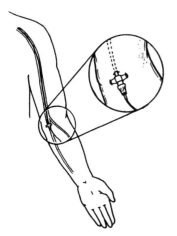

Peripherally inserted central catheter.
(Drawing by Mel Drisko; courtesy of
Educational Support Services, University
of Colorado Health Sciences Center.)

outside the operating room if maximal barrier precautions are used (e.g., sterile gloves, gown, drape, masks). After insertion in a central vein, the catheter is tunneled several centimeters under the skin and brought out through the skin to a suitable exit site (anterior chest between the sternum and nipple, upper abdominal wall). Unlike most nontunneled catheters, the subcutaneous portion of the tunneled catheter includes a Dacron cuff that adheres to scar tissue, forming an internal anchor and barrier against the inward spread of microorganisms. A second antimicrobial cuff also may be present (e.g., Vita Cuff, which releases silver ions as a deterrent to infection). The tunneling of the catheter offers the theoretical advantage of reducing the rate of infection, although recent studies reported no difference in rates of infection in tunneled vs. nontunneled catheters. Disadvantages include site care with dressing changes for the first few weeks, activity restrictions, and regular flushing. Once the exit site of a tunneled catheter has healed (approximately 3–4 weeks), the sterile dressing change is modified to a clean technique, which decreases cost and time.

Peripherally inserted central catheters (PICCs) are generally indicated for short-term use (weeks to a few months); however, some catheters have successfully remained in place over 300 days. Insertion costs are lowest (about $300) of all CVCs. They are easily placed by a trained nurse or physician into the cephalic or basilic veins of the antecubital space and are available with one or two lumens. Advantages include reduced insertions risks (e.g., pneumothorax) and decreased rates of infection in comparison with other nontunneled CVCs. Disadvantages include daily flushing (weekly for the Groshong PICC), sterile dressing changes, and activity restrictions. Self-care may be difficult or impossible because the patient is required to change the dressing and flush the catheter with one hand.

Implanted ports (e.g., Mediport, Portacath, Infusaport, Cathlink) are made of stainless steel, titanium, or plastic. They are indicated for long-term use. Port implantation is usually done in the operating room at costs similar to those for tunneled catheters. Single- or double-lumen and low-profile (preferable in thin patients) ports are available. Ports are implanted entirely under

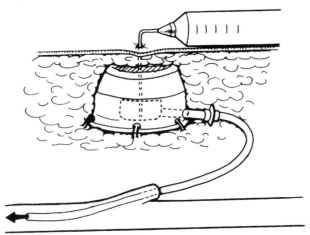

Implanted port. (Drawing by Mel Drisko; courtesy of Educational Support Services, University of Colorado Health Sciences Center.)

the subcutaneous tissue and attached to a catheter that is threaded into the SVC. Smaller ports also may be implanted peripherally, like a PICC, in the forearm with the catheter threaded into the SVC. Advantages of the port include minimal site care with no dressing when not accessed and infrequent flushing (once per month when not accessed), which may decrease costs and infection rates. Many patients prefer ports because they preserve bodily image and require no restrictions on activities, such as bathing or swimming. Disadvantages include discomfort related to accessing the port with a noncoring needle, and the need for a surgical procedure for removal when the port is no longer needed or becomes infected.

7. How is a Groshong catheter different from other catheters?

A Groshong catheter is a silastic catheter with a two-way valve at the tip; infusion of fluid opens the valve outward, and aspiration of blood opens the valve inward. When not in use, the pressure-sensitive two-way valve remains closed to prevent back flow of blood or air into the catheter. The closed valve results in a potentially lower incidence of fibrin sheath formation and eliminates the need to clamp the catheter when injection caps are removed. Groshong valves are available for tunneled catheters, PICC lines and implanted ports. Because blood clotting may be of less concern, normal saline is used instead of heparin for flushing; however, there is no incompatibility between heparin and the material used to make Groshong catheters.

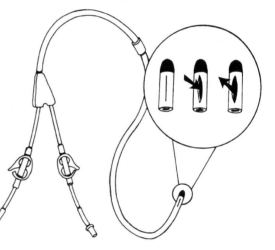

Groshong catheter and valves. (Drawing by Mel Drisko; courtesy of Educational Support Services, University of Colorado Health Sciences Center.)

8. How is a central line selected?

The choice depends on many factors, including:

- Costs
- Length of therapy
- Treatment schedule (daily, continuous, intermittent)
- Type of drug or fluids to be infused (vesicant)
- Frequency of blood tests

- Benefits and risks
- Patient preference (cosmetic appearance, activity/work limitations, anxiety associated with needlesticks)
- Site care and flushing requirements
- Capability of patient or significant other to care for a central line at home

9. What are the insertion risks when a central line is placed?

Risks involved with insertion of central lines include:

- Bleeding and hematoma
- Malpositioned tips and migration
- Pneumothorax

- Air embolus
- Nerve injury
- Dysrhythmias

Rare complications of PICC placement are nerve injury and arterial puncture, most commonly of the ulnar artery.

10. The nurse observes bloody drainage at the insertion site of a newly placed central line. Is this a worrisome finding?

It is common for blood to saturate the dressing of a new exit site. Patients with a low platelet count should be monitored for increased bleeding, and bloody dressings should be changed as frequently as needed to prevent infection. Application of manual pressure or use of a sandbag helps to prevent development of a hematoma.

11. What are the signs and symptoms of malpositioned tips?

Malpositioned tips are common and may be especially problematic with PICCs (4–38%). Catheters may be coiled in the superior vena cava, malpositioned in the jugular vein when the basilic vein is used, or malpositioned in the axillary vein when the cephalic vein is used. In general, malpositioned catheters need to be removed and replaced. One may first try to reposition the catheter by guidewire under fluoroscopy, snare manipulation from a femoral vein, or rapid jet injection with normal saline.

Site of Malpositioned Catheter	Symptoms
Internal jugular (ipsilateral or contralateral)	Sensation of ear gurgling, headache, swelling or neck pain
Axillary vein	Hand and arm swelling, with arm and shoulder pain
Azygos vein	Vague back discomfort
Innominate or contralateral subclavian	Shoulder pain or swelling of contralateral arm
Internal thoracic	Anterior chest pain or tenderness
Right atrium or ventricle	Thrombosis, arrhythmia, or perforation, of catheter leading to pulmonary embolus

12. Should a PICC be removed for signs of phlebitis?

No. Immediate removal is not necessary. Sterile mechanical phlebitis is the most common complication of PICCs (12.5–23%), occurring within 1 week after insertion. It may be caused by trauma to the endothelial lining of the vein during insertion and consequent vasoconstriction. Powdered gloves also may irritate the vein and should be avoided. A warm pack should be applied at the first sign of reddening and swelling along the vein, palpable venous cord, skin temperature change, or tenderness. Rest, elevation of the affected arm, and nonsteroidal antiinflammatory drugs (NSAIDs) may be of benefit. If symptoms do not improve within 24 or resolve in 72 hours, the catheter may need to be removed.

13. How can the risk of malpositioned PICCs be decreased?

A newer technique, which may reduce the incidence of misplaced PICCs by up to 13%, involves pulling the guidewire back a few centimeters during insertion. This makes the tip more pliable and allows blood flow from the subclavian and jugular veins to push the tip downward into the SVC. The patient should be sitting or semireclining to take advantage of gravity while the PICC is advanced slowly. The patient's head does not need to be in any special position. The guidewire is gently reinserted, if needed, to determine placement by x-ray, provided that the guidewire tip cannot penetrate the catheter.

14. What is considered routine care and maintenance of a central line?

Routine care of a central line catheter includes cleansing the exit site, changing dressings and caps, and flushing the lumens to prevent clotting. Cleansing solutions, type of dressing, and frequency of dressing changes or flushing are controversial issues. Site care protocols vary from hospital to hospital.

Common Maintenance Procedures

VAD	DRESSING	FLUSHING[1]	CAP CHANGE[2]	BLOOD WITHDRAWAL DISCARD (ml)
Central (Subclavian)	Transparent dressing every 5–7 days; gauze dressing on alternate days or with catheter change	Heparin, 100 U/ml, 3 ml/day or 2 ml/day per each lumen	Weekly	1–2
PICC lines	24 hr after insertion, then transparent dressing every 5–7 days or gauze dressing on alternate days	Heparin, 100 U/ml, 3 ml/day or 10 U/ml, 3 ml 3 times/wk	Weekly	1–2
Tunneled	Transparent dressing every 5–7 days; gauze dressing on alternate days, then clean technique unless myelosuppressed	Heparin, 100 U/ml, 3 ml/day or every other day	Weekly	3–5
Implanted port	For continuous access, change noncoring needle and transparent dressing every week or gauze dressing on alternate days	Heparin, 100 U/ml 5 ml/month	Weekly	5
Groshong (Bard Access Systems, Salt Lake City, UT)	Transparent dressing every 5–7 days; gauze dressing on alternate days, then clean technique unless myelosuppressed	Normal saline, 5–10 ml weekly	Monthly	3–5

[1] Heparin solution may be 10 U/ml concentration.
[2] Change caps more frequently if damaged or used frequently.
From Oncology Nursing Society: Access Device Guidelines, with permission.

15. How should the exit site be cleaned?

Common features of all protocols include removal of the old dressing, inspection of the exit site for signs of infection, cleansing the skin, and covering with a sterile dressing. The site should be cleaned with an appropriate antiseptic, using friction and working outward in a circular pattern from the exit site. Hospital personnel should wear gloves when cleaning the site or changing dressings. The 1996 Centers for Disease Control (CDC) guidelines make no recommendation for use of sterile vs. nonsterile clean gloves during dressing changes. Clean technique may be used by the patient at home.

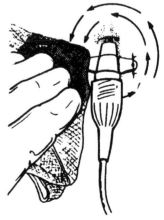

Proper technique for cleansing the exit site. (Courtesy of University Hospital Biomedical Services, Denver.)

16. What solutions or agents are recommended for cleaning the exit site?

The following antiseptic solutions are effective for skin antisepsis:

- **Isopropyl alcohol** (70%) removes skin oils and squamous skin cells and provides the most rapid and greatest reduction in microbial counts on the skin. However, it has no residual antimicrobial activity. Alcohol should be applied before iodine.
- **Povidone-iodine** (10%) or **tincture of iodine** (1–2%) should be allowed to remain on the skin for at least 2 minutes to enhance antimicrobial activity while drying. To prevent skin irritation, it may need removal with alcohol after drying. It is effective for use before catheter insertion but has not been thoroughly evaluated in decreasing catheter colonization and infection.
- **Aqueous chlorhexidine** (2%) has the advantage of residual antibacterial activity (up to 6 hours). One study showed that it was superior to alcohol or povidone-iodine in prevention of CVC infections; however, this concentration is not commercially available in the United States. A recently introduced, sustained-release chlorhexidine gluconate patch for use in dressing the catheter insertion site holds promise for decreasing VAD infections.

17. Should antimicrobial ointments be used?

The answer is not yet resolved. Iodophor ointments have been shown to be ineffective, whereas polymicrobial ointments have some benefit but may increase the frequency of candidal infection.

18. Are gauze dressings better than transparent dressings?

The answer to this question is unresolved and controversial. Some studies report no difference in infection rates between transparent and gauze dressings, whereas others show increased infection rates with the use of transparent dressings. Ideal dressings should minimize the buildup of skin microorganisms, provide protection against external contamination, keep the exit site dry, be nonirritating and easy to apply and remove, and permit convenient examination of the site.

Commonly used exit site dressings include sterile gauze and tape or transparent semipermeable coverings with or without gauze. Transparent dressings with gauze are considered equivalent to gauze dressings. A gauze and tape dressing with tape covering all edges is preferred for diaphoretic or fragile skin. Disadvantages include limited visualization of the site and an increased risk of potential contamination. Transparent dressings permit continuous inspection of the site, adhere well, provide protection against external moisture, and assist in stabilizing the catheter. In patients undergoing bone marrow transplants, transparent dressings were reported to be comfortable and more cost-effective (less nursing time and less dressing frequency) than gauze dressings. The major limitation of the transparent dressings has been moisture retention underneath the dressing, which may significantly increase colonization of the site and potentially lead to an increased risk for catheter-related infections. However, preliminary studies show that newer, moisture vapor permeable transparent dressings have colonization and infection rates similar to those of gauze dressings.

19. How often should dressings be changed?

The frequency of dressing changes is controversial and variable (see table on p. 375). Gauze and tape dressings need to be changed every 24–72 hours. Transparent dressings are usually changed every 72 hours or once a week. (It is not known how long a transparent dressing can remain safely in place.) All types of dressings should be changed after showering or when damp, loose, or soiled. Tunneled catheters may not need a dressing after several weeks of healing. In fact, no dressings have been associated with a low risk for infection, and some health care professionals prefer not to use a dressing.

20. How are central lines usually flushed?

Heparin, in concentrations varying from 10–10,000 U/ml, is the accepted flush solution for all CVCs except the Groshong, which uses saline. Frequency of flushing ranges from once per week to as often as twice per day. The Intravenous Nursing Society (INS) recommends that the flushing volume be equal to two times the internal volume of the catheter. Positive pressure should be maintained during flushing, and every effort should be made to remove blood from the injection cap. A different syringe and needle should be used for each lumen that is flushed.

21. Is saline as effective as heparin for routine flushing?

Recent studies report that 0.9% saline solution is as effective as heparin in preventing phlebitis and maintaining patency in peripheral lines; however, it is not yet routine practice to use only saline for flushing central venous catheters (CVCs). Flushing the catheter with heparin not only prevents thrombosis but also may reduce infection because thrombi and fibrin deposits are potential sites of microbial growth. CVCs are usually flushed once a day with heparin with intermittent flushes of normal saline, e.g., between antibiotics. There is a concern that even low doses (250 to 500 units) of heparin may be associated with thrombocytopenia and bleeding problems. Sodium chloride is cheaper than heparin and may cause less interference with laboratory tests. If only sodium chloride is used as a flush for central lines, there could be an increased potential for occlusion, phlebitis, and formation of small clots or fibrin strands. Low-dose warfarin, 1 mg/day orally, may be used prophylactically to decrease the incidence of thrombus.

22. Can a registered nurse remove a central line?

In accordance with hospital policy and specific State Board of Nursing Practice Acts, nurses may discontinue a central venous catheter with a physician's order. The nurse should remember the following points when removing a catheter:
- To prevent pulmonary embolus, instruct the patient to perform a Valsalva maneuver while the catheter is being withdrawn, or pull the line during expiration for patients unable to bear down.
- Because air may enter a subcutaneous tract into a vein, apply ointment and an occlusive dressing for at least 24 hours.
- Contact the physician immediately if difficulty is encountered with removing the catheter or the Dacron cuff. A cutdown procedure by the physician may be indicated to remove the cuff, particularly if a tunnel infection is suspected. A chest x-ray or venogram is recommended if there is any question about incomplete catheter removal.

23. What should be done if a PICC is resistant to removal?

Resistance to removal may be caused by thrombus, fibrin sheath, or venospasm. The following tips may facilitate removal of a resistant PICC:
- Remove the catheter at a moderate rate, using gentle traction. **Aggressive pulling is contraindicated.**
- Do not apply pressure at or near the course of the vein.
- Use warm compresses to distend the vein.
- Attempt removal again in 20–30 minutes after the spasm has abated.
- If spasm is still present, wait an additional 12–24 hours.
- Infuse warm normal saline over 5–15 minutes via a distal IV line to increase blood flow.
- A warm or alcoholic beverage also may help to relieve the spasm.

24. How are implanted ports accessed?

Using sterile procedures, locate the port by palpation. Clean the site with povidone iodine or chlorhexidine 2%, starting over the port and moving outward in a circular motion. Using the fingers of one hand to stabilize the port, insert the needle through the skin, and push through the septum until the needle lightly touches the bottom of the port. Needle position is verified by blood return. If neither irrigation nor aspiration is possible, the needle may need to be pushed further into the septum or repositioned.

25. Are Huber needles necessary to access implanted ports?

Except in emergencies, a Huber (noncoring) needle should be used to access an implanted port because it preserves the life of the septum. A port septum is good for 1,000 (using a 19-gauge needle) or 2,000 (using a 22-gauge needle) punctures. The gauge and length of the needle are determined by the viscosity of the infused solution, depth of port placement, and type of implanted port. Huber needles (90°) with extension tubing, wings, and foam pad attached are frequently used for continuous infusion. The cathlink, however, is accessed with a straight angiocath. A straight Huber needle may be used for withdrawing blood samples or giving bolus injections. All needles and extensions should be primed with normal saline before use.

26. How often should Huber needles be changed?

To prevent skin breakdown, change the needle at least every 7 days. In the case of intermittent injections, some patients prefer that the port be accessed daily. Before needle removal at the end of the infusion, flush with normal saline followed by heparin.

27. How is discomfort decreased when ports are accessed?

Topical anesthetics, such as Emla cream (Lidocaine 2.5%, Prilocaine 2.5%) covered with a transparent dressing, may be applied to the skin over the port at least one hour before needle placement. Application of ice over the site or ethyl chloride spray also may be helpful.

28. How much blood should be discarded prior to blood sampling?

Approximately 5 cc of blood from adults and 3 cc from children is discarded prior to drawing the sample. There is no need to discard any blood when drawing blood cultures. All infusions should be stopped temporarily, and blood should be drawn through the proximal lumen via the catheter hub or through the injection cap. Pulling back slowly on the syringe prevents catheter collapse; a Vacutainer may be used to decrease needlestick risk. Because heparin adheres to the catheter and may result in prolonged prothrombin time or partial prothrombin time, samples for these particular tests may be drawn from a peripheral vein. Flush with 10–20 cc (20 cc for Groshong) of normal saline after blood withdrawal. If there is concern about wasting blood, the mixing method can be used. Prior to drawing the sample, blood is aspirated and then infused back into the patient four times without removing the syringe.

29. What are the complications associated with central lines?

- Infection
- Sepsis
- Occlusion
- Migration
- Pinch-off
- Extravasation

30. What are of the signs of central line infection?

Erythema, pain, and purulence at the exit site or along the tunnel are the most consistent indicators of infection. Immunosuppression may diminish or completely mask these signs. Infection of central lines may present as sepsis without another apparent source or as thrombosis alone. Risks for infection include:

- Type of catheter material
- Longer duration of use
- Emergent vs. elective placement
- Skill of the operator
- Absence of maximal barrier precautions during placement (sterile gloves, gown, drape, masks)
- Increased number of lumens
- Age (< 1 year or > 60 years)
- Failure to maintain sterile technique during routine care
- Altered host defenses (dermatitis, burns, HIV infection, neutropenia)
- Sepsis at time of placement

31. What is the difference between local (exit site, port pocket, and tunnel) and systemic infections?

Catheter-related infections can be grouped into local (at the exit site, port pocket or tunnel) or systemic. An **exit site infection** is suggested by erythema that extends approximately 2 cm from the exit site, with warmth, tenderness, swelling, or purulence. A **tunnel infection** is defined as inflammation along the subcutaneous tract of the catheter extending > 2 cm from the exit site. A **port pocket infection** is characterized by inflammation or necrosis of the skin over an implantable device or purulence in the pocket containing the device. Port pocket infections closely resemble tunnel infections in their treatment and response to therapy. Do not cannulate an implanted port if a port pocket infection is suspected.

A **systemic catheter-related infection** may or may not involve the soft tissue around the catheter and refers to the presence of signs and symptoms of bacteremia (presence of bacteria cultured from the blood) or sepsis. Sepsis is defined as clinical evidence of infection plus two or more of the following systemic responses: body temperature > 38° C or < 36° C, tachycardia, increased respiratory rate or $PaCO_2$ < 32 mmHg, leukocytosis (WBC > 12,000 cells/mm^3), impaired peripheral leukocyte response (< 4000 cells/mm), and/or > 10% immature (band) forms. Sepsis syndrome, severe sepsis, and septic shock are terms representing increased degrees of the severity of sepsis when altered organ function or compromise occurs (e.g., hypotension, hypoxemia, lactic acidosis, oliguria, altered mental status). A **systemic catheter-related blood stream infection** (CR-BSI) is defined as isolation of the same organism from a catheter segment culture and a peripheral blood culture with clinical symptoms of a blood stream infection and no other apparent source of infection. Criteria that implicate the catheter as the source of infection include: semiquantitative cultures showing greater than 15 colony-forming units (CFUs) of the same organism or quantitative cultures showing that the number of organisms cultured from the central line is 5–10 times the number cultured from the peripheral blood.

32. What are the sources of catheter-associated infection?

There are potentially four sources of infection:
1. Skin insertion site (most common)
2. Catheter hub
3. Secondary catheter infection with bloodstream seeding
4. Infusate contamination (rare)

33. How is infection in central lines treated?

Management depends on the causative organisms and extent of infection. Empiric treatment consists of an antimicrobial effective against gram-positive and gram-negative organisms. Specific antibiotic therapy is directed against organisms recovered from culture. Local site infections may be treated by aggressive site care and oral antibiotics (ciprofloxacin) in the absence of neutropenia. Outpatient management may be successful for people with intact immune systems whose infection is localized to the exit site without fever or hypotension. Tunnel infections may require catheter removal. Sepsis requires parenteral antibiotics and possible catheter removal. Septic syndrome and septic shock are indications to remove the catheter.

34. What organisms commonly cause catheter-related infections? Which infections require catheter removal?

The most common organisms have been coagulase-negative staphylococci, *Staphylococcus aureus*, enterococci, and *Candida* sp. Exit site infections, tunnel infections, and even bacteremia due to coagulase-negative staphylococci usually can be treated without catheter removal, although the rate of recurrence is decreased if the catheter is removed. Because *S. aureus* is associated with serious complications, removal of the catheter is suggested. Fungal infections occur less frequently but require catheter removal. Gram-negative organisms, including *Pseudomonas* sp., *Klebsiella* sp., *Acinetobacter* sp., and *Serratia* sp., may respond to medical therapy when causing exit site infections but usually require catheter removal with involvement of the tunnel. Catheter removal is indicated for infections with gram-positive bacilli and atypical mycobacteria.

35. What can be done to prevent catheter infections?

Prevention strategies include hand-washing, strict aseptic technique, and patient education. Special catheter designs include antimicrobial substances to prevent colonization, heparin coatings that may decrease formation of fibrin sleeves and thereby colonization of bacteria, or use of a collagen cuff impregnated with silver ions, which exerts an antimicrobial effect for 4–6 weeks and serves as a barrier to organisms that migrate down the catheter. Prophylactic use of antibiotics as a flush solution is under investigation with vancomycin alone and in combination with heparin or urokinase.

36. What should be done if there is no blood return with aspiration?

If there is no blood return, the catheter may no longer be in the venous system. The site should be assessed for:
- Drainage due to catheter rupture, obstruction, or fibrin sheath
- Subcutaneous swelling due to catheter damage or infusate exiting backward out of the vein
- Stricture of sutures
- Swelling of the neck, throat, or arm
- Loops of tunneled catheter under the skin

Patients should be encouraged to change position (e.g., the Trendelenburg position) to increase venous flow and to cough or breathe deeply to help move the catheter away from the vein wall. Injection caps should be removed and aspiration attempted; the needle should be repositioned if it is an implanted port; 10–20 cc of normal saline should be infused while assessing the site for swelling. If catheter placement is still in doubt, placement of the CVC may be confirmed with chest radiograph or dye study. Instillation of urokinase may be considered if a clot is suspected.

37. What causes central line occlusion?

Occlusion should be considered when the ability to infuse is lost and blood return is absent with aspiration. Partial obstruction is indicated by resistance to flushing and/or absence of blood return with aspiration. Causes include:
- **Intraluminal thrombus** may result from injury to the vein wall during insertion, contact with the catheter tip, or hardened blood in the catheter lumen.
- **Extraluminal fibrin sleeve** formed at the catheter entry site into the vein may impair ability to flush but not to withdraw, because it acts as a flap that blocks the tip when withdrawal is attempted but opens with injection.
- **Drug precipitate** may be formed by incompatible solutions, inadequate flushing, or calcium phosphorus complexes (as with total parenteral nutrition).
- **External occlusion** may occur when a catheter is clamped, twisted, or constricted by sutures or by a nonpatent Huber needle.

38. How is an occluded line treated?

Instillation of **urokinase** into a central line has been highly successful in dissolving clots. Approved by the Food and Drug Administration (FDA), urokinase is a nonantigenic, nonpyrogenic enzyme. Administration consists of placing 5,000– 10,000 units (1 or 2 cc) into a clotted lumen with a 10-cc syringe; smaller syringes may exert too much pressure on the catheter. Make sure to label the syringe or tape the syringe to the catheter so that it is not accidentally disturbed. The syringe is kept in place for 5–60 minutes; then an attempt is made to aspirate the urokinase and the dissolved clot. A 5,000-unit dose costs the pharmacy approximately $30–40. An alternative procedure consists of dissolving 25,000 units of urokinase in 150 ml of D5W and infusing over 90 minutes.

Streptokinase may be used if urokinase has not cleared the catheter. It is also approved by the FDA but causes fever. The recommended procedure is to inject 250,000 units of streptokinase into an occluded line and allow it to dwell for 1–2 hours before attempting to aspirate the dissolved clot. Patients with a recent history of streptococcal infection may have developed antibodies that render streptokinase ineffective.

Hydrochloric acid (HCl) **0.1%** has been reported to dissolve mineral deposits without serious adverse effects. The recommended procedure is to dissolve 0.2–1 cc of 0.1% HCl in normal saline (amount determined by catheter volume), allow to dwell for 1 hour, and then aspirate. Febrile reactions have been reported if large amounts are used.

Although limited information is available, **sodium bicarbonate** may be used to dissolve clots due to medications with a high pH, such as phenytoin sodium. In addition, **70% ethyl alcohol** can be used to dissolve fat associated with lipid occlusion. The alcohol is left in the catheter for 1–32 hours, and the procedure is repeated if the first trial is not successful. Side effects include dysgeusia.

Warning: During use of declotting agents or even during routine flushing, the nurse should be alert to the potential release of an infected clot or septic emboli. Patients have demonstrated signs of hemodynamic instability (hypotension) and sepsis within a few minutes after flushing.

39. Is extravasation a common complication of CVCs?

Although more common in peripheral IV access, extravasation is a potential complication of CVCs. Symptoms of extravasation may include pain, burning or stinging, and perhaps swelling or leaking. Blood return may or may not be present. If extravasation is suspected while infusing a vesicant, the nurse should stop the infusion and aspirate residual. If symptoms are present, a chest radiograph or dye study should be performed to confirm placement in the venous system.

40. What are the major causes of extravasation?

1. Needle dislodgement from ports
2. Backward flow of infusate due to fibrin sheath formation where the catheter enters the vein
3. Catheter damage (overvigorous flushing may weaken or even perforate the catheter wall)
4. Dislodgement or migration of a catheter tip from the venous system (although the mechanism for spontaneous migration is unclear, coughing or sneezing may be factors, especially with softer catheters).

41. What is "pinch-off syndrome"? How is it recognized?

A catheter may become fragmented as a result of "pinch-off," which occurs in about 1% of patients due to compression and shearing of the catheter between the clavicle and first rib. "Pinch off" should be suspected with intermittent lack of blood return or intermittent inability to infuse. It is made worse by sitting and relieved by raising the arms overhead. "Pinch off" is recognized on chest radiograph by a narrowing of the catheter between the clavicle and first rib. It may result in embolization and is an indication for catheter removal and replacement.

BIBLIOGRAPHY

1. Baranowski L: Central venous access devices: Current technologies, uses and management strategies. J Intraven Nurs 16:167–194, 1993.
2. Brandt B, DePalma J, Irwin M, et al: Comparison of central venous catheter dressings in bone marrow transplant recipients. Oncol Nurs Forum 23:830–836, 1996.
3. Brown JM: Polyurethane and silicone: Myths and misconceptions. J Intraven Nur 18:120–122, 1995.
4. Camp-Sorrell D (ed): Access Device Guidelines: Recommendations for Nursing Practice and Education. Pittsburgh, Oncology Nursing Society, 1996.
5. Eastridge BJ, Lefor AT: Complications of indwelling venous access devices in cancer patients. J Clin Oncol 13:233–238, 1995.
6. Hadaway LC: Comparison of vascular access devices. Semin Oncol Nurs 11 (3):154–166, 1990.
7. LaQuaglia MP, Caldwell C, Lucas A, et al: A prospective randomized double-blind trial of bolus urokinase in the treatment of established Hickman catheter sepsis in children. J Pediatr Surg 29:742–745, 1994.
8. LaQuaglia MP, Lucas A, Thaler HT, et al: A prospective analysis of vascular access device-related infections in children. J Pediatr Surg 27:840–842, 1992.
9. Lucas A: A critical review of venous access devices: The nursing perspective. Curr Issues Cancer Nurs Pract 1:1, 1993.
10. Maki DG, Ringer M, Alvarado CJ: Prospective randomised trial of povidone-iodine, alcohol, and chlorhexidine for prevention of infection associated with central venous and arterial catheters. Lancet 338:339–342, 1991.
11. Pearson ML, for the Hospital Infection Control Practice Advisory Committee: Guideline for prevention of intravascular device-related infections. Part I: Intravascular device-related infections: An overview. Am J Infect Control 24(4):262–277, 1996.

12. Pearson ML, for the Hospital Infection Control Practice Advisory Committee: Guideline for prevention of intravascular device-related infections. Part II: Recommendations for the prevention of nosocomial intravascular device-related infections. Am J Infect Control 24(4):277–293, 1996.
13. Young LS: Sepsis syndrome. In Mandell GL, Bennett JE, Dolin R (eds): Principles and Practice of Infectious Disease, 4th ed. New York: Churchill Livingstone, 690–705, 1995.
14. Ryder MA: Peripherally inserted central venous catheters. Nurs Clin North Am 28:937–971, 1993.
15. Wickham RS: Advances in venous access devices and nursing management strategies. Adv Oncol Nurs 25:345–362, 1990.
16. Wickham R, Purl S, Walker D: Long term central venous catheters: Issues for care. Semin Oncol Nur 8:133–147, 1992.
17. Winslow MN, Trammel L, Camp-Sorrell D: Selection of vascular access devices and nursing care. Semin Oncol Nurs 11(3):167–173, 1995.

54. BLOOD COMPONENTS

Beth E. Mechling, RN, MS, OCN,
Lowell Anderson-Reitz, RN, MS, ANP, OCN, and
Rocky L. Billups, RN

1. What are the four ABO blood types?

The four blood types are A, B, AB, and O. A and B are antigens present on the RBC membrane. A person may have both antigens and be AB or neither antigen and be O. Individuals who lack these antigens on their RBC membranes may make antibody to the antigens when exposed to the A, B, or AB antigens. Individuals with a particular antigen on their RBC membrane will not make antibody to that antigen. Thus, people with the blood type O are known as universal donors. Conversely, people with the blood type AB are universal recipients. The population distribution is as follows: O, 47%; A, 41%; B, 9%; and AB, 3%.

2. What is the Rh system?

The Rh system refers to the presence or absence of Rh antigens. The six most common Rh antigens are C, D, E, c, d, and e. Presence of the D antigen means that a person is Rh-positive. Absence of the D antigen denotes an Rh-negative person. Expression of the Rh D antigen can occur by transfusion of an Rh-positive blood product in an Rh-negative person or through pregnancy in an Rh-negative woman carrying an Rh-positive fetus. Such exposure of an Rh-negative person to Rh-positive RBCs will result in the production of antibodies to the Rh antigen. The main difference between the two classes A, B, O and Rh is that antibodies may randomly develop to A and/or B in a person who lacks these antigens but the Rh-negative person will not develop antibodies to Rh without exposure to Rh.

3. What are the acceptable donor blood types for the eight ABO/Rh blood types?

Patient Blood Type	Acceptable Donor Blood Type
A positive	A positive, A negative, O positive,* O negative*
A negative	A negative, O negative*
B positive	B positive, B negative, O positive,* O negative*
B negative	B negative, O negative*
AB positive	AB positive, AB negative, A positive,* A negative,* B positive,* B negative,* O positive,* O negative*
AB negative	AB negative, A negative,* B negative,* O negative*
O positive	O positive, O negative
O negative	O negative

* If plasma is incompatible, reduce volume to 200 ml.

4. What are the primary components of whole blood?

Whole blood components include red blood cells, platelets, fresh frozen plasma, cryoprecipitate, factor concentrates, and white blood cells.

5. What are the common indications for transfusion of whole blood and primary components?

Whole blood is used primarily for intravascular volume expansion when critical patients require massive transfusions for hypovolemic shock. Whole blood is rarely, if ever, used in the oncologic setting.

Packed red blood cells (PRBCs) are commonly administered to oncologic patients for intravascular volume expansion, support during hemorrhage, and treatment of symptomatic anemia.

Platelets are transfused for significant thrombocytopenia and hemorrhage. A designated platelet count ≤ 10 thousand in the absence of active bleeding is a common transfusion parameter in oncology centers.

Fresh frozen plasma (FFP) has many uses in the oncologic setting. The main indications are intravascular volume expansion; replacement of coagulation factors II, V, VII, IX, X, and XI; reversal of the anticoagulant effect of warfarin; antithrombin III deficiency; and thrombotic thrombocytopenic purpura.

Cryoprecipitate is most commonly used for treatment of disseminated intravascular coagulation (DIC). However, it is also used for replacement of fibrinogen, management of coagulopathy in acute liver failure, replacement of factor VIII in mild hemophilia, and factor replacement in von Willebrand's disease.

Factor concentrates replace specific factor deficiencies and assist in control of hemophilia.

White blood cell (WBC) transfusions are controversial. However, they have been used in patients with prolonged neutropenia and sepsis not responsive to broad-spectrum antibiotic and antifungal therapy.

6. Why do PRBC transfusion requirements vary among oncologic patients?

The reasons for transfusing are multifactorial. Experience of the practitioner, understanding of the literature, and individual patient presentations (including symptoms) guide medical and nursing judgment about transfusion decisions. Religion and personal patient preferences also must be discussed in regard to transfusions of blood products.

7. Which intravenous solution is used to prime blood tubing for administration of all products?

Normal saline, 0.9%, is the only intravenous solution that is compatible with blood products. Agglutination or hemolysis may occur with use of other intravenous solutions.

8. What premedication is commonly administered before infusion of PRBCs and platelets? Why?

Acetaminophen and diphenhydramine are commonly used as premedication. The doses prescribed may vary depending on the patient's clinical status. Common doses are 650 mg or 10 grains of acetaminophen and 25–50 mg of diphenhydramine. Both drugs are used to prevent nonhemolytic febrile transfusion reactions.

9. What are the acceptable parameters for transfusion time of blood products?

Generally PRBCs are infused over 1.5–4 hours. The time of infusion depends on the age of the patient as well as clinical status. For rapid volume expansion, PRBCs may be infused in as little as 5–10 minutes with telemetry and intense nursing monitoring.

Platelets are infused rapidly over 15–45 minutes. Platelets can be infused as a continuous drip, no longer than 4 hr/U. The longer platelets hang after being dispensed from the blood bank, the less effective they become. Platelets can be infused over less time in emergent situations such as exsanguination in thrombocytopenic patients.

FFP and cryoprecipitate may be infused as quickly as possible. It is important to evaluate the pulmonary status of each patient before rapid infusion of any blood product.

Factor concentrates may be given as an intravenous bolus or as a continuous infusion.

10. Most institutions have designated parameters for monitoring of vital signs during transfusion of which two blood products?

PRBCs and platelets. The rationale for such policies is the increased risk of transfusion reactions associated with blood products. The frequency of vital sign monitoring depends on the institution's standard of care. According to common guidelines, complete vital signs should be monitored before beginning administration, 15 minutes into the administration, and immediately after infusion is complete.

11. Why should PRBCs and platelets be leukopoor for patients who receive multiple transfusions?

Patients who receive multiple transfusions may develop a clinical disorder called alloimmunization. This disorder results when antibodies are developed against HLA antigens expressed on white blood cells. When alloimmunization develops, patients have a minimal increase in posttransfusion platelet count with random or single donor platelets. The risk of developing alloimmunization decreases with the use of leuko-reduced blood products.

12. What are the three types of platelet concentrates?

The three types of platelet concentrates are random-donor, single-donor, and HLA-matched. Random-donor platelets are obtained from several different donors and pooled into a single pack for administration, whereas single-donor platelets are obtained from a single donor and dispensed for administration. HLA-matched platelets are obtained from a single donor who has a partial HLA match with the recipient.

13. What are the advantages of using single-donor platelets?

Use of single-donor platelets decreases sensitization of the recipient, otherwise known as alloimmunization, and the risk of transfusion-transmitted diseases.

14. What techniques are used for leukocyte depletion?

The methods available for leukocyte depletion are washing, centrifugation, freezing, and filtration. Leukocyte filtration is the most common method of leukodepletion in current use. Leukofiltration can be accomplished during transfusion with the addition of a commercially available filter that is attached to the blood product and intravenous tubing. Several commercially available filters consistently remove 95–99% of the leukocytes. Filtration also can be done at the blood bank before blood products are released for transfusion.

15. What are the benefits of leukodepleting blood products?

The primary benefits are the prevention or delay of alloimmunization in frequently transfused patients, decreased risk of transmitting cytomegalovirus, and decreased nonhemolytic febrile transfusion reactions. Patients with hematologic malignancies and bone marrow transplant candidates should receive leukodepleted blood products.

16. Why are blood products irradiated?

Irradiating blood products with a low dose of ionizing radiation (approximately 2500 cGy) decreases the incidence of developing transfusion-associated graft-vs.-host reactions (TA-GVHD). The radiation destroys lymphocytes, which are the mediators of graft-vs.-host reactions. The following patients are at greatest risk of developing TA-GVHD: patients with Hodgkin's or non-Hodgkin's lymphoma; patients with congenital immunodeficiency syndromes; patients undergoing high-dose chemotherapy; and patients receiving transfusions from relatives.

17. Name the six types of transfusion reactions.

Acute intravascular hemolytic reaction	Nonhemolytic febrile reaction
Delayed intravascular hemolytic reaction	Allergic/anaphylactic reaction
Acute extravascular hemolytic reaction	Delayed intravascular hemolytic reaction

18. What is the most common transfusion reaction in the oncologic setting?

Nonhemolytic febrile transfusion reaction. Signs and symptoms include fever, chills, nausea, and vomiting. Hemolytic transfusion reactions present similarly to nonhemolytic transfusion reactions in the early stages. Hemolytic transfusion reactions account for 0.5–1% of all transfusion reactions and are due to the destruction of donor red cells by the recipient's antibodies. This type of reaction contributes to 70% of transfusion-related deaths. Hemolytic transfusion reactions may be associated with chills, fever, flank pain, chest tightness, hypotension, disseminated intravascular coagulopathy, hemoglobinuria, shock, and feeling of impending doom expressed by the patient. Allergic/anaphylactic transfusion reactions present with classic signs and symptoms of an allergic response, including urticaria, pruritus, rash, bronchospasms and anaphylaxis.

19. What are the appropriate steps when a transfusion reaction is suspected?

1. Stop the blood component infusion immediately and notify the physician and blood bank.
2. Maintain intravenous access with 0.9% normal saline solution.
3. Maintain adequate airway.
4. Monitor blood pressure and heart rate. Notify physician of systolic blood pressure changes > 20 mm/Hg or heart rate change of > 20 beats/minute.
5. Administer antihistamine.
6. Institute diuresis.
7. Perform a blood-band work-up according to institutional policy. This commonly includes rechecking of paper work, repeat cross-match, direct antiglobin test, urine test for hemoglobinuria, and return of the unused portion of the blood product to the laboratory or blood bank for evaluation.
8. Monitor renal status for hemoglobinuria. The patient may require hydration to ensure adequate renal perfusion.
9. Monitor coagulation status. This may entail drawing a screening panel for disseminated intravascular coagulopathy.
10. Monitor for signs of hemolysis. Serial laboratory tests may be ordered, including a complete blood count, full chemistry panel, urinalysis, and bilirubin with fractionation to evaluate levels of indirect and direct bilirubin.
11. Culture the patient for a septic event.

20. What is the risk of transfusion-associated transmission of hepatitis C virus (HCV), hepatitis B virus (HBV) and human immunodeficiency virus (HIV)?

The risk of transmission for HIV is 1:400,000 units transfused; for HCV, 1:103,000 units transfused. HBV has the highest risk of transmission associated with transfusion: 1:63,000 units transfused.

21. What should be the nurse's response to the patient who is fearful of receiving blood products?

The nurse should clarify the patient's fears and reassure the patient that blood is screened for hepatitis virus and HIV. If the patient is concerned about risk of infection, the nurse should provide current statistics about the incidence of infection after receiving blood products. It is important to inform the patient that, although complications of receiving blood products are uncommon, every procedure involves risks. In the process of informed consent, a patient has the right to refuse any treatment or procedure.

22. Are there any benefits to receiving blood products from relatives?

The only benefit to receiving blood products from family members is psychological well-being. Although a family member may have the same blood type as the patient, the cross-match may not be compatible. Patients who are platelet-refractory at times get a significant response with related donor platelets. However, no published data support the use of related donor platelets vs. HLA-matched unrelated donors.

23. Can patients donate autologous red cells before a scheduled procedure?

Yes. Patients can donate a unit of blood every week. PRBCs can be stored for 42 days before reinfusion. A person may donate blood up to 8 days before the scheduled procedure. The patient must have a hematocrit of 38 or greater before donation of the first unit of PRBCs. For subsequent donations the hematocrit must be 33 or greater. Some physicians may order iron supplementation for auto-donating patients to help prevent anemia.

24. What do the patient and family need to know about donating PRBCs or platelets for a relative?

The above criteria for donating autologous PRBCs also apply to family members wishing to donate blood for a patient. Platelets can be donated by family members every 72 hours. There is often an additional charge to the patient for designated donations.

25. What are the factors that may render a person ineligible for donating blood?

Every blood bank has general guidelines for assessing blood donor eligibility. These may vary depending on the institution. The following persons may not be eligible to donate blood:
- Persons who have had acupuncture, electrolysis, ear/body part piercing (for 12 months) unless sterile, disposable needles were used
- Persons on antibiotics (may be eligible 48 hours after completion or if using for acne)
- Persons with hepatitis, HIV
- Persons receiving hepatitis A and B vaccines are deferred for 2 weeks after injection
- Persons with lyme disease
- Persons with malaria are eligible 3 years after becoming symptom-free
- Women who are pregnant or who have delivered within 6 weeks
- Persons who have received tattoos are deferred for 12 months
- Persons who have received a transfusion of blood or blood products are deferred for 12 months
- Persons with diabetes controlled with insulin may be acceptable, if free from infection and have physician permission

(Bonfils Blood Center Medical Guidelines for Volunteer Blood Donors. Denver, Colorado, revised July 1996.)

26. Can PRBCs be infused through an infusion pump?

Infusion pumps must be designated as compatible with infusion of blood products. If information cannot be found about pump compatibility with blood products, the pump should not be used for infusion because it may cause lysis of blood cells.

27. Can blood products be administered in the home setting?

Yes. Home care agencies with blood product infusion services have policies and procedural guidelines that direct blood product administration in the home. Common criteria for home administration of blood products include the following: (1) the patient has a physical limitation that makes leaving the home a taxing effort; (2) the patient is alert, cooperative, and able to respond to bodily symptoms; (3) the patient's medical condition allows safe transfusion at home; (4) the patient has access to a telephone; (5) the patient has a hemoglobin < 10 gm/dl and a platelet count < 20,000. Reimbursement of blood product administration in the home depends on the patient's insurance policy.

28. How much of an increase in hemoglobin should be expected in the patient who is not losing blood following a transfusion of 1 unit of PRBCs? How long after a transfusion do you need to wait before an accurate posttransfusion hemoglobin can be obtained?

In the patient who is not losing blood by bleeding or destruction, an increase in the hemoglobin of approximately 1 gm/dl for each unit of PRBCs transfused can be expected. Contrary to what might be intuitively expected, the fluid that is administered with PRBCs quickly equilibrates with the extravascular space. Thus a posttransfusion hemoglobin can be obtained 15 minutes past the completion of the transfusion. The value will be comparable to a hemoglobin obtained 24 hours later, and the time saved in not having to bring the patient back for a followup posttransfusion hemoglobin is obvious.

BIBLIOGRAPHY

1. Armitage JO, Antman KH (eds): High-Dose Cancer Therapy: Pharmacology, Hematopoietins, Stem Cells, 2nd ed. Baltimore, Williams & Wilkins, 1995.
2. Benson K, Fields K, Hiemenz J, et al: The platelet-refractory bone marrow transplant patient: Prophylaxis and treatment of bleeding. Semin Oncol 20:102–109, 1993.
3. Coffland F, Shelton D: Blood component replacement therapy. Crit Care Nurs Clin North Am 5:545–556,1993.
4. Ewald G, McKenzie C (eds): Manual of Medical Therapeutics: The Washington Manual, 28th ed. Boston, Little, Brown, 1995.
5. Forman S, Blume K, Thomas ED (eds): Bone Marrow Transplant. Cambridge, Blackwell Scientific Publications, 1994.
6. Freedman S, Haisfeild M, McGuire D, et al: Nursing considerations in the administration of blood component therapy. Semin Oncol Nurs 6:155–162, 1990.
7. Hoffman R, Benz E, Shattil S, et al (eds): Hematology: Basic Principles and Practice. New York, Churchill Livingstone, 1991.
8. Jetter EK, Spivey MA: Noninfectious complications of blood transfusion. Hematol Oncol Clin North Am 9:187–203, 1995.
9. Mummert TB, Tourault MA: Transfusion-related fatality reports—a summary. Nurs Manage 25:801–803, 1994.
10. Visiting Nurse Support Services of Denver, CO: Policy and Procedure. Home Blood Transfusion Therapy. Denver, Visiting Nurse Support Services, 1993.
11. Wiesen AR, Hopenthal DR, Byrd JC, et al: Equilibration of hemoglobin concentration after transfusion in medical inpatients not actively bleeding. Ann Intern Med 121:278–280, 1994.

55. PATIENT EVALUATION

Rebecca Hawkins, MSN, ANP, AOCN

1. What are important points in evaluating a cancer patient?

Obtaining a careful history for any cancer patient is crucial to guiding assessment and physical examination. Knowing and asking the right questions are essential to determining what is wrong. Evaluation of patients with cancer is complex because they have multiple symptoms with multiple possible causes. For example, a complaint of back pain may indicate a vertebral metastasis or spinal cord compression. Mental confusion may be due to opioids, sepsis, brain metastasis, hypercalcemia, or a combination of causes. The patient's complaints need to be assessed for recurrent or metastatic disease, infection, side effects and complications of therapy, and oncologic emergencies. Preexisting conditions, chronic illnesses, and new noncancer-related conditions and drug effects also need to be considered in the differential diagnosis. For example, acute abdominal pain may be related to constipation or tumor, but it also could be appendicitis. Other points to remember in evaluating the cancer patient include:

- Do not discount any sign or symptom
- Attempt to find the cause and refer the patient as needed for further diagnostic examinations
- Assess the duration of symptoms and rate of progression; be alert to the potential for an oncologic emergency
- Obtain the patient's input and ask what the symptom means to the patient or significant other
- Be attentive to the patient's anxiety or worry. Each new symptom may cause fear of recurrence or disease progression
- Know the drugs and treatments that the patient is receiving, and be aware of potential side effects, complications, and interactions
- Evaluate the *whole* patient, not just the physical complaint
- Constantly assess and reassess

2. What questions should be asked of the cancer patient who recently had chemotherapy?

- When was your last chemotherapy treatment, and what drugs were used?
  In general, blood counts fall to the lowest level (nadir) at 7–14 days after chemotherapy. Knowing the time frame of the last chemotherapy treatment alerts the nurse to potential signs of neutropenia, anemia, and thrombocytopenia.
- What side effects are you experiencing?
  Be sure to follow this question with specific questions, such as, "Did you feel sick to your stomach or vomit? Are you having loose stools? When was your last bowel movement, and was it normal? Are your fingers or toes feeling numb?" Knowing the chemotherapeutic agents given guides the nurse in looking for side effects during both examination and history taking. Often patients are reluctant to report side effects of chemotherapy in fear that the treatment will be discontinued. Side effects differ according to the chemotherapeutic drugs and doses. Explain to patients that side effects can and will be managed. Stress that it is the patient's responsibility to report side effects for adequate symptom control.

3. What should be considered if an enlarged lymph node is palpated?

Determine how long the lymph node has been present; lymphadenopathy that has not decreased in size and has enlarged in 4 or 5 weeks is significant. Isolated lymph nodes < 1 cm are usually not significant in the normal adult population. An enlarged tender lymph node may indicate an inflammatory process, and other symptoms of infection should be elicited. Fixed, immobile lymph nodes are suspicious for malignancy or metastatic cancer. The enlargement of lymph nodes in metastatic cancer is characterized by discrete, nontender, firm or hard nodes with an irregular shape. Lymphomas are characterized by large, discrete, nontender nodes of a firm, rubbery consistency.

4. What are the signs and symptoms of carcinomatous meningitis?

Carcinomatous (leptomeningeal) meningitis refers to diffuse metastatic seeding of cancer in the meninges and cerebrospinal fluid (CSF) pathways of the central nervous system (CNS). The major diagnostic clue is the presence of signs and symptoms suggestive of a multifocal process. Most patients present with headache (which may be accompanied by nausea and vomiting), cranial nerve palsies, and cranial nerve deficits (e.g., diplopia, hearing loss, facial numbness). Lethargy and decreased memory are common. Back pain and spinal cord compression also may be present. Classical signs of meningitis, such as neck rigidity and pain with leg-raising, are absent in most patients. Neurologic symptoms range from subtle symptoms of several weeks' duration to acute seizures, mental confusion, and coma. CSF studies reveal malignant cells, elevated CSF pressure, increased protein content and white cell count, and decreased glucose. Other diagnostic studies include CT and MRI scans. MRI scanning of the entire spine should precede lumbar puncture in patients with back pain and neurologic signs based on the assumption that epidural metastases are involved. If untreated, carcinomatous meningitis leads to progressive neurologic decline and death within 4–6 weeks. Treatment consists of steroids, intrathecal chemotherapy, or radiotherapy. The most common primary cancers associated with carcinomatous meningitis include breast and lung cancer (small-cell), non-Hodgkin's lymphoma, adult acute leukemias, and malignant melanoma. Primary brain tumors (e.g., medulloblastomas, glioblastomas) are less commonly involved.

5. What do the heart sounds represent?

The **first heart sound (S1)** results from closure of the mitral and tricuspid valves. These atrioventricular valves close immediately after the atria have contracted and emptied the remaining blood into the ventricles. It is best heard on examination at the apex of the heart, where the left ventricle is closest to the chest wall

The **second heart sound (S2)** is produced by the closing of the aortic and pulmonic valves immediately after the ventricles have emptied the blood into the aorta and pulmonary artery, which also begins the period of ventricular expansion or diastole. It is best heard by placing a stethoscope diaphragm at the aortic area. In patients with tachycardia, differentiating between S1 and S2 by auscultation may be difficult. The best way to make this distinction is to feel the carotid pulse, which occurs immediately after S2. You can watch the stethoscope move in response to the apical impulse. With the other hand feel for the carotid pulse; the heart sound you hear at almost the same time is S1.

The **third heart sound (S3)** can be heard in children and young adults and is considered a normal finding. It represents the period of rapid ventricular filling and is best heard with the bell of the stethoscope, using light pressure. An S3 heard in a person over 40 years is usually pathologic and may represent myocardial failure or volume overload of the ventricles. The third heart sound is sometimes referred to as a gallop.

6. What causes pericardial friction rubs? How are they assessed?

Pericardial friction rubs result from inflammation or tumor involvement of the pericardial sac. They may be heard with effusions due to lymphoma and breast and lung cancer. Pericardial friction rubs are not confined to one portion of the heart and are usually best heard in the third interspace to the left of the sternum, with little radiation to other areas. The intensity varies, increasing when the patient leans forward. It may be described as a high-pitched, scratchy, or scraping sound or sounds.

7. What are the signs and symptoms of congestive heart failure?

Symptoms, which are caused by intravascular and interstitial volume overload and inadequate tissue perfusion, include paroxysmal nocturnal dyspnea; orthopnea; dyspnea on exertion; decreased exercise tolerance; fatigue and weakness; dry, hacking cough; unexplained confusion;

and abdominal discomfort (nausea, anorexia, pain, and tenderness). Clinical signs include elevated jugular venous pressure, positive hepatojugular reflux, third heart sound, laterally displaced apical impulse, rales and peripheral edema.

8. What cardiac toxicities are related to chemotherapy?

Chemotherapeutic drugs have a wide range of cardiac toxicities, including dysrhythmia, transient left ventricular dysfunction, and long-term cardiomyopathy. Doxorubicin in doses > 550 mg/m² is known to cause cardiomyopathy. The risk is greater for patients who have previously received mediastinal radiation. Cyclophosphamide may cause hemorrhagic cardiac necrosis in doses > 120 mg/kg; it also may cause transient pericardial effusion, dysrhythmia, and heart failure. Drugs such as 5-fluorouracil, biotherapeutic agents, and paclitaxel may cause electrocardiographic changes.

9. How do I distinguish among rales, rhonchi, wheezes, and pleural rubs? What do they indicate in patients with cancer?

Rales are light crackles, often described as the sound made by rubbing hair between the fingers or crinkling cellophane. Rales are produced when fluid, pus, or mucus is present in the small airways or alveoli; they are usually heard in the lung bases during inspiration. Rales may clear when the fluid is mobilized by coughing or taking a deep breath. In patients with cancer rales may indicate left-sided heart failure, pneumonia, or pulmonary edema.

Rhonchi are deeper-pitched and coarser than rales, often described as a hoarse moan, deep snore, or musical breath sounds. Rhonchi result from fluid or secretions in the larger airways and can also be cleared by coughing. They may be heard throughout the respiratory cycle as well as during inspiration. In patients with cancer, rhonchi may indicate bronchitis or pneumonia.

Wheezes are high-pitched, musical sounds heard on both inspiration and expiration. They result from narrowing of airways, such as constriction or spasm. In contrast to rales or rhonchi, wheezes do not clear with coughing. Usually wheezes are associated with conditions such as asthma or bronchospasm.

Pleural friction rub is an abnormal breath sound described as squeaky shoes, creaking floor boards, or two pieces of leather rubbing against each other. The rub is heard best during auscultation of the anterior lung fields with the patient in an upright position. Rubs do not clear with cough. Often heard during inspiration, rubs are associated with pain due to inflammation. They may indicate pneumonia, pulmonary infarction, pulmonary infection, tumor, or pleural effusions.

Decreased or absent breath sounds indicate a potentially serious problem that requires prompt attention and diagnostic work-up. Decreased or absent breath sounds may be noted in atelectasis and pneumothorax. Absent or decreased vesicular breath sounds may indicate pleural effusions or thickening. Malignant pleural effusions indicate that cancer cells are present in the pleural fluid and effusion (e.g., lymphoma, cancers of the breast and lung).

10. What findings are significant in examining a mastectomy site?

Along with normal breast examination, the mastectomy site should be inspected and palpated. Erythema and palpable nodes are suspect for recurrent local breast cancer. Biopsy or confirmation by an oncologist is indicated in determination of recurrence.

11. What are the possible causes of hepatosplenomegaly?

Hepatomegaly and splenomegaly (enlargement of the liver and spleen, respectively) are abnormal findings requiring prompt attention and further work-up. Cancers that commonly metastasize to the liver include breast, lung, colon, pancreas, and stomach cancer. Splenomegaly may be seen in lymphomas, chronic lymphocytic leukemia, hairy-cell leukemia, and chronic myelogenous leukemia.

12. How are patients assessed for abdominal ascites?

Ascites is common in patients with ovarian, breast, gastrointestinal, and primary or metastatic liver malignancies. It should be considered in patients with increasing abdominal girth, protuberant abdomen, and flank bulges. Ascitic fluid settles with gravity and can be detected by listening to the change in percussion sounds. Dullness is heard in the dependent parts of the abdomen and tympany in the upper parts where the bowel is located. The clinical test for ascites is to assess for shifting dullness to ascertain the presence of fluid. Begin by percussion for dullness and tympany and mark the borders. Then lay the patient on one side, and again percuss for dullness and tympany and mark the borders. In patients without ascites, the borders are similar. In patients with ascites, the border of dullness shifts to the dependent side or is more midline as the fluid resettles through gravity.

Another method is to test for a fluid wave. Because this method requires three hands, the patient or another health care provider must offer assistance. The primary examiner asks the patient to lie supine. An assistant presses the edge of one hand and forearm firmly along the vertical midline of the abdomen. The primary examiner places a hand on each side of the abdomen and strikes one side sharply, feeling for the impulse of a fluid wave. The presence of a fluid wave suggests ascites. This method is not always reliable. Ascites should be confirmed by abdominal ultrasound, CT scan, or MRI; sometimes it can be seen on plain film.

13. What information is obtained from the complete blood count and differential?

The complete blood count (CBC) and differential are a series of tests that provide information about the hematopoietic system.

1. **White blood cells** (WBCs) **and differential.** The major function of the WBCs or leukocytes is to fight infection or foreign bodies. Five types of WBCs can be identified on the CBC. The total white count is the total percentage of each of these types. The percentage of each type of leukocyte is reported in the differential. The leukocytes include neutrophils, lymphocytes, monocytes, eosinophils, and basophils. *Neutrophils*, the most abundant leukocytes, are responsible for phagocytosis and digestion of bacterial microorganisms. Acute bacterial infections and trauma stimulate neutrophil production and result in an increased WBC count. Often when neutrophils are stimulated, the immature forms (bands or stab cells) enter the circulation. The process of overproduction of immature neutrophils, referred to as a left shift, indicates an acute bacterial infection or recovery from chemotherapy. *Lymphocytes* are divided into T cells and B cells. T cells are involved in cellular type immunity, whereas B cells are active in humoral immunity and antibody production. The primary function of the lymphocytes is to fight chronic bacterial infections and acute viral infections. The differential does not report the number of T and B cells but rather the combination of the two. *Monocytes* are phagocytic cells that can kill bacteria much like neutrophils. The primary difference is that monocytes last longer in the circulation than neutrophils. *Basophils* and especially *eosinophils* are involved in the allergic response. Parasitic infections also may raise the eosinophil count.

2. **Red blood cells and indices.** *Hemoglobin* (Hgb) serves as a vehicle for transport of oxygen and carbon dioxide. The Hgb value is a measure of the concentration of hemoglobin in the peripheral blood. Normal values differ according to sex and age. The Hgb value may be altered by dehydration (which causes a higher value) or overhydration (which causes a lower value). Anemias, hemorrhage, hemolysis, cancer, and cancer treatments may cause a decrease in the Hgb. Abnormal increases in the Hgb may be seen in chronic obstructive pulmonary disease (COPD), congestive heart failure (CHF), polycythemia vera, and congenital heart disease. *Hematocrit* (Hct) is a measure of the percentage of red blood cells (RBCs) in the total blood volume. This value closely reflects the status of the RBCs and Hgb. The Hct is usually about three times the value of the Hgb. Normal values vary according to age and sex. *Mean corpuscular volume* (MCV) is a measure of the average size and volume of a single RBC. When the MCV is increased, the RBC size is abnormally large or macrocytic (e.g., megaloblastic anemias, vitamin B_{12} deficiency, chronic liver disease, alcoholism, chemotherapy). When the MCV value is decreased, the RBC is abnormally small or microcytic (e.g., iron deficient anemia). *Mean corpuscular hemoglobin* (MCH) is a measure of the average weight of hemoglobin in an RBC. Macrocytic RBCs generally have more hemoglobin, whereas microcytic RBCs generally have less hemoglobin. Therefore, the MCH value follows the MCV value. *Mean corpuscular hemoglobin concentration* (MCHC) is a measure of the average concentration or percentage of hemoglobin

within an RBC. When the cell is deficient, it is said to be hypochromic and the value is usually decreased (e.g., iron deficient anemia and thalassemia). When the value is normal, the anemia is said to be normocytic (e.g., hemolytic anemia).

3. **Platelets.** Platelets are responsible for the initiation of blood clotting. Because platelets may clump together, counting by automation gives a level that is 10–15% inaccurate. A platelet count > 400,000/mm^3 constitutes thrombocytosis. Vascular thrombosis with organ infarction is a major complication of thrombocytosis. Patients with marked thrombocytosis (> 1 million/mm^3) in fact may bleed. Thrombocytopenia is indicated by a platelet count < 100,000/mm^3. Low levels are usually hand-counted. Counts falling below 20,000/mm^3 place the patient at serious risk for spontaneous bleeding. A platelet count > 40,000/mm^3 poses little risk for spontaneous bleeding but may cause prolonged bleeding in the case of trauma or surgery.

14. Define ANC. How is it calculated?

The absolute neutrophil count (ANC), also called the absolute granulocyte count (AGC), is important for assessing the patient with cancer who has received chemotherapy. The ANC, which helps to determine whether to give or withhold further chemotherapy, is a measure of the mature white blood cells within the total white count. Usually an ANC above 1,000 poses little risk of infection for the patient. Neutropenia is generally defined as an ANC below 1,000. Patients with an ANC below 500 are at especially high risk for infections that may be life-threatening. ANC is calculated by multiplying the percent of granulocytes (neutrophils + bands) by the total WBC:

Total WBC = 3.5
Neutrophils = 28%
Bands = 3%
28% (neutrophils) + 3% (bands) = 31%
ANC = 3.5 × 0.31= 1,085, or approximately 1,000

15. How do the presenting signs and symptoms of infection differ in patients with cancer?

The typical signs of infection may not be present in patients with cancer. Patients with decreased neutrophils (neutropenia) do not have the same clinical response to infection as patients with a normal white count. Neutropenic patients exhibit minimal or no signs of inflammation (e.g., pus, erythema, pain, swelling). In addition, infiltrates associated with pulmonary infection may not be evident on radiographs. Sites of infection that need to be considered include the blood, lungs, urine, skin, and especially venous access devices. Typical signs and symptoms of infection in these sites include fever, erythema and increased warmth of the skin, cough, dysuria, pain (any location), and possible elevation of the total WBC or neutrophil count. Neutropenic fever is an oncologic emergency requiring prompt medical attention and initiation of broad-spectrum antibiotics. Neutropenic patients who become febrile are considered infected until proved otherwise. Cultures are obtained from the sputum, urine, blood, and other areas of concern (spinal fluid, venous access device site).

16. What is the significance of liver function tests in patients with cancer?

Liver function tests (LFTs) are important for detecting metastasis to the liver and determining the functioning of the liver for further cancer therapies. Elevated LFTs indicate an increase in intracellular liver enzymes with liver inflammation or dysfunction.

Alanine aminotransferase (ALT). ALT is found primarily in the liver and to a lesser extent in the kidneys, heart, and skeletal muscles. Damage to the liver parenchyma causes release of hepatocellular enzymes, resulting in an elevated serum ALT. ALT is a sensitive index of hepatocellular injury and liver malfunction. A rise in serum ALT is rarely seen without liver involvement.

Aspartate aminotransferase (AST). AST is found in high concentration in the heart, liver cells, skeletal muscle cells, and to a lesser degree in the kidney and pancreas. AST is a non-organ, nonspecific enzyme; however, damage to the liver and hepatocytes results in release of AST and a rise in the serum AST level. The AST can be compared with the ALT. A ratio of AST to ALT > 1.0 is an indicator of alcohol-induced liver injury, liver congestion, and metastatic tumor of the liver.

A ratio < 1.0 may be seen in acute hepatitis, viral hepatitis, or infectious mononucleosis. A rise in AST also maybe seen in patients with RBC abnormalities, such as hemolytic anemia, and severe burns.

Lactate dehydrogenase (LDH). LDH is an enzyme widely distributed in tissues and is thus non-organ- and non-tissue-specific. It is found in the kidney, heart, skeletal muscle, brain, lungs, and liver. Elevation of LDH is seen with pulmonary diseases, hepatitis, hemolytic anemias, renal infarction, skeletal injuries, and some cancers (e.g., lymphomas, testicular cancer). Frequently LDH is used in the diagnosis of myocardial infarction.

Alkaline phosphatase (ALP). ALP is found in many tissues, but the highest concentrations are in the liver, biliary tract (Kupffer cells), epithelium, and bone. It is used as an index of liver and bone disease when correlated with other clinical findings. Elevated serum ALP is associated with obstructive biliary disease, metastatic liver cancer, primary liver cancer, cirrhosis, and new bone growth. Pathologic new bone growth occurs with osteoblastic lesions of the bone, as seen in metastatic breast and prostate cancer. Ingestion of hepatotoxic drugs may also elevate serum levels of ALP and AST.

17. A patient complains of burning with urination. What should be considered?

In general, burning with urination is a possible sign of urinary tract infection, including cystitis (inflammation of the bladder). Symptoms of a urinary tract infection (UTI) include urinary urgency and frequency as well as dysuria (painful urination). Some patients also complain of fever, hematuria (blood in the urine), and flank pain. In elderly people, dysuria is often absent, but there may be complaints of incontinence, confusion, and anorexia. UTIs are suggested by an abnormal urinalysis (presence of white cells and/or bacteria) and confirmed by urine culture. The absence or presence of bacteria is reported in the microscopic portion of the urinalysis. Gram stains of the urine may be performed prior to the culture results (which take 24–72 hours).

Hemorrhagic cystitis also may be indicated by burning urination in a patient with cancer who is receiving cyclophosphamide. Symptoms of hemorrhagic cystitis are similar to those of UTI; the diagnostic difference is the absence of organisms in the urinalysis. Hemorrhagic cystitis related to chemotherapy is a result of bladder mucosal irritation and inflammation from contact with acrolein, the metabolic byproduct of cyclophosphamide and ifosfamide.

18. A 73-year-old man with a history of lymphoma develops lower extremity edema. What are the possible causes?

To help identify the cause of peripheral edema, the first step is to determine whether it is unilateral or bilateral. Unilateral edema can be caused by (1) increased hydrostatic pressure from deep venous thrombophlebitis (DVT), venous insufficiency, or popliteal (Baker) cyst; (2) increased capillary permeability due to cellulitis or trauma; and (3) lymphatic obstruction. Patients with cancer, especially lymphoma, should be carefully evaluated for DVT (higher incidence in patients with cancer) and lymphedema caused by prior lymph node dissection or progression of disease. Bilateral edema can be classified into four main causes: (1) decreased oncotic pressure (e.g., malnutrition, hepatocellular failure, nephrotic syndrome, protein loss); (2) increased hydrostatic pressure (e.g., CHF, renal failure, salt retention, venous insufficiency, menstruation, pregnancy); (3) increased capillary permeability (e.g., systemic vasculitis, idiopathic edema, allergic reactions); and (4) lymphatic obstruction (rare, but may be seen with retroperitoneal or generalized lymphatic obstruction).

BIBLIOGRAPHY

1. Dowd TR, Stewart FM: Primary care approach to lymphadenopathy. Nurse Pract l9(l2):36–44, 1994.
2. Glick JH, Glover D: Oncologic emergencies. In Murphy GP, Lawrence W, Lenhard RE (eds): American Cancer Society Textbook of Clinical Oncology. Atlanta, American Cancer Society, 1995.
3. Goroll A, May LA, Mulley AG (eds): Primary Care Medicine, 3rd ed. Philadelphia, J.B. Lippincott, 1994.
4. Powel LL, Fishman M, Mrozek-Orlowski M (eds.): Oncology Nursing Society Cancer Chemotherapy Guidelines. Philadelphia, Oncology Nursing Society Press, 1996.
5. Shuey KM: Heart, lung and endocrine complications of solid tumors. Semin Oncol Nurs 10:177–188, 1994.

56. BREAST CANCER SCREENING

Mary Alice Browning, RN, MSN, OCN

1. What screening procedures are used to detect breast cancer?

Screening is the procedure of assessing presumably healthy people with no symptoms to detect disease before it has a chance to progress. The underlying concept is that early detection of disease can save lives and prevent unnecessary suffering. The three components of breast cancer screening are breast self-examination (BSE), clinical breast examination, and mammography. The general consensus is that the three techniques should be combined to ensure the earliest detection of breast cancer.

2. How compliant are women about performing breast self-examinations?

Although women currently discover approximately 90% of all breast lumps, it is estimated that BSE is practiced by only one-third of adult women in the United States. Primary barriers to consistent BSEs are lack of proficiency, lack of confidence in skills, and fear associated with finding a lump.

3. When should BSE be performed?

The BSE ideally should be done monthly. The best time for premenopausal women is 5–7 days after menses stops when breasts are least lumpy and tender. Postmenopausal women, women who menstruate irregularly, and pregnant women can select a specific date each month for their examinations.

4. What are the components of BSE?

The three essential components of BSE are (1) visual examination using a mirror, (2) palpation in the shower, and (3) palpation in the supine position on the bed. Visual examination should assess changes in appearance, including changes in shape, size, or symmetry; skin discoloration or dimpling; sores or scaling of the skin in the areola or on the nipple; nipple retraction; and discharge or puckering of the nipple. During visual examination, the arms initially should be relaxed at the side, then raised above the head, ending with the hands pressed downward into the hips. Visual inspection also should include an assessment of the breasts while bending at the waist.

5. How small of a lesion can a mammogram detect?

Currently, mammography can detect lesions in the breast as small as $\frac{1}{2}$ cm or one-fifth of an inch. To be palpated during self-examination, a lesion must be at least 1 cm or two-fifths of an inch.

6. What are the limitations of a mammogram?

A mammogram can take a picture only of the portion of the breast that protrudes. Breast tissue in the periphery is not caught on film. Malignant and benign lumps both appear white on mammography. Breast tissue is very dense and appears white on the mammogram, whereas fat is not dense and appears gray. Therefore, a lump in an area of dense breast tissue will be hidden and not readily apparent on the mammogram. For this reason mammograms are not very helpful in adolescents, whose breasts are predominantly dense. In premenopausal women under the age of 30, lesions can be difficult to identity; the possibility that a breast lesion may be missed is 9–20%.

7. What is digital mammography?

Digital mammography is an imaging method that computerizes the breast image and records it in computer code rather than on film. The radiologist can manipulate the computer image, focus on areas of concern, block the breast tissue so that only fat is visible, or block the fat so that only breast tissue is visible. Other advantages include greater accuracy in women with dense breasts and electronic transmission of the image to other health care providers, which facilitates consultation among experts.

8. Should patients be concerned about the amount of radiation used with mammography?

X-ray techniques have been refined so that little radiation is now used in mammography. The federal government has set standards that limit the amount of radiation to one-tenth of a rad for each two views of one breast. It is now commonly said that the radiation exposure received from mammography is equal to the amount of radiation received in an airplane flying over Denver.

9. How affordable is mammography?

The cost of a screening mammogram depends on the area of the country and the type of facility that is used. Most mammograms cost between $100–$150, although it is important to remember that high cost does not always indicate high quality.

Many insurance companies pay for all or part of the cost of screening mammograms. In fact, some states have passed legislation that requires that a portion or, in some cases, all mammography fees be paid by the insurance company before the deductible is met by the insured. For women 65 years or older, Medicare pays for a part of the cost every 2 years. This policy is unfortunate because increased age means increased risk and mammography has been shown to reduce deaths from breast cancer by 30% in older women.

10. Should women with breast implants have a mammogram?

Yes. However, special techniques must be used, both in taking the mammogram and in reading the films. First, because silicone implants are very dense on mammography and can block the view of the soft tissue behind them, proper breast positioning is particularly crucial to detect abnormal areas. Secondly, the mammographer must take care to avoid rupturing the implant when compressing the breasts. Finally, because interpretation is more difficult with implants, the mammograms should be reviewed by experienced radiologists.

11. What instructions about mammography should be provided to all women?

Women should be instructed about how the mammogram is performed and advised to schedule appointments after their menstrual period when the breasts are less tender. It is also important to remind women not to wear deodorant, perfumes, powders, ointments, or other preparations in the underarm or breast areas on the day of the procedure because they may either block the image or cause artifacts on the films.

12. What are the screening guidelines for having a mammogram?

Mammography has been shown to reduce breast cancer mortality by 30–39% in women aged 50 and older; however, there is debate over the benefit of screening mammography in women aged 40–49. The American Cancer Society based its guidelines on two studies (1962 Health Insurance Plan and Breast Cancer and Cervical Detection Project) suggesting that a baseline mammogram be taken at age 35 with a regular mammogram every 1–2 years in women under 50 years of age and every year in women over 50. In 1993 the National Cancer Institute (NCI) withdrew its support for regular mammograms in women aged 40–49 years. The NCI also changed its guidelines for women over 50 from annual to biennial mammograms. Some investigators believe that the mortality from breast cancer in women aged 40–49 could be reduced by 35% with annual mammograms (2 views per breast). In light of conflicting data about when to obtain screening mammography in women aged 40–49, the National Institutes of Health Consensus Development Program met in January 1997 to review updated results from recent studies of the role of breast cancer screening in women ages 40–49. Controversies still remain about screening guidelines. Women and their physicians will decide on a case by case basis.

13. Are there imaging alternatives to mammography?

Other imaging tests—such as ultrasound, magnetic resonance imaging (MRI), positron emission tomography (PET), 2-methoxy isobutyl isonitral (MIBI) scan, computerized tomography (CT), thermography, transillumination, and diaphography—have both advantages and limitations compared with mammography. However, because of factors such as cost and accuracy, none has been found to be an effective replacement for mammography in screening for breast cancer.

Ultrasound uses high-frequency sound waves delivered in pulsations to detect abnormalities in the breast. Ultrasound is appealing because no radiation is involved and it can distinguish a cyst or fluid-filled lesion from a solid lesion. Because a technician is holding and moving the transducer, it is also easier to examine the harder-to-reach areas and periphery of the breast, which is not imaged in mammography. There are two major limitations: efficacy depends on technician proficiency, and microcalcifications or other lesions may be less identifiable than with mammography.

When **MRI** was initially used in a study in Texas to detect breast lesions, it was hailed as the replacement for mammography. However, as a screening test, MRI is much too expensive and, as yet, not accurate in locating the lesions that it reveals. Needles and wires currently used for localization of a lesion in the breast cannot be used because of magnetization. An important advantage of MRI is that it can sometimes depict more accurately than mammography the extent of an identified cancer.

PET scans assess the amount and utilization of glucose in the breast. Because rapidly growing cancer cells use more glucose than normal tissues, malignant and benign lesions can be distinguished by glucose usage. PET scans may be used to assess the effectiveness of chemotherapy in slowing tumor growth. They have been successful in identifying metastatic disease and malignant nodes in the axillary region; however, sensitivity has not been reliably tested.

MIBI is a nuclear medicine imaging technique in which gallium is injected intravenously and a scanner determines whether the gallium is taken up by a suspicious breast lesion more readily than by the surrounding tissue. Cancer cells are more likely than benign cells to pick up gallium. Because radioactive material must be injected, MIBI is not particularly useful for screening. It also does not localize lesions well, and the results have far less resolution than mammography.

CT scanning is not acceptable for screening because the amount of radiation necessary to make cross-sections in the breast is not considered safe.

Thermography visualizes the interior of the breast by utilizing the principle that certain breast cancers and other breast abnormalities generate more heat than normal tissues. Unfortunately, this technique has not been accurate, primarily because not all cancers give off heat and some cancers are insulated from detection because they are wedged between areas of fat.

Transillumination is an old technique using equipment called diaphography to determine the amount of light transmitted in a lesion. If light showed through a lesion, it was assumed to be cystic; if not, it was considered solid and possibly malignant.

14. What is the role of genetic screening in the identification of breast cancer?

In 1994, BRCA1, an unusually long gene containing about 10 times the DNA found in the typical gene, was isolated on chromosome 17, region q12-21. When mutated, this gene has been connected to a susceptibility to breast and probably ovarian cancers. BRCA1 mutations are transmitted in an autosomal-dominant fashion. Approximately 1 in 200–400 women carries a susceptible allele of BRCA1. Fifty percent of the carrier's children will inherit the gene. The probability of carriers developing breast cancer is approximately 60% by age 50 and 82% by age 70. In 1995, a second breast cancer gene, BRCA2, was isolated on chromosome 13, region q. Mutations of BRCA2 may be responsible for about one-half of all cases of inherited breast cancer.

Another important discovery, the p53 antioncogene located on chromosome 17, region p13, seems to act as a regulator of the progression of the cell through the cell cycle. When the DNA is damaged, p53 commands other genes to halt cell division. If the damage is serious, p53 activates other genes to cause the cell to self-destruct. If damage to the cell is not evident, p53 allows the cell cycle to continue. Alterations in p53 have been identified in 50% of breast cancers. The effects of p53 mutation and inactivation are evident in families affected by Li-Fraumeni syndrome, which is also associated with an increased risk of many malignancies, including breast cancer. Affected persons often develop neoplasms before age 30.

Located on chromosome 9, region p21-2 is the multiple tumor suppressor-1 antioncogene (MTS-1), which directs the cell to make a protein called p 16. This gene may be particularly important because its mutation has been implicated in the genesis of many cancers, including breast cancer. HER-2 neu, a gene located on chromosome 17, band q21, is an intensively studied proto-oncogene. This protooncogene encodes a protein that is normally present in cell membranes. HER-2 neu amplification is found in 10–40% of breast cancers, with up to a 20-fold amplification found in 25–30%.

Although only an estimated 5–10% of all breast cancers are inherited, the identification of susceptibility genes will allow a more precise evaluation of the incidence of inheritance of breast cancer, as well as identification of women at highest risk for the disease. Genes and gene markers may provide tools for improving cancer diagnosis and treatment. By identifying a mutated gene in cells that may be shed into stool, urine, saliva, or tissues biopsies, health care professionals may be able to detect cancer years earlier than with conventional techniques in current use. The evaluation and development of cancer drugs may be refined through an understanding of genetics. If a gene is found to produce an antitumor protein, it may be possible to synthesize the protein as a cancer medication. It may even be possible to overcome cancer by inactivating or replacing an altered gene. Genetic screening is likely to play a significant role in the future; however, the initiation of such screening before vital questions about its impact are answered may cause more harm than good.

15. What are the limitations of genetic testing?

1. Current genetic testing cannot provide a satisfactory answer for everyone who seems to be at risk for inherited breast cancer. In some families, multiple cases may reflect a shared environmental exposure rather than inherited susceptibility. Even when an inherited gene is responsible for breast cancers in a family, it may not be the test gene. For example, BRCA1 is found in only about one-half of the families with hereditary breast cancer.

2. Despite major advances in genetic testing, identifying mutations remains a great challenge. BRCA1, for example, is one of the largest genes being tested. It contains many bases in long stretches of DNA that may contain one or many mutations anywhere within the gene. With this fact in mind, a positive test for a mutated gene does not necessarily mean that breast cancer is imminent. In addition, a negative result cannot completely rule out breast cancer because the test evaluates only the most common mutations.

3. Even if the breast cancer gene is absent, the woman is still not safe from developing breast cancer. Over 90% of breast cancers are sporadic and not associated with the currently identified gene.

4. Predictive genetic tests deal in probabilities, not certainties. A person with a dominant gene, such as the hereditary breast cancer gene, may develop the disease, whereas another person with the same gene remains healthy.

5. Mutations of a specific gene may not be the only important factor. The breast cancer gene may respond to the commands of other genes or gene markers, or it may respond to a factor within the environment.

6. Finally, the most significant limitation to genetic screening for breast cancer is that no interventions have been definitely identified to prevent breast cancer in the event of a positive genetic test result. The ethical question is raised: Should the ability to predict precede the ability to prevent or cure?

16. Is there a role for preventive mastectomies?

One drastic solution used over the years to prevent breast cancer is preventive mastectomy. Contrary to popular belief, this procedure does not eliminate the risk of breast cancer. Breast tissue extends from the clavicle to below the rib cage and from the sternum around to the spine, with no obvious distinction from surrounding tissues. Therefore, it would be impossible for any surgeon to eliminate all breast tissue from the body. Preventive mastectomies probably remove some of the risk of breast cancer, but it is impossible to quantify the risk. Currently, participation in routine screening, with detection of breast cancer at an early stage, offers women the best chances of successful treatment and survival.

BIBLIOGRAPHY

1. American Cancer Society: Breast Cancer Facts and Figures 1996. Atlanta, American Cancer Society, 1996.
2. Carlson K J, Eisenstat SA, Ziporyn T: The Harvard Guide to Women's Health. Cambridge, MA, Harvard University Press, 1996.
3. Carroll-Johnson R M (ed): The genetic revolution: Promise and predicament for oncology nurses. Oncol Nurs Forum 22:1–37, 1995.
4. Feig SA: Estimation of currently attainable benefit from mammographic screening of women age 40–49 years. Cancer 75:2412–2419, 1995.
5. Groenwald SL, Frogge MH, Goodman M , Yarbro CH (eds): Cancer Nursing: Principles and Practice, 3rd. ed. Boston, Jones & Bartlett, 1995.
6. Henderson LC: Breast cancer. In Murphy GP, Lawrence W, Lenhard RE (eds): American Cancer Society Textbook of Clinical Oncology. Atlanta, American Cancer Society, 1995, pp 198–219.
7. Kneece JC: Finding a Lump in Your Breasts: Where to Go, What to Do. Columbia, SC, EduCare, 1996.
8. Love S M, Lindsey K: Dr. Susan Love's Breast Book, 2nd. ed. New York, Addison-Wesley, 1995.
9. Morra M, Poots E: Choices: Realistic Alternatives in Cancer Treatment, 2nd. ed. New York, Avon Books, 1994.
10. National Cancer Institute: Understanding Gene Testing. NIH publ. no. 96-3905. Washington, DC, U. S. Department of Health and Human Services, 1995.

57. CANCER AND PREGNANCY

Linda U. *Krebs*, RN, PhD, AOCN

1. How common is cancer associated with pregnancy?
Although generally considered to be a rare event, the incidence of cancer associated with pregnancy is increasing. Cancer is one of the most common diagnoses and the second leading cause of death during the reproductive years. Approximately 1 of every 118 pregnancies will be complicated by a cancer diagnosis.

2. Why is the incidence of cancer associated with pregnancy increasing?
As women delay childbearing until later in life (into their 30s and early 40s), the likelihood of having concomitant pregnancy and cancer has increased. In addition, the incidence of some of the more common types of cancer (e.g., breast cancer, cervical cancer) appears to be increasing in younger women. The combination of delayed childbearing and younger incidence of specific cancers has led to the increase.

3. What is the time frame for pregnancy associated with cancer?
Most authors include not only the 9 months of pregnancy but also the 6 months (some include up to 1 year) before becoming pregnant or after delivering as the time frame for a pregnancy-associated cancer.

4. What are the predominant types of cancer diagnosed during pregnancy?
In descending order, the cancers most commonly diagnosed during pregnancy are breast cancer, cervical cancer, ovarian cancer, colorectal cancer, lymphoma, and leukemia. Malignant melanoma, although rare, is often included in any discussion of cancer associated with pregnancy because its incidence is rising and it is frequently found during the reproductive years. Breast cancer occurs in approximately 1 of every 3000 pregnancies. Cervical cancer occurs in approximately 1 of every 400 pregnancies; the majority of cases, however, are not invasive but rather carcinoma in situ. Ovarian masses are a common finding during pregnancy. Between 1 in 9,000 and 1 in 25,000 will be malignant. Pregnancies associated with colorectal cancer, Hodgkin's disease, non-Hodgkin's lymphoma, leukemia, and malignant melanoma are even less common.

5. Is cancer arising during pregnancy more aggressive than the same type of cancer in a nonpregnant woman?
Cancer arising during pregnancy was previously believed to be more aggressive because the stage of disease was more apt to be advanced (stage III or IV) at diagnosis. However, indepth review of the stage of disease at diagnosis, treatment regimens, and overall survival statistics has shown that woman of equivalent stages and treatments have similar survival statistics regardless of pregnancy. What appears to be the most likely cause for advanced disease is delay in making the diagnosis. This delay is due, in part, to the difficulty of recognizing the signs and symptoms of cancer in pregnant women.

6. Is therapeutic abortion of benefit in the management of cancer associated with pregnancy?
Scientific studies have not shown therapeutic abortion to be of any benefit in controlling disease or prolonging survival. In general, the pregnancy does not affect the outcome of the cancer, and the cancer does not affect the pregnancy. Therapeutic abortion may be of benefit if the planned treatment would be detrimental to the fetus and altering treatment to spare the fetus would have a negative impact on the mother's survival. The decision to have a therapeutic abortion should not

be made until the risks of maintaining the pregnancy during delivery of optimal cancer treatment have been thoroughly explained and discussed with the pregnant woman and her significant others.

7. Is it difficult to differentiate between body alterations found with routine pregnancy and signs and symptoms of cancer?

Making the diagnosis of cancer during a pregnancy may be difficult because of similarities among common symptoms associated with pregnancy and the signs and symptoms often associated with cancer. Nausea and vomiting, constipation, breast changes, changes in moles, fatigue, backache and other constitutional symptoms are common to both cancer and pregnancy. A breast mass is often believed to be related to a plugged milk duct, whereas the changes in the size and pigmentation of a mole may be believed to be part of normal changes in the skin during pregnancy. Patient concerns must be fully evaluated. In addition, the patient's history and current risks for cancer must be taken into consideration.

8. Are there any specific contraindications to the use of x-rays, radioisotopes, or other diagnostic methods in pregnant patients?

X-rays should be used sparingly, if at all, in pregnant patients. When they are necessary, adequate fetal shielding must be used. Chest x-rays deliver minuscule doses of radiation and, with appropriate shielding, appear to be safe during pregnancy.

Mammography may be safely undertaken if the abdomen is adequately shielded. Mammography is not considered to be highly reliable, however, because of increased breast density, decreased fatty tissue, and increased water content of the breasts during pregnancy.

Ultrasound and magnetic resonance imaging may be safely used. Computerized tomography and isotope studies are not recommended.

Tumor markers (e.g., alpha-fetoprotein, beta-human chorionic gonadotropin, lactate dehydrogenase, CA-125) are of limited benefit because many markers are routinely elevated during pregnancy.

Fine-needle aspiration, Papanicolaou smear, and colposcopy are considered safe. Biopsy under local or general anesthesia is also safe if adequate fetal oxygenation and circulation are maintained. Although cone biopsy may be undertaken, complication rates may be as high as 30%; specific complications include infection, hemorrhage, and premature delivery.

9. How should cancer associated with pregnancy be treated?

As a general rule, a woman diagnosed with cancer during pregnancy should receive the same treatment options as a nonpregnant woman with the same malignancy. Some modifications may be necessary to minimize fetal exposure to chemotherapy or radiation. In some instances, definitive therapy may be delayed until after delivery with little or no risk to the patient. In other instances, therapeutic abortion may be undertaken to provide aggressive therapy that could be potentially lethal to the fetus. In all cases, therapeutic decisions should be individualized. Recommendations for specific cancer types include the following:

Breast cancer. Modified radical mastectomy with lymph node sampling is the standard treatment. Lumpectomy with lymph node sampling also may be undertaken. Radiation therapy is not generally recommended for pregnant patients and is usually delayed until after delivery. Adjuvant chemotherapy may be safely given after the first trimester or may be delayed until after delivery.

Cervical cancer. For carcinoma in situ, the pregnancy can be allowed to continue, with definitive therapy delayed until after delivery. Close follow-up with intermittent biopsy is imperative. For invasive disease, radical surgery or radiation therapy, without therapeutic abortion, is recommended. If the patient is near delivery, viability can be awaited, the infant delivered by cesarean section, and definitive therapy then completed.

Ovarian cancer. Early-stage disease may be safely managed by unilateral oophorectomy and biopsy of the contralateral ovary. The pregnancy can be continued. For advanced disease, treatment consists of a radical hysterectomy, omentectomy, node biopsies, and peritoneal washings. The uterus is removed without prior evacuation of the fetus.

Colorectal cancer. Definitive therapy with a colectomy or abdominoperineal resection can generally be undertaken in the first 20 weeks of gestation without hazard to the fetus. For more advanced disease, involving the uterus or impeding access to the rectum, radical hysterectomy may need to be included. For the second half of gestation, viability is awaited, if possible, with definitive therapy after delivery. If an obstruction is present, a colostomy may be performed in the interim.

Lymphoma. Combination chemotherapy is generally the treatment of choice. In the first 20 weeks of gestation a therapeutic abortion is recommended. In the second half, chemotherapy may be given or, if the fetus is near viability, treatment may be delayed until after delivery.

Leukemia. Treatment with chemotherapy should be instituted without delay. If the fetus is viable, delivery should occur as soon as possible. Therapeutic abortion is suggested for patients in the first trimester.

Malignant melanoma. Primary treatment consists of wide local excision with skin graft, if necessary. Lymph node dissection remains controversial. The benefits of adjuvant therapy are unclear.

10. Is the survival rate of pregnant patients diagnosed with cancer different from that of nonpregnant patients?

A stage-for-stage comparison reveals no difference in survivorship between pregnant and nonpregnant patients diagnosed with cancer, regardless of the type of cancer.

11. What are the effects of cancer treatment on the fetus?

Surgery. Maternal surgery involves minimal risk to the fetus if hypotension is prevented and adequate oxygenation is ensured. General anesthesia is well tolerated after the first trimester. Pelvic surgery is more easily achieved after the first trimester.

Radiation therapy. Fetal damage is unlikely at doses < 50 cGy. Radiation doses > 250 cGy have been associated with fetal damage, including spontaneous abortion, mental retardation, microcephaly, sterility, cataracts, and skin changes. Radiation exposure during the first trimester is of greatest concern. Even with adequate shielding, radiation scatter may be sufficient to cause harm or fetal demise. Radiation therapy should be avoided if at all possible.

Chemotherapy. Chemotherapy during the first trimester has been associated with low birth weight, fetal malformations, and fetal demise. The incidence may be minimized or avoided by careful selection of agents or combinations of agents and/or delaying chemotherapy until after the first trimester. Unexpected or more severe toxicities may occur in the fetus because of alterations in individual drug pharmacokinetics due to the normal physiologic changes associated with pregnancy. This is of particular importance if chemotherapy is administered close to delivery. The neonate's metabolism and excretion of chemotherapeutic agents may not be sufficient when its primary mechanism of drug excretion, the placenta, is no longer present; thus, increased exposure to drugs and enhanced toxicities may result.

12. What is the incidence of malformation in fetuses exposed to chemotherapy during gestation?

Fetal malformation is estimated to be < 10%. Examples of malformation include skeletal malformations, hydrocephalus, atrial/septal defects, cranial dysostosis, various limb deformities, and cerebral anomalies. Methotrexate and aminopterin (a folic acid antagonist developed before methotrexate) have been most commonly implicated. The incidence is higher when combination therapy is given. The incidence is highest when chemotherapy is given in the first trimester and lowest when chemotherapy is given in the second or third trimester. The incidence of major congenital malformations in all births is approximately 3%, whereas it may reach 9% in minor malformations.

Fetal Abnormalities Associated with Exposure To Chemotherapy

AGENT	ABNORMALITY/MALFORMATION
Aminopterin	Spontaneous abortion Aminopterin syndrome: cranial dysostosis, hypertelorism, wide nasal bridge, micrognathia, external ear anomalies Skeletal malformations Cerebral anomalies
Methotrexate	Spontaneous abortion Skeletal malformations Intrauterine growth retardation
5-Fluorouracil	Spontaneous abortion Intrauterine growth retardation
Cyclophosphamide	Spontaneous abortion Intrauterine growth retardation
Busulfan	Spontaneous abortion Skeletal malformations
Procarbazine	Atrial/septal defects

13. Does the mother's cancer ever spread to the fetus?

Maternal-to-fetal spread is extremely rare, although scientific reports have included malignant melanoma, non-Hodgkin's lymphoma, leukemia, breast cancer, lung cancer, and gastrointestinal malignancies. A variety of single case reports also can be found in the literature. In all instances, the mothers had widely disseminated disease. In most reported series, malignant melanoma is the most common form of cancer associated with fetal spread. In some instances only the placenta is involved; in other instances, the cancer spreads to the fetus. Some infants have died of the disease.

14. What are the specific recommendations about delivery?

The type of delivery, vaginal vs. cesarean section, is controversial for women with cervical cancer. Some health care professionals are concerned that, in the presence of active disease, vaginal delivery will spread the cancer or cause infection or hemorrhage; thus cesarean section is recommended. Others report that vaginal delivery does not increase risk of disease dissemination, hemorrhage, or infection and in fact may be associated with increased maternal survival. Four cases of recurrence of disease in the vaginal episiotomy have been reported. The definitive answer for cervical cancer remains unclear. Careful follow-up for recurrence is mandatory in all women who have vaginal deliveries. Cesarean section is the method of choice if the woman is to undergo radical hysterectomy after delivery.

For all other cancer types, the type of delivery depends on disease status, fetal gestation, immediacy of delivery, and whether definitive treatment, requiring an abdominal incision, is to be done after delivery. For ovarian cancer, treatment is often undertaken at delivery; thus, a cesarean section is performed, followed by radical hysterectomy.

If possible, delivery should be timed so that patients receiving chemotherapy will have recovered from bone marrow suppression and other therapy-related toxicities. A complete blood count and other appropriate laboratory parameters should be evaluated before delivery, and extra precautions to minimize bleeding and infection should be taken as necessary.

15. What types of neonatal monitoring should occur at delivery?

The fetus exposed to chemotherapy may be premature and also may weigh less than expected for gestational age. Because of the potential for increased toxicities, particularly if treatment is given close to delivery, laboratory evaluation should include a complete blood count. The neonate should be evaluated carefully for chemotherapy-induced malformations, including skeletal and internal organ abnormalities. The placenta and neonate also should be evaluated for signs of metastatic involvement, particularly if the mother has disseminated disease.

16. Is it possible to breastfeed an infant during or after treatment for cancer?

Breastfeeding is contraindicated when the mother is receiving chemotherapy or undergoing tests that use radioactive materials; these agents or their metabolites can be found in breast milk and may be detrimental to the infant. Breastfeeding can be safely recommended for all other patients. Women with breast cancer who have received breast radiation may have diminished or absent lactation on the radiated side. They are generally discouraged from attempting to breastfeed on the radiated side because of an increased risk of developing mastitis.

17. Are future pregnancies possible or recommended after a diagnosis of cancer?

The ability to become pregnant after a diagnosis of cancer depends on the primary site, stage of disease, type and extent of therapy, and age of the woman. For women who wish to conceive and remain physically capable of doing so, there are no known contraindications. Most authors recommend a waiting period of 1–5 years after completion of therapy, depending on stage of disease. This recommendation minimizes the possibility of recurrence during the future pregnancy and allows the woman to regain physical and emotional health before undergoing the rigors of pregnancy.

18. What are the specific recommendations for prevention and early detection of cancer while a woman is pregnant?

All initial prenatal visits should include a Papanicolaou smear and a thorough breast examination. Women should be instructed to do breast self-examinations (BSE) monthly throughout pregnancy. In addition, women should be taught self-examination techniques for skin and encouraged to complete them on a monthly basis. A thorough history for cancer risks should be obtained, and special precautions and evaluations should be included in prenatal care as appropriate. Pregnant woman should be encouraged to discuss all abnormal findings or concerns with health care providers. All concerns should be evaluated thoroughly.

19. What is known about the long-term survival and future cancer risk of children exposed to cancer treatment in utero?

There appear to be no alterations in longterm survival and no increased risk of cancer, beyond that which is related to heredity, in children exposed to cancer treatment in utero. Rare abnormalities with no obvious pattern have been shown in long-term studies of children exposed to chemotherapy. Long-term effects of low-dose radiation are currently unknown. Follow-up of children exposed to higher doses of radiation is limited. Concerns for such children remain, and follow-up over many generations will be necessary to determine the exact effects.

20. Is nursing management of pregnant women with cancer any different from management of a woman who has cancer or a woman who is pregnant?

Nursing management for pregnant women with cancer is much more complex. Primary nursing roles include assessment, physical care, emotional support, and provision of information and education. The team approach, involving oncology, obstetrics, neonatology, and various support services, is essential. In addition to routine medical and nursing management strategies, educational, psychosocial, and ethical interventions need to be incorporated into the plan of care. Because of disease, treatment, fears for the fetus, concerns about survival, and numerous other anxieties, normal activities of pregnancy may be deferred or prevented. Ethical dilemmas may occur as treatment needs are weighed against fetal survival. Emotional support is essential and can take its toll on the health care provider as well as on the patient and family.

21. What are the risks to the health care professional who mixes, administers, or handles chemotherapeutic agents while pregnant, breastfeeding, or attempting to conceive?

Risks vary, depending on whether one is mixing or administering chemotherapy or handling chemotherapy-contaminated excreta. The highest risk occurs when admixing drugs, the lowest when handling excreta. The Occupational Safety and Health Administration notes a lack of in-depth information available to quantify exact risks. Previous studies showing increased risk to women handling chemotherapeutic agents were conducted when adequate guidelines were not available or recommendations for protection had not been followed. Possible risks include spontaneous abortion and an increased incidence of ectopic pregnancy. Adequate protection should minimize, if not eliminate, potential risks.

22. Do special precautions in the mixing, administration, and handling of chemotherapeutic agents apply only to women who are trying to conceive?

Both women and men who are attempting pregnancy should minimize exposure to chemotherapeutic agents through the use of appropriate protective equipment.

BIBLIOGRAPHY

1. Brant J: Is it safe for pregnant nurses to be exposed to chemotherapy agents? ONS News 10(3):5, 1995.
2. Caligiuri MA: Leukemia in pregnancy. Adv Oncol 8(3):10–17, 1992.
3. Doll DC: Chemotherapy in pregnancy. In Perry MC (ed): The Chemotherapy Sourcebook. Baltimore, Williams & Wilkins, 1992, pp 703–709.
4. Dow KH, Harris JR, Roy C: Pregnancy after breast-conserving surgery and radiation therapy for breast cancer. JNCI Monographs 16:131–137, 1995.
5. Krebs LU: Sexual and reproductive dysfunction. In Groenwald SL, Frogge MH, Goodman M, Yarbro CH (eds): Cancer Nursing: Principles and Practice, 4th ed. Boston, Jones & Bartlett (in press).
6. Mott-Smith ME, Stolberg L: Sexual function and pregnancy. In Casciato DA, Lowitz BB (eds): Manual of Clinical Oncology, 3rd ed. Boston, Little, Brown, 1995, pp 575–582.
7. Oncology Nursing Society: Safe Handling of Cytotoxic Drugs. Pittsburgh, Oncology Nursing Society, 1989.
8. Shapiro CL, Mayer RJ: Breast cancer in pregnancy. Adv Oncol 8(3):25–29, 1992.
9. Ward FT, Weiss RB: Lymphoma in pregnancy. Adv Oncol 8(3):18–22, 1992.

58. CANCER IN THE ELDERLY

Deborah McCaffrey Boyle, RN, MSN, OCN

1. Why is cancer in the elderly an issue in cancer care?

Cancer in the elderly is an issue for two critical reasons. First, cancer is prominent in this age group. More than one-half of all cancers occur in the elderly, despite the fact that the elderly represent only approximately 12% of the United States population. Thus, most cancers occur disproportionately in relatively few Americans.[6] Second, despite the prevalence of cancer in this age group, there has been little investigation of cancer and its treatment in the elderly. Studies need to be done to explain the heightened risk of cancer in the elderly, their response to treatment, incidence, and severity of toxicities.

2. How can we explain the lack of research?

Ageism, or societal prejudice against the elderly, is most likely responsible for a lack of interest in addressing the special needs of the elderly who face cancer. There is no dedicated subspecialty in elder cancer care similar to pediatric oncology, which was initiated over two decades ago. Yet children with cancer represent less than 10% of all Americans who develop cancer. Our culture places higher value on children than on the elderly, which has been described as the social worth phenomenon. We perceive the actual or potential loss of a child to be significant not only to the immediate family but also to society as a whole. Related to this phenomenon is the tendency to establish loss rationales; health professionals and the public alike can justify the potential diagnosis and death of an elder from cancer as due to longevity, which is not the case with a child. Identification with the younger patient and family is also a consideration, for the majority of the oncology workforce is drawn from the baby boomer generation that first emerged in the mid 1970s.

3. How has the lack of attentiveness to the elderly affected what we know and do not know about cancer?

Of most significance is the fact that historically we have not treated cancer among the elderly aggressively, based on the assumption that they could not withstand the rigors of aggressive therapy. Until recently, the elderly have been excluded from participation in clinical trials on the basis of chronologic age, with age 65 as the cutoff point. This exclusion has resulted in two important phenomena. First, by not allowing the elderly to be entered in clinical trials, we have minimal quantitative data to substantiate how in fact the elderly fare in a variety of cancer treatment regimens. This lack of information then perpetuates the practice of treating the elderly based on assumption and speculation rather than on the results of vigorous research. Second, the lack of research facilitates the elderly receiving substandard treatment when, in fact, they may have benefited from a more aggressive regimen. An important article published in *Lancet* in 1990 by European oncologists states the following:

> There is widespread misconception that the elderly are always poorly tolerant of chemotherapy or radiotherapy, with the inevitable result that many elderly patients with cancer are undertreated. In current practice the elderly, disenfranchised as they are from entry to clinical trials, receive either untested treatments, inadequate treatment or even none at all, at the whim of their clinician. Any novel therapy, if only used for those aged less than 70 years, will have a reduced effect on population mortality statistics because only half of those with that disease will receive adequate treatment.[5]

Inadequate treatment affects not only statistics about the elderly, but also how these statistics impact overall success in reducing cancer mortality in a more global fashion. The war on cancer initiated in the early 1970s has few major success stories in terms of mortality reduction. Perhaps the inadequate treatment of the elderly over the years has contributed to this reality.

4. How should the elderly be treated for cancer?

The elderly individual's physiologic age should be a major determinant of appropriate cancer therapy recommendations rather than the patient's chronologic age. The patient's baseline function—in particular, the presence or absence of comorbid disease—is an important consideration in the planning of a treatment regimen for the elderly with cancer. Comorbid diseases such as cardiovascular, pulmonary, renal, and diabetes conditions often interfere with an aggressive approach to an antineoplastic regimen. These conditions often preclude the administration of regimens with possible organ toxicity or dose-intensive treatment schema.

5. Why is cancer so prevalent in the elderly?

There are nine major theories about why cancer is so prevalent in the elderly. These theories are, in most respects, complementary and highly interrelated. They include the likelihood that cancer in the elderly is due to the following factors:
- Longer duration of carcinogen exposure
- Accumulation of somatic mutations with longevity
- Decreased ability to repair DNA
- Oncogene activation or amplification
- Tumor suppressor gene loss
- Decreased immune surveillance
- Increased cell-mediated immune senescence
- Increased sensitivity to oncogenic viruses
- Increased tendency toward hormone imbalance[3,4]

6. What are the major cancers in the elderly?

The major cancers in the elderly are primarily solid tumors that have a long latency period. Along with prolonged tumor doubling times (which are characteristic of most solid tumors), there is the heightened possibility for metastases. Often, the cancers that occur most often in the elderly population are difficult to treat regardless of the age of the patient at diagnosis. The major tumors in the elderly are the following:

Male	Female
Prostate	Breast
Lung	Lung
Colorectal	Colorectal
Bladder	Uterine

7. Are other cancers prominent in the elderly?

Yes. Other malignancies that do not represent the highest overall incidence rates are significant because they occur almost exclusively in the elderly. Examples include gastric malignancies, cancers of the vulva and gallbladder, multiple myeloma, and chronic leukemias. Approximately two-thirds of these malignancies occur in the elderly population. Additionally, the incidence of acute nonlymphocytic leukemias (variants of acute myelogenous leukemia) is rising in the above-60-year-old population.

8. How does this heightened incidence rate relate to mortality rates in the elderly subset of cancer patients?

Until recently, it was thought that the elderly always fared poorly in regard to treatment outcomes, based primarily on the variable of advanced age. However, close scrutiny of major clinical trials in which the elderly were allowed entry reveals that the stage of disease at initial diagnosis is an important determinant of treatment outcome. Many elderly are initially staged with higher levels of malignant involvement at diagnosis than their younger counterparts. Greater tumor burden, then, may be responsible for poorer outcomes from treatment rather than the variable of chronologic age alone.

9. Who is responsible for the lack of early detection, health professionals or the patient?

The responsibility may lie with both parties involved at the time of initial diagnosis. The patient may allocate potential suspicious symptoms of cancer to factors related to advancing age or to other comorbid diseases, as may the health professional. Cohen[4] outlined these factors as the phenomenon of cancer symptom confusion in the elderly.

Symptom or Sign	Possible Malignancy	Aging Explanation
Increase in skin pigment	Melanoma, squamous cell	Age spots
Rectal bleeding	Colon or rectal cancer	Hemorrhoids
Constipation	Rectal cancer	Old age
Dyspnea	Lung cancer	Getting old, out of shape
Decrease in urinary stream	Prostate cancer	Dribbling—benign prostatic hypertrophy
Breast contour change	Breast cancer	Normal atrophy, fibrosis
Fatigue	Metastatic or other	Loss of energy due to aging
Bone pain	Metastatic or other	Arthritis: aches and pains of aging

10. What is the best approach to deal with this problem?

Despite the fact that cancer is primarily a disease of the elderly, few public education programs target the elderly who are at greatest risk for cancer. Public education programs should take into consideration barriers to community education specific to the elderly. Examples include problems with transportation (can they get to the programs and screening?), neurosensory impairment (can the person read, see, and hear the information?), misperceptions (does the individual understand the varieties of cancer and the many factors that influence outcome?), and acknowledgment of the benefit of early detection in terms of treatment outcome (does the elderly individual have a fatalistic attitude, assuming that all cancer is a death sentence and viewing screening and early detection as useless?).

11. Which cancers should we target in terms of elderly education and early detection?

The two most problematic cancers now and certainly in the future are breast and prostate cancers. The majority (> 50%) of these malignancies occur in the elderly; hence, they should be the focus of major efforts in public awareness and screening. Lack of knowledge of risk based on advanced age and embarrassment due to the nature of the examinations associated with these cancers may preclude willingness to participate in early intervention programs and educational offerings. Monthly breast self-examination and yearly mammograms are recommended for women over age 50. Annual digital rectal examination and prostate-specific antigen (PSA) evaluation are recommended for men over age 50.

12. Is surgery usually problematic for older cancer patients because of advanced age?

Normative changes in physiologic function occur with advancing age. The major changes include reductions in the following parameters:

- Cardiac index
- Standard glomerular filtration rate
- Vital capacity
- Standard renal plasma flow
- Maximal breathing capacity[3]

These changes, however, are highly variable based on genetic, nutritional, and self-care practices. Yet in looking at factors that appear to contribute to morbidity, factors associated not only with surgery but also with the prominence of toxicities associated with radiation therapy and chemotherapy, it appears that the presence of comorbid conditions is the most important predictor of problems associated with treatment tolerance.

13. What are the most important comorbid conditions affecting outcomes of treatment for elderly patients?

Comorbid conditions (sometimes referred to as intercurrent illnesses) that are most problematic include cardiovascular conditions (i.e., cardiac and cerebrovascular disease, hypertension, thromboembolism), pulmonary compromise, diabetes, renal problems, and malnutrition. These problems rather than chronologic age alone may contribute to the incidence and severity of toxicities associated with cancer therapy, and thus place the older patient at heightened risk for poorer outcome from treatment.

14. Do the elderly in general have more problems with medication tolerance than younger counterparts?

Important pharmacologic parameters of medication tolerance in the elderly include consideration of pharmacokinetics (i.e., how the elderly person activates, metabolizes, distributes, and excretes drugs) and pharmacodynamics (how the drugs affect the elderly person's target organs in terms of toxicity prevalence).[1] Despite acknowledged changes in both processes with advanced age, there is little information to help with dose titration guidelines compared with what is available for pediatric dosing recommendations. The exception is information about renal toxicity and dose modification in the elderly when a renally toxic drug is prescribed. In general, however, drugs with bone marrow toxicity are most problematic in the elderly. Limited bone marrow reserve and cellularity may preclude the older cancer patient's ability to bounce back from bone marrow compromise caused by chemotherapeutic agents. This is of particular concern when the older patient has a hematologic malignancy in which bone marrow dysfunction predates administration of antineoplastic therapy.

15. What other problems may be medication-related in the elderly?

An important medication-related issue in the elderly is polypharmacy or multiple drug therapy. When multiple drugs are prescribed to treat a variety of ills (which may be the case in the elderly with numerous comorbid conditions), several phenomena may relate to compliance. First, the elderly may not take the drug(s) as prescribed because of confusion, forgetfulness, or the fact that pill-taking becomes an overwhelming expectation on an ongoing basis. On the average, two drugs are prescribed per chronic illness, and many elderly may be dealing with multiple chronic conditions other than cancer. Evidence suggests that when we ask the elderly to take more than three drugs on a routine basis, at least one of the drugs will be mishandled. Hence, the clinicians should think of the medications that they ask patients to take for pain, emesis, bowel alterations, infection, and hormonal control as well as what they may be expected to take for other chronic illness(es). Polypharmacy in the elderly is a critical consideration in the assessment of untoward effects during cancer treatment, yet it remains a predominantly unstudied and unacknowledged area of concern.

16. Is confusion often related to problems with drug therapy?

Acute confusion in elderly cancer patients is often related to problems with drug therapy as well as metabolic factors. Infection, hypoxia, hypercalcemia, and hyponatremia are just a few common physiologic factors to consider. Additionally, the use of drugs with central nervous activity, particularly those with central anticholinergic effects (drugs with atropine), are most troublesome to the elderly. Concurrent administration of these drugs to the elderly often escalates the likelihood of acute confusion. When assessing the nature of confusion in an elderly patient, it is critical to ask key family members, "Is the confusion new, or is it a gradual worsening of an insidious problem?" If the confusion is new and unlike any prior change in the patient, then an acute confusional state must be considered and a metabolic or drug-related etiology should be evaluated. Once the source of the confusion is determined and treated, the confusion should clear and be reversible. A history of ongoing and progressive mental status changes reported by the family over time, however, may indicate the presence of an organic dementia rather than an acute confusional state.

17. Why are bowel problems of concern in elderly patients?

Like acute confusion, there are multiple causes of bowel alterations, most specifically constipation, in the elderly. Just as multiple factors may contribute to the problem, so must multiple factors be considered in treatment. Alterations in mobility, changes in eating patterns, decreased fluid and insufficient fiber intake, and use of drugs that may cause constipation are factors to consider. In particular, opioids and vinca alkaloid chemotherapeutic agents (vincristine, velban, etoposide) cause constipation because of peripheral neurotoxic effects in the elderly. When these drugs are prescribed, a prophylactic bowel regimen should be started immediately to counter the likelihood of constipation.

18. What about depression in the elderly?

Many nurses and other health professionals expect depression to be a major corollary to cancer in the elderly. It is indeed true that the older adult has many losses to adapt to. Examples include loss of work or financial independence, change in living arrangements, and loss of health, spouse, significant others, or physical stamina. Hence, much of what the elderly must contend with is normal sadness rather than a major depressive event. The most important predictor of a major depressive response in elderly cancer patients, however, is a premorbid history of depression. Thus, just because patients are elderly, we should not expect the majority to suffer from significant depression. A careful precancer history is paramount.

19. Overall, what are the major areas I can learn more about to provide better care for older patients with cancer?

All of us would be well served to learn more about general principles of gerontologic nursing and then to apply them to what we know about cancer nursing. For example, six conditions linked with aging have implications for nursing care of elderly cancer patients: falls, acute confusion, altered nutrition, bowel and bladder dysfunction, skin integrity, and sleep disturbances.[2] Applying knowledge gained from the gerontologic literature to the clinical practice of cancer nursing will improve the quality of nursing care delivery to elderly patients with cancer.

20. Do elderly patients ever fare better than younger patients?

Indeed yes. Many of us can cite numerous occasions in which older patients with cancer in fact did much better than anticipated and even seemed to run circles around younger counterparts. Again, the patient's physiologic age is a better determinant than chronologic age. The fact that someone is elderly does not mean that he or she has significant diminished capacity. In fact, many elderly may be in better physiologic condition than some middle-aged patients. In emphasizing the resiliency of many elderly to overcome many obstacles put before them, a patient once poignantly reminded me, "If your time hasn't come yet, not even a doctor can kill you!"

BIBLIOGRAPHY

1. Balducci L, Parker M, Sexton W, Tantranond P: Pharmacology of antineoplastic agents in the elderly patient. Semin Oncol 16:76–84, 1989.
2. Boyle DM, Engelking C, Blesch KS, et al: Oncology Nursing Society position paper on cancer and aging: The mandate for oncology nursing. Oncol Nurs Forum 19:913–933, 1992.
3. Boyle DM: Realities to guide novel and necessary nursing care in geriatric oncology. Cancer Nurs 17:125–136, 1994.
4. Cohen HJ: Oncology and aging: General principles of cancer in the elderly. In Hazzard WR, Bierman EL, Blass JP, et al (eds): Principles of Geriatric Medicine, 3rd ed. New York, McGraw-Hill, 1994.
5. Fentiman IS, Tirelli U, Monfardini S, et al: Cancer in the elderly: Why so badly treated? Lancet 335:1020–1022, 1990.
6. Monfardini S, Yancik R: Cancer in the elderly: Meeting the challenge of an aging population. J Natl Cancer Inst 85:532–538, 1993.

59. SURVIVORSHIP

Susan A. Leigh, BSN, RN, and
Debra Thaler-DeMers, BSN, RN, OCN, PHN

> From the time of its discovery and for the balance of life, an individual diagnosed with cancer is a survivor.
>
> *F. Mullan*

1. Why should nurses who care for patients in a hospital or clinic be interested in survivors of cancer?

Historically, a diagnosis of cancer has elicited feelings of fear, dread, terror, doom, mutilation—all words that describe the underlying notion that the person will surely die of the disease. This myth about cancer can psychologically paralyze the individual who receives the diagnosis; it can also evoke negative reactions from nurses and other caregivers. Negative reactions from nurses can decrease the sense of hopefulness and future orientation that is vitally necessary during the early stages of survival.[2] The knowledge that people do survive different types of cancer—many are actually cured, and others live with cancer as a chronic illness—helps nurses to introduce the potential for survival, to decrease the sense of helplessness, and to transform a passive acceptance of fate into a proactive sense of control. Thus quality of life is improved for both survivor and caregiver.

2. How long after diagnosis is a patient considered to be a survivor?

The traditional medical definition is survival for 5 years beyond the cancer diagnosis. The National Coalition for Cancer Survivorship, an organization founded in 1986, has crafted a definition that focuses on the qualitative aspect of survival. According to this definition, "From the time of its discovery, and for the balance of life, an individual diagnosed with cancer is a survivor."[5]

3. What does cancer survivorship mean?

Cancer survivorship, as defined above, is a process rather than a fixed point in time. It is the experience of living with cancer, adapting to it as a part of the individual's life process, and incorporating the experience into the broader perspective of the person's entire life experience. Many survivors have provided valuable insight into the experience of living with cancer by writing about the impact of cancer on their lives. These books and stories indicate that the experience of living with cancer can have profound positive repercussions. It is important for newly diagnosed cancer survivors as well as the nurses and physicians who care for them to understand the importance of quality of life to the survivor.

4. How many cancer survivors are there in the United States?

Currently, it is estimated that 9–10 million people in the United States have histories of cancer. Approximately one-half of this population are long-term survivors (5 or more years). Taking into consideration all types of cancer, the relative 5-year survival rate (the ratio of observed survival rate for survivors vs. the expected survival rate of the general population) has reached 51%. Although this percentage is much higher for some and much lower for others, depending upon the specific type and stage of cancer, it means that approximately one-half the number of people diagnosed with cancer today will be long-term survivors.

To put these statistics in perspective, consider the fact that the number of cancer survivors in the United States has more than tripled over a 10-year period. With recent advances in the ability to detect cancer early, in the development of supportive therapies, and in genetics that have identified specific cancer-causing genes, it is expected that the number of cancer survivors will continue its rapid growth.

5. Do survivors go through known phases or stages?

Llke any life-changing event, cancer survival involves stages. Two obvious stages are B.C. (before cancer) and A.D. (after diagnosis). Each survivor will have different issues to deal with, depending on life circumstances B.C. The stages of coping with death, as first described by Elisabeth Kubler-Ross, can be applied to almost any situation involving loss. As with any life-altering event, cancer survivors are dealing with the loss of their life as they knew it before cancer. They may experience shock, anger, denial, bargaining, and acceptance. It is important for nurses to keep in mind that no one progresses through these stages in the same way. An individual may move back and forth between stages or may not experience one or more of the stages at all. As with any model, the stages act essentially as guidelines. The continuum of cancer survivorship also has been described in terms of the seasons of survival: acute, extended, and permanent.

Acute stage. Acute survival begins with the cancer diagnosis. It is a period when the survivor's life is dominated by the illness. The focus is on treatment, whether it be surgery, radiation, chemotherapy, or biotherapy. It is a time when survivors may be feeling sick and considering their mortality. It is also a time when the survivor has more access to support services. Physicians, nurses, social workers, and many community resources are available through the hospital, clinic, physician's office, or local cancer agencies to assist the survivor and family members in dealing with the immediate needs surrounding diagnosis and treatment.

Extended stage. During the season of extended survival, the individual enters remission of the cancer or discontinues routine treatment. At this time, the survivor makes a transition from life as a patient to a reintegration into everyday activities. The focus shifts from the medical environment to the community. Survivors may return to work, school, or the responsibility of managing a household. It is important that survivors be supported during this transition time. Nurses should continue to be available as a source of information, reassurance, and support. Survivors may benefit from a referral to community support groups, legal services, counseling services, or programs such as I Can Cope, Reach to Recovery, CanSurmount, National Coalition for Cancer Survivorship, or Wellness Community.

Permanent stage. The season of permanent survival is equated with the word "cure"; cancer is no longer a major focus of the survivor's life. During this extended remission, the cancer experience is integrated into the broader experience of the survivor's entire life. It is important that cancer survivors remain in contact with the medical community during this season. Long-term follow-up of survivors, with at least annual examination, is important for screening for long-term and late effects of cancer treatment. Legal, economic, and insurance issues may also arise during this season of survival.

6. What issues are of primary importance to someone entering the acute stage of survival?

During the acute stage of survival, patients focus on issues related to treatment options. This entails gathering information about the disease process, methods of treatment (surgery, radiation, chemotherapy, brachytherapy, bone marrow transplant, stem cell procedures, biotherapy), and survival statistics related to their particular type of cancer. During this stage nurses must assist survivors in communicating their needs to the health care team. Survivors are entering the environment of the medical community, where a foreign language is spoken— "medicalese." It is a language filled with abbreviations (CBC, CT, MRI, ABVD, HCT) and words that may be unfamiliar to the survivor. The problem becomes more difficult if the survivor's primary language is not English. A survivor may not know what questions to ask, particularly during the initial consultation with the oncologist. Excellent resources are available through the National Coalition for Cancer Survivorship and the National Cancer Institute to assist survivors during the acute stage. In addition, support groups in which newly diagnosed survivors can meet veteran survivors may be of benefit.

7. What can nurses do to help survivors make informed decisions about treatment during the acute stage of survival?

A newly diagnosed survivor is faced with gathering information quickly to make critical life-altering decisions and receives a great deal of information during a time when the ability to concentrate may be impaired. During this confusion, nurses can do many things to help survivors make informed decisions about treatment. Because people learn in various ways—through either visual or auditory input or through a written format—nurses can use a variety of teaching methods to convey information. Videotapes, written information, audiotapes, pictures, and verbal communication can be used to share important information with survivors and their significant others. The following hints may be helpful:

1. Repeat information numerous times; less than 50% of what is conveyed is usually retained by the survivor.

2. Use a variety of different settings and contexts, both to reinforce the information and to elicit questions from the survivor.

3. Encourage survivors to bring a family member or friend to consultations and conferences to take notes and help recall information.

4. Always assess the person's ability to read and understand the language of printed material.

5. Encourage survivors to keep a journal or a log of their experiences, questions, and concerns. The journal can be kept at the bedside so that if questions or concerns arise during the night, the survivor can write them down and deal with them later.

6. Suggest using a tape recorder. Teaching sessions, consultations, and conferences with survivors and/or caregivers can be recorded. If questions arise later when the survivor returns home, the recorded information can be used as a reference. It is possible that the question was answered during the conference, and listening to the tape saves additional telephone calls to the physician's office. In addition, family members who may not have been able to attend the conference will be able to hear the information. The tape becomes a resource for both survivors and their families.

8. Who else is available to help the multidisciplinary health care team deliver support, information, resources, and treatment?

It is helpful to have the survivor's insurance company assign a case manager to the survivor. The case manager's name and office number should be available to both the treatment team and the survivor. Ideally, the insurance company also should provide a way to reach the case manager outside normal business hours. Family, friends, and community support groups can provide support and help the survivor to gather and process information.

9. What problems or barriers do survivors face that may cause them to discontinue treatment?

Treatment for cancer is difficult and takes its toll in many different ways. Any number of problems—physical, psychological, social, financial, cultural—can prompt survivors to interrupt or stop their therapy.

Problems Prompting Discontinuation of Therapy

Physical	Social
Uncontrollable or unacceptable acute effects (e.g., nausea and vomiting, fatigue, pain)	Lack of transportation
	Fear of losing job
	Inadequate or unaffordable child care
Chronic or long-term effects of treatment (e.g., peripheral neuropathy)	Insufficient support with family responsibilities
	Decreased social interactions (e.g., dating, marriage)
Inability to concentrate or think clearly	**Financial**
	Unable to miss work or survive on reduced paycheck
Increasing disability or dependence	Un- or underinsured
Psychological	Unaffordable out-of-pocket expenses
Fear of disfigurement (e.g., scarring, hair loss)	Ineligible for government assistance (e.g., Medicaid, Medicare, Social Security Disability)
Fear of permanent disabilty, including impotence	**Cultural**
	Language barriers
Fear of late effects (e.g., infertility, second malignancies)	Lack of understanding
	Erroneous information or belief in myths
Decreased quality of life	Conflicting attitudes, beliefs and values

10. What resources are available to assist survivors and their families with problems and barriers?

After specific problems or barriers are identified, nurses must find the appropriate resources to help deal with them. Consultations with other professionals within the hospital or community may involve the following: specially trained nurses, attending physician, social workers and social services, translators, psychologists, chaplains, legal assistance, and financial and government consultants. Other resources include written publications, cancer-related videos, educational programs, on-line services (Internet), and support groups. Local cancer organizations also may be accessed (e.g., American Cancer Society and Leukemia Society). The important point is to be aware of what resources are available.

National Resources for Cancer Survivors (Limited List)

National Cancer Institute (NCI)	
Cancer Information Service (CIS)	800-4-CANCER
Physician Data Query (PDQ)	800-4-CANCER
CANCERFAX	301.402.5874
National Coalition for Cancer Survivorship (NCCS)	
General Information	301-650-8868
Fax	301.565.7650
Candlelighters Childhood Cancer Foundation	
General Information	800-366-2223
Local (Washington, DC)	301-657-8401
Fax	301.718.2686
American Cancer Society	
General Information	800-ACS-2345
Leukemia Society of America	
Educational Materials	800-955-4LSA
General Information	212-573-8484
Fax	212.856.9686
Cancer Care, Inc.	
General Information	800-813-HOPE
Local (New York)	212-302-2400
Fax	212.719.0263
Y-ME National Breast Cancer Organization	
General Information	800-221-2141
24-hour Hotline	312-986-8228
Fax	312.986.0020
US TOO International, Inc. (Prostate)	
General Information	800-808-7866
Local (Hinsdale, IL)	708-323-1002
Fax	708.323.1003
National Brain Tumor Foundation	
General Information	800-934-CURE
Local (San Francisco)	415-284-0208
Fax	415.284.0209
National Alliance of Breast Cancer Organizations (NABCO)	
General Information	800-719-9154
Fax	212.689.1213

11. What issues are specific to the survivor who is an adolescent or young adult?

Nurses should be aware of issues important to younger cancer survivors, such as fertility, cognitive deficiencies, and growth problems. Chemotherapy protocols that may preserve the survivor's fertility should be used whenever possible, and young men should be encouraged to bank their sperm before treatment.

The delivery of therapy involving the brain or central nervous system of a child should attempt to minimize cognitive problems after treatment. Such children may need long-term follow-up, which includes assessment for learning disabilities, memory deficit, distractability, and decreased verbal ability and IQ scores. If children are treated before puberty, they should receive long-term follow-up with specialists who can address potential growth problems.

12. Are treatment options that are less toxic to the reproductive system available for younger survivors?

In some types of cancer, such as Hodgkin's disease, it is possible to shield the reproductive tissue from direct radiation. Oophoropexy is a procedure in which the ovaries are surgically placed midline in front of or behind the uterus. This procedure reduces ovarian exposure in women receiving pelvic irradiation. Testicular shields can reduce testicular exposure to less than 10% of the prescribed dose. When a male patient undergoes retroperitoneal lymph node dissection, nerve-sparing techniques should be used to preserve fertility. When there has been nerve damage, techniques such as electroejaculation and sperm banking can be used to preserve fertility options for the future. Furthermore, in female patients with Hodgkin's disease, ovarian suppression during therapy, cyclic estrogen replacement, and alternative chemotherapy protocols have been used to preserve fertility. The standard MOPP (nitrogen mustard, vincristine, procarbazine, prednisone) chemotherapy has been found to cause infertility in a significant number of long-term survivors. Use of the ABVD (Adriamycin [doxorubicin], bleomycin, vinblastine, dacarbazine) protocol has proved to be less toxic to ovarian function and equally effective in inducing long-term remissions. Long-term follow-up of young survivors is important to identify long-term or late physiologic effects or psychosocial problems. Continued research to develop effective and less toxic teatment protocols is an essential component of cancer treatment.

13. As the initial phase of treatment is completed, the extended stage of survival begins. Does life automatically return to normal?

Anticipating the end of treatment provokes an array of mixed emotions. Ambiguity defines this stage as survivors experience a mixture of joy and fear, relief and anxiety, security and uncertainty. Although no longer a patient, the survivor is not entirely healthy and tries to balance both physical and emotional recovery. This stage encompasses learning to live with the fear of recurrence, uncertainty about the future, and loss of treatment-based support systems. The survivor must also learn to assess and trust his or her body again and to resume prior family and social roles and relationships. In general, this period is characterized by a feeling of being in limbo. The sense of "normal" has changed; it will never be the same as before the cancer. A "new normal" specific to the individual must be created gradually. This process takes time; it will not happen overnight. For many survivors, this new normal is better than the original.

14. How can nurses prepare survivors for potential problems once therapy is completed?

Knowledge helps to decrease the fear of the unknown. As survivors complete treatment, an individualized exit interview assists with the transition into life after therapy. Components of this interview should include information about medical follow-up appointments with specific diagnostic tests; possible late effects from therapy; symptoms that require attention or symptoms that may be expected; cancer prevention, health promotion, and wellness education; referrals for physical, psychological, and social rehabilitation; support networks, educational programs, and survivor publications; and continued access to specific individuals on the health care team.

15. When does permanent or long-term survival begin?

No one really knows when this stage of survival begins because it is different for each individual. Much depends on the type and extent of the original disease and the risk for recurrence. Athough no specific time frame or event defines this stage, freedom from disease for 2 or more years begins to yield a certain level of trust, and a sense of comfort gradually returns. This stage could be labeled sustained remission or possibly cure, although the definition of cure is controversial (see question 16). Some survivors can breathe a little easier after two years, such as those who are diagnosed with testicular cancer or Hodgkin's disease. Others who have non-Hodgkin's lymphoma or ovarian cancer may need 5 or more years to feel "out-of-the-woods." Survivors of breast cancer are now watched closely for recurrence for up to 10 years. All of these numbers are arbitrary and act only as guidelines for increased vigilance; they are not meant to hinder survivors from living life to the fullest.

A lack of guidelines to optimize disease-free survival continues to be a major problem for long-term survivors. Although many survivors have no physical evidence of disease and appear fully recovered, the life-threatening experience of having had cancer takes its toll in many ways. Physically, the survivor is at risk for other malignancies and organ system failures; psychologically, the survivor must live with the constant fear of recurrence; socially, the survivor frequently encounters employment and insurance discrimination; and spiritually, survivors struggle with the meaning of life and the identification of new goals and priorities. Although survivors are often praised for overcoming adversity, identification of real problems can be hampered as they are reminded how lucky they are to be alive. And in this age of managed care and cost-containment, the new population of long-term survivors needs continued access to appropriate specialists and guidelines for systematic follow-up.

16. Is there any guarantee of "cure" for survivors who remain disease-free for 5 years?

The concept of cure implies successful treatment of disease or restoration to health. Surely this is the ultimate hope for anyone treated for cancer. Yet no one can say for sure that a disease as ruthless and secretive as cancer will never return; thus, guarantees are not realistic. Yet probabilities for cure can be estimated and are available in the American Cancer Society's annual publication, *Cancer Facts & Figures*. The 1960s and 1970s brought a new sense of hopefulness to researchers and clinicians who treated people with cancer. With the development of potentially curative therapies, specialists carefully followed patients for signs of disease recurrence. Many believed that if a person could live disease-free for 5 years, the chance of cure and a normal life-span would be greatly increased. So many patients "walked on egg shells" or "held their breath" anxiously waiting to reach the magic 5-year landmark. They were not considered survivors until they reached this point. Unfortunately, many survivors have recurrence of disease even after 5 years, or they are diagnosed with other cancers. Because there are multiple types of cancers with different stages of disease, a wide variety of treatment options, and circumstances unique to each survivor, it is literally impossible to guarantee cure.

17. Do survivors face any form of discrimination due to their history of cancer?

Approximately 25% of people with histories of cancer are estimated to experience some type of employment discrimination. Examples include not being hired for a particular job, being selected for layoff, demotion or cut-back in duties, or denial of promotion or increase in salary. Some employers believe that cancer survivors are less productive and use more sick days than other employees. Studies have not supported this belief. In fact, studies have shown that survivors use fewer sick days and tend to be more productive than other workers, often because they are fearful of losing their job if they appear to be sick.

Cancer survivors may experience "job lock"; that is, they feel unable to apply for a change in employment because of a fear of losing health insurance benefits attached to their current employment. Survivors also may feel that they cannot accept employment from a company that does not provide adequate health insurance benefits. For this reason, they may accept employment in a position for which they are overqualified to obtain needed health insurance. Federal legislation has recently been enacted that will allow cancer survivors to obtain health insurance when they change jobs without having to endure a long waiting period.

Insurance companies also tend to give survivors a higher rating for purposes of setting insurance premiums. This practice applies to both health and life insurance. Some life insurance carriers will not insure cancer survivors until they have been disease-free for 5 years or more. Others will insure the cancer survivor but charge high premiums. Cancer survivors should be encouraged to check with a number of insurance providers before agreeing to a premium amount. A financial planner may be able to present options other than life insurance that will serve the same purpose for survivors and their families.

Another situation finds survivors dependent on their spouse for health insurance benefits. In most states, survivors are no longer able to obtain insurance benefits from their former partner once a divorce takes place. Survivors may feel locked into a marriage because of the need for insurance coverage. Along with an insurance consultant, an attorney specializing in family law may provide the survivor with options for obtaining individual or group insurance. Organizations such as university alumni associations, American Association of Retired People, professional associations, fraternal organizations, and other special interest groups also may provide insurance to members at group rates.

18. How long should cancer survivors be followed by an oncologist after termination of treatment?

The "how long" question is of major concern in the changing health care delivery system. Before managed care and cost containment, long-term follow-up was left to the discretion of the oncologist and survivor. Many oncologists wanted an ongoing relationship with people whom they had treated, even if it was once a year. Furthermore, many survivors felt bonded to the specialists who had helped them overcome a life-threatening disease. The establishment of trust over the years made the yearly follow-up examination easier to bear, and many oncologists still believe that they know best how to assess survivors for potential treatment-related problems.

The current system of managed care and cost containment has changed this once sacred, ongoing relationship by decreasing both utilization of services and referrals to specialists.[2] Oncologists now are more inclined to see the survivor for a limited number of years after therapy as prescribed by the individual plan. They then refer the survivor to the primary care provider—a family practitioner or internist—for long-term follow-up.

Because little systematic long-term follow-up has been done in adult cancer survivors, there are no guidelines for continued care. It becomes imperative for researchers and clinicians in oncology to develop standards of care that can be shared with the generalist physicians who see and assess survivors. Survivors are best served through cooperation among oncologists, primary care providers, and other specialists; education of primary care providers about the special needs of this expanding population; and timely referrals to the appropriate specialist when complicated or unusual problems arise.

19. What are the physical aftereffects of cancer therapy?

Even as we celebrate successful therapy, we must also be cognizant of long-term and late effects of treatment or disease. Surgery, radiation therapy, chemotherapy, biotherapy, or combinations of therapy may cause chronic or delayed problems that impede full recovery from the original diagnosis. These problems or effects fall into three categories: system-specific, cancer-related, and general related problems. The following are examples of these patterns:

System-specific

Organ damage or failure	Cardiomyopathy, pulmonary fibrosis
Premature aging	Cataracts, muscle atrophy
Compromised immune system	Increased infections
Damaged endocrine system	Reproductive problems, thyroid dysfunction

Cancer-related

Increased risk of recurrence	Primary malignancy
Increased risk of other malignancy	Related to primary cancer (e.g., breast cancer after ovarian cancer)
	Related to therapy (e.g., sarcoma after Hodgkin's disease)

General problems

Functional changes   Lymphedema, pain syndromes, fatigue
Cosmetic changes   Amputations, ostomies, scars
Chronic illness   Osteoporosis, arthritis

Although physical aftereffects of therapy are a reality, they do not preclude the necessity of the original therapy. But they validate the need for research into long-term and late effects, improvements in therapy, continued medical surveillance, and survivor education.[2]

20. As access to physicians and medical plans vary, how can survivors optimize their health care follow-up?

The era of personal responsibility has arrived. Consumers of health care can no longer stand by passively and allow others to make unilateral decisions about cancer care and follow-up. Cancer survivors must learn to make informed choices, to understand treatment options, and to request changes or alternatives when their needs are not met. To ensure optimal long-term follow-up care, survivors are encouraged to do the following:

1. Keep all medical records, including types and doses of chemotherapy, sites and amounts of radiation.

2. Develop a personalized health maintenance plan with oncology caregivers that covers time frames of check-ups, specific diagnostic tests, rehabilitation practices, and healthy behavioral modifications.

3. Carefully study and select, if possible, health insurance plans that offer flexibility and choice.

4. If warranted, negotiate a price for an annual follow-up visit outside one's insurance plan, and pay out-of-pocket if the rate is affordable. Survivors must decide for themselves whether this added expense is worth the peace of mind it may bring.

5. Learn to identify and communicate needs, and obtain assertiveness training if necessary.

6. Know individual rights as a health care consumer and how to take appropriate legal action if warranted.

7. Advocate insurance reform and standardized guidelines.

BIBLIOGRAPHY

1. Clark EJ: You Have the Right to be Hopeful. National Coalition for Cancer Survivorship (NCCS), Silver Springs, MD, 1996.
2. Clark EJ, Stovall EL, Leigh S, et al: Imperatives for Quality Cancer Care: Access, Advocacy, Action, and Accountability. National Coalition for Cancer Survivorship (NCCS), Silver Springs, MD, 1996.
3. Hoffman B: Working It Out: Your Employment Rights As a Cancer Survivor. National Coalition for Cancer Survivorship (NCCS), Silver Springs, MD, 1993.
4. Leigh S: Cancer survivorship: A consumer movement. Semin Oncol 21:783–786, 1994.
5. Mullan F: Seasons of survival: Reflections of a physician with cancer. N Engl J Med 313:270–273, 1985.
6. Swartz CL, Hobbie WL, Constine LS, Ruccione KS (eds): Survivors of Childhood Cancer. St. Louis, Mosby, 1994.

60. PATIENT EDUCATION

Kimberly A. Rumsey, RN, MSN, OCN

1. What is the purpose of patient education?

The major goal of patient education is to help patients maintain quality of life and to empower them to participate actively in their health care. Patient education can be implemented for promotion of health, adherence to prescribed regimens, maintenance of independence, provision of basic information, or improving ability to cope.

2. Why is patient education a nursing function?

In 1972, the American Hospital Association (AHA) first published *A Patient's Bill of Rights*, which delineated 12 rights of patients. Included in this list is the right for patient education regarding diagnosis, prognosis, treatment options, and side effects. Several regulatory agencies, such as the Joint Commission on Accreditation of Healthcare Organizations (JCAHO) and the Health Care Financing Administration (HCFA), specify health education of patients as a requirement for accreditation.

Nurses have a legal responsibility to teach. State nurse practice acts discuss the role of the nurse in patient education. The *Standards of Oncology Nursing Practice* and *Standards of Oncology Education: Patient/Family and Public* specify that the oncology nurse at both the generalist and advanced practice levels is responsible for patient/family and public education related to cancer.

3. Who are the target populations for education?

Potential target populations include patients and their significant others, school children, employees on the work site, and community organizations (e.g., church groups, Boy Scouts, Girl Scouts). The media also may be the target of teaching endeavors, thereby providing a means of educating the community at large.

4. What is the first step in the process of patient education?

The nursing process provides a familiar and practical framework for teaching patients. Assessment, diagnosis, planning, implementation, and evaluation compose the teaching process. Documentation also should be included as the sixth step in the process. During the first stage of the teaching process, ability to learn, readiness and willingness to learn, and knowledge deficits are assessed. Assessment of the learner is an integral step of the education process because it forms the basis for the development of the entire teaching plan and facilitates a successful teaching session.

5. What is included in a learning needs assessment?

Data for the learning needs assessment for patients can be gathered from three major sources: the medical record; the patient, family member, or significant other; and other members of the health care team. A comprehensive learning needs assessment includes assessment of ability to learn, readiness and willingness to learn, and potential topics for teaching. The target audience should be assessed for sensory impairment (visual or auditory) and other physiologic barriers to learning. Ability to communicate verbally in English and literacy level also should be considered in assessing ability to learn. In addition, the manner in which the target audience learns best (through visual, auditory, or tactile stimuli) should be identified to ensure appropriate use of teaching materials. Assessment of readiness and willingness to learn includes information about sociocultural background, emotional state, and goals related to the health care situation. Finally, potential topics for instruction should be assessed, including previous knowledge and experience, topics of concern, and specific information and skills needed. Although laborious, a comprehensive learning needs assessment helps the nurse to formulate an appropriate teaching plan.

An assessment also should be done before teaching in the community setting. The nurse should talk with the person requesting the presentation and assess the same areas as with individual clients.

6. What should be included in the teaching plan?
The teaching plan is an organized, written document that specifies learning needs and how those needs are to be met. The plan should be mutually agreed upon by the target audience, the nurse, and other members of the health care team. Components of the teaching plan include the goals and objectives of learning, content to be presented, and teaching strategies to be implemented. In addition, comprehensive plans specify resources, teaching aids, and personnel responsible for the actual teaching.

7. What are the essential elements of effective goals?
Goals provide structure for the teaching session and serve as a guide for evaluation of teaching. There are five essential characteristics of effective goals:
1. Mutually acceptable to learner and teacher
2. Realistic and achievable
3. Measurable
4. Centered on the learner
5. Written and placed in an identified, consistent location

8. What is the best teaching technique?
Factors to consider in selecting teaching techniques include the target population (group or individual), learning style of the target population, content to be included, resources available, and the nurse's preference. Commonly used strategies include lecture; discussion; demonstration; modeling; programmed instruction; simulated environment; games; activities; role playing; and team teaching. Advantages and disadvantages of each are listed in the table that follows. It is helpful to include several techniques to target different types of learners.

Teaching Strategies

STRATEGY	ADVANTAGES	DISADVANTAGES
Lecture	Easier to organize and transfer a large amount of information Predictable, efficient, good for a large group and quicker Allows teacher control over presented material Easiest method for focusing	Lacks client feedback Information overload Difficult to sustain interest Difficult to tailor material for the group
Discussion	Allows continual feedback, attitude development, and modification Changes according to motivation of the audience Picks up confusion and helps resolve difficulties Serves as a vehicle for networking	Increases the chance of getting off focus Easy for discussion to become pointless Allows some participants to be dominant and others passive Takes a lot of time
Demonstration	Activates many senses Clarifies the "whys" of a principle Commands interest Correlates theory with practice Allows teacher to see learning and diagnose the problem Helps learner get well-directed practice	Takes a lot of time Does not cover all aspects of cognitive learning

Table continued on following page.

Teaching Strategies (Continued)

STRATEGY	ADVANTAGES	DISADVANTAGES
Modeling	Facilitates affective learning Bypasses defenses Effective with children	Ineffective without rapport Does not always make what is learned visible Allows learner ambivalence

Programmed instruction	Allows students to go at their own pace
	  and repeat a section at will
	Breaks material down into manageable
	  increments
	Saves the teacher's time
		Depends on motivation of learner
		Does not account for unplanned
		  feedback, which can
		  distance clients

Simulated environment, games, activities, role playing	Promotes the greatest transfer of learning
	Helps client learn what she or he needs
	  to cope with specific problem or
	  environment
	Allows practice that is most transferrable
		Facilitates unpredictable occurrences
		Appears threatening for clients
		Takes a lot of time
		Makes achievement of outcomes
		  difficult

Team teaching	Enhances teaching by using compe-
	  tencies of more than one teacher
	Allows teachers to learn from each
	  other
	Accentuates divergent points of view
		Lacks continuity and internal
		  consistency
		Requires more planning time
		Makes group processing slower
		Forces teachers to give up autonomy

9. What resources are available to help with patient education?

Teaching aids provide visual stimuli, allow hands-on demonstration, invite emotional involvement, supply variety and interest to the teaching session, give meaning to abstract concepts, and make complicated explanations more understandable. Various teaching aids are readily available, and each has its own advantages and disadvantages (see below).

Resources for Teaching Aids

American Cancer Society
    1599 Clifton Road N.E.
    Atlanta, GA 30329
    404-320-3333 or call your local ACS office

Leukemia Society of America
    600 Third Avenue
    New York, NY 10016
    212-573-8484 or call your local office

National Cancer Institute
    9000 Rockville Pike
    Bethesda, MD 20892
    800-4-CANCER

Oncology Nursing Society
    501 Holiday Drive
    Pittsburgh, PA 15220-2749
    412-921-7373

Features of Teaching Materials

TYPE	ADVANTAGES	DISADVANTAGES	HELPFUL HINTS

Chalkboards and whiteboards	Widely available
	Useful for spontaneous
	  illustration at the time
	  of client's concern
	Offer reinforcement to
	  respondents
	Erasable
	Allow the teacher to
	  add to and take away
	  from illustrations
	Good backups
		Two-dimensional
		Messy
		Require chalk or pen
		  and eraser
		Can be time-
		  consuming
		Require a teacher with
		  good writing skills
			Require teacher to supply
			  chalk and eraser
			Can be messy and get on
			  dark clothing
			Require the teacher to start
			  high on the board and to
			  refrain from writing
			  below the viewers' line
			  of vision
			Should be divided in half to
			  accommodate lengthy lists

Table continued on following page.

Features of Teaching Materials (Continued)

TYPE	ADVANTAGES	DISADVANTAGES	HELPFUL HINTS
Pamphlets and posters	Portable, attractive Can be used before, during, and after a presentation Can be studied at client's pace Readily available Often free	Time-consuming to make Provide limited viewing Need a prop Bulky to carry and store Useful only to readers Too many pamphlets may overwhelm client No auditory component	Pamphlets must be checked for currency and passed out at the best time Should contain few words and lots of space
Photographs and cartoons	Easily personalized Can elicit emotions Can portray many more thoughts than words alone Allow the client to control the pace	Inappropriate for large groups Distracting if passed during talk Yellow with age Cartoons may inadvertently offend or confuse	Should be tried out on clients of similar ages and backgrounds Look more lively in color May require explanations
Bulletin boards	Attract browsers	Can get cluttered and outdated Unsuitable for long or complex messages	Should be changed often and kept attractive and lively Should contain a minimal number of messages
Computer-assisted intruction (CAI) programs	Allow the client to control the pace Reinforce correct responses immediately Good for sequential thought processes Allow the client to repeat the lesson if necessary	Depend on client initiative Time-consuming to monitor Of limited value if the teacher is not available Require clients who are visual learners and computer literate Can be boring	Teacher should select the most user-friendly software available Work best if the teacher spends enough time with the client to ensure that he or she is comfortable with the program
Public address systems	Augment teacher's voice to any size audience	Can be ineffective if faulty equipment is used	Microphones should be tested before clients arrive and adjusted to the correct height Should be held in front of teacher's mouth Step back and aside if squeals are produced Be sure the audience can hear the teacher
Flip charts	Versatile, portable, used like a chalkboard May be prepared before the presentation or spontaneously during presentation	Require artistic talent and good handwriting Provide clients with a limited view	Teacher should have a good supply of black and colored pens and should use masking tape or soft, gummy adhesive to affix flip charts to wall

10. What topics concerning cancer risks, prevention, and detection need to be discussed?

Nurses should assume responsibility for teaching the public about the risk of cancer and techniques for prevention and detection. The *Standards of Oncology Education: Patient/Family and Public* specifies that public education programs should include the following:

1. Accurate and current information about principles of carcinogenesis and genetic, environmental, and lifestyle risks for cancer

2. Methods to modify health behaviors and practices for cancer prevention and health promotion

3. Signs and symptoms of common cancers

4. Strategies to improve the accessibility, use, and evaluation of cancer prevention, detection, and control programs

5. Criteria to evaluate unproven and alternative cancer therapies

6. Community resources for health promotion and cancer-related information and services

7. Legal and ethical rights of persons at risk for cancer

8. Religious, ethnic, and cultural values and beliefs that influence health

11. What is a readability test?

A readability test measures the approximate grade of education needed to understand written information. Most tests involve an evaluation of word complexity and length of sentences. The National Cancer Institute's Office of Cancer Communication uses the SMOG grading system to test its materials. The SMOG formula is valid, accurate, and easy to use. It predicts difficulty of reading material based on sentence length and number of polysyllabic words found in a total of 30 sentences (10 consecutive sentences near the beginning, 10 near the middle, and 10 near the end of the text). All the words containing 3 or more syllables are counted and totalled; then a SMOG conversion table is used to approximate the reading grade level. For example, a total of 3 to 6 polysyllabic words in a total of 30 sentences equals a fifth grade reading level.

12. What is the average reading level of adults in the United States?

The average reading level is between the fifth and eighth grade level. This presents a challenge to oncology nurses because studies show that common cancer patient literature has reading levels ranging from grade 5.8 to 15.6, with a mean grade level of 11.9. Patient education materials written before 1985 are written at higher grade levels.

13. What can nurses do to simplify written patient education materials?

In addition to doing a readability test, other guidelines to develop easier reading materials include the following: use short words with two or less syllables; use simple, lay language; write short sentences and paragraphs; use large print, especially for the elderly patient and children; provide visual appeal with bold colors, cartoons, and pictures; and highlight or boldface important points. Remember that readability tools only estimate the reading difficulty of the material and that an assessment of the material for individual patient acceptability and appropriateness is still necessary.

14. What topics need to be discussed once cancer has been diagnosed?

The newly diagnosed patient initially should be given only essential information; misconceptions about cancer also should be corrected. This patient generally is anxious, and the information may need to be presented several times before the goals are attained. The *Standards of Oncology Education: Patient/Family and Public* outlines a comprehensive education program for patients diagnosed with cancer, including the following:

1. Accurate and current information about cancer prevention, detection, diagnosis, treatment, rehabilitation, and supportive care

2. Accurate and current information about alternative treatment methods

3. Criteria to evaluate unproven cancer therapies

4. Cognitive, psychomotor, and affective skills needed for problem-solving, decision making, and self-care

5. Methods to modify health behaviors for health promotion, cancer prevention, detection and control

6. Signs and symptoms of potential physical and psychosocial responses related to cancer or treatment

7. Signs and symptoms of potential responses related to cancer and/or treatment that should be reported to the health care team

8. Psychosocial strategies to facilitate adaptation of the patient/family to the cancer experience

9. Legal and ethical rights of persons with a diagnosis of cancer

10. Community resources available to the patient/family for health promotion and cancer care

Whether teaching individuals with cancer or the community, the nurse should focus on one or two learning needs at each teaching session. Too much information at once may prove overwhelming for the learner and frustrating for the educator.

15. What is the best way to ensure that all important concepts are covered?

Have a complete, written teaching plan, and ensure that each teaching session is documented. In this way, health care professionals can communicate with each other about topics that have been covered and topics that still require teaching. A list of the key points to be covered is a simple and effective way to organize the content and can be kept handy for quick reference during the teaching session so that topics are not omitted. The nurse should bear in mind, however, that what the patient wants to know first may not be the first point in the teaching plan. For example, in learning self-injection, most patients are anxious about the injection procedure. Therefore, the nurse may want to have the patient demonstrate the injection procedure before demonstrating reconstitution or drawing up the medication. The nurse should be attentive to the changing needs of the target population and make appropriate changes during the teaching session.

16. How much time should be allotted for each teaching session?

Generally, most one-to-one teaching sessions with individual patients last 10 or 20 minutes. If a skill is involved, several short sessions are better than one or two long sessions. A specific time for teaching should be established with the patient, taking into consideration when family members are available to learn the information. The nurse should then make arrangements to ensure that other patient care responsibilities do not interfere. The nurse also should incorporate teaching into every patient encounter. A presentation in the community generally lasts 1–2 hours, depending on the needs and time constraints of the participants.

17. What are the most common barriers to optimal teaching, and how can they be overcome?

Physiologic barriers include visual or hearing deficit, increased age, or brain metastasis. Other barriers to learning include anxiety, learning disabilities, language barrier, and medications that change sensorium. The use of a translator or material with large print for the elderly may be indicated. Another technique is to teach the client *and* a significant other, whenever possible, and to reinforce the material as often as possible.

18. What strategies can be used to evaluate learning?

Evaluation is the continuous and systematic review of the learner's progress during and after the teaching session. Evaluation should occur at the time of teaching and be repeated later. Evaluation should relate to the goals outlined in the teaching plan. If goals were appropriately written, the nurse can evaluate learning realistically. Effective methods of evaluation include verbal feedback, return demonstration, and role-playing for specific situations.

19. Why is documentation of patient education important?

All teaching sessions with individual patients must be documented in the medical record to facilitate communication with other health care team members. In addition, documentation provides a legal record of education provided, documenting compliance with state practice acts, standards of nursing practice, and requirements of accreditation agencies. Nurses also may wish to keep information about community education for future reference.

20. What information should be included in the documentation?

One way to ensure accurate documentation of education is to use a multidisciplinary tool for the plan and documentation. This approach minimizes repetition of the learning needs and appropriate teaching plan. A checklist may be helpful for the documentation and communication of teaching sessions (see attached form).

Department of Patient Services
Patient Education Teaching Standards
MR#2100.195 (Rev 8/95)

CANCER CHEMOTHERAPY

*Teaching Method Code

A = Audiovisual   G = Group Class
E = Explanation   W = Written Material
D = Demonstration

Pt = Patient   S.O. = Significant Other

PATIENT OUTCOME

	Taught to: PT/S.O.	* Teaching Method *	States/Identifies	Return Demonstrates	Routinely Performs	No Evidence of learning	Reinforced	Reinforced	Reinforced	Reinforced	COMMENTS
I The Patient/Significant Other will verbalize understanding of the following:											
Cancer Packet											
"Chemotherapy and You" book											
Eating Hints											
Drug Sheets											
II Describes expected side effects and methods to prevent/manage them:											
Nausea/Vomiting											
Antiemetic Side Effects											
Stomatitis											
Mouth Care											
Diarrhea											
Constipation											
Dysuria/hematuria											
Myelosuppression											
Infection											
Anemia											
Bleeding											
Weight Loss/Gain											
Anorexia											
Fatigue											
Alopecia											
Effects related to specific organs											
Cardiotoxicity (SOB, increased fatigue, orthopnea)											
Neurotoxicity (Numbness/tingling in hands/feet, constipation, jaw pain).											
Skin Reactions											

MR#2100.195 (Rev 8/95)   ptedcemo.cnc < pted2 > (8/95) rmf

Example of documentation of chemotherapy patient education form. *(Continued on following page.)*

*Teaching Method Code A = Audiovisual G = Group Class E = Explanation W = Written Material D = Demonstration Pt = Patient S.O. = Significant Other **PATIENT OUTCOME**	Taught to: PT/S.O.	* Teaching Method *	States/Identifies	Return Demonstrates	Routinely Performs	No Evidence of learning	Reinforced	Reinforced	Reinforced	Reinforced	COMMENTS
Ototoxicity (decreased hearing, tinnitus, vertigo)											
Renal Toxicity (increased CR/BUN, decreased urine output, weight gain, edema)											
Pulmonary Toxicity (SOB, dry cough)											
Reproductive (sperm banking, barrier contraceptive)											
III DESCRIBES POSSIBLE METHODS OF CHEMO ADMINISTRATION											
A. SUB-Q Injections											
Drugs/Side Effects 1. 2.											
Technique for giving											
Other:											
B. Ambulatory Infusion Pump											
Type											
Troubleshooting											
Who to call with problems											
IV Verbalizes signs/symptoms of chemo related toxicities for which to notify RN/MD											
1. Burning with injection											
2. Temperature > 100.5											
3. Vomiting which lasts more than 1 day											
4. Feeling nervous, jittery, can't sit still											
5. Chills, sore throat, productive cough, burning with urination											
6. Constipation/diarrhea not relieved within 48 hours using over the counter or prescribed medications.											
7. Bleeding, excessive bruising											
V Who to contact with problems											

Pt/Significant Other Signature:

Signature	Init	Signature	Init	Signature	Init.

Example of documentation of chemotherapy patient education form *(Continued)*. (From University Hospital, Denver, Colorado, with permission.)

The following should be included in documentation of individual patient or community education:

1. Learning needs listed and prioritized with target date for completion identified
2. Who was present during the teaching
3. Resources and teaching aids used
4. Outcome of the teaching session
5. Unresolved goals with a follow-up plan identified
6. Learner signature

BIBLIOGRAPHY

1. American Hospital Association: A Patient's Bill of Rights. Chicago, American Hospital Association, 1992.
2. American Nurses Association and Oncology Nursing Society: Standards of Oncology Nursing Practice. Kansas City, MO, American Nurses Association, 1987.
3. Anderson C: Patient Teaching and Communicating In an Information Age. Albany, NY, Delmar Publishers, 1990.
4. Babcock DE, Miller MA: Client Education: Theory and Practice. St. Louis, Mosby, 1994.
5. Cooley ME, Moriarty H, Berger MS, et al: Patient literacy and the readability of written cancer educational materials. Oncol Nurs Forum 22:1345–1351, 1995.
6. Meade CD, Diekmann J, Thornhill DG: Readability of American Cancer Society patient education literature. Oncol Nurs Forum 19:51–55, 1992.
7. Oncology Nursing Society: Standards of Oncology Nursing. Education: Patient/Family and Public. Pittsburgh, Oncology Nursing Society, 1989.
8. Stephens ST: Patient education materials: Are they readable? Oncol Nurs Forum 19:83–85, 1992.

61. COMMUNICATING, CARING, AND COPING

Rose A. Gates, RN, MSN, and
Patricia W. Nishimoto, RN, MPH, DNS, LTC, AN, USAR

> When there is love of man (philanthropia), there is also love of the art [of healing] (philotechnia).
>
> *Hippocratic Praecepta (quoted by Entralgo)*

1. How do patients respond to the diagnosis of cancer?

Each person responds to the diagnosis of cancer in various individual ways. The diagnosis may lead to a crisis or turning point in which past methods of coping do not work. Some patients claim no problems, whereas others experience many. Responses vary along the continuum of disease:

Work-up. The work-up period is often described as the most difficult time because it is filled with uncertainty and a new world of medical jargon (e.g., MRIs, adenopathy, neutropenia) and procedures. It may take several weeks of anxious waiting before patients know their diagnosis. Some patients try to pretend that nothing is wrong and keep everything to themselves. Others get irritated easily and lash out at friends or family without realizing why. Patients may increase alcohol use or start taking antianxiety medications or sleeping pills. Often they tell you that "the not knowing is the worst."

Diagnosis. After they are given the diagnosis, patients may respond with fear, shock, disbelief, denial, anger, sorrow, bargaining, or "why me?" For some, the diagnosis is a confirmation of their worries, and they almost seem to take it in stride. Others nod their heads, ask pertinent questions, and then five minutes later seem to have forgotten the entire conversation. Some respond with anger or believe that the "doctor made a mistake" or begin doctor-shopping. Many express a feeling of vulnerability or helplessness, "feeling out of control," "being alone," and feeling that "no one understands." A few may feel hopeless and even contemplate "ending it all."

Recurrence. Many patients respond as when they were initially diagnosed; however, news of an unexpected recurrence may result in more feelings of disappointment, despair, or sense of failure that they or others "did not fight hard enough." Other patients are glad for the extra time that they had and are more accepting of their prognosis. Depending on the diagnosis and stage of disease, patients may be required to adjust from curative to palliative goals. Distress may be more evident as patients come to the realization that their time is limited or that death is close. They may start worrying about their last days and wonder if they will be a burden. Patients may become more spiritual or religious and seek resolution of conflicts and meaning in their living and/or dying.

2. What is coping?

Coping refers to problem-solving efforts to overcome a risky or threatening situation. Many equate coping with cancer as fighting on the front lines of a battlefield. Patients have to cope with the diagnosis, its effects, and treatment. The goal of coping is emotional acceptance or resolution of a problem. Nurses facilitate patients' coping to promote healing and to ensure compliance with necessary therapies. Patients cope in their own ways, which are affected by many variables. There is no right or wrong way to cope. Most of all, coping depends on the meaning of cancer to the patient and how the patient usually deals with life stresses.

3. How do you assess patient coping?

An assessment of coping considers the patient's emotional responses and problem-solving activities as well as the phase of the patient's illness (before diagnosis, initial diagnosis, treatment, rehabilitation, follow-up, recurrence, dying). The nursing history helps to identify the patient's past and current stressors, prior or present substance abuse, and current medications. It is important to assess coping abilities, mood, availability of support, physical symptoms, and how the future looks to the patient. Patients who are coping well can verbalize their feelings and concerns, use available resources, actively participate in care and decision making, identify alternative solutions or resources, and state realistic goals. Effective coping is also measured by the patient's ability to return to usual activities. According to the patient's stage of illness, questions to ask in the coping assessment include:

- What do you think or understand about your diagnosis, treatment, and goals of treatment?
- What information would you like at this time?
- What do you expect to happen over the next few weeks or months? How does the future look?
- How do you feel about your diagnosis? What does it mean to you?
- Has anyone close to you ever had cancer?
- Describe a stressful event or crisis in the past. How did you deal with it? How do things usually turn out for you?
- How are you feeling physically? What kind of problems or symptoms do you have now? (Ask specific questions about pain, constipation, insomnia, fatigue, anorexia, and nausea.)
- How do you feel emotionally? Are your spirits low or high? Is anything bothering you now? Describe your attitude (hopeful, discouraged).
- What bothers you most about your illness? About therapy? Can anything be done to help?
- Tell me about any experiences you have had with anyone else with cancer.
- How well are you coping now? What is helping you to cope? What is keeping you from coping? What are you doing about your problems?
- Are you able to keep up with your activities—work, chores, recreation?
- How are you getting along with your spouse or partner? How is your interest in sex?
- Are you getting along with your family or friends? How supportive are they?
- Are you having any thoughts about not wanting to live?
- Do you have any unfinished business? What do you need to accomplish?

4. What commonly used medications may affect mood or cause depression in patients with cancer?
- Glucocorticoids
- Interferon and interleukin-2
- Barbiturates
- Propranolol
- Amphotericin B
- Chemotherapy drugs: vincristine, vinblastine, procarbazine, L-asparaginase

5. How do patients cope with cancer?

Patients with cancer must face all kinds of changes, health care providers, diagnostic tests, symptoms, losses, and uncertainties. Strategies or responses of patients adapting to a diagnosis of cancer include the following:

Denial may be protective or detrimental. The nurse's role is to evaluate how long the denial lasts, how often it is used, and its intensity. From the beginning, it is important to establish what and how much information a patient wants and can handle at any one time. Denial can give the patient time to absorb and adapt to distressful or overwhelming information. Patients should not be forced out of denial if it helps them to cope. However, denial is detrimental if it prevents a patient from understanding consequences or if it potentially hurts others.

Search for meaning often begins with the question, "why me?," when patients attempt to make sense of their illness. Anxiety may be reduced by having an explanation or reason.

Spirituality identifies what is purposeful and valuable in life. Prayer and religion help many patients to find peace and meaning in their illnesses.

Downward comparison helps patients to feel better by comparing their condition to someone who is worse off or less fortunate. Patients may express relief that their condition is not as bad as another patient's.

Sense of mastery gives the patient a sense of control over the cancer or side effects related to therapy. Techniques that provide mastery include imagery, self-hypnosis, distraction, meditation, exercise, and dietary changes.

Reappraisal of life clarifies what is most important in a patient's life since the diagnosis of cancer. Patients often conclude that family and/or friends and health are more important than money and work.

Cognitive restructuring redefines or reframes the situation by finding positive aspects of the diagnosis, such as improvement in a patient's marriage since the diagnosis.

Emotional expression uses humor or talking with others to help with coping.

Wish-fulfilling fantasy wishes the cancer would go away or that it was not as advanced.

Self-blame is feeling responsible or guilty for cancer. Patients may express regret for failing to get regular exams.

Information-seeking involves self-help and active engagement in learning about the disease and treatments.

Threat minimization is an attempt to focus on aspects of life other than cancer or to put cancer out of mind with distracting activities or simply talking about the cancer.

6. When should a patient be referred to a psychiatric clinical nurse specialist, psychiatrist, or psychologist?

Patients should be referred whenever the health care provider is uncomfortable with treating the patient's psychological problems and when the patient does any of the following:

- Asks for additional help.
- Exhibits dysfunctional behaviors (e.g., extreme anxiety or depression, substance abuse, suicidal ideation, paranoia).
- Is not responsive to current treatment for depression or anxiety.
- Has multiple stressors and may benefit from additional support.
- Symptoms prevent the patient from cooperating with medical treatment.
- Other specific therapy is offered, such as hypnosis, that may benefit the patient.

7. How do you respond to patients who ask, "Why did I get cancer?"

Almost all patients and families want to know what caused the cancer. Casual attribution may or may not be beneficial to the patient's adjustment. When patients ask "why?" they may just want a simple answer about risk factors, or they may be seeking a sense of meaning in their illness. Cancer takes on different meaning according to age, culture, religion, and previous experiences.

Although a good reason may be suspected for a patient's cancer, you should avoid telling the patient with certainty what caused the cancer. There simply is no way to be sure. It may be helpful to answer the patient's question in theoretical terms, such as discussing recognized risk factors for a particular type of cancer. It may be helpful to point out that although smoking is a known cause of lung cancer, many people who never smoke get lung cancer and many people who smoke do not develop the disease. Attention should not necessarily focus on attempts to isolate a single factor as the cause but instead on efforts to point out that cancer is a complex disease and that so much more needs to be learned.

8. What is therapeutic use of self?

Therapeutic use of self is the use of one's personal identity or personality to show caring and to promote the patient's healing. The nurse offers caring within a "transpersonal" relationship in which both nurse and patient are mutually growing or changing. To be therapeutic, the nurse must have self-awareness and be healthy (physically, psychologically, socially, and spiritually). In other words, it is difficult to meet someone else's needs if you do not meet your own.

9. What are some tips in listening?

- Listen to what the patient is saying or not saying. Be alert to nonverbal cues; sometimes what is unsaid is just as important.

- Physically place yourself at the patient's level. If the patient is lying in bed, do not stand above the patient; sit down, lean forward to show interest, and face the patient to maintain eye contact.
- Maximize privacy.
- Learn to be good at "active listening." Attempt to "tune in" or to understand the other person's feelings or concerns and then "reflect them back." For example, the patient may say, "Nothing is bothering me," but you notice that he is wringing his hands. With active listening, the nurse may say, "I know you say things are okay, but it seems like you really are concerned about your test results."

10. What does hope mean in patients with cancer?

Hope is an inner force that motivates and enriches a person's life. Hope holds promise that problems can be overcome or that something positive will occur. Hope varies with time, experience, and personal interactions. When patients feel hopeless, they may be easily overwhelmed, feel exhausted, not comply with therapies, or be grouchy with friends or family. Threats to hope include physical deterioration, negative attitudes or interactions with others, side effects of therapy, lack of information, and spiritual distress. Sources of hope include family, friends, and religious beliefs. As cancer progresses, goals change and patients hope for different things. Patients with cancer can remain hopeful despite limitations in activity or approaching death. Initially the patient may hope for a cure, but as the cancer becomes terminal, he or she may hope for short-term goals such as relief of pain or seeing another sunrise.

Hopefulness is essential to successful coping, good quality of life, and spiritual healing. Hope enables a patient to believe in a reason for living. Therefore, it is important to nurture hope by conveying your care and helping patients to focus on realistic and achievable goals.

11. How do you respond to difficult questions?

Nurses are often faced with difficult questions posed by cancer patients, such as "Am I going to die?" "When am I going to die?" "Should I take this treatment?" or "How should I decide about resuscitation?" When patients ask such questions, they usually do not want a long, involved answer. There are no magic answers to difficult questions. It may not be as important to give answers as it is to listen, understand, and discover the patient's meaning. Your responses should be direct and honest. If a patient is trying to make a decision, offer guidance in looking at the positives, negatives, and alternatives. Before giving an answer, it is helpful to ask patients, "What has your doctor told you about that?" Patients may already know the answer and are testing to see how honest you are going to be. It is also helpful to ask patients to tell you what they think the answer is. Ask them to help you understand what information they are really seeking or want. Your objective and focus should be to decrease fear or anxiety and to reassure patients with honest information and accurate facts.

12. How do you respond to a mother who says, "I have heard that leukemia in cats is contagious. I was just diagnosed with leukemia. Can I give this to my kids?"

Start by saying, "That's a good question, and I'm glad you asked it." Because many fears are universal, patients need to be reassured that they are not abnormal and that their questions are not "stupid." Convey the sense that you respect their questions. For patients who are not reassured by the facts that you offer, provide a good cancer resource book or Internet sources so that they can gather their own information. For patients or family members who are afraid that cancer is contagious, try the following answer:

> It was not that long ago that many people thought that cancer was contagious. When I first became an oncology nurse [for old-timers] or at one time [for younger nurses], it was not uncommon for cancer patients to be given paper plates and plastic utensils to use when they went to visit friends or family. We have learned a great deal about cancer since that time and have found that, although it is contagious among cats, it is not contagious among humans. If it were, every single oncology nurse, oncologist, or radiation oncologist would get cancer.

13. What do patients perceive as the most important nursing care behaviors?

According to Leininger, "Caring is one of the most crucial and essential ingredients for health, human development, human relatedness, well-being and survival." Caring, as the essence of nursing, may not mean the same to patients as it does to nurses. For example, the nurse's willingness to listen may be ranked by patients as the most caring behavior or well below other behaviors. Whereas nurses place high value on psychosocial skills, in one study patients with cancer ranked competency of skills above the need to be listened to by the nurse. Listening and talking skills became more important only after the patient's "getting better" needs were met. Other studies of nurse caring behaviors indicated that patients valued "being accessible," "monitoring and following through," physical care, and professional knowledge. The bottom line is that nurses should not assume that caring has the same value to the patient as it does to them.

14. What interventions may help to cope with anxiety?

Normal or situational anxiety is common among cancer patients. It arises out of attempts to make sense of things. Situational or initial anxiety is managed by clarifying information about the cancer or its treatment and providing emotional support and reassurance. Antianxiety agents, such as short-acting benzodiazepines, may be used along with stress management modalities to "take the edge off" or help patients to feel calmer (see chapter 42). Patients exhibiting signs of anxiety disorders (responses to real or imagined threats) should be referred to an appropriate mental health care provider. Abnormal anxiety reactions generally include disorders related to panic, phobias, posttraumatic stress, and obsessive-compulsive behaviors.

Patients may be interested in learning about stress management modalities, such as keeping a journal or stress awareness log, deep-breathing exercises, visualization, guided imagery, progressive relaxation, meditation, Yoga, exercise, therapeutic touch, autogenic training, biofeedback, and thought stopping. Music or humor therapy also may be used to decrease anxiety.

15. How is imagery used to reduce anxiety?

Relaxation and imagery techniques help reduce anxiety by altering environmental awareness and decreasing muscle tension. The following imagery script from Stephens may be useful in reducing anxiety as well as other symptoms, such as pain or nausea. During the relaxation phase the script counts down from 5 to 1; however, in actual practice, it is more helpful to count from 10 to 1.

> Imagery is a fast way to connect body-mind-spirit by quieting the busy mind and allowing the mind to focus on a particular event. It is one way to learn to use your "wise self" to promote healing . . . . I will start with a relaxation technique . . . . You can communicate with me by raising your right index finger for yes and your left index finger for no . . . . You are in complete control at all times during this session and you may stop the session at any time by simply opening your eyes.
>
> I want to ask you, if you will, to allow yourself time to withdraw within . . . to take time for you . . . to rejuvenate and refresh yourself . . . . And to begin I would like to ask you to count backwards with me from five to one . . . . And as I count backwards I would like to ask your subconscious mind to go back into comfort at the rate of one-fifth at a time . . . . So that by the time we get to one, you can be as deeply relaxed as possible at this point in time . . . and as you breathe in and out, ask your body to allow the relaxed feelings to flow all the way through . . . *five.*
>
> And as we go down [pause], ask your subconscious mind to release any unnecessary tensions in muscle groups like your eyes, eyelids, forehead, scalp . . . [pause], nostrils, lips and cheeks . . . . Releasing unnecessary tension that you don't wish to keep . . . . It is not a requirement, simply an invitation that you are welcome to accept . . . . Give up any tension around your cheeks, chin, and jaw . . . . And as you do this, you may find your mouth opening . . . . It is a sign that your muscles are letting go . . . *four* . . . . This is an internal exercise for your education, for your comfort.
>
> Letting go of any excess tensions across your neck and throat, down your biceps, triceps, past your elbow, forearm, wrist . . . . Breathing—calm, regular . . . . Even letting go of the tension of the little muscles between your ribs . . . . Each time you let go of air, you might want to, if you wish,

imagine blowing out tension with it. So that each and every breath becomes more relaxing . . . . Calm regular breathing . . . . *three* . . . . Just letting go of the tensions down your spine . . . Each individual vertebra, each muscle in your vertebrae . . . . Almost as if warm water is being poured down the inside of the vertebrae and radiating warmth and comfort throughout your torso . . . . All the way down . . . . Letting go of the tensions along your sides, abdomen, hips and seat . . . . Very good . . . . You're halfway there.

Deeper and deeper into comfort you can go, at your own pace in your own way . . . . Thighs, letting go . . . knees . . . Letting go of tension along your calves and ankles . . . . Breathing and relaxing . . . *two* . . . . Heels letting go . . . . And as you get down to your toes, you might want to continue letting your mind empty itself, much like that water, that warm water, going down your spine . . . Releasing the cold tension . . . . It's coming from your head and just emptying itself . . . . Cool forehead . . . *one* . . . . As deep and comfortable as you wish, fully relaxed . . . . That's right . . . nothing to do.

Now let your imagination take you to a place that feels safe and comfortable.

Imagine a smooth white beach . . . .

You walk through a garden filled with flowers to reach the beach . . . . The air is filled with the gentle fragrance from the flowers . . . . As you reach the beach you see a hammock tied between two trees . . . . You go over to the hammock and lie down . . . . The texture of the hammock is soft and nubby . . . . You can feel the warm sun against your skin . . . . You can feel a gentle breeze . . . . Notice the sea gulls as they dip and glide on the wind currents . . . hear the faint sounds of laughter in the background.

You have not been this comfortable for a long time . . . . The hammock swings gently back and forth . . . back and forth.

Nothing to do but relax and enjoy your special place . . . . You look out over the crystal, clear, aquamarine waters and notice a sail boat slowly moving off in the distance.

Enjoy the differences in hues, as the light plays on the water . . . . Swinging, comfortably swinging in the hammock, with a breeze that keeps you at just the right temperature . . . . Hear the water as it laps on the shore and the wind as it ripples through the palm trees . . . . And now, if you wish, get up and move to the water . . . . Feel the cool water as it reaches your toes . . . . Feel the sand on your feet as you slowly enter the water . . . as you swim through the water, each individual water molecule touching you, in its own way, finding a way to soothe and calm you. . . . . You are finding that new and ever-emerging more comfortable you . . . . It is nice to swim freely, comfortably through the water . . . . Finally, you get out of the water and return to the hammock and lie down . . . . You are relaxed and pleasantly tired . . . . As the hammock moves slowly back and forth, you think back over the last few minutes . . . . You enjoy your newfound freedom, your complete sense of comfort . . . . You can retreat to this place of comfort whenever you wish . . . . It is a place especially for you . . . . You can change it.

And enjoy it as much as you wish . . . . Use this relaxation/imagery technique to escape the difficulties and pressures of daily life . . . . And when you are ready to return from your special place, count slowly from one to five . . . . Open your eyes and stretch your arms and legs . . . . Move around in your chair . . . . You are awake and alert . . . . Feeling rested and comfortable.

(From Stephens RL: Imagery: A strategic intervention to empower clients, part II—A practical guide. Clinical Nurse Specialist 7:235–240, 1993, with permission.)

16. Do support groups really help?

Cancer care was founded on the premise that life does not end when cancer begins. Families and friends are necessary for support, but it is also helpful for patients to talk to others outside their immediate circle. Experienced patients can describe what it was like to go down the cancer path and provide the "light at the end of the tunnel" perspective of life after cancer. They can provide an outside third ear that can empathize, not sympathize. Studies show that support groups or talking to others can complement medical therapy and may accelerate recovery or enhance outcome.

Support groups are not for everybody. For patients who are unable or do not want to attend support groups, other helpful options include telephone support groups, internet chat groups, books written by other patients, and videotapes. For patients who do not like to interact with other people, human–animal bonding or pet therapy programs offer great support.

17. Give examples of statements from friends that patients find unhelpful.

Family and friends are often at a loss when they learn that a loved one has been diagnosed with cancer. At times relatives, friends, or perfect strangers may suffer from the common ailment of "foot-in-mouth" disease caused by putting the mouth into gear before engaging the brain and making terribly inappropriate or thoughtless comments. Good advice to patients' friends: it is more important to listen than to worry about what to say. Nurses cannot protect the patient from such often well-meant comments, but they can listen, provide factual information, and help patients strategize meaningful responses. Prepare patients to hear the following types of outlandish comments:

- "My Aunt Harriet had the same types of cancer and she took that chemo poison and suffered and died screaming with pain at the end."
- "If you hadn't smoked so much and had changed your diet, you wouldn't have this."
- "What did you do to cause this?"
- "I heard that shark cartilage and coffee enemas three times a day really help."
- "The medical establishment found a cure for cancer years ago. They keep it only for their families because they want to make money off of us."
- "Get a grip on yourself. It's not that bad. You've had this for two months already; it's time to move on with your life."

18. Give examples of helpful and unhelpful comments from health care providers.

It is inevitable that sometimes you will say the wrong thing, but it is important to recognize such incidents and to find an alternative therapeutic response. Avoid excessive questioning or giving too much advice without taking time to hear the patient's concerns and viewpoints. Let the patient's reactions guide the discussion. Center your attention on the patient while he or she is talking. Listen, instead of focusing on what you are planning to say next. Don't feel that both of you have to talk all the time; make use of silence to absorb what the patient has said. If the patient did not understand your explanations, clarify and validate your statements. Examples of statements that promote communication include the following:

Tell me about yourself. Go on . . . tell me more . . . Give me an example. Describe that further. Please explain. Help me to understand that. What do you mean? What was the importance of that event? What do you see as the reason? What would you say was the problem? Is that what you meant? If I hear you correctly, you are telling me . . . Let me restate. Is this what you were saying? What would you do if a situation like this comes up again?

At the end of an interaction, it is helpful to summarize what has been said. The table below gives examples of barriers to therapeutic communication.

Barriers	Not Helpful	Helpful
Giving advice	"Why don't you . . . ."	"I understand what you are saying."
	"If I were you . . . ."	"What do you think would work?"
Giving false reassurance	"Don't worry."	"What worries you most?"
	"Everyone feels like that."	"Tell me what you are thinking."
	"Things always look worse before they get better."	"I realize this must be a bad time for you."
Changing the subject	"Let's talk about that later."	"That sounds important, so tell me more."
	"I wanted to tell you about . . . or I want to ask you about . . . ."	"I know this is painful to talk about, but try to tell me how you're feeling."
		"Let's talk about that more."
Being judgmental	"You're wrong."	"Your understanding is different. How do you see the situation?"
	"You shouldn't think like that."	
	"We know what's best for you."	"I don't agree with your decision, but I can understand where you're coming from."
Giving directions	"This is the way it should be done."	"Which way works best for you?"
	"You have to/you must follow these directions."	"Let's look at the different options."
		"How would you handle the situation?"

Continued on following page.

Barriers	Not Helpful	Helpful
Using emotionally charged words	"Your wife makes you very angry."	"How do you feel about what she did?"
	"You feel guilty about what happened."	"I wonder if you feel responsible about what happened?"
	"You describe your husband as being mean."	"You describe your husband's behavior changing."
Challenging	"You can't stay home by yourself."	"It sounds like you think you could be okay by yourself."
Making trite or stereotypical comments	"You're looking chipper today."	"I notice you're smiling more today; does that mean you're feeling better?"
	"Keep your chin up."	
	"Things always look better in the morning."	"How hard is it for you to keep up with this chemotherapy?"

Adapted from Haber J: Barriers to therapeutic communication. In Haber J, Krainovich-Miller B, McMahon AL, Price-Hoskins P: Comprehensive Psychiatric Nursing, 5th ed. St. Louis, Mosby, 1997, pp 136–140.

19. Give examples of important ways to help patients cope with cancer and to show that you care.

- Listen to patients. Hear their stories. Don't be hurt if the patient chooses to confide in the janitor—as long as you know the patient has someone with whom to share personal feelings.
- Practice self-awareness. Know what you are thinking and allow yourself to have feelings and be compassionate.
- Take care of yourself so that you have good energy to share. A nurse can help a patient cope better if he or she is able to cope well. Balance the need to "be there" with your own needs.
- Try to be empathetic. Put yourself in the patient's place, or imagine that the patient is a friend or relative. Discover what the patient did or looked like before cancer.
- Allow time. Don't avoid offering support because you think you're too busy, or don't have enough time. It may only take a few seconds or a few kind words to show empathy and caring. For example, a hug—if acceptable to the patient—takes only a few seconds. If you only have five minutes, inform the patient of your time limit and you will be surprised at how much can be accomplished in a short time.
- Don't make promises you cannot keep. Don't say you're coming back within a certain time unless you mean it.
- Try to find something unique and human about every patient. Accept patients for who they are, and learn from them. The most difficult and challenging patient may turn out to be your favorite. Accept that you cannot like everyone, but you can still be therapeutic or find someone else who can.
- Be sensitive to patients from different cultural, ethnic, or religious backgrounds. Learn what is appropriate in caring for them, but avoid stereotyping.
- Always know your facts and be competent in what you are doing. Technical proficiency is just as important as caring.
- Pay meticulous attention to basic nursing care. Good patient hygiene promotes comfort and prevents infections. Clean linens, fresh water, and neat bedside areas reflect good nursing care to patients and their families.
- Use touch to convey caring and support; however, be aware that touch is not acceptable to all patients.
- Prevent and treat distressful symptoms. All dimensions of quality of life are affected by pain or discomfort.
- Collaborate and coordinate with other members of the team. Be a team player; it will ultimately help your patients.
- Facilitate the patient's empowerment to take responsibility for health by providing accurate information and education.
- Don't forget to involve the family and significant others. Give them feedback and reassurance about how they are doing.

- Reassure patients that they will not be abandoned and that someone will "be there" to help them. Let them know when and who to call for problems.
- Be creative. Individualize what works for a particular patient, not just what is in the books or guidelines. Examples of creative caring include allowing a loved pet in the hospital, rolling a patient's bed to a window to see fireworks on the Fourth of July, putting a sign up for "intimate time" between a young couple, and providing special badges of honor after completion of chemotherapy.

20. What resources are available to help patients with coping?

Cancer Care Counseling Line (800-813-HOPE or 800-813-4673)

Immediate professional counseling. Publishes *The Resource Guide for People with Cancer*, which lists support and educational resources for all types of cancers.

E-mail: cancer@aol.com

Web page: http://www.cancercareinc.org

Cancer Information Service–National Cancer Institute (800-4-CANCER or 800-422-6237)

E-mail: cancernet@icib.nci.nih.gov

Current medical information on cancer and therapies.

American Cancer Society (800-ACS-2345 or 800-227-2324)

Cancer-related community resources.

Web page: http://www.cancer.org

Coping Magazine

E-mail: copingmag@aol.com

Well Spouse Foundation

E-mail: wellspouse@aol.com

Patient information books such as:

Dollinger M, Rosenbaum EH, Cable G: Everyone's Guide to Cancer Therapy: How Cancer is Diagnosed, Treated, and Managed Day to Day. Toronto, Somerville House, 1991.

Morra M, Potts E: Choices. New York, Avon Books, 1994.

ACKNOWLEDGMENT

The authors wish to thank Linda U. Krebs, RN, PhD, for her thoughtful review of this chapter.

BIBLIOGRAPHY

1. Berckman KL, Austin JK: Casual attribution, perceived control, and adjustment in patients with lung cancer. Oncol Nurs Forum 20:23–30, 1993.
2. Hagopian GA: Cognitive strategies used in adapting to a cancer diagnosis. Oncol Nurs Forum 20:759–763, 1993.
3. Haber J, Krainovich-Miller B, McMahon AL, Price-Hoskins P: Comprehensive Psychiatric Nursing, 5th ed. St. Louis, Mosby, 1997.
4. Herth K: Fostering hope in terminally ill people. J Adv Nurs 15:1250–1259, 1990.
5. Larson PJ: Important nurse caring behaviors perceived by patients with cancer. Oncol Nurs For 11(6): 46–50, 1984.
6. Leininger M: Caring: A central focus of nursing and health services. In Leininger MM (ed): Care: The Essence of Nursing and Health. Thorofare, NJ, Slack, 1984, p 46.
7. O'Berle K, Davies B: Support and caring: Exploring the concepts. Oncol Nurs Forum 19:763–767, 1992.
8. Post-White J, Ceronsky C, Kreitzer MJ, et al: Hope, spirituality, sense of coherence, and quality of life in patients with cancer. Oncol Nurs Forum 23:1571–1579, 1996.
9. Roth AJ, Holland JC: Psychiatric complications in cancer patients. In Brain MC, Carbone PP (eds): Current Therapy in Hematology–Oncology, 5th ed. 1995, pp 609–621.
10. Spiegel D, et al: Effect of psychosocial treatment on survival of patients with metastatic breast cancer. Lancet 2(8668):888–891, 1989.
11. Stephens RL: Imagery: A strategic intervention to empower clients, part II—a practical guide. Clinical Nurse Specialist 7: 235–240, 1993.
12. Watson J: Nursing: Human Science and Human Care. East Norwalk, CT, Appelton-Century-Crofts, 1985.
13. Zacharia DR., Glilg CA, Foxall MJ: Quality of life and coping in patients with gynecologic cancer and their spouses. Oncol Nurs Forum, 21:1699–1706, 1994.

62. RELIGION AND SPIRITUALITY

Julie R. Swaney, MDiv

1. What is the difference between religion and spirituality?

Spirituality is not necessarily religion. Many more people are spiritual than religious. Religion is a type of spirituality that refers to a disciplined, dogmatic set of beliefs usually set forth in writings (Koran, Bible, Creeds and Confessions) and institutions (synagogues, churches). Spirituality refers to patterns or habits that human beings practice "for the purpose of grounding their ordinary lives in a life of the spirit which has meaning for them and to which they commit and re-commit themselves."[5] Spirituality has to do with meaning-making.

Some people find meaning in religion; others find or make meaning in their own spirituality. Spirituality asks and helps to answer crucial questions: How does this illness make sense in my life? How does my life make sense with this illness? What meaning does this cancer have for me? What meaning do I have with this cancer? What meaning do I have to my family? To God? To myself? What is spiritual has to do with what is essential; that is, what is of essence. We often think of spirituality as an external relationship with God—"out there"—rather than the more accurate notion of God within us.

2. What is the importance of religion and spirituality in illness?

Religion and spirituality provide the interpretive lens or framework within which persons make sense of living and dying. Being left to the whim of fate is universally terrifying. Patients with cancer and their caregivers often believe in something that helps to maintain hope. Patients may believe in chemotherapy, radiation, doctors, vitamins, macrobiotic diets, God's faithfulness to them, superstitious ritual, or their immune system. What they believe in provides a way of making sense of themselves and their experiences. As one patient stated, "believing in my immune system is everything . . . . It's the peg to hang my hat on." When people are coping with cancer, what they believe about themselves—what they hold in their spirits—profoundly affects their experience.

3. How do religious beliefs help people to cope with terminal illness?

People with healthy faith are better able to face reality, maintain hope, tolerate uncertainties, and retain their self-esteem and dignity. Religious beliefs that promote the constancy of God's presence help patients to realize their significance and permanence and to accept the ambiguity of God's ways. Prayer and meditation can reduce anxiety and strengthen coping skills. Certain beliefs answer the question "why?," whereas others provide comfort in the midst of the question itself.

The crisis of cancer prompts questions of meaning and existence: How much do I want to live? How much time do I have? Why did this happen to me? What did I do or not do? Why does God allow this? Why do I have to suffer? Am I a good person? Is God punishing me? Where is God? If I promise to go to church, will God heal me? Many people understand their existence in relation to God, whereas others do not. These existential questions of the human spirit are significant because they affect coping skills. "Being religious" does not guarantee survival, but it does guarantee a qualitative difference in the experience of cancer.

4. Can beliefs impede the healing process?

What people believe to be true may be what they will experience. Belief systems centered around punishment and guilt or even satanic forces may impede the healing process. Such beliefs lead people to think that they "deserve" the cancer and cannot be well again, whereas beliefs centered on forgiveness and hope facilitate healing and wholeness. Unhealthy faith provides an escape from reality and hinders adaptation to the experience.

5. How does hospitalization affect religion and spirituality?

Impressive human changes may occur during illness and hospitalization. During hospitalization, patients journey along a path with hope and healing on one side and terror and tragedy on the other. In a 1985 study of changes in hospitalized patients,[3] 90% of the patients claimed to use their hospitalization to review and reorder their central values. Over 50% reported major shifts in their perception of the importance and quality of their relationships. Other changes reported in the study included the following: 71% reported that illness had changed their understanding of the purpose of their lives; 85% reported being more aware of the passing of time; 81% reported a decreased sense of being in control of their lives; 58% reported that illness had deprived them, to some extent, of the sense of being like other people; and 70% reported changes in their religious faith and practice.

6. What are the common religious beliefs and rituals related to illness and death?

Because a religion's stated positions may influence individual medical decisions, it is important to be familiar with some of the beliefs of particular religions, as outlined below. The nurse may ask patients about their beliefs and make use of religious authorities to assist the patient.

Buddhism (Tibetan)

Illness rituals	Prayer and meditation
Meaning of illness	Natural part of life
Faith healing	Possible through prayer and meditation
Sacraments	Respect intermediate state; preparation for death very important. Death signals entry into intermediate state of great intensity. Do not interrupt period of great concentration as deceased travels through intermediate state. Environment to be peaceful, focused, and intimate for terminally ill or deceased. Do not move body for 72 hours after death. Spiritual goal: extinction.
Autopsy	Permissible
Burial	Cremation
Meaning of death	Enlightenment

Roman Catholicism

Illness rituals	Baptism, confession, Sacrament of the Sick, Eucharist, Prayer
Meaning of illness	Natural part of life; preserve dignity of patient; some suffering considered meaningful.
Faith healing	Possible through prayer, Sacrament of the Sick (anointing)
Sacraments	Sacrament of the Sick
Autopsy	Permissible
Burial	Burial or cremation
Meaning of death	Release to God

Christian Science

Illness rituals	Prayer
Meaning of illness	Mental concept that can be destroyed by altering thoughts and discovering "spiritual truth." Use Christian Science practitioners.
Faith healing	Primary means of healing; emphasize spiritual healing.
Sacraments	None
Autopsy	Unlikely, but permissible
Burial	Burial or cremation
Meaning of death	Return to God

Mormon (Church of Jesus Christ of Latter-day Saints)

Illness rituals	Prayer
Meaning of illness	Natural part of life; revelation of meaning through individual visions
Faith healing	Laying on of hands for divine healing
Sacraments	Adult baptism essential, even after death; preach gospel. Wash body; dress body in white robe.
Autopsy	Permissible
Burial	Burial; no cremation
Meaning of death	Death a blessing; return to God

Hindu

Illness rituals	Prayer
Meaning of illness	Punishment
Faith healing	Possible through prayer and meditation
Sacraments	Tie thread of blessing. Pour water in mouth. Washing of body. Particular about who touches body.
Autopsy	Permissible
Burial	Cremation (Ganges)
Meaning of death	Death an endless passage through cycles of life; natural part of life. Hope for better existence in next life. Death is liberation.

Jehovah's Witness

Illness rituals	Prayer
Meaning of illness	Natural part of life; strong sanctity of life
Faith healing	Possible through prayer
Sacraments	None
Autopsy	Acceptable; body intact
Burial	Burial or cremation
Meaning of death	Natural part of life

Judaism (Orthodox)

Illness rituals	Prayer
Meaning of illness	Natural part of life; strong sanctity-of-life ethic requiring all possible medical care to preserve life.
Faith healing	Demand medical attention; possible through prayer
Sacraments	Goses, Shiva, Yetziat Neshamah, Kevod Hamet
Autopsy	Rarely permissible; consult rabbi.
Burial	No cremation, quick burial
Meaning of death	Natural part of life; no afterlife

Presbyterian (Protestant)

Illness rituals	Baptism, communion, anointing, prayer
Meaning of illness	Natural part of life; quality of life valued over quantity of life
Faith healing	Prayer, communion
Sacraments	Prayer
Autopsy	Acceptable
Burial	Burial or cremation
Meaning of death	Resurrection into afterlife

7. How do religious beliefs affect ethical decision-making?

At times of uncertainty, people often turn to their moral or religious community for guidance in ethical decision making. What is "right" or "beneficial" or "futile" to a patient may be defined by the religious community or doctrine to which they belong. A Muslim patient may demand "futile" treatment because the tenets of Islam dictate the sanctity of life; life must be prolonged regardless of its quality. A Jehovah's Witness patient may refuse blood, even if the outcome is death, because of religious tenets. Suicide is generally not allowed by religions and denominations; however, religious authorities should be consulted if suicidal ideation or suicide becomes an issue with any patient. Other common religious beliefs that affect ethical issues are outlined below.

Buddhism

Drugs, blood, artificial life support	Acceptable
Organ donation	Allowed if enhanced possibility of enlightenment
Termination of treatment	Allowed
Withholding/withdrawing life support	Allowed. Death is natural, to be accepted. Avoid unnatural intrusion of dying process
Active euthanasia	Prohibited

Roman Catholicism

Drugs, blood, artificial life support	Acceptable
Organ donation	Justified

Termination of treatment	Allowed except in cases of pregnancy
Withholding/withdrawing life support	Allowed. "Ordinary but not extraordinary" duty to prolong life. Importance of dignity. Exception: pregnancy.
Active euthanasia	Prohibited

Christian Science

Drugs, blood, artificial life support	Unacceptable
Organ donation	Unlikely
Termination of treatment	Allowed. Rely on faith healing.
Withholding/withdrawing life support	Allowed. Unlikely to accept in first place; unlikely to prolong dying process.
Active euthanasia	Prohibited

Mormon (Church of Jesus Christ of Latter-day Saints)

Drugs, blood, artificial life support	Acceptable
Organ donation	Individual decision
Termination of treatment	Allowed
Withholding/withdrawing life support	Allowed. Inevitable death viewed as a blessing.
Active euthanasia	Prohibited

Hindu

Drugs, blood, artificial life support	Acceptable
Organ donation	Permissible
Termination of treatment	Allowed
Withholding/withdrawing life support	Allowed. Death is liberation.
Active euthanasia	Prohibited

Jehovah's Witness

Drugs, blood, artificial life support	Some drugs; *no blood or blood products*; life support acceptable
Organ donation	Forbidden
Termination of treatment	Allowed
Withholding/withdrawing life support	Allowed. Rely on individual conscience in this decision. Duty not to accept blood or blood products.
Active euthanasia	Prohibited

Judaism (Orthodox)

Drugs, blood, artificial life support	Acceptable
Organ donation	Consult rabbi.
Termination of treatment	Not allowed. Consult rabbi.
Withholding/withdrawing life support	Not allowed. Consult rabbi.
Active euthanasia	Prohibited

Presbyterian (Protestant)

Drugs, blood, artificial life support	Acceptable
Organ donation	Acceptable
Termination of treatment	Allowed
Withholding/withdrawing life support	Allowed. Quality of life valued over quantity of life. Importance of dignity.
Active euthanasia	Prohibited

8. How do I understand a belief system different from my own?

Listen intently. *Ask* with sincerity. *Respect* what you hear. Some people have specific religious views to fashion their understanding, whereas others have their own theology, which may not fit any particular religious tradition. Even if you do not agree with all of a patient's beliefs, you can still help the patient by allowing him or her to articulate personal beliefs. It is not appropriate to try to convert patients to your belief system during vulnerable times. It is important to remember that beliefs exist for a reason.

9. How does one make a spiritual assessment?

The first step is to assess one's own view of the role and importance of spirituality and religion in health and illness. Person-centered nursing requires tending to the human spirit. The second step is to assess personal comfort level with addressing spiritual issues. The nurse who is uncomfortable with such issues should refer the patient to someone else. The third step is to offer one's self in a genuine, honest, empathic way. Empathy and respect for the patient's questions and views are more important than providing answers. One may help the patient simply by listening. The final step is to ask questions such as the following:

- Were you raised in any religious tradition? If so, do you still follow that religion?
- Are you active in a congregation?
- What religious stories and rituals have particular meaning to you?
- What does your religion or spirituality mean to you? Is it helpful? How?
- How does religion or spirituality give meaning to you now?
- Are you allowed to question God?
- Are you allowed to question your faith?
- Do your religious beliefs affect your morality? How so?
- What was an "organizing crisis" of your life? What theologic framework was used for answering your dilemma?
- What does your faith do for you?
- Do you pray? How often? When?
- Do you ever feel like God has abandoned you? If so, what do you do?
- What is important for me to know about your religion or spirituality ?

10. What are key nursing interventions to promote the spiritual well-being of patients?

Perhaps the most important nursing intervention is to offer genuine concern and empathy in eliciting the patient's spiritual strengths, beliefs, doubts and confidences. Nurses should not impose their beliefs on patients; instead, they should assist patients in discovering and utilizing their own beliefs.

A 1985 study[6] asked Protestant, Catholic, and Jewish respondents if they thought that nurses could be helpful to them in establishing or maintaining a relationship with God. Only 5 (20%) of Jewish subjects said "yes," whereas 42 (91%) of Protestant respondents and 26 (72%) of Catholic respondents said "yes." The table below summarizes Protestant and Catholic views of specific nursing activities thought to be most helpful.

Nursing Activity	Catholics Responding Yes	Protestants Responding Yes
Read to me Bible passages I have chosen	15/20 (75%)	36/41 (88%)
Read or recite Bible passages of nurse's choice	12/22 (55%)	31/40 (78%)
Listen to me talk through my problem	22/24 (95%)	32/40 (80%)
Pray with me at my bedside	20/24 (83%)	37/40 (93%)
Tell me that the nurse is praying for me (when not with me)	23/24 (96%)	36/39 (92%)

Adapted from Murray R, Zentner J: Spiritual and Religious Influence on the Person. Nursing Assessment and Health Promotion Strategies Through the Life Span. New Jersey, Prentice-Hall, 1989.

11. What is spiritual distress?

Spiritual distress is a condition in which a person experiences or is at risk of experiencing a disturbance in a belief or value system that provides strength, hope, and meaning to life. Spiritual distress or faith crisis, as a nursing diagnosis, refers to "a disruption in the life principle that pervades a person's entire being and that integrates and transcends one's biological and psychosocial nature."[7] Spiritual distress occurs when religious ideology or accepted beliefs suddenly hold no integrity for an individual. Such a faith crisis is generally accompanied, if not precipitated, by anger and distress. Ways of interpreting life ("I always thought God would protect me"), of making sense, of finding meaning, fall apart. Sources of spiritual distress may be the crisis of illness, suffering, or death itself; the inability to practice spiritual rituals; or conflict between beliefs and treatment regimen.

12. List common signs of spiritual distress.

Signs of spiritual distress range from obvious expression to subtle clues:
- Statement of spiritual distress or crisis
- Withdrawal, depression
- Anger
- Crying
- Loneliness, loss of self-esteem
- Hopelessness, helplessness
- Changes in reading or not reading religious literature
- Expression of feeling abandoned by persons and God
- Inability to cope with illness or treatment
- Refusal of or demand for treatment
- Praying for a miracle
- Tenacious grip on a rigid set of beliefs

13. What are nursing interventions for spiritual distress?

If spiritual distress is related to the inability to practice spiritual rituals, the nurse may help by addressing the disruptive factors and enabling the patient to engage in important (health-aiding) rituals. When spiritual distress is related to the crisis of illness, suffering, or dying, the nurse can help the patient verbalize the sense of meaning, sense of forgiveness, and sense of belonging and love. Such distress may be expressed in such questions as "Why is this happening to me?" (meaning), "What did I do to deserve this?" (forgiveness), or "Why do I feel so alone?" (love/relatedness). The nurse can help patients use their own inner resources to address such questions and may also enlist the help of external resources (clergy, family, friends, literature, health care professionals). Spiritual distress related to conflict between religious or spiritual beliefs and the prescribed health regimen can be relieved by providing thorough and accurate information for informed consent or informed refusal. The health care team should support the patient in his or her stated wishes and goals.

14. Why do people with faith tend to suffer less than those without it?

"Being religious" offers a qualitative difference in one's experience of cancer. People with healthy faith are generally more able to remain centered, to come to terms with their suffering, if not their death, because they seek to know themselves as God knows them. Their sense of significance, permanence, and self-esteem is determined in this larger context.

People suffer less when they are able to maintain a sense of personal worth, dignity, significance, even permanence in the wake of death. "Being religious" does not guarantee positive self-regard but does reduce sources of suffering. Religious individuals may suffer less from fear of dying because of their belief in spiritual permanence. Discovering themselves as God knows them makes people aware that they belong to a greater order in which they matter and in which attachment to God is fundamental. Patients with healthy faith believe that "in life and death, we belong to God;" thus, they are more able to accept the ambiguity of God's ways and to maintain hope in the midst of uncertainty.

15. What is the difference between suffering and pain?

Bodies do not suffer; people do. Pain refers to a physical sensation, whereas suffering refers to the quest for meaning, purpose, and fulfillment. Although pain is often a source of suffering, suffering may occur in the absence of pain. For example, a nuclear physicist with malignant melanoma metastasized to his brain is paralyzed on the left side of his body and dying. He describes suffering over the perceived lack of meaning in his life and death with cancer: "My life has meant nothing. It ends here." He is suffering because he has lost his centeredness and feels himself to be fragmenting and disintegrating in terms of personal significance. Suffering may occur when a person perceives death as meaningless or as a form of personal disintegration. People who have not made the most of their lives have a hard time facing death.

Other sources of suffering are the effects of disease and treatment, such as change in identity, loss of control, isolation, not feeling understood, perception of a foreshortened future (i.e., "nothingness," death), and threats of losing relationships, mobility, independence, finances, control, self-worth. Theologically and existentially, suffering occurs when we are threatened by something not in our control. In this sense, some suffering is inevitable, because we are always facing things we cannot control. Suffering is more bearable when we remain centered, when we can plumb the depths of our suffering to discover life's ultimate meaning for us.[2]

16. What difference does faith make in the experience of pain and suffering?

How persons view their pain and suffering affects their healing or dying process. The early Greeks and Romans emphasized the practice of euthanasia as an honorable way to manage pain. *Euthanatos* translates as "a good death." For the ancients, it was important to die a good death with self-control. Plato, Socrates, and many Greek and Roman physicians who administered poisons claimed that when a person became "useless to society," dying decently was a measure of the final value of life. Pain and suffering were meaningless.

The Judeo-Christian tradition transformed pain and suffering into meaningful experiences. After the second century A.D., this influential tradition in western thought and culture emphasized the importance of enduring suffering. Pain and suffering were believed to be the sign of God's presence in one's life. Suffering meant that one belonged to God and had to endure the life that one was given. The goal, then, was not to alleviate suffering but to endure it.

Many people still believe that pain and suffering are meaningful signs of God's presence and must be endured. Others are outraged by the pain and suffering that they endure and demand alleviation. Both positions may be more than simple attitudes; they may be deep religious convictions. The nurse may verify patient's beliefs and give the patient permission to verbalize personal points of view. When in doubt, the nurse should err on the side of alleviating pain and suffering.

17. How does spiritual care contribute to healing?

The most powerful healing emotion is expectant faith. Healing is the product of a human bond between caregiver and patient. Faith, hope, respect, compassion, trust, and empathy are essential elements of that bond that contribute to healing. The heart of nursing or caring is a healing relationship, and the heart of healing relationships is trust, acceptance and empathy.

To cure (Latin: *curare*) means to take care of, to take charge of. It implies successful medical treatment. To heal (Anglo-Saxon: *haelen*) means to make or become whole, to recover from sickness, to get well. Helping someone to become whole is accomplished through a healing relationship as well as technical competence. Both are important. Healing is a process and comes from the same root word as holy. Both refer to wholeness. To facilitate healing is to facilitate greater wholeness. Through relationships and skills, the nurse can facilitate healing, wholeness, and even that which is holy in patients. It is hoped that nurses can experience the same processes in themselves.

18. What is the connection between prayer and healing?

"The science of prayer" has generated much debate and controversy. Prayer seems to be effective, but how and why? Why does prayer "work" for some people and not for others? To answer this question, as well as to define the relationship between prayer and healing, we must remain open to the mystery and ambiguity of healing, and perhaps of God.

Both theologians and physicians are enlarging their frameworks for understanding the connection between faith and healing. Historically, all physicians were priests, and religious orders ran hospitals. Spiritual and physical healing were recognized as intimately connected. Early 19th century rationalism, with its mechanical view of the body, increasingly separated the body from the mind and spirit. Religion left medicine, and medicine left the church. Yet there remained a holistic notion of persons that emphasized the integration of body, mind, and spirit.

Prayer is one way of attending to the spirit. Prayer grounds people in what gives them meaning and in their relationship with God. Prayer puts important words to their experiences. Prayer also evokes important feelings for healing—safety, hope, love, seeing oneself as one is seen by God, personal worth and self-esteem, and feeling cared about and "not alone." Prayer helps people to face reality; to tolerate ambiguity and uncertainty; and to confront the unknown, which is so constant in illness. At the very least, prayer helps to reduce anxiety, to remain centered, to remember that one is part of God's greater order; it helps patients to relax. And at the very most, prayer is an expression of a profound and empowering relationship with God.

Positive effects of prayer have been reported in patients with high blood pressure, wounds, heart attacks, headaches, and anxiety. One study showed that intercessory prayer (prayer for others) was a contributing factor to the healing of cardiac patients. The positive effects of prayer have also been indicated on nonhuman subjects such as water, enzymes, bacteria, plants, yeast, mice, and red blood cells.

19. Is prayer magic?

Prayer is not magic, religion is not magic, and God is not a magician. Many people use prayer and religion as a way of invoking "divine magic"; they are likely to be disappointed. One cannot manipulate God through piety or ritual. The adage, "there are no atheists in foxholes," is especially true when the foxhole is cancer. It is not wrong to pray when one is frightened, regardless of one's relationship with God. But it is wrong to try to manipulate God. The power to affect the outcome of prayer is in God, not in the person praying.

Miracles are not magic. Many people say that they are "praying for a miracle." A miracle is a purposeful intervention from God that is often a process and not an instant. "Praying for a miracle" does not relieve one of continuing personal responsibility, such as pursuing treatment or making difficult decisions. Miracles happen as part of God's order, not our magical wishes for situations to change. It is fine for people to pray for miracles as long as they also face the reality before them.

20. When should a chaplain be called?

Chaplains are frequently called for deaths, although religion and faith are not just about death. The goal of pastoral care is healing of the spirit, whether a person is living or dying. As nurses become acquainted with the hospital chaplain, they come to know how he or she approaches the nuances of a patient's concerns. Very often this is accomplished through an empathic relationship that encourages and allows patients to use their own inner resources to affect healing and strength.

Chaplains generally represent all denominations and faith traditions—Protestant, Catholic, Jewish, Hindu, Islam. Staff chaplains can assist the nurse in finding a representative from a particular faith. Chaplains are available for sacramental purposes such as baptism, communion, anointing, weddings, funerals, and confession. They are also available for pastoral purposes such as counseling, prayer, support, and assistance in decision-making. Although there are many times and reasons to call a chaplain, some of the most common are when the patient:

- uses religion as a source of support
- is withdrawn, depressed, restless, complaining, or irritable
- is anxious (notably preoperatively)
- worsens, becomes terminally ill, or dies
- expresses interest or curiosity about religious questions or issues
- reads scripture and other religious literature
- is struggling with loss or grieving
- exhibits spiritual distress
- has ethical dilemmas, decisions to make
- asks to see chaplain, asks about worship services, desires a Bible
- has no visitors, cards, or flowers in room
- expresses a desire for sacraments

21. What does a chaplain do during a visit?

Chaplains respond to the presenting need (e.g., fear of dying, anxiety about procedures, grief over a diagnosis, hopelessness of ongoing treatment, need for prayer and reassurance, anger at God). One of the most valuable pastoral interventions is to offer an empathic relationship. This means entering into the world of the patient and listening to his or her experience, conflict, dilemma, or fear. Chaplains should not try to convert people unless requested to do so by the patient. Chaplains encourage a person's inner strengths. They assist persons in finding hope when they feel hopeless and help persons to recover or discover for the first time who they are in relationship with God. Because of the intimacy of the process of illness, dying and death, many chaplains perform funerals and memorial services for patients who have died. Chaplains also assist in discussions about code status, requests for organ donation, and mortuary arrangements.

22. Are chaplains available to staff?

Most chaplains are available to staff members as well as patients and families. Oncologic nurses must take care of themselves, allow themselves to suffer with their patients, acknowledge their own pain and losses, and utilize supportive people around them. Chaplains are also available for support, clarification, encouragement, and hope. Chaplains may offer periodic memorial services for the staff to gain closure in regard to patient deaths.

BIBLIOGRAPHY

1. Baumann A, Johnston N, Antai-Otong D: Decision Making in Psychiatric and Psychosocial Nursing. Philadelphia, B.C. Decker, 1990.
2. Cassell E: The nature of suffering and the goals of medicine. N Engl J Med 306:639–645, 1982.
3. Gibbons J, Miller S: An image of contemporary hospital chaplaincy. J Pastor Care 43:355–361, 1989.
4. Marty M, Vaux K (eds): Health/Medicine and the Faith Traditions: An Inquiry into Religion and Medicine. Philadelphia, Fortress Press, 1982.
5. Mitchell K: Spirituality and pastoral care. J Pastor Care 43:93–95, 1989.
6. Murray R, Zentner J: Spiritual and Religious Influence on the Person. Nursing Assessment and Health Promotion Strategies Through the Life Span. New Jersey, Prentice-Hall, 1989.
7. Taylor EJ, Amenta M, Highfield M: Spiritual care practices of oncology nurses. Oncol Nurs Forum 22:31–39, 1995.

63. HUMOR

Lynn Erdman, RN, MN, OCN

1. What are the benefits of laughter for nurses and patients?

Benefits may be physiologic or psychologic. **Physiologically** laughter increases heart rate, quickens breathing, increases oxygen intake, improves circulation, and works the muscles in the face and stomach. William Fry, M.D., of Stanford University has studied the effects of laughter for more than 30 years. He says that laughing 100 times/day is the cardiovascular equivalent of 10 minutes on a rowing machine. Laugher also releases enkephalins and endorphins, which are pain killers, and thus it is a natural way to reduce pain ranging from headaches to bone pain. Laughter also aids digestion by massaging the intestines. The last physiologic effect is probably the best: the body enters a relaxed state in which vital signs drop and tension eases. Unlike chemical tranquilizers and antidepressants, laughter is natural. It is also free.

Psychologically laughter reduces tensions, provides an outlet for release of negative feelings, softens personal interactions, helps to put matters into perspective, and lifts the spirit. As one patient put it, "I found that when I caught myself laughing, I realized I was beginning to enjoy life again." Often laughter helps to defuse anger or ease tensions so that difficult issues can be discussed. Laughter is a bonding emotion. It has been said that laughter is the shortest distance between two people. Think how good it feels to be around someone who makes you laugh. Patients and their families feel the same way, and the use of humor can make the health care environment much more friendly. As one nurse put it, "Laughing is a mini-vacation, an escape from reality, even if it lasts only 30 seconds. When I return to reality, I am able to look at things from a different perspective."

2. What are the benefits of using humor in the health care setting?

Humor has the following benefits:
- Feels good physically
- Offers emotional release
- Provides defense mechanism
- Releases stress and anxiety
- Relieves boredom
- Breaks down barriers between staff and patient
- Builds group cohesion
- Heightens productivity
- Improves decision-making and negotiating abilities

3. How do you know if the time is right to use humor?

If the patient initiates humor, you know it is safe. Otherwise, assess three factors before initiating humor: timing, content, and receptivity. Is the time appropriate? (i..e, Did the patient just receive bad news?) Is the context of the humor appropriate? And is the patient receptive to humor? The nurse can determine the answers by asking a few questions:
1. Do you laugh?
2. Before you became ill, did you laugh?
3. What makes you laugh?
4. Do you feel better after you laugh?
5. Would you like to select a humorous video to watch while receiving your treatment today?

If you decide that humor is an appropriate intervention, jump in and remember something that most nurses have learned over the years: if it comes from the heart, you cannot go wrong.

4. Is humor appropriate in dealing with dying patients?

Yes. Dying is not death—it does not mean that life has ceased, and it certainly does not mean that emotions have stopped. The use of humor that produces laughter can be beneficial by releasing the tension and diffusing the anger that surrounds death. It can break the sadness even if just momentarily. I remember two daughters who were sitting patiently by their mother's bed, waiting for her to die. The mother had uttered no words during the past 24 hours and slept most of the time. Finally, one daughter turned to the other and asked in a loud whisper, "How much longer is this going to take?" At that moment the mother opened her eyes, looked at her daughters, and said in a clear voice, "A watched pot never boils." Everyone in the room began to laugh, and the whole tone of the room changed. Often humor occurs spontaneously and when we least expect it—so go with it! Most people agree that a good belly laugh makes them feel better. Now evidence shows that the benefits of humor may be even more powerful and longer-lasting.

5. Is there an inappropriate type of humor?

Yes. "Put-down" humor or humor with sexual overtones is inappropriate. Humor that can hurt someone else's feelings should never be used. Much health care humor is appropriate only for other health care workers and should be kept behind closed doors so that patients and visitors do not hear.

6. How can you add humor to your work setting?

Try some of the following tips in the outpatient chemotherapy setting, radiation treatment room, inpatient unit, home care bag, or break room for staff:
1. Make a bulletin board or file of funny cartoons.
2. Create a basket of humorous items that the patient can borrow: bubbles, Play Doh, coloring books and crayons, finger paint, funny hats or wigs, water guns, humorous gadgets (e.g., big glasses, large noses, reflex hammer that squeaks when you tap it, mirror that laughs), and humorous books, audiotapes, and videotapes.
3. Make a laughter first-aid kit for your personal use or for patient use. (Develop your own—whatever makes you or the patient laugh.)
4. Show home movies.
5. Make funny pictures and display them.
6. Have dress-up day or theme day when staff and/or patients dress in funny outfits.
7. Create funny songs.

7. How can you add humor to your own life?
- Look for humor—try to see the amusing side of situations, and learn to laugh at yourself first!
- Keep a humor first-aid kit. Stock it with items that you think are funny, and pull it out when you need to laugh.
- Brighten your surroundings—use posters, cartoons, bumper stickers, pictures, or anything to make the workplace appear brighter and thus happier.
- Make time for fun—schedule some humor time each day (10 minutes).
- Be playful—spend time with a child or bring some of that childlike behavior into your life.
- Encourage laughter—laughter is contagious.

8. Give a few examples of humorous stories from oncology nursing.
- One day a young woman in her early thirties named Diane was admitted to our medical oncology unit with acute leukemia. She was a newlywed, and her husband, Joe, stayed by her side as she underwent induction chemotherapy. After several complications, the days turned into weeks, and she entered her seventh week with us. During her stay, when she and her husband wanted private time to share intimate moments together, they would place a "Do Not Disturb" sign on her door. This was continually ignored by the health care workers, who sould simply knock and enter anyway. One night Diane and Joe decided to make sure they had privacy. Joe placed a sign on the door that read "SEX IN PROGRESS." That sign was *not* ignored; no one bothered them at all. The staff laughed until their sides hurt. Diane and Joe laughed too.
- Elsie was going to her plastic surgeon for a follow-up visit after having undergone a bilateral mastectomy and reconstruction 8 weeks earlier. When she arrived she was wearing a

T-shirt that read, "Boobs by Dr. Smith, phone #333-8201." This message was painted on both sides of her shirt. When Dr. Smith saw Elsie, his first statement was, "I hope you haven't been sitting in the waiting room very long." Elsie responded, "Oh no, but I went to the mall shop for an hour or two before I came here!" Dr. Smith's face turned bright red, and then he and Elsie burst into laughter.

- I was riding through a cemetery one day and saw a sign that read, "Pick flowers *only* from your own grave!" It made me laugh. I wondered whether anyone obeyed.
- Sophie was a patient in our inpatient hospice unit. She told her nurse Sally she was dying. She asked Sally to call her minister and the rest of her family to come quickly. Everyone arrived, and Sophie wanted to have a prayer service. She asked that candles be lighted in her room. On her table beside the candles, she had two pictures: one of her family and one of Jesus and his disciples. The candles were lit, and everyone bowed their heads as the minister began to pray. After a few seconds there was a burning smell that caused the group's eyes to open. To everyone's surprise, the picture of Jesus and his disciples had gone up in flames. Sophie's eyes got big, and she said, "Oh no, what am I going to do? The first thing Jesus is going to ask me is why I burned his picture?" Then Sophie began to laugh. The tension in the room eased as everyone joined in the laughter. Sophie died peacefully a few minutes later.

Remember, humor helps to balance our lives. It can occur in the most unexpected places and at the most unexpected times. Welcome it!

9. What humor resources are available to nurses and patients?

American Association for Therapeutic Humor
> Networking source for practical applications of humor in all therapeutic modalities. Excellent newsletter and annual conference. Send $50 per year to: A.A.T.H., 222 S. Meramec, Ste. 303, St. Louis, MO 63105. Phone: 314-863-6232; fax: 863-6457; WWW site: http://www.callamer.com/itc/aath

Hair by Chemo
> T-shirts and hats with this logo and "Not by Choice" on backside. Box 216, Wauzeka, WI 53826 or call to order 800-729-9713.

Humor and Health Journal
> Bimonthly newsletter featuring interviews with humor experts, review of latest research and books published on humor and laughter. Send $22/yr to: Humor and Health Journal, PO Box 16814, Jackson, MS 39236. 601-957-0075.

Humor Project
> Publishes *Laughing Matters*, an excellent quarterly journal, large catalog of humor books, annual humor conference. 110 Spring St., Saratoga Springs, NY 12866. 515-587-8770.

Journal of Nursing Jocularity
> A hilarious quarterly publication about the funny side of nursing. For annual subscription, send $14.95 to J.N.J., 5615 W. Cermak Rd., Cicero, IL 60650-2290. For catalog and conference information, telephone 602-835-6165. Fax: 835-6922. E-mail: laffinm@neta.com WWW site: http//www.jocularity. com

Too Live Nurse
> Tape of funny songs about nursing, cardiac arrhythmias, and drugs. Send $17 each to PO Box 201, Cannan, NY 12029. Telephone 518-781-4943.

Whole Mirth Catalog
> Access to many humorous items, toys, gags, books. 1034 Page Street, San Francisco, CA 94117.

A Little Book of Nurses' Rules
> This book presents over 400 tips, helpful observations, and useful do's and don't's for nurses, offering insight into interactions with physicians, patients, and other nurses. It is a 128-page paperback book. Send $9.95 to Hanley & Belfus, 210 S. 13th Street, Philadelphia, PA 19107. Phone: 215-546-7293; fax 215-790-9330; internet: http://www.hanleyandbelfus.com.

The Best of Nursing Humor: A Collection of Articles, Essays, and Poetry Published in the
Nursing Literature

> This hardcover $8\frac{1}{2} \times 11$ book presents the best pieces of creative, humorous writing to
> appear in the nursing and related literature over the last 20 years. Addresses the funny side
> of interrelationships and communication between nurses and their colleagues, physicians,
> patients, and patients' families. Send $27.00 to Hanley & Belfus, 210 S. 13th Street, Phila-
> delphia, PA 19107. Phone: 215-546-7293; fax 215-790-9330; internet: http://www.han-
> leyandbelfus.com.

10. What are some funny books that may appeal to patients and health care professionals?

> Barry D: Stay Fit and Healthy Until You're Dead. Emmaus, PA, Rodale Press, 1985.
>
> Bonhom TD: The Treasury of Clean Jokes. Nashville, TN, Broadman, 1988.
>
> Brillian A: I Want to Reach Your Mind—Where Is It Currently Located? Santa Barbara, CA,
> Woodbridge Press, 1994.
>
> Klein A: Quotations to Cheer You Up When the World Is Getting You Down. New York,
> Sterling, 1991.
>
> Metcalf CW: Lighten Up: Survival Signs for People Under Pressure. Reading, MA, Addison
> Wesley, 1992.
>
> Mickie S, Hillman R: Death Is—A Lighter Look at a Grave Situation. Saratoga, CA, R & E
> Publishers, 1993.
>
> Saltzman D: The Jester Has Lost His Jingle. Jester Company, 1995.
>
> Wooten P: Heart, Healing and Humor. Salt Lake City, Commune A Key Publishing, 1994.

BIBLIOGRAPHY

1. Buxman K (ed): Nursing Perspective on Humor. Staten Island, NY, Power Publishers, 1995.
2. Cousins N: Anatomy of an Illness. New York, W.W. Norton, 1979.
3. Erdman L: Laughter therapy for patients with cancer. J Psychosoc Oncol 11(4):55–67, 1993.
4. Klein A: Healing Power of Humor. Los Angeles, Tarcher, 1989.

64. CARING FOR THE CAREGIVER

Anne E. Belcher, PhD, RN, FAAN

1. Why is caring for the caregiver such an important topic?

Caring for the caregiver has to be viewed within the context of health care and nursing. Current changes in health care generate both stresses and challenges for nurses. Such changes include accelerating technology, competition among delivery systems, pressures for cost containment, changes in access to care, declining quality of care, and downsizing and reengineering. Nursing trends and issues that affect the caregiver include sicker patients with a shorter length of stay in the hospital; fewer if any clinic or home visits covered by third-party payers; perceived lack of autonomy and accountability; multiple role requirements; stereotyping of nurses by other health care providers; role encroachment from allied health care providers; conflicting personal and professional responsibilities; and internal and external pressures for additional education, specialization, or certification.

All of these issues and changes can be stressful for nurses and may have a negative effect on patient care. Thus, it is important for nurses to take care of themselves.

2. Briefly define the term stress.

Stress is the response of the individual to the demands placed on him or her. Adaptation is required to avoid short- or long-term damage to the body, mind, and spirit. Stress may be viewed as an opportunity for personal growth or as a risk factor for further disorganization and distress. Stress is viewed as a major determinant of a nurse's level of job satisfaction.

3. What is burnout?

Burnout is a syndrome of emotional exhaustion, depersonalization, and reduced personal accomplishment that may occur in response to the demands of the job and work environment. Burnout occurs frequently among individuals who work with people and are confronted with circumstances that are difficult to change. Burnout is not simply caused by hard physical work; it results more from a feeling of futility or not being able to accomplish anything meaningful. It is a response to the chronic emotional strain of dealing with other people, especially if they have problems. The first sign for many nurses is physical fatigue, which they presume is a result of working longer hours and more shifts. Only when other signs and symptoms appear do they realize that they may be developing burnout.

Some nurses use burnout as a copout. If they lose enthusiasm for their job or the profession in general, they blame decreased motivation and unhappiness on stress. In reality, they may be unwilling to devote the time, energy, and caring that excellence in professional nursing requires. Hence the expression, "How can you experience burnout if you have never been on fire?"

4. What are the key aspects of burnout?

Emotional exhaustion is evident when the nurse feels that he or she can no longer give of the self to others. Examples include dealing with patients or colleagues "strictly by the book," "pigeonholing" people, or carrying out tasks in a routine manner. Depersonalization is present when the nurse is negative, cynical, or even callous in dealing with both patients and peers. A decreased sense of personal accomplishment is reflected in the tendency to evaluate the self negatively, to describe low self-esteem, and to react in a "mea culpa" manner (tendency to blame oneself for whatever goes wrong).

5. What factors commonly contribute to overall stress and burnout in the oncology work environment?

Among the factors that have been identified are complex technology; long-term continuous contact with acutely ill patients; heavy workload, often combined with a shortage of staff; conflicts with or lack of support from other nurses, physicians, and other members of the health care team; patient dependence; ethical dilemmas; excessive time spent in non-nursing tasks; and lack of positive feedback and other rewards for "a job well done."

Stressors identified as unique to oncology nurses are death and dying; conflict between the goals of curing and palliation; search for meaning in the patient's illness; and effects of the disease and its treatment on the patient and family, including pain, disfigurement, and depression.

6. What are the consequences of stress and burnout?

A partial list of the many consequences of stress and burnout includes the following:

Job dissatisfaction and turnover	Fatigue
Absenteeism	Sleeplessness
Low morale	Boredom
Personal and family problems	Resentment
Deterioration in quality of patient care	Failure to contribute to unit or organization
Numerous or repeated errors	Lack of professional growth
Decreased productivity	Loss of idealism
Frequent use of poor judgment	Decreased commitment to service
Expressions of negativism or subversive activity	Emotional detachment from patients and others
Increased frequency of physical or psychological illness, with decreased resistance to infection	Feelings of powerlessness
	Urge to avoid or escape patients and job

7. Identify personal characteristics of oncology nurses who are susceptible to burnout.

Characteristics that are known to predispose an oncology nurse to burnout are lack of assertiveness, impatience, intolerance, and lack of self-confidence. Burnout is prevalent among younger, less experienced, and less educated nurses.

8. What characteristics of oncology nursing make stress and burnout so prevalent?

The meaning of oncology nursing, as defined by Cohen and Sarter,[1] helps to explain both its rewards and stresses:

> working with patients with cancer is analogous to being on the front lines of a war against death, disfigurement and intense human suffering. It requires the performance, prioritization, and coordination of multiple complex tasks. It involves handling frequent, unexpected crises, both physiologic and psychological. It carries the rewards of reversing a fatal illness, balanced by the ever-present reality of death. Working with persons with cancer requires constant vigilance in monitoring for sudden problems and life-threatening errors. The cancer nurse's empathy is sharpened by the awareness that 'this could be me or my loved one' . . . . working with persons with cancer means 'being there' for people in their most private moments of suffering and responding to the heights and depths of their responses to this suffering (p. 1485).

9. What strategies may be helpful for managing stress in the oncology work environment?

1. Set realistic goals for self, patient, and family.
2. Define success in terms of realistic outcomes.
3. Avoid feeling like you have lost if the patient dies.
4. Feel like you have won if the patient had the best quality of life or a dignified death.
5. Use short-term objectives and take pride in small gains.
6. Work smarter instead of harder.
7. Break away ("downshift") at intervals by going for a walk, running errands, doing paperwork.
8. Be good to yourself: praise yourself, develop positive self-talk skills and positive attitudes.
9. Enjoy pleasure both on and away from the job without guilt.
10. Compliments should be given and accepted without qualification.

11. Place events in their proper perspective; avoid overreacting.

12. Accept criticism objectively, and use evaluation as a potential for growth; take issues less personally.

13. Actively seek collaboration and assistance from peers.

14. Take risks when ideas come to mind, when experiences with patient care should be shared, when creativity is needed to solve a problem.

15. Identify rewards and incentives, which may come from within.

16. Develop a support network, which may include coworkers as well as interdisciplinary colleagues and managers.

17. Request mental health days, vacation, and sabbatical when the need is felt.

10. How can an oncology nurse manage stress whenever it occurs?

1. Take one day at a time. Live for the moment. Do not dwell on past failures. Do not worry obsessively about the future. Avoid second-guessing and stereotyping.

2. Focus on job satisfaction, which includes becoming actively involved in governance, participating in scheduling and other potentially frustrating aspects of the job, chairing committees that address areas of professional concern, organizing educational and support sessions for self and peers.

3. Consider a job change, perhaps within the specialty but in another setting (e.g., ambulatory, home care, hospice), with a different population (children vs. adults vs. elderly), or with a different focus (prevention, screening and detection, palliative care). One of the joys of oncology nursing is the opportunity for new and different challenges.

4. Maintain positive health habits, including a balance between exercise and rest; balanced diet; "looking good;" decompression between work and home; volunteer activities; and hobbies such as music and reading.

5. Use simple breathing exercises and other relaxation techniques.

6. Practice assertiveness rather than aggression or passive behavior.

7. Utilize time management skills.

8. Cultivate and maintain a sense of humor, which is contagious.

9. Use audiotapes and videotapes, movies, books, articles, and cartoons to stimulate laughter and to relieve tensions.

10. Set boundaries between job and personal life. Set aside private time. Develop and maintain inner strength and spiritual well-being.

11. Use the imagination to relive the past and rehearse the future.

BIBLIOGRAPHY

1. Cohen MZ, Sarter B: Love and work: Oncology nurses' view of the meaning of their work. Oncol Nurs Forum 19:1481-1486, 1992.
2. Maslach C: Burnout: The Cost of Caring. Englewood Cliffs, NJ, Prentice-Hall, 1982.
3. Schaufeli WB, Maslach C, Marek T (eds): Professional Burnout: Recent Developments in Theory and Research. Washington, DC, Taylor & Francis, 1993.
4. Schulmeister L: Burnout in oncology nursing. Innovat Pract 4(2):4-5,9,15, 1980.

65. HELPFUL HINTS

Judy Kadlec-Fuller, RN, MSN, OCN, AOCN

1. What types of interventions may help a patient through a transient depressive reaction to a cancer diagnosis or treatment?

Depressive symptoms that are not severe enough to warrant psychiatric or pharmacologic intervention may be helped by various interventions:

- Encourage the patient to talk with a "veteran" who has been through a similar situation. Credibility is often greater and advice more influential when coming from someone who has actually been there. Veteran patients should be screened carefully and matched with the cancer patient's age, diagnosis, and personality as closely as possible.
- Encourage the patient to talk with a social worker or chaplain. Often professionals who are one step removed from the physical treatment can build a rapport with the patient and family and focus on the emotional impact of the situation.
- Encourage the patient to attend a support group. Even the patient who is reluctant to talk in a group can sit and listen to others' experiences and successful coping mechanisms. Often this helps the patient to gather ideas about how to cope and lessens the feeling of aloneness.
- Give the patient permission to take a "mental vacation." Tell patients it is okay to forget about the cancer, dream of the future, or talk about goals and dreams. Providing distraction through a movie, visit from a pet, or relaxing drive in the country may help the patient escape the cancer for a short time. Many health care providers believe that this is a form of denial; however, temporary denial can be a healthy coping mechanism.

2. What techniques are helpful for starting an intravenous line in a patient with "bad" veins?

Venous access in oncologic patients can be a challenge. Here are a few tips:

- Apply heat. Heat causes vasodilation, which makes it easier to locate and access the vein. Hot packs can be applied by placing a warm moist towel around the patient's arm. Cover the towel with a plastic bag to contain the heat and to prevent linens and clothes from getting wet. You can also have the patient soak his or her arm in a basin of warm water. Heat should be applied for approximately 10 minutes before attempting venipuncture.
- Use a blood pressure cuff instead of a tourniquet. A blood pressure cuff produces greater vasodilation than a tourniquet and is less painful for the patient. The blood pressure cuff should be pumped up to approximately 100 mmHg—enough to decrease venous return but not to occlude arterial flow.
- Place a folded towel under the patient's elbow for maximal extension of the arm. This pushes the veins in both the upper and lower arm to the surface for easier access.
- Have the patient squeeze a tennis ball or folded wash cloth in one hand. The muscle contraction from squeezing will push the veins to the surface of the arm for easier visualization, palpation, and access.

3. What do you tell patients who say that no one seems to know how to care correctly for their central line?

Care of central lines is highly controversial. Research results are inconclusive as to the best type of dressing (gauze, transparent, or no dressing); frequency of dressing change; type, volume, and frequency of flush; and procedure for drawing blood. Patients may become anxious and confused and lose confidence in the knowledge of the health care providers when they see and learn a variety of methods to care for the catheter. The best solution is to encourage standardization of catheter care among hospital staff, physicians, and home care providers involved in the patient's care. If this is not possible, it is important to teach patients that various methods of catheter care are acceptable and that a different technique does not mean that the caregiver is unskilled. In addition, the patient should receive clear written instructions for home care of the catheter to prevent confusion. These interventions help to prevent additional stress on the patient and family who are already struggling to endure cancer treatment.

4. Why is the internal volume of a central line important for giving medications?

If you are giving a small volume of concentrated medication by intravenous push through a central line, it is important to understand how the internal volume of the catheter may affect the administration. Most central lines range from 0.3–2.5 cc in internal volume. Many nurses use the **SASH** method (i.e., **s**aline flush, **a**dminister medication, **s**aline flush, **h**eparin flush) when giving medications by intravenous push. For example, if you are giving the patient 1.0 cc of lorazepam (Ativan) by intravenous push through a subclavian lumen with an internal volume of 0.9 cc, first you flush the line with saline, then slowly administer the lorazepam, then flush with saline again, and end with the heparin flush. Most nurses administer the lorazepam slowly and follow with a rapid saline flush. However, in this situation, 0.9 cc of the 1.0 cc dose of lorazepam is still in the catheter (and not yet in the bloodstream) when you give the next saline flush. If you give the second saline flush rapidly, you also rapidly administer the 0.9 cc of lorazepam that still remains in the catheter.

A second situation in which it is important to know the internal volume of the catheter is when you are administering urokinase to unclot a catheter. The goal is to fill the catheter with urokinase. If you administer too much, the patient gets an unnecessary dose of a strong anticoagulant. If you administer too little, the entire catheter will not be filled and the clot may not be dissolved.

The internal lumen volume is written on the outside of some catheters. If it is not, this information can be obtained from an instruction booklet from the manufacturer. Keeping the internal volume of the catheter in mind when working with central lines helps to ensure safe administration of medications.

5. What is the safest way to prevent dislodgment of a catheter when you are removing an adhesive dressing?

It is sometimes difficult to remove a transparent adhesive dressing without dislodging the catheter, especially true when working with a peripherally inserted central catheter (PICC) or epidural catheter that is not sutured in place. When removing a dressing from any tube or catheter, pull the dressing toward the exit site (see figure below.) This technique tends to push the tube/catheter toward the skin rather than pull it out. Second, try using sterile steri-strips over the catheter/tube before you apply the dressing. Then, when you remove the dressing, the steri-strips help to anchor the tube/catheter to the skin. Third, if you are using a transparent dressing, place a 2 × 2 gauze pad over the catheter just proximal to the insertion site. The gauze will cover the catheter but leave the exit site exposed. This technique prevents the transparent dressing from sticking to the catheter but still allows visualization of the exit site through the transparent dressing.

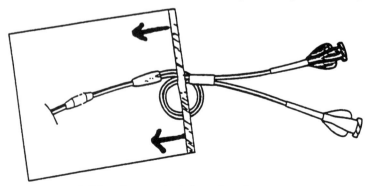

Pull dresssing toward exit site as shown by arrows.

6. What options are available to anchor a dressing in a patient who is allergic to plastic and adhesive tapes?

This situation often takes nursing creativity. A few ideas include:

- Try paper tape, to which most patients are not allergic. However, paper tape does not always stick, especially if the patient is diaphoretic, and you may need to try other options.
- Try placing a thin hydrocolloid dressing, such as Duoderm or Restore, at the periphery of the dressing site. Many patients who are allergic to tape are not allergic to the hydrocolloid dressings. You can then place the tape on top of the hydrocolloid dressing. You should remove the hydrocolloid dressing after 24 hours to check for an allergic reaction. If no reaction is seen, the hydrocolloid dressing needs to be changed every 3 days.
- Depending on the location of the dressing, you can try snug fitting socks or underwear to hold the dressing in place instead of tape.
- To secure dressings on the neck, trunk, or extremities, try using a piece of tube-shaped net mesh, such as Surginet, that can be cut to the appropriate size and slipped over the body part holding the dressing in place.

7. How do you keep a dressing intact on a patient who is highly diaphoretic?

This challenge also requires creativity. Some of the suggestions in question 6, such as the hydrocolloid dressing, socks, underwear, or Surginet, may work. In addition, Montgomery Straps can be applied with the laces holding the dressing in place. To get the Montgomery Straps or hydrocolloid dressing to stick, first clip (do not shave) the hair from the area. Then clean the area with alcohol, and apply a protective barrier (such as Skin Prep). Dry the protective barrier with a blow dryer on the cool setting, making sure that it is completely dry, and then apply the Montgomery Straps or hydrocolloid dressing. Preparing the area in this manner usually keeps the Montgomery Straps or hydrocolloid dressing in place for several days even in a diaphoretic patient.

8. Do egg-crate mattresses and sheepskins prevent the development of pressure ulcers?

Egg-crate mattresses and sheepskins do not help to prevent the development of pressure ulcers. They should be used as comfort devices only. Turning and repositioning are the best ways to prevent development of pressure ulcers. Various pressure-reducing and pressure-relieving mattresses are available commercially. A pressure-reducing mattress should be used for patients at high risk for skin breakdown or with minor (stage 1 or 2) pressure ulcers. Pressure-relieving mattresses should be used for patients with severe (stage 3 or 4) pressure ulcers. The appropriate mattress should be used because insurance will not pay for a mattress that is not indicated. Even with use of specialty mattresses, the basic interventions of repositioning and maintaining clean, dry skin must be provided.

9. How should nasogastric (NG) tubes, gastrostomy (G) tubes, jejunostomy (J) tubes, Jackson Pratt drains, and Foley catheters be stabilized?

All of these tubes should be stabilized to prevent dislodgment, unnecessary pressure on the skin, and development of an ulcer at the exit site. It is especially important to stabilize G-tubes and J-tubes because continual movement may cause enlargement of the track during healing and eventual reflux of stomach and intestinal secretions onto the skin.

Heavy tubes, such as **NG tubes** and **Jackson Pratt drains**, should be supported to prevent pulling and dislodgment. A piece of tape may be placed around the tube and fastened with a safety pin to the patient's clothing, with some slack in the tubing to prevent pulling.

G-tubes and **J-tubes** can be secured with a baby-bottle nipple. Make a hole in the end of the nipple so that the tube can fit through but is still held securely. Push the nipple down over the tube until the base of the nipple sits on the skin surrounding the exit site. The base of the nipple should then be taped securely to the skin. Be sure to remove the tape and clean under the nipple at least daily.

Foley catheters should be taped securely to the abdomen. When taped to the leg, the Foley catheter is moved each time the leg is moved, causing irritation and pressure at the urinary meatus.

10. What methods can be used to control gingival bleeding?

Gingival bleeding is a common problem in oncologic patients. A low platelet count (< 50,000), stomatitis, and preexisting dental problems contribute to gingival bleeding. Use of a sponge toothbrush (Toothette), avoidance of hard foods (such as fresh fruits and vegetables), and discontinuance of hydrogen peroxide rinses help to prevent further irritation to the oral cavity. To control minor bleeding, try the following tips:

- Have the patient suck on ice chips, gently irrigate with ice water, or place partially frozen saline-soaked gauze pads between the cheek and gum. Application of cold (cryotherapy) causes vasoconstriction and reduces bleeding.
- Place moist tea bags between the cheek and gum for 30–60 minutes. The local pressure of the tea bag and vasoconstriction produced by the caffeine decrease the bleeding. Decaffeinated tea may not produce the vasoconstrictive effect. Tannic acid, contained in the tea, may cause mild decalcification of the teeth with prolonged use.

11. How can sedation, often seen as a side effect of narcotics, be minimized?

The sedation produced by narcotics can greatly diminish a patient's quality of life. In most patients, sedation is a transient side effect lasting 2–3 days after initiating or increasing a narcotic. If the sedation is persistent, consult the physician about adding other nonsedating analgesics to the pain medication regimen so that the narcotic dose can be decreased while still maintaining pain control. In addition, assess whether the patient is getting adequate sleep at night. Suggest an afternoon nap and planning of activities during the time of greatest energy, usually in the morning. Caffeine may be adequate to counteract the sedation. Suggest caffeinated beverages during the day. Make sure that the patient also drinks plenty of other fluids, because caffeine causes diuresis and can lead to dehydration. If these interventions are inadequate, talk with the physician about use of stimulant medications, such as methylphenidate or dextroamphetamine. These medications, usually administered in the morning and afternoon to prevent interference with nighttime sleep, help patients to maintain activity and independence while still controlling their pain.

12. What special precautions should be taken when fentanyl patches are used?

Fentanyl patches (Duragesic) should be placed on smooth skin surfaces. Hair may be clipped but should not be shaved. The skin should be washed with water and dried thoroughly. Avoid use of soaps, lotions, or powders that may affect drug absorption and adhesion of the patch. The location of the patch should be changed with each application. If the patch falls off, it may be reapplied and held in place with a transparent dressing. Patches should be applied on the trunk of the body.

When the patch is first applied, it takes 9–15 hours for the fentanyl to get through the skin and into the bloodstream. The patient will need short-acting pain medication until the fentanyl reaches the bloodstream. Conversely, when the fentanyl patch is discontinued, a depot of fentanyl remaining in the skin will be absorbed for approximately 17 hours after the patch is removed. Additional pain medications should be given cautiously during this period. Medication remains in the patch after removal. The patch should be folded in half and flushed down the toilet for disposal.

If the patient has been overmedicated with a fentanyl patch, the risk of respiratory depression remains after the patch has been removed. In addition, absorption of fentanyl through the skin is increased when the temperature of the skin is increased. Patients with a fever (> 102° F) should be watched closely. Use of a heating pad over the patch, sitting in a hot tub, or sleeping on a heated bed (waterbed or electric blanket) should be discouraged.

13. How does chewing ice (cryotherapy) reduce fluorouracil-induced stomatitis?

Stomatitis, a common side effect of fluorouracil (5-FU), can be diminished or even eliminated through the use of cryotherapy. Cryotherapy works by causing local vasoconstriction, which results in reduced volume of blood flow—and thus reduced exposure to chemotherapy.

Cryotherapy can be effective during 5-FU boluses or intermittent infusions. The patient should start sucking on ice chips 5 minutes before the infusion is started, then continue through the infusion and for approximately 15–30 minutes after completion. Alternatives to ice chips are frozen grapes or sugarless popsicles.

Cryotherapy can be considered controversial because it diminishes the delivery of chemotherapy to the area of vasoconstriction. Theoretically, this effect could allow cancer cells to remain in the area. For this reason, cryotherapy should not be used near tumor sites. If you are unsure, check with the physician.

14. During the course of a day, a nurse often draws many syringes of saline and heparin and goes through numerous single or multi-dose vials. Would it be more cost-effective and quicker to use a 250-cc bag of saline or premixed heparin solution to fill the syringes?

No! This practice may seem like a smart idea, but it is very risky. Bacteremia, caused by the same organism, has been reported in numerous patients as a result of contamination of the bag and continued use from patient to patient. The more times a system (bottle or bag) is entered, the greater the chance of contamination. Using the same bag to draw medications for different patients has the potential for spreading infection.

15. What can be done to ensure safe administration of opioid infusions?

There are many different types of opioid infusions, with or without local anesthetic—for example, intravenous, epidural, intrathecal, and infraclavicular. A color-coded labeling system ensures safety. Three different-sized labels can be made—one for the infusion bag or syringe, one for the tubing, and one for the Kardex or medication administration sheet. Five different types of infusions can be differentiated with a separate color—patient-controlled analgesia, continuous opioid infusion, epidural, intrathecal (spinal), and infraclavicular. Using this system, the type of infusion for a specific patient is brought **immediately** to the nurse's attention.

16. What can the nurse do to minimize complications with epidural catheter tubing?

Epidural catheters, tubing, and connections may easily become kinked or disconnected. A padded tongue blade can be placed at the connection site and secured with tape to decrease the chance of disconnection while maintaining a safe mode of epidural infusion. Labeling the tubing and the connection with a sticker to identify the type of catheter also lessens confusion.

17. What influences the accuracy of pulse oximeter measurements of oxygen saturation in arterial blood (SaO_2)?

The pulse oximeter is a helpful assessment tool, but the nurse must be cautious when interpreting the reading. Many conditions can affect the accuracy of the pulse oximeter reading:
- Conditions causing low peripheral perfusion, such as hypovolemia, hypotension, or peripheral vascular disease (false low reading)
- Carbon monoxide bound to hemoglobin, as occurs with smoking. It is usually considered acceptable to monitor oxygen saturation as soon as 20 minutes after smoking, but the reading can stay falsely elevated for as long as 8 hours.
- Hyperbilirubinemia (false high reading)
- Colored fingernail polish (false high or false low reading)
- Severe anemia. Oxygen saturation reading may be within normal limits (suggesting that an adequate percent of hemoglobin is saturated, or carrying oxygen), but the patient may still be hypoxemic because there is not enough hemoglobin to carry enough oxygen. Anemic patients may not look cyanotic because the hemoglobin is bound with oxygen, making it red rather than the dark bluish color of desaturated hemoglobin.

18. What are some tips for incorporating cultural aspects into a patient's plan of care?

Culture not only encompasses ethnic background, but also subcultures such as religion, rural vs. urban environment, gender, sexual orientation, and professional vs. blue collar employment.

Because culture may influence how an individual interprets and responds to illness, dying, and symptoms such as pain, nurses need to be aware of and to respect cultural traditions and practices. The following suggestions may help nurses to care for culturally diverse patients:

- Avoid stereotyping. It is wrong to assume that two people from the same culture will react the same to a like situation. It is as wrong as assuming that one family member will react the same as another family member.
- For language barriers, use interpreters. Exercise caution in using a family member to translate because the patient may not be totally open. If a translator is unavailable, call the 24-hour AT&T Language Line (800-628-8486). A translator is provided for most languages within 60–90 seconds at a cost from $4.15 to $7.25 per minute.
- Obtain information about a patient's religious beliefs from an appropriate religious figure (priest, rabbi, etc.).
- Contact community representatives from specific ethnic/cultural groups to educate health care providers about their beliefs and practices.
- Develop a resource manual with information about commonly held beliefs and rituals of major cultural/ethnic groups in your area.
- Form a Multicultural Patient Care Team with staff members from various cultures to educate and liaison with community groups to promote culturally-oriented health care.
- Provide educational materials in different languages.
- At the bedside, keep individualized care statements on cards in various languages for non-English-speaking patients to use in communicating their needs or complaints; e.g., I am having pain; I am feeling sick in my stomach; I am constipated; I am scared; call my family, etc.

Editor's note: Interested in more practical tips? *Oncology Nursing Forum* has a Practice Corner that compiles tips from nurses monthly.

BIBLIOGRAPHY

 1. Coull A: Making sense of pulse oximetry. Nurs Times 88:42–43, 1992.
 2. Krasner D: The 12 commandments of wound care. Nursing 92 22:34–41, 1992.
 3. Levy M: Pharmacologic management of cancer pain. Semin Oncol 21:718–739, 1994.
 4. McKiernan P: Practice corner: Translation service helps nurses to overcome language barriers for patients in the home. Oncol Nurs Forum 21:1738, 1994.
 5. Nishimoto P: Venturing into the unknown: Cultural beliefs about death and dying. Oncol Nurs Forum 23: 889–894, 1996.
 6. Pies R: Psychotropic medications and the oncology patient. Cancer Pract 4:164–166, 1996.
 7. Rivera LM: Practice corner: Language and culture provide challenges to nursing care. Oncol Nurs Forum 21:1737, 1994.
 8. Smith J: Practice corner: Multicultural patient care team ensures quality care for all cultures. Oncol Nurs Forum 21:1737–1738, 1994.
 9. Whedon M, McAtee N: Cryotherapy reduces fluorouracil related side effects. Oncol Nurs Forum 22:1287, 1995.
10. Whedon M, Steele S: Controlling gingival bleeding with tea bags. Oncol Nurs Forum 19:663, 1992.
11. Whedon M, Burmylo S: Tips ease IV access and chemotherapy administration. Oncol Nurs Forum 21:922. 1994.

66. FAMILY ISSUES

Priscilla Ingebrigtsen, MSW, and Meribeth Wallio Smith, MSW

1. What is the typical family response to a diagnosis of cancer?

There is no typical patient or family response to cancer. Families are as individual as patients. No two families or patients respond to the same cancer in the same way. Disbelief or denial is a common first reaction, often followed by shock and fear. Many families describe feeling as if they were riding on an emotional roller coaster and need extra reassurance and time to regain equilibrium. Some families are distrustful of physicians and/or other members of the health care team and should be given information to reassure them of the medical team's credibility.

2. How do you deal with a family that is in denial or refuses to talk about cancer?

Unfortunately, health care providers are critical of persons who deny or refuse to accept information about diagnosis, treatment needs, or prognosis. Denial is a genuine defense mechanism to fend off or delay overwhelming data. Denial protects family members' emotions until they are ready to ask for information about what to do and how to deal with the cancer. Forcing patients or family members to accept a cancer diagnosis or prognosis before they are ready strips them of defenses necessary for coping with vulnerability. Unconscious denial cannot be broken through, and conscious denial seems to be a pacing of adjustment to feared realities. Undoubtedly, families avoid talking about the patient's cancer for many reasons, but a common motive is the wish to protect the patient. This motive is most likely a projection; they wish to avoid the reality themselves.

Gentle "course corrections" are recommended, along with acceptance of the family and patient's perceptions and coping style. In talking to the family, use normalizing statements to prevent defensive responses, such as "I have worked with many families who could not mention cancer, but now they are finding it helpful to . . . ." It may be helpful to point out to the family that silence is isolating. Families should be encouraged to share their feelings with one another about the experience of cancer in order to enrich each other's lives. Active intervention in denial mechanisms is necessary only when they interfere with treatment and healthy coping.

3. How can families be encouraged to listen and respond to patients' needs to talk?

Remember that families are also undergoing loss. They also need to feel that someone is listening to their concerns. Strange and uncomfortable emotions may surface in family members as they try to listen and encourage. Many people fear that discussion of such feelings constitutes "negative thinking" and can somehow impair the effectiveness of therapy. Families need encouragement to take care of their own needs, to participate in activities that may rejuvenate and restore them, to remember there is no "right way" to talk about cancer, and to give themselves permission to try and fail. There are many unspoken ways to communicate caring, and all of them can be powerful. Sometimes the presence of a third party, such as a trusted friend, spiritual advisor, or therapist, allows a sense of safety to begin communicating.

4. Is it possible to predict a family's coping ability?

Because each family is unique, it is not possible to predict how the members will cope with the patient's illness, but there are clues. Every family (the word encompasses a wide range of social relationships) has deeply embedded "rules" or dynamics that are not readily apparent, even to the members themselves. The health care provider quickly becomes a pivotal person in the family system and needs to learn the family's rules and culture to communicate and intervene effectively.

Family functioning is affected by educational background, cultural and ethnic beliefs, and past experiences with illness or loss. If a family did not cope well with a past crisis, they may require more assistance in coping with the present one. Healthy families respond with flexibility, independence, and even humor when problems occur. They can tell when communication is impaired and even offer suggestions for improvement. In contrast, stressed families are inflexible. Communication among family members may be poor or nonexistent. The health care provider may become part of a triangle to diffuse tension between family members.

5. What are the indicators of the need for intervention in families experiencing stress, anxiety, and depression?

Every patient is not fortunate enough to have a supportive, nurturing family. Although the patient has the cancer, the family also suffers or responds to the diagnosis. Some relationships will not survive the illness. Each person in the patient's life has different skills for coping with the ambiguity of cancer. It is normal for family members to be fearful at first, but appropriate referrals and assistance may be required for the following indicators:
  • Persistent and unremitting negative emotions such as anger
  • Apparent conflicts between patients and caregivers that spill over into the health care setting
  • Signs of caregiver burden, such as depression and physical complaints. This is a high-risk time for health problems in spouses or primary caregivers.
  • Inability of the patient to comply with medical treatment, including significant weight loss, poor hygiene, inappropriate use of medications, or substance abuse.
  • Inability of the patient to provide self-care or to make competent decisions. If no reliable family member is available to assist, a report needs to be given to the local social services agency.
  • Physical abuse or patient reports of financial exploitation, neglect, or other serious problems. Occasionally, situations become so stressed that the physical and mental health of the patient or caregivers is jeopardized. Many states have mandatory reporting laws that require health care providers to report elder abuse and neglect to a designated agency. Obviously, this intervention is a last resort, when all other attempts to educate and provide resources have failed or when there is grave danger. Detailed descriptions required in the report include physical injuries, amount of weight loss, and specific accounts of statements of harm or threat.

6. Give examples of ways to help families organize and adapt to the abrupt changes of a cancer diagnosis.

  • Help families to prioritize the many tasks that need to be accomplished. Provide a checklist of things that need to be done and who can be called for help. Getting organized can help families to feel more competent and capable of managing the stresses of the patient's illness.
  • Encourage and support family members to delegate tasks.
  • Check financial and insurance benefits and assist with necessary paperwork.
  • Ensure that physical and emotional needs of children are met.
  • Assist with tracking or initiating legal documents such as wills, powers of attorney, living wills, and advance directives.
  • Keep long-distance family and friends informed of progress.
  • Refer to outside help such as home health care, community resources, legal aid, or special transportation.
  • Help patients to research treatment options and obtain second opinions, if necessary.

7. Give examples of the typical issues and stressors encountered by patients in significant relationships.

The impact of cancer usually results in some restructuring of relationships:
  • Spouses or partners may have to cope with redelegation of family roles, chores, and tasks.
  • Patients may be involved in bad relationships that are further stressed by cancer. They may require assistance in recognizing healthy relationships and in moving away from bad ones.
  • Parents may struggle to be honest and not overprotective with their children about the parent's cancer; they must learn to assess the child's need for information and ability to cope emotionally.

- Elderly parents may forget to honor the patient as an adult and tend to treat the patient as a child again.
- Siblings of patients may overidentify and needlessly intensify feelings.
- In-laws may be isolated from information as "not really relatives" or blamed for complications in family relations.

8. What are ways to help patients who continue to work during cancer treatments?

Many patients need or desire to continue working during cancer therapy. In addition to income, working may bring structure and a sense of normalcy. It is important to ask whether patients are aware of benefits to which they are entitled. Patients or a delegated family member should contact the employee benefits office for an explanation of regulations in the Consolidated Omnibus Budget Reconciliation Act (COBRA), which allow employer-based health insurance plans to continue when employment is terminated. Social Security (800-772-1213) also should be contacted to explore options. For patients in extreme need, emergency resources may be available through county social service or welfare departments.

The health care team should give a realistic assessment of the time and energy required for therapy and a honest appraisal of the patient's potential for working. The oncology team can contribute to the patient's work performance by providing optimal symptom management and flexible appointment scheduling. Expected changes in appearance, body image, and energy level need to be discussed. The American Cancer Society sponsors a program, called Look Good Feel Better, through a national cosmetology organization that provides cosmetic and head covering expertise.

If work becomes impossible, patients need emotional support to grieve the loss of an important part of their identity. Often, the patient's spouse may need to return to work, resulting in further role changes. It should be a priority to assist the patient to find a meaningful replacement or diversional activity.

9. How can families be assisted to deal with inevitable role changes and other losses?

Families of patients with cancer grieve not only the potential loss of a loved one, but also the loss of the normal health and functioning of the family system. Often the simple process of naming the change and validating families' feelings of loss helps them to accept the impact of cancer. Family members' understanding may be enhanced by normalizing their experiences and providing information about realistic expectations, common adaptations, and predictable changes. Families may be helped to grieve by frank discussions of losses and step-by-step goal setting.

10. How can families extend their support network?

Reaching out to established friends is more likely to succeed than striking up new friendships during a crisis. Friends sincerely want to help and can do so with concrete guidance. Families should be encouraged to overcome their reluctance to use friends and to let friends help with tasks such as sitting with the patient to give the family a break, driving children to activities, running errands, picking up prescriptions, grocery shopping, and transporting the patient to the hospital. Meals on Wheels may be available to provide food. The American Cancer Society and home health agencies are excellent contacts for local resources.

Family members, as well as patients, should be informed about appropriate support groups to dispel isolation and assist coping. Telephone support lines and the Internet can also provide convenient networking and information. Cancer Care, Inc. (212-221-3300) publishes a resource guide that provides listings of many support and educational resources specific to the type of cancer and offers a counseling line (800-813-HOPE).

11. How does the health care team balance the patient's need for privacy against the family's need for information?

Always ask the patient's permission before sharing information with family members. It is helpful to arrange a family meeting to clarify communication issues. The family should be encouraged to elect a spokesperson or one family contact who will communicate with health care providers and then share the information with the rest of the family.

12. How may nurses talk to families about the transition from treatment to comfort or hospice care?

Hopefully, communication about the course and effectiveness of treatment has been open and honest from the beginning. Discussion of hospice care is a critical turning point and needs to be handled in a sensitive manner. Patients and families cannot be expected to make the leap of optimistic hoping and efforts for cure to the quiet acceptance of ending treatment in a single office visit. As the patient and family are able, they will hear and accept information that is given honestly and gently.

Sometimes it is a relief to everyone to acknowledge that a cure is not possible and that the treatments are not working. Often the fear that the patient will be abandoned may be expressed by comments from patient or family that "nothing more can be done." It is important to address the subject directly by saying many things will be done to maintain comfort and quality of life. Hope should not be taken away but reframed or redefined to include goals other than cure. Patients and families need to share hope and recognize together that miracles can be neither ruled out nor counted on.

13. What can be done to help the family of a terminally ill patient?
- Remember the concept of anticipatory grief, and honor individuals' unique, gradual adjustments to a poor prognosis.
- Encourage the expression of difficult questions and offer information to counter anxiety.
- Discover family members' previous experiences with death, especially from cancer.
- Provide appropriate reassurance that pain and other symptoms can be managed; pain and suffering are often more feared than dying.
- Assist physicians in talking honestly with the family.
- Ensure contact with religious or spiritual figures in the family's life.
- Offer hospice support early.
- Help the family to discuss its future and the place of the loved one in its history.
- Prepare to make referrals to professionals who handle concrete issues such as life insurance or mortuaries.

14. What is the ongoing role of health care providers when treatment ends?

Treatment may end with successful control of cancer, hospice referral, or death of the patient. Health care providers are often invited to survivor's celebrations or included in family's anniversary remembrances. Patients and/or families need to honor the enormous role that the medical caregivers have played in their experience with cancer. Unique social norms and boundaries help to decide the nature of the follow-up contact. Sympathy cards with bereavement resources, phone calls, or attendance at funerals may be appropriate. Most frequently, patients or families express gratitude for the role of the medical care team and need reconnection to commemorate the intimacy encountered in cancer care and to complete the episode in their lives.

BIBLIOGRAPHY

1. Blanchard C, et al: The role of social support in adaptation to cancer and to survival. J Psychosoc Oncol 13(1 and 2):75–95, 1995.
2. Cancer Care, Inc: A Helping Hand: The Resource Guide for People with Cancer. New York, Cancer Care, Inc., 1996.
3. Cordoba CS, Fobair P, Callan DB: Common issues facing adults with cancer. In Stearns N, et al (eds): Oncology Social Work: A Clinician's Guide. Atlanta, American Cancer Society, 1993, pp 43–78.
4. Hermann J: Children of cancer patients: Issues and interventions. In Stearns N, et al (eds): Oncology Social Work: A Clinician's Guide. Atlanta, American Cancer Society, 1993, pp 151–164.
5. Hull MM: Coping strategies of family caregivers in hospice homecare. Oncol Nurs Forum 19:1179–1187, 1992.
6. Jansen C, Hailiburton P, Dibble S, Dodd MJ: Family problems during cancer chemotherapy. Oncol Nurs Forum 20:689–696, 1993.
7. Schultz R: The psychological, social, and economic impact of illness among patients with recurrent cancer. J Psychosoc Oncol 13 (3):21–45, 1995.

67. HOME CARE

Ida Sansoucy, RN, MS, OCN

1. What factors contribute to the increase in home care services, particularly for patients with cancer?

The increased shift of patient care from the hospital to the home setting can be attributed to the following factors:

- Shortened hospital stays mandated by economic constraints, prospective Medicare payments for hospitalization, and reimbursement limitations set by insurance companies and managed care programs
- Downsizing of hospitals
- Increasing population of elderly patients and patients with chronic disease, including patients with cancer who are surviving longer
- Technologic advances that facilitate the delivery of medical care in the home (e.g., infusion pumps, venous access devices, portable medical devices)
- Consumer preference; patients desire the convenience of home for chemotherapy treatments, antibiotic administration, and other procedures

2. What are the advantages of home care?

As Dorothy says in *The Wizard of Oz*, "There's no place like home, there's no place like home." Home is where a person feels safe and more in control. Patients avoid hospitals because they are often cold and impersonal. At home they have privacy and are surrounded by familiar items, comfortable furniture, pets, and loved ones. Patients may feel dehumanized by hospital rules, institutional clothing, strange routines and noises, and references to the patient as a room number or disease type (e.g., "the breast in room 711"). At home patients may have an increased sense of control and independence to direct their care and follow their own pace and schedules. Patients can participate in home chores and routines with the closeness and support of family members instead of simply occupying the "sick role." Finally, home care for patients with cancer may be less costly than inpatient care. Direct expenses may be decreased; however, out-of-pocket expenses may be increased. Because home care is not always cheaper, each situation is individually assessed based on patient needs, family abilities and availabilities, and insurance benefits.

3. Why is home care not an option for everyone?

Everyone is not fortunate enough to have family members and resources to manage care at home. Home care has the disadvantages of complicating a family's daily routine, increasing demands on family roles, indirect costs (e.g., a family member who must miss work to provide care), and emotional and physical strain. Home care may be difficult or not possible in the following circumstances:

- Patient lives alone with no close or competent support systems. Episodic visits from the home care agency may not be enough to provide safe care for the patient who is alone.
- Significant others in the home are unwilling, unable, or too anxious to assist with care.
- The patient's condition is so demanding that even if the family members are willing, the care would be too physically or emotionally burdensome.
- Home care is too costly. Investigation must be done with the insurance company to evaluate the financial impact of home care. If a frequent technical procedure is involved and no able caregiver is available, the skilled nursing services may not be cost-effective. In another scenario, the patient prefers to receive chemotherapy at home, but the insurance company may pay for the durable medical equipment at home (e.g., the pump) but not the chemotherapy drug.

• Symptoms, such as pain, are uncontrolled and intolerable. Admission to the hospital for a short period may be necessary for closer monitoring and for initiation of new interventions or evaluation of the patient's response to treatment.

4. What are the types of home care agencies?

• Public health agencies: official agencies affiliated with city or county health departments, Veteran's Administration, or public medical centers; funded by state and local tax revenues.
• Medicare-certified home health agencies, which include voluntary or nonprofit agencies (usually community-based, funded with private fund endowments), or private for-profit agencies that are financed by fee-for-service payments, and hospital-based agencies (clients are usually captured from hospitals and clinics, with reimbursement dependent mostly on third-party insurers).
• Private duty for-profit agencies: owned by stockholders; contracted by patient and financed on fee-for-service basis.
• Combination agency: nonprofit services and proprietary (or profit) services.

5. Can multidisciplinary care be provided in the home setting?

Yes. Multidisciplinary care can be provided in the home as directed and ordered by the physician. Home health agencies are expanding to provide infusion therapy, medical equipment and supplies, hospice care, rehabilitation, and even prevention and screening care. The services rendered depend on the patient's needs and ability to pay (insurance, self-payment, or indigence). Services available for home care include the following:

Skilled nursing	Physical therapy
Occupational therapy	Speech and audiology
Social work	Home health aide
Respiratory therapy	Pastoral care
Nutritional support	Pharmaceutical support
Laboratory services	Medical therapies

6. What medical therapies can be provided in the home setting?

Examples of medical or home infusion therapy include peripheral intravenous (IV) catheter insertion; maintenance of central venous and peripheral access devices; administration of intravenous antibiotics, opioids, chemotherapy drugs, colony-stimulating factors, and other medications; hydration and electrolyte replacement; enteral or parenteral nutrition; transfusion of blood products; and administration of spinal opioids and local anesthetics.

7. What factor has the greatest effect on the cost of home care?

The patient's functional status or level of independence, not necessarily the diagnosis, dictates the complexity and costs of home care. Other factors to be considered in assessing the cost-effectiveness of home care include direct and indirect costs to the patient and family (e.g., transportation, drugs, and respite care; physical and emotional burden; disruption in family lifestyle and roles); complexity of treatments and nursing care; competence and willingness of family to provide care; necessary resources to provide care at home; and financial reimbursement by insurance plans. Insurance companies will reimburse for home care services provided that the need for skilled nursing is well documented. For example, dressing changes or wound care may be considered unskilled nursing care, whereas skilled nursing care is required for the evaluation of the wound or assessment of the patient's response to interventions.

8. What is the the role of a home care nurse?

Home care nurses utilize the nursing process to help patients reach various outcomes, ranging from cure, symptom control, and rehabilitation to peaceful death. In contrast to hospital nursing, home care nursing is intermittent instead of continuous, and in most cases, a primary caregiver is needed to help foster the outcomes and goals. Motivated patients and caregivers are necessary for effective home care. The home care nurse must tailor care to meet the needs and well-being of the primary caregiver as well as the patient.

The foremost skills needed by home care nurses are physical assessment and evaluation, knowledge of safety issues, and problem-solving abilities. The nurse must be able to function autonomously and coordinate services and community resources. Cancer patients often have high-acuity, complex needs that require the home care nurse to be especially proficient in high-technology skills and documentation. A realistic assessment of the patient and family is essential for planning care and setting goals. Specific elements include the following[7]:

1. Patient history: tumor site and stage; treatment, previous and current; prognosis; other health problems; chief concerns.

2. Physical examination: general assessment of all body systems, operative site, radiation ports (if applicable).

3. Self-care abilities: performance of activities of daily living; return demonstration of treatments, medication administration; ability to assume usual roles.

4. Physical care requirements: need for assistance with care or help with equipment; pain management; nutrition counseling; management of treatment- or disease-related problems.

5. Psychosocial assessment: social supports, coping mechanisms, emotional status, usual diversional activities.

6. Family and caregiver assessment: composition of family; who makes decisions; values; communication patterns; health of family members; family's knowledge of patient's disease, treatment, and prognosis; family's ability to provide care, physically and emotionally.

7. Environment: assess for cleanliness; barriers in home that may impede care (e.g., no telephone); availability of emergency care

8. Financial situation (e.g., ability to pay, coverage by health insurance, federal assistance).

9. Are there any tips for reducing the costs of care or adapting care in the home?

Home care nurses, patients, and their families can become quite creative when providing care in the home as shown by the following examples:

- No shower bench? Use a plastic lawn chair.
- No intravenous pole? Use a hanger on a door frame or a standing lamp.
- Try to reuse or recycle equipment as much as possible; instead of disposable equipment, use equipment that can be cleaned or sterilized and reused.
- Teach the primary caregiver clean technique for dressing changes or wound care; for example, after a Hickman catheter site is healed and no longer draining, instruct the patient to use a clean wash cloth and mild soap to wipe around the site instead of alcohol or Betadine.
- Use household products for disinfection. A 1:3 dilution of white vinegar in water can be used for equipment that comes in direct contact with mucus membranes. A 1:9 dilution of chlorine bleach is effective in cleaning blood-contaminated surfaces.
- Need a nutritional supplement to increase the patient's caloric intake? Instead of products such as Ensure or Sustacal, suggest Carnation Instant Breakfast with ice cream, which is less expensive and may even taste better.
- For patients who are having problems with chewing, use a blender or food processor to liquefy solid food.
- Uninfected PEG tube site with normal drainage? Cut up clean linen towels or cotton handkerchiefs into 2×2 size and cut a slit like a drain sponge. Change the "bandage" as needed. Wash by hand or in a net bag in the washing machine with soap and hot water.
- Walker doesn't move well over carpet? Place cut tennis balls over the bottom of the back legs of the walker and glide away.

10. Has a common problem for patients with cancer been identified in home care?

Yes, constipation. Prevention is the best treatment. Assess the patient's normal bowel regimen and develop an early plan of action. Identify contributing factors, such as opioid use, decreased activity, or inadequate nutrition and hydration.

11. Describe how chemotherapy can be safely administered in the home.

Each home nursing care or infusion agency should have policies and guidelines specifying patient eligibility; types of chemotherapy agents; preparation, transport, administration, and disposal of drugs; criteria for withholding chemotherapy; monitoring parameters; and qualifications and education for nurses administering the drugs. Safety considerations are as follows:

1. Close attention must be given to the accuracy of administering chemotherapy in the home. No first doses should be given in the home because of the risk of severe adverse reactions.

2. The body surface area, drug dosing, and administrative technique should be double-checked with a pharmacist or oncology clinician.

3. The registered nurse should be knowledgeable of the physician's standing orders for drug reaction and have ready access to the necessary equipment and drugs. For example, if doxorubicin (Adriamycin) is given in the home, be sure that diphenhydramine (Benadryl) is available for a flare reaction and a cold pack for extravasation.

4. An emergency kit for anaphylaxis should be in the home as well as a rebreather in case of respiratory arrest.

5. The nurse should adhere to the Cancer Chemotherapy Guidelines developed by the Oncology Nursing Society for proper protection and administration of chemotherapy (e.g., clean environment, use of latex gloves). Handle supplies on disposable surfaces, and use only syringes and intravenous sets with Luer-lock fittings, if possible.

6. Carefully anchor and tape all tubing to avoid disconnection or extravasation.

7. If possible, have pharmacy preprime tubing to minimize drug aerosolization. Drugs should be transported in sealed, labeled containers.

8. Make sure a chemotherapy spill kit is available.

9. After the procedure is completed, chemotherapy items should be placed in a labeled chemotherapy waste disposal bag or container and picked up from the home by the pharmaceutical company that initially delivered the supplies. In rural settings where this is not always feasible, secure the waste items carefully and transport them to the nearest facility with a safe waste disposal system for cytotoxics. Sharp objects may be disposed of in a purchased container or a coffee can with a reinforced lid.

10. Instruct family members about (1) important phone numbers and who to contact for problems; (2) self-care responsibilities, such as changing the battery of an infusion pump and venous access site care; (3) side-effect management; and (4) proper disposal of excreta. In the home setting, the toilet should be flushed twice. Clothing, towels, or sheets contaminated with excreta should be washed separately. Family members should wear latex gloves when handling excreta (urine, stool, vomitus, and blood).

12. Discuss the needs of the primary caregiver.

The primary caregiver is "the individual responsible for the majority of caregiving tasks, including the emotional support and supervision of the person with cancer."[6] Caregiver needs vary according to the patient's condition and phase of illness. Studies have shown that the major areas of caregiver needs are categorized as informational and psychological. Identified needs and suggestions for assistance include the following:

1. Initially, the primary caregiver may experience "information overload." Repeat instructions, using language the caregiver can understand. Ask the caregiver to verbalize what is understood. Provide written or audiovisual references (videotapes, cassette tapes). Pharmaceutical companies often furnish free videotapes that demonstrate how to administer parenteral drugs and other aspects of medicinal care. The American Cancer Society and the National Cancer Institute are excellent sources of free patient educational materials.

2. Caregivers are often concerned about their own health and how well they can manage in providing emotional support and physical care for the patient. Caregivers do not want to burden the patient with their own concerns. Consider spending some time alone with primary caregivers to query how they are coping. Are additional resources needed? Is respite care needed? Assess whether other family members, friends, or church members can help in the care of the patient.

Encourage development of supportive social relationships. Provide information about community resources, such as the American Cancer Society or the Ostomy Association. Alert the primary caregiver to hotlines such as 1-800-ACS-2345. Provide reassurance that help is accessible. Ideally, help should be available to the caregiver 24 hours/day via telephone triage or episodic home visits.

3. Caregivers may have additional financial strains and employment limitations imposed by having the patient at home. Assist the family by locating appropriate resources and community support services (American Cancer Society and American Red Cross) for additional funding, particularly free transportation and equipment loans.

13. What kinds of problems do home care agencies face? How can nursing care be monitored?

Home health care agencies face the following challenges: capitation, maintenance of adequate service populations, broadening range of services to meet consumer demands, development of successful mergers and alliances, and fraud and abuse. Until recently, home care agencies were not very accountable to insurance and federal regulators. Public and private insurers are now beginning to dictate the services allowed in the home as well as the number of home care visits to accomplish the goals of the medical regimen. Medicare will be conducting more focused medical reviews, and the Office of Inspector General continues to investigate home care providers for unethical practices such as illegal kickbacks, ghost billing, and falsified patient care interventions. The prevalence of fraud in the oncology home care industry is not known; however, nurses should be aware of such problems as well as the laws and regulations regarding costs and reimbursements.

Nurses need to help develop and follow quality improvement and risk management plans. Definitions of quality of care and outcomes of health care services, such as patient satisfaction, morbidity, and quality of life, are being developed by the National Association of Home Care. Record reviews, patient and caregiver surveys, and monitoring forms, such as the home health agency utilization review form developed by The City of Hope National Medical Center,[2] can assist nurses in identifying and monitoring care at home.

14. Give an example of a home treatment with potential involvement of the primary caregiver.

The patient is a 34-year-old man recently discharged after an allogeneic bone marrow transplant. Home care includes intravenous administration via a Hickman catheter of vancomycin, 1 gm every 12 hours. The patient lives with his wife and two small children. The wife works from 8 A.M. to 5 P.M. as a computer programmer. A home nursing assessment reveals that the wife is capable and willing to administer the medication. The administration hours will be 6 A.M. and 6 P.M. Arrangements have been made with a pharmaceutical company to deliver the necessary supplies to the home. An initial home care visit is made. The wife is instructed how to safely store the drug and supplies, with special consideration of the children in the home. Teaching also begins with the steps necessary to prepare the medication and to deliver the drug through an infusion pump. Written instructions with pictures are reviewed with the wife and left in the home. The registered nurse will remain in the home throughout the entire infusion and teach the wife how to discontinue the drug, flush the Hickman, and safely dispose of used supplies. Instructions are also given about catheter complications, troubleshooting ideas, and potential complications with vancomycin. Home visits will continue to be made every 12 hours until the wife can demonstrate the entire procedure correctly and safely. For potential problems, the patient and his wife are made aware of the availability of contact with a registered nurse on a 24-hour basis.

BIBLIOGRAPHY

1. Caie-Lawrence J, Peploske J, Russell J: Training needs of home healthcare nurses. Home Healthcare Nurse 13(2):53–61, 1995.
2. Chapman AH, Sebastian W: Selected issues in quality improvement and risk management. Semin Oncol Nurs 12:231–237, 1996.
3. Dollinger M, Rosenbaum EH, Cable G: Everyone's Guide to Cancer Therapy: How Cancer is Diagnosed, Treated, and Managed Day to Day. Toronto, Somerville House Books, 1991.

4. Groenwald SL, Frogge MH, Goodman M, Yarbro CH: Delivery Systems for Cancer Care: Part VII. In Cancer Nursing: Principles and Practice, 2nd ed. Boston, Jones & Bartlett, 1992.

5. Haylock P: Home care for the person with cancer. Home Healthcare Nurse 11(5):16–28, 1993.

6. Laizner A, et al: Needs of family caregivers of persons with cancer: A review. Semin Oncol Nurs 9:114–120, 1993.

7. Lowdermilk DL: Home care of the patient with gynecologic cancer. J Obstet Gynecol Neonat Nurs 24:157–168, 1995.

8. McEnroe LE: Role of the oncology nurse in home care: Family-centered practice. Semin Oncol Nurs 12:188–192, 1996.

9. Powell LL, Fishman M, Mrozek-Orlowski M (eds): Oncology Nursing Society Cancer Chemotherapy Guidelines. Philadelphia, Oncology Nursing Society Press, 1996.

10. Seeber S, Baird SB: The impact of health care changes on home health. Semin Oncol Nurs 12(3): 179–187, 1996.

68. HOSPICE CARE

Janelle McCallum Betley, RN, BSN, MSM

1. When is hospice care appropriate?

A person is ready for hospice care whenever he or she chooses palliative, noncurative holistic care instead of aggressive, curative medical care for a life-limiting illness. Typically hospice care has been available for people with a prognosis of 6 months or less. More recently patients have been referred close to the week of death. Unfortunately, such late referral precludes much of the benefit offered by the interdisciplinary team. To meet the needs of people and physicians who are reluctant to accept hospice care earlier in the course of illness, many hospices offer pre-hospice services. Pre-hospice services are for patients who are clearly terminal but who choose aggressive palliative care such as second- or third-line chemotherapy.

Historically, the majority of hospice patients have had cancer. Now patients with non-cancer diagnoses are using hospice services. Other hospice-appropriate diagnoses include:

- Organ cancers (e.g., pancreas, liver)
- Cancers with metastatic processes
- Life-threatening congenital defects
- Massive cerebrovascular accidents (CVAs)
- Endstage chronic diseases, such as acquired immunodeficiency syndrome (AIDS), chronic obstructive pulmonary disease (COPD), multiple sclerosis (MS), amyotrophic lateral sclerosis (ALS)
- Failure to thrive or significant weight loss
- Discontinuation of treatment or medications that prolong life (e.g., dialysis, antirejection medications, ventilators)
- Bone marrow transplant failure
- Patients with a do-not-resuscitate (DNR) order in a home health system
- Patients with complex pain symptoms who need expert management
- Patients with repeat hospitalizations
- Patients with social, psychological, or spiritual challenges dealing with terminal illness and disease process
- Patients in whom aggressive treatment is less useful
- Patients with frequent changes in treatment plan
- Patients who decline treatment or diagnostic interventions

2. Where can a patient receive hospice care?

Hospice care can be provided in almost any setting: home, apartment, assisted living facility, nursing home, hospital, specialized inpatient hospice unit, or prison.

A 1992 Gallup poll revealed that 9 of 10 Americans surveyed would choose the services offered by hospices if faced with a terminal illness. Most people prefer to remain in their homes as they die. A Medicare expenditure report for 1982–1986 showed that 80–84% of Medicare hospice beneficiaries remained in their homes to die.[3]

Some people, however, need or choose an inpatient setting, including (1) patients who have no family or caregivers, (2) patients and families who desire an inpatient setting for personal reasons, and (3) patients with extreme medical or social conditions that make it necessary to transfer to an inpatient setting.

3. Who should bring up the subject of hospice care?

This can be a tricky area in which intuition and diplomacy are warranted. As the patient's nurse, you can do the following:

1. Begin your discussion and assessment with the patient's physician.
2. Offer to be present for the physician's discussion with the patient and family.
3. Offer to present the hospice option yourself. (In many hospitals discharge planners may be given the role of discussing hospice care.)

Often a hospice referral comes abruptly in the eyes of the patient and family. They believe that an aggressive curative course is under way, and the next day everything changes. The patient needs hospice care and, if hospitalized, must leave the hospital that same day. Proactive public education about hospice philosophy is the key to diminishing the frequency of this scenario.

4. What if hospice care is clearly appropriate, but the physician refuses to discuss it with the patient or family?

First, discuss your concerns with the patient's physician. Try to follow Covey's axiom, "Seek first to understand, then to be understood." Perhaps more information or a more complex dynamic is involved than is readily apparent. After exhausting all proper channels of communication, you may decide to approach the patient or family yourself. In this case it may be helpful to begin by asking the patient:

1. How are things going with your body?
2. What do you think is going on with your medical condition?
3. What do you think the future holds for you?

Depending on the patient's answer, follow the appropriate path. Let the patient know that you are open to hearing and discussing the unthinkable—dying.

5. What do I say when patients ask me if they are dying?

Always be truthful. Chances are good that the patient has already been told that he or she is dying but may need to hear it again as conditions change. Approaches to answering this question include:

• What does it seem like to you? Then confirm the answer, if appropriate.
• What has your doctor told you? Then build or expand on what the patient already knows.

Reassure the patient that symptoms will be controlled. One hospice nurse emphasizes that someone given a "terminal diagnosis" often has time to do and say anything they want to before they die. Many people do not have this gift of time and die without saying and doing what they may have wanted. The bottom line is to follow the patient's lead. Ask, "Do you think you are dying?" Then take the conversation from there. This question helps to discover what the person really wants to know.

6. What promises should I never make to a dying person?

The premise is simple: Don't make promises you can't keep. Remember that the dying person has less time in which to have the promises fulfilled. Examples of key promises not to make include:

• I promise I'll be with you when you die.
• I promise I'll see you before you go.
• I promise I'll help you die.
• I promise I won't be depressed after you die.

It is also helpful to encourage family members not to make promises that they cannot keep.

7. What if I'm not sad when every patient dies?

One hospice nurse recalls that when she first started taking care of hospice patients, she expected that she should be sad when every patient died. Then she realized that she was connected to some patients and families and not so connected to others. Another hospice nurse says, "It's okay not to be sad. We don't like everyone we meet in life, so we won't like everyone we meet in death." Death is the natural conclusion of life. Hospice nurses strive to make the final hours or day a period of quality time for patient and family. Hopefully when they look back on that time, the actual death will be only a small part of a greater event.

8. How can I show respect for life after the patient has died?

Handle the patient in death as you did in life—with respect and care; make no distinction. Specific interventions include:

- Allow families private time with the body, and respect families' wishes, traditions, and customs.
- Be gentle and caring when removing lines and tubes and washing the body.
- Close the patient's eyes. Cover the patient to the neck; there is no need to cover the face.
- Brush the hair off the forehead and touch the face of the deceased in a gentle, loving manner.
- Reminisce with the family about the patient.
- From a chaplain's perspective: touch the body by laying on hands in blessing and talk as if their spirit is still present in the room. Sit in silence and reverence with the body.

9. What matters to families immediately after the death of the patient?

Ask the family what matters to them. Each family is different, and we must give them space to tell us what would be helpful. For example, some families want to spend lots of time with the dead body, whereas other families want the body removed as soon as possible. For some, the patient's appearance is of great concern (e.g., hair, make-up, clothing, position). However, families seem to have some fairly universal needs:

1. Show them that someone cares about them and the patient.
2. Let them know that you will take care of necessary details (e.g., with the physician, coroner, mortuary, equipment company, medications).
3. Provide a time and a place to make phone calls.
4. For deaths that occur in a private residence, it is important to have the medical equipment (e.g., bed, wheelchair, oxygen) removed as soon as possible.

Be sure to ask about rituals and spiritual needs. Be sensitive to cultures unlike your own. Most families want reassurance that their loved one will be treated with respect even in death.

10. What is anticipatory grief?

In the context of hospice care, anticipatory grief refers to emotions of loss and grief and even relief before the person's death. Many people expect profound anguish, but they feel guilt as they find themselves planning for the future—before the person actually dies. Hospice workers encourage anticipatory grief and help to normalize such emotions. Planning for the future is a healthy sign of anticipating life after the death of a loved one. It does not mean the survivors do not love the dying person or wish that the person would die sooner. It is what healthy people do when facing such life-changing circumstances as losing a loved one to terminal illness.

11. What can I do to help during the grieving process?

Simply stated, listen to the person's fears, ask about strategies to deal with the fears, and assist as appropriate. Ask about future plans. If the person has none, encourage thinking about the future. Reassure the person that future planning is normal and may cause some feelings of guilt. If a severely depressed survivor speaks of having no plans or future, this may be a red flag. Refer the person immediately to a social worker or chaplain.

Not all people who die are "loved ones." Be open to relief in family members or friends, who may make such statements as "He was so abusive," "We had a terrible marriage," or "I hated her." We tend to expect everyone to be sad about the patient's death, but this is not always the case. Know that even though a person may be relieved that the patient died, the associated guilt must be resolved eventually.

12. Is it professional to go to the patient's funeral and maintain contact with the family?

In an inpatient setting, if scheduling allows and you feel a need to attend the funeral for your own closure, it is appropriate to do so. Continued contact with the family is generally *not* appropriate. Refer the family to a local hospice for bereavement assistance.

In a hospice setting, staff are encouraged to attend the patient's funeral and to make bereavement follow-up. Generally the staff who knew the patient attend the funeral, and a grief counselor does the follow-up bereavement work. The goal of follow-up is to assist the grieving person to heal in a healthy way.

Continued contact by direct care staff is discouraged because it continues a relationship that was begun during a time of crisis and death. The nurse's job is to assist the patient and family along the journey to death. The journey after death is equally important and may be assisted by another caregiver (e.g., bereavement counselor). There are always exceptions to this advice, however. Be careful to consider whose needs are primary—yours or the family's? Your goal in caring for the family after death is the same as when the patient was alive: *Do what is best for the patient and family first; meet your own emotional and social needs secondarily.*

Furthermore, it is known that morbidity and mortality increase significantly after a spouse's death. A recent study by Connor and McMaster evaluated the impact of psychosocial intervention on the use of inpatient and outpatient health care services by bereaved spouses. The results showed that spouses treated with hospice services used hospitals and clinics significantly less than spouses in the nonintervention and limited intervention groups. This study helps to describe the positive health and economic benefits provided by hospice bereavement services.

13. What is the role of the hospice in discontinuation of life-sustaining treatments?

Unfortunately, hospice staff are not consulted enough in such situations. The interdisciplinary hospice staff can be of great assistance in discussing options and supporting choices from many perspectives. They can help in determining the patient's decision-making capacity and ensuring that all parties are informed and advised. Whereas the medical model typically addresses only the physical domain, hospice staff consider the physical, emotional, social, and spiritual domains as the patient and family struggle with the decisions to end life-sustaining treatment.

For example, Emily was a patient whose family had made the decision to remove her from the ventilator. But they wanted her to die at home. They wanted to dress her in her prettiest nightgown, play her favorite country music, and have the smell of apple pie coming from the kitchen. After much negotiation, the hospice was able to assist the family to bring Emily home in the ambulance with an ambu bag. When she arrived home, the whole family was there. Her husband, who needed a wheelchair, was able to sit next to her on the couch and hold her hands as the ambu bag was discontinued. The sounds of country music mixed in with the clatter of kitchen noises. Emily died smelling apple pie and the other familiar scents of her own home. The family was touched and felt that they had influenced her life as well as her death. They were proud of themselves.

14. What questions should be asked in assessing a patient's decision-making capacity with regard to discontinuation of life-sustaining treatments?

- Is the patient able to communicate feelings and desires clearly to others?
- Is the patient clearly stating (via his or her method of communication) the desire for discontinuation of technical support?
- Is the patient able to articulate (via his or her method of communication) various options and consequences of actions?
- Is the patient depressed? Have antidepressant therapy and counseling been attempted?
- What are the patient's and family's spiritual concerns or understanding about discontinuation of treatment?
- Has the patient talked with others outside the health care team about this decision? If not, would this be helpful?
- Does the patient require more time for a thoughtful decision?
- Does the patient have an advance directive consistent with this decision?

15. What areas of agreement or disagreement should be addressed before discontinuing life-sustaining treatments?

- Are family and friends in agreement?
- Are current health care providers in agreement?

- Is there a physician's order for discontinuation?
- Which physician will preside at removal of the ventilator?
- Does the decision seem reasonable to staff who have assessed patient and family?

16. Is it true that it does not matter whether a terminally ill person is addicted to narcotics?

No. The point is that less than 1% of people who need narcotics for terminal pain actually display symptoms of true addiction. To alleviate the patient's and family's fears, it is helpful to understand and be able to teach the three components of the addiction scenario (tolerance, physical dependence, and psychological dependence.) As Foley points out, "The truth is that addiction is not the issue for cancer patients, and informing health care professionals and patients about the distinctions between tolerance, physical dependence, and psychological dependence is crucial."

Challenge the statement, "Who cares if he is addicted in the last months of his life anyway?" It is important to explain the following points:

1. In most cases the patient is not addicted.

2. Thinking that the family member was addicted to narcotics may be a stumbling block in the bereaved person's road to recovery.

3. The myth of addiction serves only to continue the public's misunderstanding of narcotics and appropriate pain management.

17. How can I remain compassionate yet not go crazy caring for dying patients and their families?

Here is how several hospice workers answer this question:

Ed: Take care of yourself. If you don't, you can't care for others. Cherish your life and all who are in it. Nurture your spiritual being to sustain you in times of need. Be aware of how this vocation can affect you. Talk about your feelings with your co-workers, and don't be afraid to seek outside help.

Jean: I get energy from the courage and love of so many of the families. I get two hugs for every one I give.

Micki: I maintain the philosophy that everyone dies, and if I can in any way facilitate meeting the patient's needs and wishes surrounding this one-time event, it is rewarding. Educating, reassuring, and guiding families is great.

Phyllis: When I close the door of the hospice inpatient unit, I am symbolically closing that part of my life until the next day. Recipe for success: do fun things, let the inner child out.

Janelle: If you're going to work with people who die, you had better learn how to live, decide what's important to you, and say what needs to be said. Every now and then, someone will wrap their soul around your heart, and it hurts when they suffer or die. This then is the essence of life.

Kay: When I feel valued and supported by the people I work for, it helps me remain focused. Use the support of other team members. Talk about what is going on.

Sandi: For me the key has been finding a clear theology for this work. Theology really helped me with "What's it all about, Alfie?" This work has given me a non-anxious paradigm about death.

Sally: Working part-time helps. I take care of myself physically (exercise and rest) and especially spiritually (meditation). I nurture friendships outside of hospice, and I spend as much time as possible with people who make me laugh.

Suzette: Have a life. Do for yourself. Forget all work issues on the weekend. Get away from your normal environment. Don't be a caregiver for all the people in your life. Have a person who listens to your problems—even a therapist. Maintain inner balance. Exercise, shop, have parties.

Paula: Don't overidentify with patients and families. Know your limits. Use the support of others.

Michelle: Set limits. Take care of yourself. Have outside interests and activities. Accept the laughter and the tears. Take opportunities for closure.

18. What if the patient wants to stay at home alone, but this option really is not safe?

Our job as nurses is to assess the safety and competency of the patient in whatever setting the patient resides. At times it is hard to be objective. We often think of a preferred arrangement because it would put our minds at ease. In the case of a live-alone patient, we need to identify true safety hazards and look at our own personal tolerance for marginal situations. The following checklist may be used:

Functional, Physical, and Environmental Concerns

1. Patient residence is ( ) multiple-family dwelling ( ) single-family dwelling
2. Personal emergency response system in use: ( ) Yes   ( ) No

	Y	N	
3.	( )	( )	Bedbound
4.	( )	( )	History of falls
5.	( )	( )	Fire hazards
6.	( )	( )	Hearing and/or vision
7.	( )	( )	Home alone
8.	( )	( )	Lives alone
9.	( )	( )	Medication compliance
10.	( )	( )	Decision maker
11.	( )	( )	Transportation assistance
12.	( )	( )	Oxygen: as needed _____ continuous _____
13.	( )	( )	Smoker
14.	( )	( )	Basic utilities
15.	( )	( )	Telephone

Psychosocial concerns

	Y	N	
16.	( )	( )	Financial Management
17.	( )	( )	Psychiatric Problems: Current _____ Hx _____
18.	( )	( )	Alcohol/Drug Problems: Current _____ Hx _____
19.	( )	( )	Suicidal Ideation: Current _____ Hx _____
20.	( )	( )	Violence or Potential: Current _____ Hx _____

Y = observed and/or reported; N = not observed, not reported, or denied; Hx = history.
Adapted from Hospice of Metro Denver, Denver, Colorado.

Equally important as the safety assessment is whether the patient has the capacity to make decisions. It is important to note that capacity is situational. Generally, the patient needs only to understand the consequences of a decision to have capacity. A person may have capacity and make poor decisions. In the case of poor decision making that puts the patient or others at risk, a call to Adult Protective Services is probably the best course of action.

Unfortunately, safety assessment is not an exact science. We must try to assess objectively the social, emotional, and physical strengths, weaknesses, needs, and desires of the patient and family, then make a decision to the best of our ability. Advice: maybe a plan to stay at home can work for a while; then regroup and make a new plan.

Example: Molly is a 78-year-old woman whose primary caregiver is her daughter. The daughter works full-time and is afraid to ask for time off despite the Family Medical Leave Act. Molly is alert but bedridden. The daughter plans to leave Molly alone while she works. Certified nursing assistants will visit Molly every day for personal care and to fix lunch. The daughter leaves water and snacks. Molly has an indwelling Foley catheter and can move herself in bed somewhat. Telephone, television remote control, water, and snacks are within Molly's reach. The daughter will call to check on Molly every 2–3 hours. Molly agrees to the plan, which works for 2 months. Then Molly tells the nursing assistant that she is afraid to be alone. A family conference is held to put a new plan in place. The daughter cannot hear her mother's fears. The hospice has to advocate for the patient. Finally Molly and her daughter agree to inpatient placement.

Molly's case was not an easy one. The hospice had to define its limits and advocate for the patient and her daughter. Unfortunately, conflict around caregiving needs is not uncommon. Helping families find a tolerable middle ground is a reasonable outcome.

19. What if a hospice patient talks about suicide or tries to commit suicide?

Many people who have been told that they have a terminal illness think about suicide at some point. Most work it through and decide that suicide is not really what they want to do. However, some continue to have a strong desire to kill themselves. In talking about suicide it is important to let the patient know three points:

1. It is okay to talk about such thoughts. (In fact, it is imperative that staff ask for more details to assess the seriousness of the threat.)

2. Suicidal ideation cannot be kept a secret; other team members need to know.

3. Support and assistance will be provided to the patient to work through fears and to continue living until the illness runs its course. The patient will not be abandoned.

When a patient talks about suicide, keep the following points in mind:

1. Do not be afraid to use the "s" word. For example: "Are you considering suicide?" "Have you thought about hurting yourself?" "Do you want to do something that would end things sooner?" By speaking the words aloud, you allow the person the option of responding either yes or no. If the patient says yes, ask whether the patient has a plan and get all the details. If the patient says no, ask what keeps the patient from doing it. This information may be helpful at another time.

2. Find out what specifically is intolerable for the patient. Is it pain, fear of pain, anxiety, lack of support, worry about being a burden, worry about losing dignity, or some other concern? Often we can eliminate the issue that makes the patient want to leave life early.

3. Explain that the discussion of suicide cannot be a secret. You have to tell the social worker, who will ask further questions and assist as possible.

20. When are invasive, painful measures appropriate for a hospice patient?

Generally, invasive measures are not appropriate for hospice patients. However, there are exceptions. The goals of therapy are patient and family choice and optimal quality of life. Examples of invasive or painful treatments that may be used include:

- Intravenous fluids (when used judiciously and discontinued as fluid begins to accumulate)
- Intravenous or intraspinal pain medication
- Gastric feedings
- Rectal tubes
- Paracentesis and thoracentesis (for a limited time)
- Surgery to repair fractures (often Buck's traction and pain management are used instead)
- Certain chemotherapies (to achieve palliation of symptoms)
- Total parenteral nutrition (for a limited time)

21. What do I do when the patient insists on experiencing pain, even though I know that medications and other treatments would help?

1. Listen to the patient; hear the request to decline pain medications.

2. Ask why medications and treatments are not acceptable.

3. Ask for permission to explain pain relief measures. Describe the medications, expected actions, and side effects. Remember to explain the concept of addiction and the surrounding myths.

4. If the patient still declines, accept the answer. But check again to make sure no intervention is wanted. (Suggest starting out with a very low dose to decrease fear and build trust.)

5. Comfort the family and friends of the patient. They, too, find it difficult to watch their loved one suffer. In your conversation with the family use the term *declined*, as explained below.

6. Assess reasons why the patient declines pain relief. Often there is a spiritual component to why people choose to suffer (e.g., "I want to suffer the way Christ did").

7. In your charting and discussion about the patient, consider using the words *declined medication* instead of "refused." The simple change of wording often evokes a change in the nurse. The word *refused* conjures up the image of a noncompliant patient. By the using the word *declined* we imagine a person with dignity making an informed decision. Be sure to document the teaching you have done if indeed the patient declines the offer for pain medication.

22. What about the young patient whose body just will not die?

Younger, actively dying patients tend to linger longer than older, actively dying patients. Even though the body is full of cancer, the younger person's heart can last longer. The stage called "actively dying" is the time just before a person dies when the kidneys begin to shut down, blood pressure decreases, oral intake stops, alertness diminishes (although not always), and mottling of the extremities may occur. An older patient may be in the "actively dying" stage for 1–3 days, whereas a younger person may be "actively dying" for days to weeks. Although longer death vigils are grueling for all involved, they seem to serve an important purpose for the patient as well as the family.

23. Who makes the decision about what constitutes palliative treatment and when it is appropriate to discontinue blood transfusions, palliative radiation, total parenteral nutrition, or enteral feedings?

Generally the patient's primary physician, in conjunction with the hospice medical director, makes the decision as to what constitutes palliative treatment. Of great importance is how we talk to the patient and family about these issues. It is helpful to describe the physiologic reasons why the treatments are not effective and are probably more uncomfortable to continue. Be sure to speak with the physician about discontinuation before discussing it with the family. Here are general rules of thumb for discontinuing treatment within a hospice context:
- When the physician believes that the treatment is no longer effective.
- When the patient can no longer make the trip to the hospital or clinic (e.g., taking the patient by ambulance to receive a blood transfusion does not usually make sense. However, it is often the patient or family member who says, "You know, I'm just too tired to make the trip—even with an ambulance").
- When the patient no longer tolerates the treatment.
- When the treatment causes more pain than comfort.

24. What does normal grief look like?

Grief takes time. It often takes a year or more to regain balance in life after a loss. The following are all natural and normal grief responses, listed in "A Few Words about Grief and Loss" (published by Hospice of Metro Denver, 1996).
- Tightness in the throat or heaviness in the chest
- Hollow feeling in the stomach and loss of appetite
- Need to tell and retell the story of the events leading up to the death and its aftermath
- Restlessness and need to fill time with activity, but often with difficulty in concentrating and getting organized
- Feeling as though the loss is not real, that it did not really happen
- Sensing the deceased person's presence; perhaps expecting him or her to walk in the door at the usual time, hearing the voice, or seeing the face on a stranger in a crowd
- Aimless wandering, forgetfulness, trouble with finishing projects at work or home, or absent-mindedness
- Intense preoccupation with the life of the deceased
- Crying at unexpected times
- Feeling guilty or angry over things that happened or did not happen in the relationship with the deceased

- Intense anger at the deceased for leaving
- Taking on mannerisms or traits of the deceased
- Sense of relief, sometimes followed by pangs of guilt or regret
- Unpredictable, rapid, and sharp mood swings
- Avoidance of talking about feelings of loss around others
- Weakness or lack of energy

If any of the above symptoms persists for more than 2 years or is exaggerated to the point of bodily injury, refer the person to a mental health counselor.

25. What can be done to help the grieving person?

1. Normalize the person's grief experience. "Because grief often feels so painful and overwhelming, it can be frightening. Many people worry that they are not grieving in the 'right' way or wonder if the feelings they have are normal."[4]

2. Encourage grieving people to tell their story. Telling the story is a major part of the healing process because the death event is so important. To embed every detail in one's memory, one must tell the story—over and over.

3. Encourage grieving people to take care of their own health and nutrition.

4. Advise them to make as few major changes in their life as possible.

5. Encourage them to ask for what they need from a few friends on whom they can rely.

26. How do I respond when a patient's family member rushes from the room and says, "I think he just died!"?

Give the person your immediate attention. You may say, "Okay, let's go." It is important to attend to the situation immediately. As you enter the room, all of the family may be at the bedside, waiting. At times it is hard to be sure that the patient has really died. Take the necessary time to be sure that the heart has stopped and there are no respirations. Telling the assembled family members that their loved one has died can be difficult. Do your best to "read" their expectations in terms of the language you may use. Possible phrases for telling the news include "He's gone" or "He's passed on." Often the family will ask, "Is he dead?" or "Is she gone?" Then you can affirm the question, using the words they have chosen.

In my experience, using the "d" word (dead) has not been perceived as "sensitive" by the family. It seems that at the time of death, the word "dead" rings hollow and cold. The death of the loved one is obvious, and perhaps euphemisms are appropriate comfort at this time.

27. What do I say to a patient's wife who is upset because her husband will not eat the food she fixes?

First, realize that loss of appetite can be traumatic for the patient's family. Eating and drinking are not only physiologic acts but also important social activities. Adjusting to an ill person's lack of interest in food and fluids can make the family feel helpless. In the above example, acknowledge the wife's frustration and fear. Explain that the food she fixed probably did sound good to her husband, but the disease prevents him from enjoying the meal she prepared. Explain the following:

- Loss of appetite is normal in a terminally ill person. The body needs less food when a person has cancer and is inactive; eating less does not shorten a person's life in serious disease, and in this case, low food intake does not cause hunger.
- Eating may become a difficult activity for a very ill person. Food may be offered, but the person should eat only if he wants. In some cases, the person may eat more than he desires because he believes that it is expected and then feels sick afterward.
- The person who is ill may develop new food preferences because some foods may taste different or have no taste at all.

28. What do I do when a patient insists on believing in a cure or miracle?

First, listen to the patient's belief. Do not try to talk the patient out of it. However, it may be possible to reframe what a "miracle" looks like. Hope is always appropriate. People must be allowed to hope for a miracle that can save their life. It is *not* necessary that they go through all stages of death and dying and reach acceptance. Some people are in denial until the end.

It is our task to be present to patients wherever they are. In our love and support they may find that the miracle for which they had been hoping is the nurse who is an excellent pain manager and who is present in their time of suffering and need.

ACKNOWLEDGMENTS

The author thanks the staff of the Hospice of Metro Denver, who contributed to many of these questions. Specifically, they are Phyllis Walker, Caitlin Trussell, Michelle Taylor, Bob Severin, Sally Pyle, Micki Potter, Edward Orozco, Kay Johnson, Carolyn Jaffe, Jean Fredlund, Paula Dybinski, Vicki Dodson, Sandra Daniel, Mary Curtin, and Suzette Baca. The author also thanks the patients, families, volunteers, and other staff members who provided many life lessons as they shared the journey toward death.

BIBLIOGRAPHY

1. Conner SR, McMaster JK: Hospice, bereavement intervention and use of health care services by surviving spouses. HMO Pract 3:20–23, 1996.
2. Covey S: Seven Habits of Highly Effective People. New York, NY, Fireside, Simon & Schuster, 1989.
3. Foley KM: The cancer pain patient. J Pain Sympt Manage 3:S18, 1988.
4. Horne BK: Hospice care for the terminally ill: A logical, compassionate, and cost effective choice for case managers. NHO Newsline, November 15, 1995, pp 2–4.
5. Hospice of Metro Denver: Policy and Procedure Manual: 1996. Denver, Colorado, Hospice of Metro Denver, 1996. Specific entries include:
     • Discontinuation of life-prolonging treatments
     • Safety assessment
     • Home alone/live alone protocol flow chart
     • When eating or drinking becomes a problem
     • A few words about grief and loss
6. Jaffe C, Ehrlich C: All Kinds of Love: Experiencing Hospice. Amityville, NY, Baywood Publishing, 1997.
7. Purdue Frederick Company: Up-to-date answers to questions about pain medication. Norwalk, CT, 1986, p 7.

69. ADVANCE DIRECTIVES AND END-OF-LIFE DECISIONS

Jane Saucedo Braaten, RN, MS, CCRN, and
Paula Nelson-Marten, RN, PhD, AOCN

1. What are advance directives?

Advance directives include any kind of directions, either written or oral, by which the person makes his or her wishes for medical treatment known and/or appoints a surrogate to make decisions should he or she become unable to do so. Advance directives were created to help facilitate communication and to make end-of-life care a more positive experience. They are grounded in the principle of autonomy, or the patient's right to choose or refuse treatment.

2. What is the Patient Self-Determination Act (PSDA)?

The PSDA is federal legislation that requires all health care institutions receiving Medicare or Medicaid funds to give patients information about advance directives. It also specifies that patient preferences be queried and documented in the medical record. The PSDA specifies that a patient has the right to refuse therapy, including potential lifesaving therapy.

3. What kind of information should be provided?

Although the PSDA requires that advance directive information be given to patients, the quality of information is not specified. Frequently, advance directive brochures are given to the patient without being fully discussed. A study in 1994 found that patients in the hospital who had been given advance directive information were still not clear on the terms CPR, code (cor), and resuscitation. Thus it is important not only to give the information, but to answer questions and promote discussion.

4. Why don't more patients come into the hospital with an advance directive?

Studies have shown that fewer than 5% of patients in various settings had written advance directives. One reason is that written advance directives require a bit of formal paperwork, which sometimes deters people from completing them. Another reason is fear that with an advance directive even basic care will be denied. In addition, the public and health care providers lack a clear understanding and hold misconceptions about advance directives.

5. What is the role of the oncology nurse in advance directives?

As the patient's advocate, it is the nurse's role to help the patient make an informed decision and to ensure that the patient's wishes are followed. The nurse should provide educational material and programs, schedule time for discussion, and communicate patient wishes to all members of the health care team. Educating the community during home and office visits and through community presentations is also important, because the best time to discuss advance directives is before an acute hospitalization. Most individuals are more likely to discuss a sensitive topic when they are in a comfortable, nonthreatening environment.

6. How should the nurse bring up the subject of advance directives?

Studies have shown that most patients welcome a discussion of advance directives but are uncertain of how to bring up the subject and prefer that health care providers initiate the discussion. The subject of advance directives may be introduced with a brochure or pamphlet with an explanation that this reading is part of the standard admission process. The nurse should emphasize that he or she (or another health care provider, such as clinical nurse specialist, physician, chaplain, social worker, or patient representative) is available to answer questions after the patient has read the brochure. A time should be scheduled to discuss this issue with the primary care provider. The nurse should explain that advance directives include preferences about cardiopulmonary resuscitation (CPR) and do-not-resuscitate (DNR) orders as well as other levels of care, such as hydration, further chemotherapy, antibiotics, blood products, and analgesics. For the patient with cancer whose wishes have not yet been discussed but whose condition may be terminal, the subject of advance directives also may be brought up with a brochure or a statement that it is standard practice to query patients about their code status and other levels of care. If possible, health care providers who best know the patient should discuss the patient's wishes well in advance of a critical situation. The following examples are guidelines for a discussion in which the nurse in collaboration with the physician tries to elicit the cancer patient's desire about code status:

1. The nurse may begin by saying, "Nobody can tell you for certain how much time you have left to live, but based on past experiences and knowledge about your particular condition, we believe you have a short time left to live. In order to honor your wishes, we need to ask you some questions about your care." The nurse should ask patients what they understand about their condition, prognosis, and goals of therapy; give the patient sufficient time to ventilate feelings and questions; and continue the dialogue if the patient can acknowledge the condition and wants further discussion.

2. The nurse may begin by saying, "Knowing that your condition cannot be cured or that you may have only a short time left to live, do you want us to attempt CPR or try to bring you back when your heart stops or you stop breathing?" The nurse should be prepared to explain and clarify terms such as CPR, resuscitation, and mechanical ventilation and to discuss chances of success as well as possible complications. The nurse also should explain to the patient that CPR is most likely to be successful in generally healthy patients with sudden and reversible conditions, and that patients with serious underlying medical conditions, such as advanced cancer, have a poor chance of successful CPR and a higher chance of serious complications (see question #18). The DNR order should be clarified, and the patient should be reassured that all other levels of care, including comfort care and other therapies, will continue as the patient requests.

7. What problems related to advance directives occur in the hospital?

Many problems related to advance directives are specific to the hospital environment:

1. Paperwork may become lost during transfer to the hospital or misplaced within the hospital.

2. Patients may not be asked about their treatment preferences because of the fast-paced, cure-oriented environment or reluctance of the health care provider.

3. Misinterpretation may result from ambiguous language used in the advance directive.

4. The patient may have no advance directive and no surrogate decision maker.

8. What is an ambiguous advance directive?

Sometimes an advance directive is ambiguous because of the lack of detail needed to understand completely the wishes of the individual. An example is a verbal or written statement such as "I do not want to be kept alive on life support," with no further instructions or guidance for the health care provider. This statement is difficult to interpret because it fails to specify in what situations the individual wants it to apply and what interventions the patient considers life support. When encountering such an advance directive, the oncology nurse needs to act as patient advocate, using ethical principles to clarify the advanced directive with the patient and/or family.

9. What is SUPPORT? Why is it important?

SUPPORT (Study to Understand Prognosis and Preferences for Outcomes and Risks of Treatment), a large, 4-year, multicenter study funded by grants from the Robert Wood Johnson Foundation, examined end-of-life care in hospitals and concluded that for many patients it was less than optimal. Fifty percent of patients suffered moderate or severe pain in their last days of life; 38% of patients who died spent 10 or more days in the intensive care unit, and physicians did not accurately understand or ignored the patients preferences for advance directives. Of the

79% of patients who had a written DNR order, the DNR was written within 2 days of death. This study is important because it (1) casts a critical eye on the experience of death in the hospital, (2) depicts the problems with communication of advance directives in the hospital, and (3) finds that the problems related to end-of-life care in the hospital are not easily resolved.

10. What can be done if a member of the health care team acts contrary to the patient's wishes?

As patient advocate, the nurse has the obligation to help make the patient's wishes known and followed by the health care team. If a member of the team is not following these wishes, the member simply may not have understood the advance directive. A meeting among nurse, health care team member, and patient or family may clear this misunderstanding. If not, the nurse may request the nursing supervisor or medical director to access the hospital ethics committee.

11. What is the difference between a living will and a medical durable power of attorney?

A **living will** is a document signed by the patient stating that he or she does not want artificial life support in the event of terminal illness. The will takes effect when two physicians agree in writing that the patient has a terminal condition. A living will can be used to stop tube feeding and intravenous fluids only if this condition is stated specifically. Two witnesses need to sign the living will. Persons who cannot witness or sign include patients in or employees of the facility in which the patient receives care; any doctor or employee of the patient's doctor; the patient's creditors; or anyone who may inherit the patient's property.

A **medical durable power of attorney** is a document signed by the patient naming someone to make medical decisions in the patient's behalf. Anyone can act as a medical durable power of attorney as long as that person is at least 18 years of age, mentally competent, and willing to serve as the patient's agent. Examples include spouses, significant others, siblings, or parents. This type of advance directive covers more decisions than a living will and is not limited to terminal illness. A medical durable power of attorney can be effective immediately or when the patient becomes unable to make decisions. It is crucial to stress the importance of a thorough discussion of health care wishes between the patient and the person whom the patient has chosen.

12. What advice can the nurse give to patients who want to ensure that their wishes will be followed?

1. Encourage patients to talk to their relatives or other potential surrogates about their wishes before illness or hospitalization.

2. Encourage use of a combination of living will and medical durable power of attorney. This combination ensures that wishes are followed if the living will is unclear in a specific situation.

3. Use clear language and specific examples, such as "I do not wish to be placed on a ventilator if it is deemed that my disease process is terminal and it is unlikely that I would be able to survive without ventilator support." Do not use terms such as "artificial" or "extraordinary"; these terms can mean different things to different people.

4. Be sure that the primary care physician knows and agrees to carry out the patient's wishes.

5. Encourage patients to give copies of paperwork to their relatives and primary care physician and also to bring a copy to the hospital.

13. Why do patients with living wills receive CPR?

A living will is not an automatic DNR order. Living wills do not cover acute conditions such as infection or bleeding. The living will goes into effect only when the condition is deemed irreversible.

14. What is surrogate decision making or substituted judgment?

In the event that a patient becomes unable to make decisions and is critically ill, health care providers often ask the family or friends of the patient to inform them of what decision the patient would have made under such circumstances. This practice is based on a standard of substituted judgement and is accepted by many legal and medical authorities. The family and/or friends are the surrogate or substitute decision makers.

15. Has surrogate decision making proven to be accurate?

Studies have shown that when given hypothetical end-of-life situations, surrogates did not accurately choose what the patient would prefer. A factor that greatly increased accuracy was a prior discussion of end-of-life preferences between patient and surrogate. This illustrates two clear needs in this area, first, the patient is the only one who can predict what kind of care he/she would want at the end of life, and second, these wishes need to be clearly communicated to those who may be acting as surrogates.

16. What is a CPR directive?

A CPR directive is a document that refuses cardiopulmonary resuscitation if the patient goes into respiratory or cardiac arrest. It does not refuse other medical care. On admission to the hospital, it acts as a valid physician's order. It is available to patients from their physician, hospice, hospital, or nursing home. It must be signed by the patient or proxy and a physician. Many states now offer an outpatient CPR directive.

17. Do patients with a DNR order receive different nursing care from other patients?

The DNR order is defined simply as no CPR. Nonetheless, a DNR order is often thought to imply that other life-sustaining interventions, such as mechanical ventilation, blood products, and dialysis are not desired. In the study by Henneman et al.,[7] nurses reported that they would be less likely to perform a variety of these interventions on a patient with a DNR order, whereas they would be more likely to provide more psychosocial interventions. Because of this confusion, some health care providers and patients are reluctant to use the DNR order. In general, nursing care should remain the same for patients with or without a DNR order.

Realistically, nursing care of patients with DNR orders depends on the specific wishes of the patient and has little to do with the order itself. For example, the patient or family may request comfort care or want aggressive therapy only to a certain point. Generally, such wishes are not conveyed in a DNR order and need to be explored and documented through other more specific advance directives.

18. How successful is CPR in patients with advanced illness?

CPR was originally intended for use following acute situations in otherwise healthy individuals. It is now widely used in hospitals despite its limited effectiveness (0–28% survival rate to hospital discharge). Patients most likely to benefit from CPR are those with sudden circulatory or respiratory collapse in the setting of acute cardiovascular illness. Those least likely to survive are patients with multisystem organ failure, metastatic disease, age > 70, and severe chronic or acute conditions. These facts should be discussed when considering advance directives with patients with advanced illness.

19. Is a "slow code" ethical or legal?

A so-called "slow code" is not an ethical or legal order. An unofficial slow code order is usually an indication that the subject of advance directives has not been adequately discussed with the patient or family. Orders to resuscitate or not to resuscitate should be made clear and understandable to all hospital staff. A "slow code" is neither.

20. Are oral advance directives valid?

Oral advance directives are valid and are the most common type of advance directive in the hospital. Courts have consistently upheld decisions to withhold therapy on the basis of clear and convincing oral advance directives. However, oral directives often are vague, made long before the situation at hand, and are highly subjective, especially when being recalled by another person.

Family disagreement on the meaning of a patient's prior statement can also complicate the decision making.

21. Is legal assistance required to make out an advance directive?

A patient does not need a lawyer to make out a living will, appoint a medical durable power of attorney, or write a CPR directive.

22. Can advance directives be changed?

Advance directives can be changed at any time. The patient needs to destroy the previous advance directive and inform anyone who may have a copy that it has been changed. It is wise to revoke the advance directive in writing and to give copies of the revocation to all who may have received the original document.

23. "They can't sue me for saving their lives." Is this statement true?

Legal action can be brought against a health care provider who ignores an advance directive. Intentionally administering a treatment against a patient's wishes, such as performing CPR on a patient with a CPR directive, may be regarded as assault and battery.

24. Is there a difference between withdrawing and withholding care?

Most ethicists agree that legally and ethically there is no difference; in either case, the decision achieves the same outcome—inevitable death. However, in a hospital survey reported by Lo,[12] 57% of physicians and 73% of nurses felt that there is a difference between withdrawing treatment and not starting it in the first place. It may be that withdrawing treatment is seen as taking a more active role in the death of the patient.

25. Can treatment be withheld if the patient is not terminally ill or unconscious ?

Courts have allowed treatments to be withheld in various situations, including bleeding from trauma, gangrene, respiratory failure, renal failure, cancer, and quadriplegia. The patient may also refuse any and all treatment.

26. Can fluids and nutrition be withheld?

Courts have consistently declared that fluids and nutrition are to be handled as other medical interventions and may be withdrawn or withheld in appropriate circumstances. Patients can refuse these interventions through clear and convincing oral advance directives or through a durable power of attorney. A living will may specify a time frame chosen by the patient in which to administer and then withdraw tube feedings or fluids.

27. What is the difference between active and passive euthanasia?

Active euthanasia is administering an intervention with the intent to kill the patient. This practice is not legal in the United States. Although technically illegal in The Netherlands, it is practiced widely; approximately 2,000 patients per year receive active euthanasia or assisted suicide. Those who practice active euthanasia are rarely prosecuted as long as they follow specific guidelines that include persistent patient requests, full information on the patient's part about his or her condition, unacceptable suffering, and a second physician opinion. **Passive euthanasia** is allowing a disease to continue its natural course. Withholding and withdrawal of care fit into this category.

28. If I give pain medication that knocks out the respiratory drive, am I performing active euthanasia?

No. The intent in giving pain medication is to relieve pain and suffering, not to knock out the respiratory drive. Some clinicians undermedicate patients because of this fear. According to the ANA's Code for Nurses with Interpretive Statements, "The nurse may provide interventions to relieve symptoms in the dying client even when the interventions entail substantial risks of hastening death."

29. Why is the subject of end-of-life decision-making so difficult to discuss?

The subject of death is never an easy topic for the patient, family, or health care provider to discuss because of the overwhelming societal view that death is something to be avoided at all costs. Health care providers may not want to accept the fact that there are limits to their interventions. Furthermore, discussion about death and dying has not been a routine part of medical or nursing school curricula until recently. In addition, the patient may not want to accept the fact that death is an inevitable occurrence and that his or her disease process may result in death. Whatever the reasons for avoidance, death must be seen as an inevitable part of life. Planning and discussion can help to make death and dying more acceptable. This planning, while often uncomfortable, helps to facilitate transition to terminal illness and resolution for both patient and family.

CONTROVERSIES

30. Who determines "futility" when the family or patient wants more intervention than the health care providers think is appropriate?

Some patients and/or family members may request care that is excessive or inappropriate. A determination of medical futility can limit such requests. The problem is that medicine is not an exact science and no prognostic indicators are completely accurate. This makes futility, more often than not, a value judgment. Who makes this judgment—health care providers or patient and family—is a highly controversial topic.

Proponents of determination by clinicians or hospitals argue that futility can be judged ethically and that excessive use of scarce resources can be limited. They believe that hospitals are within their rights to create guidelines or policies for futile care that include referring the patient to a different facility or clinician for the treatment that is deemed futile. Opponents argue that determination by clinicians or hospitals is an example of paternalism (deciding for the patient) and conflicts with the principle of autonomy. Some believe that shared decision making between clinician and patient or surrogate is the ideal solution.

31. Assisted suicide: Will it soon be legal?

Approximately a dozen states have drafted legislation to legalize physician-assisted suicide. Oregon voters have passed the "Death with Dignity Act," but the act remains on hold until its legality is decided. This issue has received attention because of the common belief that patients have little control over end-of-life care. Studies such as SUPPORT further confirm this belief.

For: Right-to-die advocates (e.g., the Hemlock Society) state that society has an obligation to relieve pain and suffering if the patient wishes. They argue that competent patients should be allowed to control the time and manner of their death. They base their position on the principles of beneficence (obligation to do good) and autonomy.

Against: Opponents state that if assisted suicide is legalized, less attention will be focused on pain management and groups such as the elderly, mentally compromised, and poor patients may be coerced into this decision. In an era of managed care and emphasis on cost control, they argue that giving physicians the right "to kill" may be abused. They base their position on the principle of nonmaleficence (obligation to inflict no harm).

BIBLIOGRAPHY

1. Aiken TB, Catalano JT: Legal, Ethical, and Political Issues in Nursing. Philadelphia, F.A. Davis, 1994.
2. American Nurses Association: Code for Nurses with Interpretive Statements. Kansas City, MO, American Nurses Association, 1985.
3. Beland DK, Froman RD: Preliminary validation of a measure of life support preferences. Image 27:307–310,1995.
4. Cugliari A, Miller T, Sobal J: Factors promoting completion of advance directives in the hospital. Arch Intern Med 155:1893–1898, 1995.
5. Dautzenberg P, Brockman T, Hooyer C, et al: Review: Patient related predictors of cardiopulmonary resuscitation of hospitalized patients. Age and Aging 22:464–475, 1993.

6. Hall J: Nursing, Ethics and Law. Philadelphia, W.B. Saunders, 1996.
7. Henneman E, Baird B, Bellamy P, et al: Effect of do-not-resuscitate order on the nursing care of critically ill patients. Am J Crit Care 3: 467–472, 1994.
8. Hoffman M: Use of advance directives: A social work perspective on the myth versus the reality. Death Stud 18:229–241.1994.
9. Laffey J: Bioethical principles and care-based ethics in medical futility. Cancer Pract 4:41–46, 1996.
10. Larson D: Resuscitation discussion experiences of patients hospitalized in a coronary care unit. Heart Lung 23:53–58,1994.
11. Ledbetter N: The use of euthanasia in The Netherlands. Ethics Special Interest Group Newslett 6:1, 2–3, 1995.
12. Lo B: Resolving Ethical Dilemmas: A Guide for Clinicians. Baltimore, Williams & Wilkins, 1995.
13. Meisel A: Legal myths about terminating life support. Arch Intern Med 151:1497–1502, 1991.
14. O'Keefe S, Redahan C, Daly K: Age and other determinants of survival after in-hospital cardiopulmonary resuscitation. Q J Med 81:1005–1010, 1991.
15. Suhl J, Simons P, Reedy T, Garrick T: Myth of substituted judgment: Surrogate decision making regarding life support is unreliable. Arch Intern Med 154:90–96,1994.
16. SUPPORT Principle Investigators: A controlled trial to improve care for seriously ill hospitalized patients: The study to understand prognoses and preferences for outcomes and risks of treatment (SUPPORT). JAMA 274:1591–1598, 1995.

70. COMMON ETHICAL DILEMMAS

Paula Nelson-Marten, RN, PhD, AOCN,
and Jane Saucedo Braaten, RN, MS, CCRN

Since ethics is fundamentally a practical discipline, it is concerned with what we should do and
how we should live.

Churchill, 1989

1. Why is it important for nurses to understand ethics?

It is important for nurses to have an understanding of ethics and ethical decision making so
that they can apply this knowledge in daily nursing practice. Ethical dilemmas occur often and in
every aspect of nursing practice. Without a basic knowledge of ethics, the nurse will miss opportunities to advocate for patients and families and to enhance care. In a survey of 900 nurses from
various settings, conducted by the American Nurses' Association (ANA) Center for Ethics and
Human Rights, 43% reported that they deal with ethical issues in their nursing practice on a daily
basis and 36% on a weekly basis.[6]

2. How can the nurse use ethics in everyday nursing practice?

The nurse uses ethics in everyday nursing practice when he or she is alert to moral conflicts,
identifies ethical issues, uses the ANA Code of Ethics as a base for practice, advocates for patients, shares decision making with patients, and helps to implement moral decisions.

3. How does the nurse distinguish a dilemma from an ethical dilemma?

A dilemma occurs whenever a situation requires a choice between two equally desirable or
undesirable alternatives. All people are confronted by daily dilemmas that involve choice. A
dilemma acquires moral qualities when an individual can justify alternative courses of action
through use of fundamental moral rules or principles. An ethical dilemma arises when moral
claims conflict with one another.

4. What is the difference between the terms *morals* and *ethics*?

The terms *morals* and *ethics* are often used interchangeably. Each word, however, has a distinct derivation and meaning. The word *morals* is derived from the Latin word *mores*, which
means custom or habit and refers to a set of values or rules that are peculiar to each individual.
These values and rules are based on an individual's conscience and cultural or religious beliefs;
they serve as a guide in personal decision making regarding right and wrong. The word *ethics* is
derived from the Greek word *ethos*, which means customs, conduct, and character. Ethics is the
study of how one determines right from wrong. The use of ethics involves a process based on the
use of principles and decision-making frameworks.

5. What ethical codes provide guidance for nursing practice?

The ANA Code of Ethics and the International Council of Nurses (ICN) Code make explicit
the ethical values of the nursing profession. The professional nurse makes a moral commitment
to practice within the expectations set by ethical codes. The ANA Code, which was first adopted
in 1950 and has undergone subsequent revisions, includes 11 statements that define ethical responsibilities of nurses in terms of the following topics: respect for human dignity, safeguarding
the client's right to privacy, client safety, responsibility for nursing judgment, competence, informed judgment, development of nursing knowledge, standards of practice, conditions of employment, protection of a client from misrepresentation, and collaboration to meet health needs
of the public. The ICN Code, which was adopted in 1973, contains statements relating to ethical
practices of the nurse in five areas—with people, in practice, in society, with coworkers, and for

the profession. For complete text of ANA and ICN Codes for Nurses, see Benjamin and Curtis, reference 3.

6. What are the major ethical decision-making processes?

The two major schools of thought in Western biomedical ethics, defined by philosophers in the eighteenth century, have resulted in two major ethical decision-making frameworks—deontology and utilitarianism. Deontology or formalism (from the work of Kant) indicates that the moral agent should consider the inherent nature of an act or rule rather than the consequences. This framework is principle-based and focuses on duties and obligations. The ethical principles used in conjunction with this framework are autonomy, justice, beneficence, and nonmaleficence. Utilitarianism or teleology (from the works of Mill and Bentham) indicates that the moral agent should consider consequences of rules and acts and seek the greatest possible balance of happiness over unhappiness for the greatest number. The two principles used in conjunction with utilitarianism are beneficence and nonmaleficence.

7. What are the major ethical principles?

Many ethical principles may be used to assist in resolution of an ethical dilemma. Basic ethical principles include the following:

1. **Autonomy.** This principle refers to self-rule, a person's right to self-determination, freedom of action, and noninterference to a degree consistent with respect for others. When an individual exercises autonomy, he or she determines what actions to take (self-determination). Freedom to act refers to a voluntary situation in which the individual is free of coercion and manipulation. The right of noninterference means that the individual's choices are respected whether or not they are in the individual's best interest. Use of this principle for major decision making requires consideration of the individual's wishes, values, and goals. It opposes the use of paternalism (see question 12), by which the health care team and/or family determine what is best for the patient.

2. **Respect for persons.** This principle is broader than the principle of autonomy. It includes respect for individual autonomy and self-determination and at the same time acknowledges the interconnectedness of individuals, i.e., that we are all members of communities.

3. **Justice.** This principle refers to fairness. In health care ethics, its meaning narrows to distributive justice, which determines equal distribution of goods and services and addresses equality of treatment in conditions of scarcity. In using this principle, the moral agent attempts to find a balance between benefits and burdens. Current health care policies and reform represent a national effort to provide distributive justice.

4. **Beneficence.** This principle asks the individual to do good and has been defined by the contemporary philosopher, Frankena,[7] as the four "oughts": (1) one ought not to inflict evil or harm; (2) one ought to prevent evil or harm; (3) one ought to remove evil; and (4) one ought to do or promote good.

5. **Nonmaleficence.** This principle asks the individual to do no harm and relates to one of Frankena's four oughts—one ought not to inflict evil or harm.

8. Is there a nursing model for ethical decision making?

Several well-known nursing models can be used in ethical decision making. One model that works well in cancer nursing is the Shared Decision Making Model of Bandman and Bandman,[1] which encourages the nurse to be a patient advocate. The model has five basic steps, each of which has several components:

Step 1: Definition of the problem
    a. Assess the situation—does a problem exist?
    b. Assess the patient's perception of the situation.
    c. Clarify the problem in relation to the patient's lifestyle, value system, resources, family, and other personal factors.
    d. Decide whether further information is needed.
    e. Identify with the patient alternatives that are appropriate to goals.

Step 2: Analysis of factors to facilitate shared decision making
   a. Is the patient competent to make a decision?
   b. Is the patient's decision fully informed and freely given?
   c. Are the ethical components of the decision clear?
   d. Does the patient/family have relevant information?
   e. Can the patient reverse his or her decision whenever wished?
Step 3: Identification of the ethical issue
   a. Discuss ethical choices with the patient.
   b. Identify sources of conflict among moral principles.
   c. Which moral principles can be justified for use in this situation?
Step 4: Decision regarding ethical choices
   a. The patient freely makes an informed decision consistent with his or her own values, moral principles, lifestyle, and goals.
   b. The nurse and health care team are supportive of the patient's ethical choice.
   c. Family and/or significant other is supportive of the patient's choice.
Step 5: Implementation of the moral decision
   The nurse as the patient's advocate supports the patient's decision.

9. What are rights vs. duties?

In ethical thought, for every right or privilege there is a corresponding duty or obligation. For example, if one considers health care to be a right, the corresponding duty on the part of the patient is to assume some personal responsibility for health and well-being. Often, one may become trapped into thinking that only patients have rights. It is important to remember that everyone in the health care arena has rights and duties, including patients, family members, nurses, and all members of the health care team.

10. To whom does the cancer nurse owe primary responsibility?

Cancer nurses, like all nurses, have many responsibilities, duties, or obligations of an ethical nature. Differing responsibilities may be of primary importance at any one time. There are responsibilities to patients, patient's families, employers, colleagues, one's own family, and self. In general, cancer nurses regard the patient as their primary responsibility. The ANA Code of Ethics outlines the nurse's responsibility to the patient.

11. What does the cancer nurse owe to the patient's family and significant other?

In order to care for the patient, the cancer nurse also may need to care for the patient's family and significant other. (In interest of space, the term *family* is used alone, but it is meant to refer to significant others that may be integral to or beyond the family unit). Often, family members are the patient's major source of social support; they need to be informed, along with the patient, about current disease and treatment status.

12. Define paternalism.

The terms *paternalism, parentalism,* and *maternalism* tend to be used interchangeably. All three terms refer to actions that override an individual's wishes or actions in order to benefit or to avoid harm to the individual. Generally, paternalism occurs when two principles—beneficence (doing good and avoiding harm) and autonomy (allowing the patient to have a voice in decision making)—are in conflict and the health care practitioner believes that he or she is making the best decision in relation to the patient's care. All members of the health care team are capable of paternalistic behavior, which often occurs daily in the oncology setting. The nurse needs to be alert so that he or she can assess when paternalism is occurring, continue to advocate for the patient, and foster self-determination (autonomy) and independence. Paternalism is not always negative, but when it occurs, it needs to be acknowledged. For example, if a patient's laboratory work and computed tomographic scan show evidence of recurrent disease, a physician may tell the patient that the cancer appears to be back but that the patient should not worry because a new course of chemotherapy will bring the recurrence under control. Nurses also need to be aware of their own actions in relation to paternalism. For example, the nurse may want to encourage the use of a pain medication that the patient rejects because of concern over the possible side effects of constipation and sedation. The nurse starts the pain medication and tells the patient, "It's important for you to get your pain under control!"

13. Why is confidentiality important?

Confidentiality, or the keeping of promises (principle of fidelity), is necessary both ethically and legally to care for the patient and to develop a relationship of trust. The ANA Code of Ethics states that the nurse will safeguard the client's right to privacy in a judicious manner that does not endanger the patient's welfare. For example, confidentiality may be violated whenever patient cases are discussed in public places or within hearing distance of others not involved in the case. The principle of fidelity needs to be considered in sharing and withholding information.

14. Discuss the principle of veracity in the care of both patients newly diagnosed with cancer and patients experiencing recurrence.

The principle of veracity (truth-telling) requires the nurse to consider whether communication is honest. At times "being truthful" may be difficult for the nurse, inconvenient for the health care team, and distressing for the patient and family. The nurse should consider four questions:

1. Does the patient have the right to know?
2. Does the patient have the right to refuse information?
3. Does the family have the right to ask the health care team not to share all of the known information with the patient?
4. Does the family have a right to know?

In general, it is assumed that the patient has the right to full and accurate information about his or her situation. Withholding information may not be beneficial and may cause the patient to distrust the health care team. In cases of cognitive impairment or mental incompetence, the patient's level of comprehension should be considered so that the information is presented in a way that can be understood. Often, patients who are not informed envision situations that are far worse than reality. Newly diagnosed patients and patients experiencing recurrence can assume no control over what is happening if they have not been told the truth. The facts may need to be restated several times in a way that promotes the truth, leads to open communication, and encourages questions. The nurse needs to be the patient's advocate. The right to information may be waived if the patient has good reason for requesting that information be withheld. The patient also may request that the family not be told. When the family requests nondisclosure, the nurse and health care team need to remember that the patient's right to confidentiality is primary.

15. What ethical issues are involved in informed consent?

Informed consent involves the principles of autonomy (allowing individuals to decide for themselves) and nonmaleficence (doing no harm). The health care team needs to make sure that the patient has access to information and that the information is understood. The term *informed* assumes that the health care team will provide as much information as possible to the patient so that the decision is based on full knowledge. The information shared with the patient needs to be truthful (principle of veracity). Informed consent is important in many areas of oncology—for any treatment (surgery, chemotherapy, radiation, clinical trials) and for participation in research. Patients must understand that they can withdraw from the treatment or research at any point and that withdrawal will not affect the level of medical or nursing care. Patients may refuse to give consent when asked, and their refusal must be respected. It is a good idea to ensure that the patient gives informed refusal as well as informed consent.

16. When resources are scarce (principle of justice), who decides which patient receives priority treatment?

When oncologic resources are scarce (e.g,. expensive chemotherapy, new protocols and medications), some patients may not have access to them. One example is bone marrow transplant (BMT). Insurance companies have variable policies regarding coverage for BMT, and not all patients are covered for this service. Another example is the use of antiemetic drugs. The drug Zofran is fairly expensive, whereas the drug Inapsine is inexpensive. The physician may prefer the use of Zofran for a patient, but the patient may not be able to afford the more expensive drug because of insurance coverage and limited ability for self-payment. The principle of distributive justice may assist the health care team in deciding which patient should get the scarce item. The team needs to consider the patient's illness, how the scarce item will or will not affect outcome, cost of the item, whether the patient can enter a clinical trial, and who will benefit most. The health care team must balance benefits and burdens. Sometimes there are no easy answers, but assessing all of the known facts and balancing outcomes, benefit, and burdens help the health care team to make the fairest decision possible.

17. What ethical issues are involved with clinical trials?

Several ethical issues inherent in clinical trials are similar to those inherent in allocation of scarce resources. All patients cannot enter the clinical trial that they might wish, and sometimes the patient dies before the trial begins. Once the patient is in the trial, another ethical issue may arise in deciding when to remove the patient from the trial. If it is obvious that the trial is not benefiting the patient, the principles of beneficence and nonmaleficence may assist the health care team in decision making.

18. When is it ethical to let a terminal patient die without violating the principle of avoiding killing?

When it becomes obvious that treatment is of no further benefit, the nurse and health care team need to consider whether active treatment should be discontinued. Palliative or hospice care may be more appropriate. The patient and family may need guidance in making this decision. The patient may not wish to quit active treatment—for example, a patient who has responded to therapy for acute myelogenous leukemia in the past but whose clinical condition and laboratory values show no improvement with current therapy. In such a patient, the doctor may be reluctant to continue aggressive treatment. In this case the physician and nurse must be open and honest with the patient and family, explaining that the situation is now terminal and that supportive care (i.e., palliative and hospice care) is more appropriate. Supportive care should be given regardless of the patient's decision. The nurse can advocate for the patient, put shared decision making into practice, and follow the principle of respect for persons. The decision to forego active treatment can be quite difficult for both patient and family, and a supportive atmosphere is of critical importance.

19. What is meant by the term *sanctity of life*?

The term *sanctity of life,* also known as sacredness of life, is similar to the principle of avoiding killing. This principle is often relevant to end-of-life decisions. According to this viewpoint, life is sacred; therefore, one ought not to do anything that may hasten death, such as removing a feeding tube or discontinuing treatment. Before putting this principle into practice, one is obligated to consider the wishes of the patient and risks/benefits of the intervention.

20. Who determines quality of life?

In the past it has been common for the physician to determine the patient's quality of life (paternalism), especially in relation to the amount of remaining physical function and the likely outcome of continued interventions. From an ethical point of view, the patient should determine his or her quality of life (principles of autonomy and respect for personhood) unless the patient is not competent to assist in this determination. The family and health care team may become involved. The nurse must advocate for the patient in this regard.

21. What is the principle of double effect?

The principle of double effect refers to a situation in which an act intended to produce a good effect also produces a bad or unintended effect. In oncology, for example, titration of medicine to the level needed to relieve pain (a good intention) may hasten the patient's death (an unintended effect). This principle states that bad consequences of an action (i.e., giving pain medicine) are morally permissible if four conditions are met:

1. The action is good or neutral.
2. The nurse intends only the good effect (i.e., pain relief).
3. The bad effect (i.e., death) must not be a means to bringing about the good effect (pain relief).
4. There must be a balance between the good and bad effects.

According to the ANA's position statement on the promotion of comfort and relief of pain in dying patients, "nurses should not hesitate to use full and effective doses of pain medication for the proper management of pain in the dying patient. The increasing titration of medication to achieve adequate symptom control, even at the expense of life, thus hastening death secondarily, is ethically justified." (See Appendix A.)

22. How does one determine ordinary vs. extraordinary means of preserving life?

Generally, the terms *ordinary means* and *extraordinary means* are used in conjunction with prolonging or preserving life. The best definition of the terms was given by Father Kelly in 1951: "Ordinary means are all medicines, treatments, and operations which offer a reasonable hope of benefit and which can be obtained and used without excessive expense, pain, or other inconvenience. Extraordinary means are all medicines, treatments, and operations, which cannot be obtained or used without excessive expense, pain, or other inconvenience, or which, if used, would not offer a reasonable hope or benefit."[2]

23. How does the nurse advocate for the patient when the nurse does not agree with the patient's decision?

Often the nurse faces an ethical dilemma if the patient decides either that he or she does not want further treatment or that he or she wants extraordinary treatment. In such situations, the nurse should follow the principles of respect for persons and autonomy. The nurse's role is to care for the patient, including advocating for the patient. The nurse or health care team must ensure that the patient is making an informed decision and that the patient and family understand the consequences of the decision. Once the patient or family has made a decision, the nurse's role is to care for the patient in a supportive manner, regardless of outcome. Three critical factors are maintenance of open communication, respect for the decision, and the patient-family's need not to feel abandoned by the health care team. In such situations, the health care team should discuss how each member feels about the patient-family decision and support one another in delivering care.

24. What happens when the nurse disagrees with the health care team about care for a patient?

When the nurse disagrees with other members of the health care team about a plan of care for a particular patient, it is critical to acknowledge the disagreement and to work toward conflict resolution. Many times conflicts occur because not everyone on the team is clear about the plan of care or the underlying philosophy. The nurse must remember his or her obligation to function as the patient's advocate and to make the patient's wishes known.

25. When are ethics committees needed? What is their role?

Institutional ethics committees provide a forum for review and discussion of ethical issues and dilemmas and share information as a guide for decision making. In general, ethics committees provide advice and consultation and do not make the final decision. Any individual involved in an ethical dilemma (health care team member, patient, family member) can request a meeting of the ethics committee.

26. How does the nurse deal with ethnic and cultural differences from an ethical perspective?

To care adequately for a patient and family from another culture, the nurse needs to be mindful of the principle of respect for persons. To avoid offending the patient or family, the nurse should recognize and respect the ethnic and cultural traditions that influence the required care. Standards and protocols of care that incorporate cultural beliefs, rituals, and religious preferences need to be developed. An example is the development of protocols for the care of Hasidic Jewish women receiving bone marrow transplants for breast cancer.

27. How does the oncology nurse care for self from an ethical standpoint? Why is self-care important?

The oncology nurse needs to work at developing an ethical sense and becoming astute at recognizing ethical dilemmas with patients, team members, and self. Although the nurse must respond to many rights, he or she also has the duty to care for self. If one does not care for self, one cannot care effectively for others. At times, the nurse has an obligation to remind others that he or she needs to care for self. Often, oncology nurses attempt to be all things to all people. Living a more balanced life will affect positively all that the nurse does.

APPENDIX A: American Nurses Association Position Statement on Promotion of Comfort and Relief of Pain in Dying Patients

Summary: Nurses should not hesitate to use full and effective doses of pain medication for the proper management of pain in the dying patient. The increasing titration of medication to achieve adequate symptom control, even at the expense of life, thus hastening death secondarily, is ethically justified.

Nursing has been defined as the diagnosis and treatment of human responses to actual or potential health problems (American Nurses Association, 1980). When the patient is in the terminal stage of life when cure or prolongation of life in individuals with serious health problems is no longer possible, the focus of nursing is on the individual's response to dying. Diagnosis and treatment then focuses on the promotion of comfort which becomes the primary goal of nursing care.

One of the major concerns of dying patients and their families is the fear of intractable pain during the dying process. Indeed, overwhelming pain can cause sleeplessness, loss of morale, fatigue, irritability, restlessness, withdrawal, and other serious problems for the dying patient (Spross, 1985, Amenta, 1988, Eland, 1989, Melzack, 1990). Nurses play an extremely important role in the assessment of symptoms and the control of pain in dying patients because they often have the most frequent and continuous patient contact. In planning nursing care of dying patients, "the patient has a right to have pain recognized as a problem, and pain relief perceived by the health care team as a need." (Spross, McGuire, Schmitt, 1990).

The assessment and management of pain should be based on a thorough understanding of the individual patient's personality, culture and ethnicity, coping style and emotional, physical and spiritual needs, and on an understanding of the pathophysiology of the disease state (Dalton & Fenerstein, 1998). The main goal of nursing intervention for dying patients should be maximizing comfort through adequate management of pain and discomfort as this is consistent with the expressed desires of the patient. Toward that end, the patient should have whatever medication, in whatever dosage, and by whatever route is needed to control the level of pain as perceived by the patient (Wanzer et al., 1989).

Careful titration of pain medication is essential to promote comfort in dying patients. The proper dose is "the dose that is sufficient to reduce pain and suffering" (Wanzer et al., 1989). Tolerance to pain medications often develops in patients after repeated and prolonged use. Thus, both adults and children may require very high doses of medication to maintain adequate pain control. These doses may exceed the usual recommended dosages of the particular drug for patients of similar age and weight (Eland, 1989, Foley 1989, Inturrisi, 1989, Schmitt, 1990).

While it is well known that pain medications often have sedative or respiratory depressant side effects, this should not be an overriding consideration in their use for dying patients as long as such use is consistent with the patient's wishes. The increasing titration of medication to achieve adequate symptom control, even at the expense of maintaining life or hastening death secondarily, is ethically justified. The nurse assumes responsibility and accountability for individual nursing judgments and actions (American Nurses Association, 1985). Nurses should not hesitate to use full and effective doses of pain medication for the proper management of pain in the dying patient.

(Reference: American Nurses Association: Position statement on promotion of comfort and relief of pain in dying patients. Kansas City, MO, ANA, 1991, with permission.)

ACKNOWLEDGMENT

The authors acknowledge the thoughtful review of chapter content and the timely suggestions of Dr. Nancy Kiernan Case, College of Nursing, Regis University, Denver.

BIBLIOGRAPHY

1. Bandman B, Bandman EL: Nursing Ethics Through the Life Span, 2nd ed. Norwalk, CT, Appleton & Lange, 1990.
2. Beauchamp TL, Childress JF: Principles of Biomedical Ethics, 3rd ed. New York, Oxford University Press, 1989.
3. Benjamin M, Curtis J: Ethics in Nursing, 3rd ed. New York, Oxford University Press, 1992, pp 216–220.
4. Benoliel JQ: The moral context of oncology nursing. Oncol Nurs Forum 20 (Suppl):5–12, 1993.
5. Davis AJ, Aroskar MA: Ethical Dilemmas and Nursing Practice, 3rd ed. Norwalk, CT, Appleton & Lange, 1991.
6. Ersek M, Scanlon C, Glass E, et al: Priority ethical issues in oncology nursing: Current approaches and future directions. Oncol Nurs Forum 22:803–807, 1995.
7. Frankena WK: Ethics, 2nd ed. Englewood Clifts, NJ, Prentice-Hall, 1973.
8. Hall JK: Nursing: Ethics and Law. Philadelphia, W.B. Saunders, 1996.
9. Veatch RM, Fry ST: Case Studies in Nursing Ethics. Philadelphia, J.B. Lippincott, 1987.

71. STORYTELLING

Regina M. Fink, RN, PhD(c), AOCN

1. What is storytelling?

Stories are narratives that provide meaning in our lives. Since the beginning of time, storytelling has been used by folk healers, gurus, shamans, priests, rabbis, ministers, witch doctors, singers, and teachers as a means to healing. Stories can be real, personal, or fictional, told to others or only to oneself. Among the different types are stories that teach us about caring; stories about our past, present, and future; stories that contribute to an understanding of ourselves and others; and stories that can heal and provide social change. Stories can have many different levels of meaning. They may deal with practical issues on the surface while exploring issues such as courage, love, grief, and hope underneath.

2. What is the value of storytelling for oncology nurses?

We learn about ourselves and others from the stories we hear and tell. By telling a story we give voice to our experiences and find meaning in who we are, who we have been, and where we are coming from. Stories can teach, heal, validate, offer reflection, and shape how we care for patients and others. Telling stories to others is a way to teach new things, to provide catharsis, to communicate more effectively while building trust, and to promote personal growth.[3] Stories can order chaotic events in the lives of patients and caregivers. They allow us to view experiences from different perspectives and provide a different lens through which a single event can be viewed. Nurses should be encouraged to share their stories with colleagues, family, friends, patients, and even themselves (self-talk).

3. Is it easy to tell a story?

We live our lives in story. Telling a story can be risky, and we may have a fear of being misunderstood. Stories can be told verbally to others, either in a group or one-on-one. A story told with affection, caring, and intensity will have an effect on others. A story has a beginning that draws the listener into its meaning or intent, a middle that builds the struggle or tension, and a closing or resolution of tension. Stories can be retold to develop meaning. Embellishments may be added, metaphors developed, and facts changed because the point of the story is to convey meaning (sometimes called a lesson or moral). This flexibility in part distinguishes a story from clinical accounts or anecdotes.

4. When is the right time to tell a story?

Storytelling can be useful during difficult and changing times. It may present new perspectives and normalize concerns. However, the successful telling of a story requires active listening, and at times active listening does not occur. Listening and hearing others' stories presupposes centering, which is key to storytelling. Being centered means being in the moment with another. Perhaps the audience is not interested, or perhaps the listener is waiting for his or her turn to speak, hurrying the storyteller. Sometimes only parts of the story are heard, and the most meaningful piece may be lost or misinterpreted. An active listener nourishes, encourages, and enters into a caring relationship with the other and finds meaning in the story.

5. How can nurses tell stories or empower their patients to share what they feel?

Nurses need to be present and in the moment with patients. Co-creation requires the physical and emotional presence of the nurse and the belief that the patient and nurse are mutually involved in development of the narrative. Through this process, the nurse and the patient are changed. Listening to the stories of patients and families helps nurses to understand the perceived meaning of the illness experience. Having patients tell their stories may be healing and reflective for the patient while providing important and sensitive information to the caregiver.

Keeping a journal or notebook is another way for patients and nurses to keep in touch with past and present selves. The journal is a form of narrative and a way to tell one's own story. Writing about experiences provides a technique to shed fears and concerns while renewing or replenishing inner resources. Photographs, mementos, videos, artwork, and music are other ways to shape stories and may provide an introduction to get the story going. Some nurses are quite adept at using psychodrama or humor to depict a particular theme. The creative use of metaphors, analogies, poetry, or songs may provide new meaning by redescribing reality.

Most patients cherish the opportunity to tell their story from the beginning (often they are not even asked to tell their story at all). How can we get patients to tell their stories if we do not share part of our own? By telling our own stories a connection is nurtured. Knowing what and how much to share is part of the art of nursing. As oncology nurses, we need to take the time to listen to others' stories. To further this goal, questions 6–10 were asked of authors of this book and other oncology nurses.

6. What are your favorite inspirational quotations?
- Nursing is a progressive art, such that to stand still, is to go backwards. (Florence Nightingale)
- What I do to today is very important because I am exchanging a day of my life for it.
- Years teach much that days never know.
- When one is a stranger to oneself, then one is out of touch with oneself, then one cannot touch others. (Anne Morrow Lindbergh)
- We are most effective as caregivers when we are centered in our own sense of well-being. (Caryn Summers, RN)

7. How do you respond to the question, "Isn't it depressing to work with cancer patients?"
- I take great pleasure helping each patient live their life to the fullest, regardless of longevity.
- At times it is very sad, but I am clear that *my job* is to make the process the best it can be. I believe that we ultimately have little control over how things proceed. My job is one of support.
- I think of depression as a process, an evolving development. Working with cancer patients can be sad, yes. There are moments you wish you weren't working that day, or moments that you wish you could change things somehow. But then there are those occasions when you have made a difference in someone's moment and that feels good. There are times when patients have done something that touched *your* moment.
- Working with persons who have cancer makes you realize that life is short so don't sweat the small stuff.
- No, it's enlightening. It's a learning experience for me. Cancer patients have much to teach about life and living. I usually tell people, "I learn more about life and living working with these patients."
- After working with cancer patients for the past 20 years, I have felt sad at times, but not depressed. I think this is because I have always been open to the energy of love and caring exchanged in each patient interaction. Yes, there have been a few difficult patients or families whom I felt were "psychic vampires," but I think I learned the most from those kinds of patients. Each patient encounter has been a lesson, challenge, or gift. From angry patients, I learned how difficult it was to let go of life. Lonely patients have taught me the value of letting the significant people in our lives know how much we care about them. Dying patients have taught me that the most important things in our lives are our families and our true friends: "Nobody ever regretted spending too much time with their families; they did regret how much time was expended by working too many hours." I believe that if you truly love what you do or accept that you can't be everything to everybody, you may get tired but not depressed. If you dread going back to work, I think then it's time for a change or to take a break.

8. **What advice may an experienced oncology nurse give to a new nurse?**
   - Trust your gut reactions. There's a reason you feel those vibes—act on them.
   - Find balance. This type of work can be all-consuming and may destroy you and your life unless you put it into perspective. Work as a team; no one person or nurse can provide everything a patient or family needs. Understand that your gift is to guide, support, and encourage. If your patient and treatment fail or even if they are cured, your job is the same. Therefore, regardless of the outcome, you are always successful. It is a wonderfully challenging profession—intellectually, emotionally, and physically. Balance your life with the not-so-serious things.
   - Listen and feel.
   - Stay centered in your own life so that when you are at home you are truly with yourself, your family, and significant others. At work you are centered on your patients at that particular moment.
   - Remind yourself and your patients to take one day at a time.
   - Find your teachers everywhere.
   - Remember that you are part of a team.
   - Everyone is human, even surgeons.
   - If you are going to be assertive, know your facts.
   - Keep an open mind. Avoid black-and-white beliefs; the truth is always changing.
   - Don't be afraid to feel; empathy is healing.
   - Always leave room for hope and time for hugs.
   - Don't be afraid to ask for advice or help.

9. **Describe special moments that you have shared.**
   - I think there is nothing more powerful than holding the hand of a person as they die or helping patients and families with the transition of life. Both birth and death are an awe-inspiring experience.
   - A 70-year-old lawyer with a total laryngectomy played "Rhapsody in Blue" for me with such emotion and intenseness. Months later, his cancer recurred. His therapy included vincristine. He could no longer play the piano because of the neurotoxicity associated with the chemo.
   - A wedding took place in the oncology unit because the grandmother was too sick to attend outside the hospital.
   - I worked with a 26-year-old man diagnosed with AML. His wife was pregnant with their second child, and he wanted to live long enough to see him born. He went into remission and was able to see his second son born. But eight months later, he relapsed. I was doing an EKG on him in the clinic before we admitted him to the hospital for more chemotherapy. I was quite saddened by his relapse. I was trying not to cry, and he looked up at me and said, "This job must be very hard for you. I don't know how you do it." I was amazed at his ability to be empathic during this time and said, "I was wondering the same thing about you. How hard this must be for you and how you find the strength."
   - Mr. M, who was doing well in the morning and was ready to be released from the hospital after receiving follow-up studies for lung cancer, had paged me immediately. He said he wanted to tell me good-bye and thanked me for all I had done for him. I reflected that he sounded like he was leaving for good instead of just going home. Then he told me that several angels had visited him during the night and were coming back for him soon. I accepted his story, and we continued sharing several more of his important life stories. I did not argue with him, even though I truly believed, as did his doctors, that he would be around for months. He died quietly and peacefully that afternoon.

10. **Describe funny moments that you have shared.**
    - A patient on vincristine came into the office and announced it was time to die. "Why now?" I asked. She responded, "When your fingers are too numb to pick your nose, it's time to go."

- A patient quoted Woody Allen: "I'm not afraid to die. I just don't want to be there when it happens."
- My 8-year-old nephew was talking to a chemotherapy patient of mine who had alopecia. After we left, he looked at me and said, "You're not a nurse, you're a barber!"
- After hearing that her leg was to be amputated, a 7-year-old with osteosarcoma said, "Gee, I wonder if I'll weigh less." She started talking about scaring her uncle by hiding her prosthesis in his bed.
- A young AML patient was feeling discouraged. On a bogus trip to radiology, the nurses decorated her room like a scene from a Hawaiian island complete with 6-foot cardboard palm trees.
- Teepeeing a patient's room was a special badge of honor on one oncology unit.

11. The following vignettes are stories of human caring, written by nurses about their patients and shared with the hope that they will encourage others to tell their stories. The names of the characters have been changed to protect confidentiality.

Al

Al was a 44-year-old man with terminal renal cell cancer metastatic to the bone and lungs. Al had failed conventional therapy and was working with a faith healer. He had much living to do. He would often say, "Gotta be around to raise those grandbabies!" He had fractured his right hip by falling at home; the orthopedic surgeons were unable to repair it because disease had destroyed the femoral head. His pain was excruciating and was not relieved by high doses of oral morphine. He was expected to live only for a couple of months, so an intrathecal catheter was placed for administration of hydromorphone and bupivicaine. Over the next year, he continued to do well and was free of pain.

One day, during a home visit, as I was changing his pain medication cartridge, I noticed a white piece of material wrapped around his infusion pump. Al asked if I could wait a moment while he unwrapped the white cloth from the pump. I asked him what the piece of material was and he replied, "It's a prayer cloth." He explained that he held the cloth every day as he prayed and that wrapping the pump with his cloth was his way of positively influencing outcome. He was hoping that the pain medication would continue to be successful. I asked Al if he wanted to pray before he unwrapped the cloth. Tears came to his eyes, and he smiled and asked, "You really want to pray with me?" Together we prayed for Al's healing, and we unwrapped the pump together. It is an experience I won't forget. Many of us are given these precious moments, but we're sometimes too busy in the daily hustle and bustle or too influenced by what others might think. Being centered and in the moment is perhaps the greatest gift we can give to ourselves and our patients.

Pearl and Isaac

When I was a little girl, I had many dolls and stuffed animals. Each night before going to sleep, I would make rounds in my bedroom, covering each doll and animal and wishing them a goodnight. If it got cold in the night, I would get up and put extra covers on my "little friends," so they wouldn't be cold either. I guess then I was preparing for my future career as a nurse.

My first rotation as a second-year student nurse was working evenings on the neurosurgical unit. In class we were told how important it was to talk to our comatose patients as we cared for them—that on some level there was always the chance that they could understand what we were saying but just could not communicate to us. Being a diligent student, I took this to heart and spent many hours having one-way conversations about the weather, sports, or anything I could think of to say.

One of my patients was Isaac. He was 65 years old and had been admitted comatose, reason unknown. An x-ray was done, and a tumor was found. Surgery was undertaken. Isaac had a Foley catheter and nasogastric tube for feeding but remained in a coma. His wife Pearl came every evening and stayed as long as she was allowed (in 1963 we were not enlightened about visiting hours; they were 6 PM–8 PM only.) She was so devoted to him and missed him so much. They had never had any children, and Isaac was her life.

It was winter, and in New York that means that it is very cold and damp. Add to that a brick building built in the 1800s with 12-foot ceilings and no insulation, and you have a picture of the neurosurgical unit. Each evening I dutifully cared for my 12 patients, feeding them, cleaning them, and turning them every 2 hours. We used large bolsters to support their limbs and keep them on their sides. The bed clothing was then draped over the bolster so that it would not chafe their skin. I could not bear the thought of all that cold air whistling down the covers. So every night before I went off duty, I would take a bath blanket and wrap it around their heads and over their shoulders and call them each by name and wish them goodnight. At the end of my rotation Isaac was still there with no sign of improvement. I had become very attached to Pearl and Isaac and hoped and prayed that he would get well.

Six months later, as I left the ER after a very long night shift, I spotted Pearl walking down the hall from rehab. She was supporting an old man who had a left-sided paresis and was shuffling as best as he could with his brace and cane. I ran to them, and Pearl and I embraced. After hugging and expressing my great delight and surprise at Isaac's recovery, I turned to Isaac to introduce myself. I said, "You don't remember me"—and that was as far as he would let me go with my introduction. He took my hand and looked into my eyes with great love and tenderness and said, "Oh, yes, I do. You were the only nurse who covered me every night so that I wouldn't be cold and called me by name as you wished me goodnight. I have never forgotten you." I was stunned, and so was Pearl. Our eyes filled with tears as Isaac and I embraced.

It was a moment I have never forgotten, a moment that changed my life. I still cry whenever I tell this story. Isaac and Pearl are always with me in my heart and mind, and I give them to you today. That experience for me was about love and caring. It was about the impact that we have on each others' lives each day. Sometimes we never know how we have positively affected someone, and sometimes we are given the gift of knowing. As you go into nursing today, please take Isaac and Pearl with you, and know that you have the opportunity now and always to co-create with your own "Isaacs and Pearls."

Back in 1963, I didn't know the term transpersonal caring occasion. It had not been conceived yet. I thank Dr. Jean Watson for putting a name on what it is that we, as nurses, do and experience each day.

Diane

This is a story about Diane, a 36-year-old woman diagnosed with non-small cell lung cancer metastatic to her spine. Understanding that the prognosis was grim, she elected to fight the cancer by starting an investigational protocol. Her clinic visits were weekly, and we all got to know Diane and her family. In a way she was a lot like me; perhaps that was why a rapport was so easy to establish. She had been a single parent to a son and daughter (both adolescents) and had recently married.

She joked, "It took a diagnosis of cancer to make Tom marry me." (Her friends had told her she needn't have been so desperate). Her sense of humor was incredible. Over the months that I had been involved with Diane's care, I rejoiced in her triumphs (the disease in her lungs was shrinking), and I cried with her heartbreaks (the pain was increasing, and she developed paraplegia due to spinal cord compression). She was having a mixed response. The treatment was not working.

Diane chose hospice care at home. She was on increasing oral doses of morphine, an anticonvulsant for neuropathic pain, and massage therapy for back pain. Diane made us promise that we would do everything to keep her pain-free. Early one snowy Monday morning, Diane was admitted to the hospital for excruciating pain. One look at Diane revealed that she was dying. Alert and oriented, she was screaming in agony, "Please do something."

New house staff that day were not comfortable with the situation; the attending physician told them to do whatever needed to be done. The pharmacist and I developed a plan of care. Over a 12-hour period, we methodically started a morphine drip, increased the dose, assessed, monitored, and communicated with Diane and her family. They were aware that she might die from increasing doses of opioids but were willing to do anything. After depleting all of the hospital's morphine supply with a dose of 2400 mg of morphine IV hourly, we finally achieved relief. Tom was saddened by how quickly Diane had deteriorated and by his inability to say goodbye. He felt comfortable expressing his frustrations and concerns to the nursing staff. He wanted the pain medication decreased so that he could say goodbye, yet hated to see Diane in so much pain. He was having a hard time letting go. We encouraged Tom to take some time to tell Diane how he truly felt. He smuggled in Diane's dog in a carpet bag. We gave them private time so they could lie beside her and be with her for the time she had left. Diane died that evening.

This story is not unusual. Oncology nurses do these things every day—helping, caring, promoting the expression of feelings, being there to support the family.

Tim

This is a story about Tim and his personal experience of being diagnosed with and treated for acute myelogenous leukemia. It is a story about his family and the many caregivers that he came to know while hospitalized for induction chemotherapy. It is a story about how one man touched the lives of so many people. (*Editor's note:* It is interesting to hear the stories of three nurses' perspectives on caring for Tim. Each nurse was affected by the experience in very different ways.)

Oncology nurse specialist. "We have a new leukemic on the floor," one of the staff nurses called to me. "Do I have the strength or energy to be involved any more?" I asked myself. "Maybe I'm burned out. These patients are so sick, they're in so long, and I wonder if I'm able to get emotionally involved. What's the matter with me? What do you say to these patients day in and day out? You can talk about blood counts, fatigue and other side effects, but it gets really hard to keep hanging in there. The staff nurses do a wonderful job. I can support them. I will meet this new patient and family to see what they need to know."

I'll never forget the day I met Tim. He had nonstop visitors, mostly house staff and medical staff continuing to quiz him about his medical history. I introduced myself as an oncology nurse specialist who would be available to talk about treatment and side effects and to answer questions. His family was one I would enjoy caring for—a supportive wife who was a nurse, a daughter in college, and a son in high school. They were all camped out in Tim's room, and listened attentively as I talked about the chemotherapy. Tim confided that this was not a new experience. He had been diagnosed with lymphoma 15 years previously and had undergone the ravages of chemotherapy. His children were very young at the time. He expressed concern about the side effects, especially nausea and vomiting. I reassured him that new drugs to alleviate nausea have changed how chemotherapy is tolerated. There were many interruptions by visiting health care professionals as we talked. His daughter just sobbed, "I'm so tired of all this medical talk. I just want to go home and live a normal life again." Everyone became teary, including Tim, and I marveled at his sensitivity and close relationship with his family. They all hugged.

I started visiting Tim every day to check in with him and his wife. His daughter and son were both in school, and Tim and his wife were concerned about how they were coping on their own. The chemo was underway, and Tim was tolerating it well. But his counts needed a heavier hit. Even after the prescribed chemo was given, his counts still had not bottomed out. The doctors were concerned about cardiac toxicity secondary to previous radiation therapy many years ago and the addition of chemotherapy now. They changed the regimen and started a second cycle of induction. Tim was concerned and obviously depressed when I visited again. This time we were alone. I asked him, "How are you really doing with all of this?" He told me a lot about himself and in doing so shared his philosophy of life.

Again with sensitivity, Tim shared his fears of death and his reality of what the future held for him. He was hoping for a long, cold winter, because he needed a frost to have a fruitful, bountiful harvest in the spring. That was his visualization and metaphor for his leukemia treatment. It was February, and it was dreary and cold outside. Tim could see the snow covering trees. He could feel the cold on the windows. And he wanted the frost to be good and long and hard, as he also wanted all of his bone marrow to die in anticipation of a bountiful, fruitful spring and remission. He shared his tears and feelings about life and death freely. He had studied theology, left the seminary, and married. He enjoyed a deep, loving, intimate relationship and read and meditated regularly.

This discussion was scary for me, and yet it awakened my soul. My soul had been dead. I had been in oncology ever since I graduated from nursing school. I had been alive at times, I must admit, but a little bit of my soul had died with the death and sadness I had encountered over the past 19 years. I shared with Tim that I was in the midst of a long winter myself but that I had been able to be present with him and that gave me hope that I, too, might have a good spring, a sense of renewal and energy. I had felt guilty that I hadn't been present for all of my patients. Tim was giving me a gift, and I was ready to receive it. Instead of running the other way, I looked forward to my visits with Tim. He had an artistic, soulful, spiritual side and was more capable of expressing his feelings than anyone I had cared for. He was giving all of us a gift.

Tim's primary nurse. Caring for Tim was a very satisfying experience. I admire people who take control of their own lives. I could give Tim suggestions or tools, and he would be appreciative and use them. On a personal level, leukemia patients are one of the more satisfying groups to take care of. Many times they go into remission; it can last a while, and they can achieve a normal lifestyle. It was difficult for me to see Tim so frustrated over losing his energy and equilibrium. I wasn't sure that he was going to be cured. I did see him crying after he was told that the chemo had not worked the first time around. Tim was the type of person who kept his milieu controlled in little ways. He was a thoughtful man who kept a journal, read, listened to music, and had lots of different experiences. He was on a long journey and was doing what he had to do to get better.

Tim was the kind of father I never had. He was so connected with his kids. That's how I want to be. I've never experienced what good parents can do. He loved to rock climb; losing energy and activity was a big loss for him. I went into nursing to be able to deal with loss, death, and all the things one fears. It was a very profound experience to see Tim's family and their dealings with loss. That makes this experience and being involved more poignant and intense.

Student nurse. When I was first assigned to care for Tim, I went to the library and looked up all the statistics about AML. No matter what I read, I felt that Tim had no chance. I felt that everyone who took care of him knew it, but nobody would admit to it. I know chemo has a chance of working sometimes, but I felt that he was not given a realistic explanation. Everyone was so optimistic—his doctors, nurses, family, friends. But I wondered if it was right to be that way.

There comes a point when we need to be realistic that someone is dying (that was my diagnosis). I was so frustrated. I wanted someone to tell him so he could do what he needed to do. Patients need this information. I was involved with my own child who, at 2 years of age, had a 100% fatal heart disease. My child was put on a respirator and died. *If only I had been told the truth.* But Tim was sick. I watched him become so weak that he couldn't talk; he lost 25 pounds because of diarrhea, nausea, and loss of appetite due to mouth sores. I wanted to protect him. I wanted to be gentle and to nurture him. I brought him some tapes (he always liked listening to music). It felt good to know that there were things I could do to try to help him. It also felt good when he asked for me to take care of him. I learned about dignity from Tim. He didn't lose his self-respect as he stood up to lean on me to urinate. He talked about the stages of life—birth, maturity, decay, and death. I could see him decaying.

Caring for Tim reinforced a beginning belief that each patient is a whole person and not a problem to be solved. One of the most important things a nurse can do is to validate the person's place and how the person is feeling at that particular time. Never separate the person from the illness. Caring for Tim also reinforced that Western medicine has a lot to offer, but we need to care for the person. We need to empower people. That's what my role is about.

Tim. Spring has been slow in coming this year. It is May already, and the trees are still stark and naked. The buds are hiding, waiting for the right time to come out. Tim is in remission, yet he had a detour along the way. Tim developed *Aspergillus* pneumonia and had a lobe of his lung removed. He was on a ventilator for $2\frac{1}{2}$ weeks and had been further weakened by weight loss. His voice was temporarily out of commission due to a tracheostomy. He slowly built himself up. Tim said, "I'm recovering as slowly as spring is coming this year." He is not anxious to start chemo again. He is living each day in the moment.

"There's a feeling of emptiness and despair that you really feel in chemotherapy and, finally, a lack of control," Tim said. "And as your resources go down and down, your disease seems bigger and in more control. You do have to find out how many bullets you have left, if any." The sense of hope gives way to a more removed "hope that you hope," he said.

Tim ultimately went into remission for over a year. He relapsed and chose not to take treatment again. He lived life to his fullest and died surrounded by his family and loved ones. It was an honor to know him. He touched many lives. Patients need to be told how they affect our lives. All involved had a chance to let him know this. Tim wrote the following poem:

The View from 8E (Oncology Unit)

I am the dark
I am the cold
I am the imageless image;
the dreamless dream
the silence that defines the rhythm.

I am a pause
in the dance of creation.
Now I embrace all that is not;
may not; the fragile; the endangered.

Yet, from the pause comes the note,
the empty allows the full.
The pause is the womb
that bears the universe.
I abide in the pause
I choose that rebirth.

Gary

I had just finished high school and left my parent's home. The high school counselor recommended I not go to college. He didn't think I would do very well. So, one morning, I left my shabby basement apartment near the Capitol Building and walked over to the "unemployment" office. A week later I had my first full-time job.

In a way, the warehouse was fascinating: shades of Upton Sinclair's *The Jungle*—concrete loading docks, a maze of mysterious pipes, banks of rectangular window panes that viewed the muddy river, slaughter houses, and rendering plants. Some days you got out of your car, grabbed your nose, and made a mad dash for the building.

I spent those first nine months of my adult youth delivering knives, aprons, and bleach to the packinghouses, where often the workers good naturedly threatened to cut off pieces of their coworkers' anatomy. I lifted 200-pound drums, ate from the catering truck and neighborhood bars, and waded through several inches of foul, nostril-tainting muck a dozen times a day. My comrades were a drug-imbibing army deserter from the Dutch East Indies and a deeply depressed recent sufferer of divorce.

One day we were joined by a new inmate, Gary. He looked to be 6'5" and 280 pounds. He could throw one of the 55-gallon drums onto the bed of a truck. He loved to talk and tell stories, absorbed all kinds of practical details, and played out some rather ornery jokes. He once sent a potato crashing into the passenger door on a chief-of-police's squad car by means of a homemade bazooka. At the end of the delivery day, we raced the three vehicles up to the second story garage in a cloud of exhaust, burnt rubber, and squealing tires, not to mention verbal assaults on each other's manhood.

I didn't see or hear of Gary for the next 22 years. Then one day I walked into a hospital room at the beginning of my shift and faced him in a different role—that of a leukemic. Complications brought him in frequently, and everyone got used to his great, pale, perpetually shirtless form wandering about the unit, always looking for a good conversation. Disease and inactivity had turned his stevedore physique to sagging flesh and a big gut. He sometimes passed out, but still managed to tell stories, go fishing, and humorously muse on the human condition.

One morning I came to work, walked into Gary's room, and encountered the strangely automaton-like respirations of someone close to death. All the muscles were working at capacity to keep the human machine going, but there was no connection with conscious struggle. Gary's feet were mottled; he made no responses; and he was alone. I bent down to his ear and softly said, "It's OK, Gary; I'm here with you." Very shortly afterward, as if he had heard me, his breathing changed and then stopped. It would never have occured to me 20 some years ago as I shot pool with him that I would someday be with him when he died.

One of the many things we have to ponder in this strange confusion called life is the interrelatedness we share. Our fates intersect, part, reconnect. As you look into someone's face for the first time, you cannot begin to fathom the role and effect that he or she will exert on your life or you on that person's life. These effects are particularly powerful when your calling is oncology nursing.

12. The following excerpts are taken from patients' stories. These are some of our patients' secrets.

- I wanted to give up, but you didn't give up on me. I never would have made it through my chemotherapy without you.
- Nurses and doctors tell you to call them when you have pain or another problem. But when you do, they come to check you and then go away. Sometimes they don't come back to tell you if it is or isn't time to have medication. If it isn't, they don't try to get another order to help. Be there. We need you.
- I want my caregivers to talk amongst themselves so they all know what is going on and coordinate my care. This would help me feel more secure about them. Knowing that they know me makes me feel better.
- Take time to know about individuals, their background, essence, and beliefs. This will help you know the person better. Everyone is unique and will act differently in different situations. This is perhaps the most important thing I want to tell you.
- Be sympathetic and helpful. I know you're busy. Be with us in the here and now. Don't rush.
- Caring goes a long way.
- A smile and a good attitude make a difference.
- When you're busy, don't lose sight of the person.
- Discover our uniqueness. Don't assume; don't stereotype. Put yourself in our shoes. That way you'll have a better understanding of what we need.
- Touching is a caring and reassuring gesture—continue to touch. Touching indicates a warmth and caring connection. It is a vital component of caring—maybe the most important aspect in my view.
- Talk with patients about their feelings.
- I want my caregiver to be someone with compassion.
- Physicians and nurses need to credit patients with the ability to take care of themselves and to think for themselves. We can be very self-reliant. Don't give me too much medication so that I'm confused. I want to take responsibility for my care. To understand pain, you need to understand people, to listen to them. People heal from the inside out. Physicians try to heal from the outside in. There are times when I think no one is listening. My health care providers are opinionated and set in many ways. Healing can happen only when trust occurs.

ACKNOWLEDGMENTS

Thanks to the oncology nurses who shared their stories with us—Mary Bloebaum, Beth Bowles, Rose Gates, Becca Hawkins, Gari Jensen, Linda Krebs, Debi McCaffrey Boyle, Cathy Pickett, Ida Sansoucy, and Mary Wilkerson—and to our patients, who always have stories to share and just need to be asked.

Two recently published books are worth knowing about and would be great additions to one's storytelling library. *All Kinds of Love: Experiencing Hospice* is written by hospice nurse Carolyn Jaffe, and *Kitchen Table Wisdom: Stories That Heal* is written by a physician.

BIBLIOGRAPHY

1. Cooper J: Telling our own stories. In Witherell C, Noddings N (eds): Stories Lives Tell. New York, Teachers College Press, 1991, pp 96–112.
2. Grumet M: The politics of personal knowledge. In Witherell C, Noddings N (eds): Stories Lives Tell. New York, Teachers College Press, 1991, pp 67–77.
3. Heiney SP: The healing power of story. Oncol Nurs Forum 22:899–904, 1995.
4. Jaffe C, Ehrlich CH: All Kinds of Love: Experiencing Hospice. Amityville, New York, Baywood Publishing Company, 1997.
5. Krebs L: Recreating harmony: Stories of Native American women surviving breast cancer. University of Colorado Health Sciences Center School of Nursing, Denver [doctoral dissertation], 1997.
6. Makler A: Imagining history. In Witherell C, Noddings N (eds): Stories Lives Tell. New York, Teachers College Press, 1991, pp 29–47.
7. Nelson GL: Writing and Being. San Diego, Lura Media, 1994.
8. Remen RN: Kitchen Table Wisdom: Stories That Heal. New York, Riverhead Books, 1996.
9. Steeves RH: Loss, grief and the search for meaning. Oncol Nurs Forum 23:897–903, 1996.
10. Watson J: Nursing: Human Science and Human Care. New York, National League for Nursing, 1988.
11. Witherell C, Noddings N (eds): Stories Lives Tell. New York, Teachers College Press, 1991.

INDEX

Page numbers in **boldface type** indicate complete chapters.

505